Symbols Summary

gf = gluten-free

 GF Lines or Facility; or
No chance of cross-contamination

 Gluten Testing is performed

 Gluten-Free based on review of ingredient label
(as no GF list was provided)

 Gluten-Free based on last year's list (use caution, as information
may be out of date)

 Procedures to mitigate Cross-Contamination are in place,
although there are shared facilities or equipment

 Cross-Contamination is possible; or, made with "gluten-free
ingredients" (with no specific mention of GF status by the
company)

No Icon. The company reported that the product is gluten-free
but provided no further context.

For the full key, see page 19 >>

Quick Reference Table of Contents

**CANNED &
PRE-PACKAGED
FOODS**

GF CERTIFIED GLUTEN-FREE

(You wouldn't know it if we didn't tell you.)

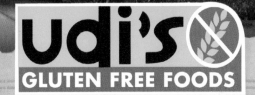

Best Tasting Gluten-Free Bread and Baked Goods

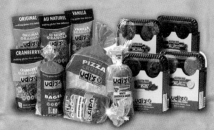

- Baked in a 100% gluten-free facility
- Gluten-Free, Casein-Free, and Soy-Free
- No artificial flavors, colors, or synthetic additives
- Looks, feels, and tastes like real bread
- No need to freeze or toast

Fresh GF New.

Free & Delivered Weekly to your email inbox

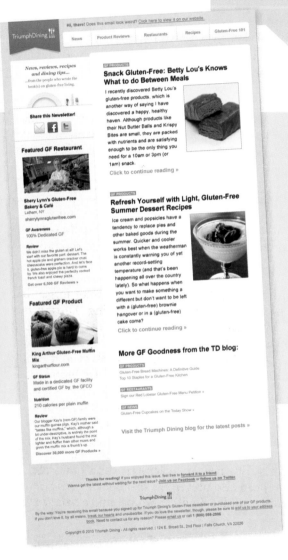

- **All the Latest GF News**

- **GF Product Reviews**

- **GF Recipes**

- **GF Restaurants**

And, check out the all-new feature, **"GF 101: A Gluten-Free Guide for Beginners."**

Sign up for free at

www.triumphdining.com

Welcome to another year of gluten-free living! Previous generations would have found this a near-insurmountable challenge. Even five years ago, this seemed like a curse. The average person had never even heard of gluten, let alone gluten-free bread. Fresh-baked gluten-free goods were a distant dream.

Now most of us can walk into our local grocery chain and find a variety of gluten-free products ranging from baking mixes to prepared meals. We have choices. We are no longer forced into buying one mediocre product because it is the only thing available. This guide covers more than 44,000 products. In other words, tonight's dinner is all but cooked.

Our hope is that this guide makes your shopping experience as pleasant and hassle-free as possible. The gluten-free market now has major brands competing to satisfy your needs. We also cover more brands than ever – regional ones, those found in national mega-chains, major national brands, and, of course, ones produced in smaller, dedicated facilities.

Despite the major strides being made in the GF world, we cannot forget that caution and common sense are still vital to our decision-making. During our editing process, we caught a few manufacturers' mistakes. The people compiling these lists are human, just like all of us, and there's a certain amount of human error expected. For this reason we have to be vigilant about reading labels even if we are told a product is gluten-free. We also have to watch out for things like brands with multiple versions of the same product (e.g. GF mac & cheese versus vegan – but not GF – mac & cheese). This can be hazardous, especially when packaging is similar. Always remember to read labels very carefully and never take anything for granted.

We must balance open-mindedness with caution so that we stay safe without sacrificing the potential to discover new and exciting foods. Our negative expectations keep us healthy, but they can also prevent us from having new dining experiences. Let common sense be your guide – in other words, find a balance that works for you.

Even with all the advancement in food labeling, product testing and food chemistry, gluten-free shopping is still a challenge. We still await the long overdue FDA regulations (but we are excited to say that we are growing closer to a ruling) and meanwhile, we sometimes find that our definitions of gluten-free are completely different from the manufacturers'. Many companies still hesitate to

WE'VE MOVED!

Triumph Dining has moved to California! We are excited to uncover new gluten-free opportunities from our new home in the Golden State.

confirm the gluten-free status of their products due to the lack of regulations and legal risks. Others are happy to share this information but only when asked. And even when the FDA regulations pass, GF labeling will still be voluntary.

This guide eliminates much of the challenge. We've already done the asking; now all you need to do is choose the products you prefer (always remembering to double-check labels). Your options are in front of you, saving you the effort of sifting through the vast amounts of products and information available. We are here to help you eat well and stay healthy while saving time and money, no matter where you choose to shop.

Our hope is that this guide becomes your most trusted shopping companion. If there is anything more we can do to make your experience easier and more enjoyable, please do not hesitate to let us know. We are always looking for ways to improve our guide and make it more useful for you. The people reading your emails and answering your phone calls are the same ones who put this publication together, and the cause is very dear to our hearts.

Happy gluten-free shopping, cooking, and eating!

Dave Morris, Bob Stamatatos, and the Team at Triumph Dining

GENERAL TIPS FOR GROCERY SHOPPING
Chapter 1

Everyone knows how to grocery shop—we've been doing it for most of our adult lives. The interesting thing is that each person approaches shopping slightly differently; some people spend hours methodically comparing prices in search of the best deal, while others race through the store as quickly as possible so they can move on to other things. There's no right or wrong way to shop, but what follows are a few basic tips and ideas to help make your gluten-free shopping trips a little more successful—no matter what your personal shopping style is.

Choosing a Grocery Store

Some grocery stores are simply better for the gluten-free shopper than others. Generally, we favor businesses that cater to gluten-free clientele in some way. It makes shopping easier and we prefer to support businesses that focus on the needs of the GF community.

A store's focus on gluten-free customers can manifest itself in several ways:

1. Grouping gluten-free goods in one section, like Kroger does.

2. Stocking an extensive selection of gluten-free products: Many smaller, specialty stores like Martindale's in Springfield, PA; Against the Grain in Salt Lake City; Gluten-Free Trading Company in Milwaukee; and Gluten Free Reviewer Grocery in our own San Francisco pride themselves on carrying hundreds or thousands of specialty gluten-free items.

3. Labeling gluten-free foods: Either in the grocery aisle like Whole Foods, or on packaging itself; Wegman's in New York marks its gluten-free private label foods with a little "G."

4. Publishing a list of gluten-free items that can be found in their stores, like the Trader Joe's chains do.

Stores that fit into these categories will tend to have more options for gluten-free customers, resulting in a better shopping experience. Try to frequent these types of stores when you can.

We understand that not everyone lives near a Trader Joe's, or can afford to buy all their groceries from premium and specialty stores. That's why this guide is designed to help you find gluten-free options in any grocery store—whether or not it specifically caters to gluten-free customers. We worked harder than ever this year to cover at least one major grocery chain in every state, and in most we have covered two or more.

COMMON PITFALLS TO AVOID

One ongoing concern for people on the gluten-free diet is cross-contamination. It can happen anywhere, there's no way to know whether it's happened to a product, and it's rarely ever flagged for us. Also, the Food Allergen Labeling and Consumer Protection Act does not set specific standards for using cross-contamination advisory statements or require manufacturers to identify the possibility of inadvertent cross-contamination. (See the next chapter for a more in-depth discussion of the FALCPA.)

Concerns about cross-contamination extend beyond grocery store shelves, to bulk bins, deli/meat counters, and the prepared foods sections.

Bulk Bins

Bulk bins are largely left unattended by grocery store personnel. There's often no way to tell if other customers have inadvertently shared serving scoops across products, potentially contaminating anything that otherwise would have been gluten-free. And, there's no indication whether products rotate through the bins or, if they do, whether the bins are thoroughly cleaned before transitions. In other words, the bin that holds a seemingly gluten-free product today could have been full of wheat flour last week. For these reasons, we recommend avoiding bulk bins and instead buying packaged items. Don't be afraid to ask your local store about its cleaning policies!

The Deli Counter

Deli counters and prepared food sections present a different challenge. Here, store personnel directly handle food products meant for your consumption. The easiest way to navigate these challenges is to think of the deli counter and prepared food section as mini restaurants. (For more information about issues to consider in gluten-free restaurant dining, please refer to *The Essential Gluten-Free Restaurant Guide*, also available from Triumph Dining.)

Before you make a purchase, you need to understand both the ingredients in the food and the preparation methods used to create it. There are many issues to consider in making a decision about these foods. Some examples include: Do gluten-containing meats go in the deli slicer? What, if any, precautions are taken in the prep area to avoid

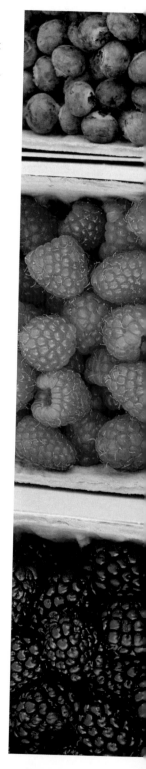

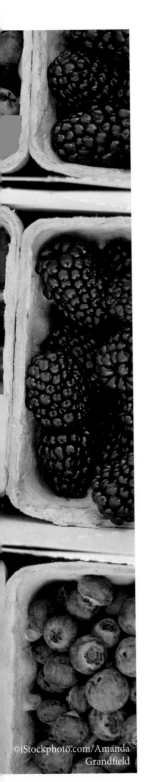

cross-contamination? Are there ingredient labels on the prepared foods? How accurate are those labels?

Often, however, it's challenging to interface with the employees who prepared these foods. At some grocery stores we've seen, the prepared foods are made off-site or by an early morning crew that's long since cleared out by the time the typical shopper gets to the store, making it hard to get questions answered about dish contents and preparation methods. For these reasons, we recommend frequenting deli counters and prepared food sections only when you've done due diligence to confirm that the products you're purchasing truly are gluten-free. Explain your issue to the employees and request cleaning of equipment or changing of gloves as needed.

Selecting Your Groceries

Despite a restricted diet, there are still many wonderful foods for gluten-free shoppers to choose from. When given a choice, we prefer to support the companies that cater to the needs of gluten-free customers. Some of these companies produce specialty products for the gluten-free market. Others have dedicated manufacturing lines and/or carefully test their products for gluten. Please consider buying their products and calling or writing in to let them know you appreciate their efforts. The more we support these businesses, the more products we'll have to choose from in the future.

Consider Your Information Source

When thinking about which products to purchase and evaluating information available to you, keep in mind that primary source information, like ingredient statements on packages and manufacturer statements, is always better and more reliable than secondary source information, like postings on message boards and compilation lists (this guide included). Think of it like a game of telephone—the more people who handle information before you receive it, or the older that information gets, the greater chance there is of it having inaccuracies or other problems. This year, for the first time, we're including a very few lists that are especially useful, but not recently updated. These are marked with a 25 symbol, which is defined on page 19.

Always Read Labels

The goal of this guide is to drastically cut your label-reading time, but the reality is that no product entirely obviates the need for label-reading. Product formulations can change without notice, companies can make mistakes on their gluten-free lists, and people compiling information can make mistakes as well. That's why you need to read labels every time you make a purchase, and regularly contact the company to confirm the gluten-free status of the products you consume.

Never Make Assumptions

When contacting companies, please keep in mind that the FDA has yet to issue a rule defining the term "gluten-free." Meanwhile, there's a lot of conflicting information on the gluten-free diet, even among dieticians, support groups and the many other experts in the field. Some believe that blue cheese is gluten-free; others do not. And the emerging question about the suitability of oats in the gluten-free diet adds even more confusion. So, don't expect a company to guess what your definition of gluten-free is. Always ask questions to make sure you understand what they mean when they say "gluten-free."

GLUTEN FREE OATS?

Ask your doctor if "gluten-free" oats may be right for you. Recent research suggests that moderate consumption of oats can be safe for most celiacs. However, there's a catch...it's only pure, uncontaminated oats.

In contrast, normal oats and oat products, like the ones found at your local grocer, are usually cross-contaminated with wheat during harvest, transport or processing. Consequently, they are unsafe for the gluten-free diet.

Pure, uncontaminated oats are available. They have to be specially grown and processed to avoid cross-contamination, so they are harder to find and more expensive than traditional oats. All the oats and oat products listed in this guide were reported to be gluten-free by the manufacturers. So if you're hankering for oatmeal-raisin cookies or a crunchy bowl of granola, you may finally have a safe option!

Where to Find More Information

This guide pre-supposes that you are familiar with the gluten-free diet. But for those just starting out, there are some excellent resources available to help you understand the gluten-free diet and make informed choices. For example, there are resources available from local and national support groups, widely available books and online materials. Doctors and nutritionists are also an excellent source of information. Even Triumph Dining's own GF 101 (which can be found on our blog) is a terrific source of information on the gluten-free diet. In short, be proactive about educating yourself. When it comes to the gluten-free diet, the educated shopper really is the only healthy shopper!

OVERVIEW OF FALCPA FOOD LABELING LAW

Effective January 1, 2006, the Food Allergen Labeling and Consumer Protection Act of 2004 (FALCPA), set requirements for the labeling of eight major allergens on packaged foods. This is a quick overview of the elements of the FALCPA that are likely to be relevant to consumers on a gluten-free diet.

Allergens Covered
The FALCPA covers eight major allergens that are credited with causing 90% of all food allergies. Those allergens include: milk, eggs, fish, crustacean shellfish, tree nuts, peanuts, soybeans and, most importantly, wheat. The FDA notes that, for the purposes of the FALCPA, wheat includes common wheat, durum wheat, club wheat, spelt, semolina, Einkorn, emmer, kamut and triticale.

Allergens Not Covered
It's important to note that the FALCPA does not cover barley or rye. Nor does it cover oats, which are likely to be cross-contaminated with wheat.

Labeling: What's Required
The FALCPA requires food manufacturers to identify allergens in ingredient lists in one of two ways:

1. In the ingredient listing, the common or usual name of the major food allergen must be followed in parentheses by the name of the food source from which the major allergen is derived. For example: "Enriched flour (wheat flour…)," or

2. Immediately following the ingredient listing, a "Contains" statement must indicate the name of the food source from which the major food allergen is derived. For example: "Contains: milk, wheat and eggs."

Allergens present in flavorings, coloring and additives must also be identified in one of the two ways listed above.

Labeling: What's Not Required
It is important to note that the FALCPA does not apply to major food allergens that are unintentionally added to food as a result of cross-contamination. Cross-contamination can result during the growing and harvesting of crops, or from the use of shared storage, transportation or production equipment.

The FALCPA also does not address the use of advisory labeling, including statements designed to identify the possibility of cross-contamination. The FALCPA does not require the use of such statements, nor does it specifically articulate standards of use for advisory statements.

Application

The FALCPA applies to all packaged foods sold in the U.S. that are regulated by the FDA and that are required to have ingredient statements.

It's important to note that the FALCPA does not apply to meat products, poultry products and egg products that fall under the authority of the USDA.

The Big Picture

What does this all mean for people following the gluten-free diet? There are three important limitations of the FALCPA to keep in mind:

- As far as gluten is concerned, the FALCPA does not cover it. The FALCPA covers wheat, but not rye, barley or other potentially troublesome grains.

- The FALCPA covers only products regulated by the FDA that require ingredient lists. For any product that does not require an ingredient list (such as raw fruits), or that falls outside the FDA's jurisdiction (such as meat, poultry and egg products that fall under the authority of the USDA), the FALCPA does not require manufacturers to identify major allergens.

- The FALCPA does not require manufacturers to identify the possibility of inadvertent cross-contamination, nor does it set specific standards for using advisory statements warning of potential cross-contamination.

The important thing to remember is that, despite improved labeling laws, hidden gluten in grocery items is still a very real possibility. Gluten can come from non-wheat sources, result from cross-contamination, or can occur in products not covered by the FALCPA. For those reasons, it's important to remain vigilant and carefully scrutinize the products you buy. It's not enough to just read labels; contacting manufacturers directly is often necessary.

In August 2011, the FDA reopened a 60-day commentary period for the proposed gluten-free labeling regulations originally required by FALCPA in 2007. These regulations have been further delayed from their previous 2008 deadline and are expected to be finalized in summer of 2012. If this law takes effect as planned, it will finally establish a uniform standard definition of the term gluten-free: "food that does not contain an ingredient that is any species of wheat, rye, barley, or a crossbred hybrid of these grains" or any ingredient resulting in the "presence of 20 parts per million (ppm) or more of gluten in the food." Although this is a huge step in the right direction, the law still has its flaws. Gluten-free labeling will remain voluntary for food manufacturers and they will have an undefined period of time to comply with the regulations. For more information, please visit the FDA at www.fda.gov.

USING THIS PRODUCT LIST

Our goal is for this guide to make your shopping trips easier, safer, and full of choices. There are a few things you need to know about this guide's content and organization to help us fulfill that goal.

PRODUCTS FEATURED

Our guide covers over 44,000 products from hundreds of different brands. The products listed are likely to be found in typical American grocery stores like Walmart, Meijer, Safeway, and others. They include brand names, as well as private label brands from many of the larger grocery chains. In cases where the grocery chain's name is different from their private label brand, we've also put the chain's name in parentheses next to the private label brand name.

When "All" are Gluten-Free

Some brands publish a list enumerating each gluten-free item, while others chose to simply say all foods in a particular category are gluten-free. In the latter case, we list the brand name in the appropriate category and sub-category, followed by a description of the products covered and the word "All" where applicable. For example, if a company, let's call it "Brand X," tells us that all its cheeses are gluten-free, it will be listed under "Brand X," followed by "Cheeses (All)." Alternatively, sometimes the brand communicates that all of their products are gluten-free, in which case they will be noted in the guide as "Brand X (All)," regardless of category.

"All BUT"

Sometimes a brand will communicate that all but a few of its products are gluten-free. In this case the items are listed by product type with the exceptions in parentheses. For example if Brand X's cheese is all gluten free except for blue cheese, it will appear as: Cheese (All BUT Blue Cheese).

PRODUCTS NOT FEATURED

This guide is far from comprehensive; there are smaller brands and new items popping up all the time. Most lists we receive are not comprehensive either – they contain whatever the company chooses to share with us. Just because a product isn't listed in these pages doesn't mean it's not gluten-free. This year, we tried to be more inclusive of smaller brands, even ones available only online, in order to give you as many choices as possible. If there's something you're interested in that's not listed in this guide, let us know, and we'll look into adding it for the next edition.

We haven't listed some items that are generally accepted and widely known to be gluten-free. For example, plain dairy milk is not listed. We have, however, listed flavored milk, sour cream and other items that often contain ingredients (e.g., thickeners or other additives) that may be of concern to some shoppers. Of course, what is generally accepted and widely known to be gluten-free is subjective.

So while one person may find an entire sub-category of items in the guide to be obviously gluten-free, some will not. We try to be as inclusive as possible for the sake of the latter audience.

For the sake of simplicity, this guide only lists items on a company's gluten-free list. We have excluded items that were not reported to be gluten-free.

Finally, there are some brands missing from the product listings because they simply do not provide or maintain lists of their gluten-free products. Unfortunately, companies are not required to maintain or share their gluten-free lists, so every company cannot be listed in this guide.

General Overview of Organization

The product catalog is organized as a three-tier system: Each item is listed first by category, then by subcategory, then by product name.

Organization by Category

The products listed in this guide are arranged like a typical grocery store. The list is organized first by master categories that align with aisles in a grocery store, like those for Dairy and Eggs, Snacks, and Frozen Foods. Our hope is that organizing the guide by grocery aisle will make your trip through the store quicker—you can follow along in the guide as you shop through the store.

There are a few exceptions to the link between master category and grocery aisle: In some cases, our consumer research found it more helpful to organize items by general category as opposed to aisle. For example, while refrigerated orange juice is often found in the Dairy and Eggs aisle, you'll find it listed here in the Beverages category.

Organization by Sub-Category

Each category is further divided by subcategories that align with the particular types of food products found in the category aisle. For example, subcategories within the Snacks category include: Chips, Cookies, Crackers, etc. Subcategories are organized alphabetically within the category. Unfortunately, not everything falls neatly into a subcategory, and it would be impractical to have a multitude of subcategories with only a few products in them. For example, Pancake Mix falls in the Baking Mixes subcategory, and Lemon juice is in Marinades and Cooking Sauces. Our index will direct you to the categories in which these products may be found.

Organization by Brand & Product

Within these subcategories, you'll find individual items listed alphabetically by brand name (in bold), then product name (not in bold). While we've done our best to organize the products into the correct category and subcategory, we hope you'll understand that it was a subjective process and there will be some variance.

Information on all items listed, except the items with the glasses symbol (more about these later) is obtained directly from the brand, manufacturer, or brand representative (we refer to these as the "company" for short). Occasionally, they also send along additional information, ranging from legal disclaimers to in-depth notes on manufacturing procedures.

AVIGATION TIP

he Easy Reference Table
f Contents on the inside
ont cover is a quick
sual reference for the
fferent categories and
b-categories. Or, use
e index in the back, if
ou prefer.

In order to make this guide portable and convenient, it's not practical to reprint all of the notes provided by a company. But, there are a few exceptions. We know that you want to know which items may pose cross-contamination concerns and, conversely, when companies go the extra mile by having dedicated production lines or gluten testing, for example. Therefore, those and other relevant situations are marked with special symbols.

We'll discuss each symbol in-depth here, but don't worry, there's a cheat sheet on Page 1 to jog your memory when you're actually at the store.

Placement of Symbols

If a symbol applies to all of a brand's listed products, we place the symbol next to the brand name. If it only applies to a particular product, the symbol will appear next to that specific product. For example, if Brand X's entire line comes with a cross-contamination warning, the disclaimer icon will appear next to the Brand X name. If the warning only applies to its Chocolate Chip flavor, we place the symbol next to the Chocolate Chip flavor listing only.

Limitation of Symbols

Another thing to keep in mind is that any information, including disclaimers like cross-contamination warnings, are provided by companies at their discretion. Unfortunately, companies are not required by law to warn shoppers of cross-contamination, so just because a company does not have a cross-contamination warning does not necessarily mean it's not an issue! We sincerely hope that the FDA will resolve this confusion in the near future.

Symbols In-Depth

Reading Symbol

Some prominent brands do not maintain or share gluten-free lists. When you're gluten-free, your choices are, by definition, limited. The goal of this book is to open up more choices.

So, in cases where brands do not have a gluten-free list but DO have a policy of accurately labeling for gluten, no matter how small the amount, Triumph Dining independently reviewed each product's ingredients (based solely on the product labeling) to determine which are gluten-free.

The information for these particular product listings did not come directly from the brand or manufacturer, as does that for the other products in this guide, so we have distinguished them with a special glasses symbol.

Calendar Symbol (New This Year!)

Some companies, for whatever reason, do not update their gluten-free information annually or do not share new lists with us for every edition. For brands with this symbol, we have reprinted the information they sent us last year in the interest of giving you the largest number of gluten-free options. It is possible that some of this information is out of date, as formulas and ingredient sources often change. Read these labels especially closely, and use caution when buying these products.

Gluten Testing Symbol

This symbol indicates that a company has tested its ingredients, finished products, machinery and/or equipment, etc. for gluten.

Gluten-Free Processing Symbol

Here's another happy symbol: this symbol indicates that the company reports any of the following:

- They use gluten-free lines, equipment, or facilities; or

- Items are produced in a gluten-free environment; or

- Cross-contamination is not an issue for whatever reason (be it because they have a dedicated facility, rigorous testing policies, etc.).

Cross-Contamination/Shared Equipment Symbol

A company may get this symbol if it reports any of the following:

- Cross-contamination may be an issue; or,

- Their products are made on equipment, lines or in a plant that also process gluten-containing items; or,

- Their products are made with gluten-free ingredients, but they would not provide information on whether the manufacturing process is gluten-free.

So, does this symbol mean that you need to avoid these products entirely? The answer is complicated, we're afraid. We don't like it any more than you're going to, but this is the world we live in and the hand the FDA has dealt us.

Some companies—too many, in our opinion—use language like the above bullet points in the hopes that it will cut down on litigation. In other words, they don't want to get sued. In these cases, it's not their Quality Control teams that are writing these disclaimers, but their legal teams.

So it's very possible that these products may be safe with little to no chance of cross-contamination, but the companies want to cover their legal bases by noting the chance, no matter how remote.

Unfortunately, there are also many cases where there may be a legitimate chance of cross-contamination. There's no surefire way to distinguish these real cross-contamination risks from an overzealous legal department. Trust us, we've tried!

Good Manufacturing Processes (Cross-Contamination Still Possible)

Something felt wrong about lumping together companies that write "cross-contamination is a possibility" and those that state "cross-contamination is a possibility but all our personnel are trained in handling allergenic materials, which are stored separately, and we sanitize and swab test shared machinery between each product run."

That's why this symbol covers companies that noted cross-contamination or shared equipment but also informed us about counter measures they have in place. Such measures may include the following:

- Special handling and/or segregation of gluten-containing ingredients or products; or,

- Scheduling equipment and machinery so that gluten-containing items are processed at different times than gluten-free items; along with,

- Thorough cleaning/sanitization procedures between gluten-containing and gluten-free product batches; or,

- Their products are made with gluten-free ingredients, but they will not claim their product are gluten-free, though they do have processes in place to minimize cross-contamination (i.e. the procedures above).

Of course, this is not an exhaustive list of the many different methods companies take to minimize cross-contamination. But we think you get the picture!

Strange Bedfellow

So you probably have this symbols thing down by now. But, then you may see ⓘ and ⚱ together. And you may rightly wonder, how can something be made on a dedicated gluten-free line or facility and still have a risk of cross-contamination? Well, a possible scenario may be that they have four lines in a plant, and three are dedicated gluten-free, but the fourth is used for gluten-containing items. So, in this case, there is both a gluten-free line (⚱) and non-gluten-free facility (ⓘ).

No Icon

When collecting gluten-free product lists, we always ask companies about cross-contamination. Not all companies, however, choose to share that information with us. And if they don't tell us about their cross-contamination status, we are unable to assign them an icon. So, when a company or product is listed without an icon, that does not necessarily mean, for example, that the products are (or are not) made in a shared facility; it just means that the company wouldn't tell us either way. Companies, unfortunately, are not required to share that information under current regulations; see Chapter 2 for more on the food labeling law.

Final Thoughts

This guide was created in response to a loose-leaf binder our company's founder used to carry. The binder was a collection of hundreds of gluten-free lists from hundreds of companies. It was a monster to carry and even worse to update. We're talking entire days spent calling companies and listening to bad hold music.

We've come a long way from loose-leaf binders and frantic calls to food companies right before dinner. And we hope that all this research we've done helps to make your life easier. We are the only guide that takes the time to give you these symbols, because we think they're relevant to good decision-making. Plus, you deserve the extra information. Please use it, and use it wisely.

LIMITATIONS OF THE GUIDE

While we hope that this guide makes gluten-free shopping easier, we do recognize that it has some limitations, which we would like to point out so that you can make informed shopping decisions.

Gluten-Free Lists

As mentioned in previous chapters, there is currently no FDA rule defining gluten-free and generally no consensus as to an exact definition. (Consider the controversies surrounding blue cheese and oats, to name a few.) So when a company reports that its products are gluten-free, there is the possibility that their definition of gluten-free may differ from yours.

In addition, the information published in this guide for each food item has been obtained directly from that item's manufacturer, the entity that licensed the manufacturing, or an affiliate, unless otherwise noted. It's impossible for us to verify the accuracy of the information companies report to us.

Always Read Labels

It's important to keep in mind that product formulations and ingredient sourcing can and do change without notice, companies can make mistakes on their gluten-free list, and people compiling and categorizing large volumes of information (like the content for this guide) can make mistakes, as well. For these reasons, Triumph Dining cannot assume any liability for the correctness or accuracy of any information presented in this guide. You should read labels every time you make a purchase and regularly contact companies to confirm the gluten-free status of the products you consume.

Contact the Company with Questions

Please contact companies directly with any questions or for updates. Any information provided in this guide was obtained from the company (unless otherwise noted), and they will always be your best source of information on their products.

A Question of Semantics

Since there is, as of this writing, no FDA regulation defining the term "gluten-free" and no requirement that companies report the possibility of cross-contamination, as consumers, we're still very much on our own. A company may claim its products are "gluten-free" and free of "cross-contamination," but since there's no universally accepted definition of either term, you may still not be getting the whole story. Therefore, a product's appearance in this guide does not mean that the product is entirely free of gluten (besides, that would likely be an impossible standard, as the most sophisticated commercially-available tests for gluten do not measure to 0 ppm). However, you may find our symbols useful in deciding whether a product is suitable for you. Please see page 19 for more details.

This guide is largely a compilation of the information provided by companies when consumers reach out to them to ask about the gluten-free status of their products. It saves you the trouble of calling or emailing thousands of companies yourself and constantly sifting through products, but it is not meant to be set in stone.

Common Sense is Your Best Guide

A guide like this should never be a replacement for your own knowledge, common sense and diligence. This guide is intended as a starting point only, and not a final determination that a listed product is gluten-free, suitable for the gluten-free diet, or safe for you personally to consume. It is not a substitute for reading labels and contacting companies. Rather, this guide is designed to help you zero in on the products most likely to be suitable for the gluten-free diet, so that you can focus your label-reading and company-contacting efforts on the most promising products, without wasting dozens and dozens of hours chasing dead ends. Always exercise caution when using any lists, even this one or ones directly from a brand. People make mistakes, so if something doesn't feel right, it probably isn't.

Some Final Notes

The information published in this guide is intended for use in the United States and with products manufactured with the intent to be sold in the United States only. Products sold or intended to be sold outside the United States may have completely different ingredients than their U.S. counterparts, and may not be gluten-free. However, this year we have included a few international companies (most of them dedicated gluten-free) that are distributed in the US or are available online. Keep in mind that other countries' regulations may differ from our own.

This guide is for limited educational purposes only and is not medical advice. If you have questions about the gluten-free diet, what ingredients are appropriate to consume, whether or not particular items are appropriate for your consumption, etc., please consult with your physician.

For the foregoing reasons, Triumph Dining cannot assume any liability for any losses or damages resulting from your use of this product listing. It's up to you to determine whether a product is appropriate based on your individual dietary needs. For more information about a particular company's testing practices, standards and thresholds, please contact that company directly.

Use of this guide indicates your acknowledgement of and agreement to these terms.

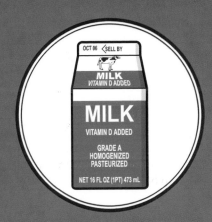

DAIRY & EGGS

BUTTER

Alta Dena
Salted Butter
Unsalted Sweet Butter

Berkeley Farms
Butter

Best Choice
Butter AA Quarters
Unsalted Butter

Cabot
Cabot Products (All)

Challenge
Butter (All)

Cub Foods
AA Butter Quarters
Butteriffic Tub
Salted Butter Quarters
Salted Whipped Butter
Unsalted Butter Quarters

Danish Creamery ⚕
Butter (All)

Darigold
Darigold (All)

Dutch Farms
Butter (All)

Fastco (Fareway)
Quarter Butter
Solid Butter

Flavorite (Cub Foods)
Butter Quarters

Food Club (Brookshire)
Butter
Unsalted Butter

Food Club (Marsh)
Butter AA Quarters
Butter AA Unsalted Quarters

Full Circle (Schnucks)
Organic Salted Butter
Organic Unsalted Butter

Garelick Farms
Salted Sweet Cream Butter

Gay Lea
Gay Lea (All)

Giant
Butter Stick
Salted Sweet Cream Butter Sticks
Unsalted Sweet Cream Butter Sticks

Grass Point Farms
Butter (All)

Great Value (Wal-Mart)
Salted Butter Quarters
Unsalted Butter Quarters

Haggen
Butter

Hiland Dairy
Butter

Horizon Organic
Butter (All)

Hy-Vee
Sweet Cream Butter Quarters
Sweet Cream Butter Solid
Sweet Cream Whipped Butter
Unsalted Sweet Butter Quarters

Jewel-Osco
Butterific

Keller's Creamery
Butter (All)

Kernel Season's ⓘ
Butter Spritzers
Kerrygold
Butter (All)
Land O'Lakes
Butter
Lucerne (Safeway) ✍
Butter - Spreadable with Canola Oil
Butter - Sweet Cream
Butter - Sweet Cream Unsalted
Meijer
Butter (Spread, Unsalted Quarters)
Organic Salted Butter Quarters
Organic Unsalted Butter Quarters
Organic Whip Butter
Meyenberg
Butter (All)
Nature's Promise (Giant)
Organic Salted Butter
Nature's Promise (Stop & Shop)
Organic Salted Butter
O Organics ✍
Organic Salted Sweet Cream Butter
Organic Unsalted Sweet Cream Butter
Oak Farms Dairy
Butter
Oberweis Dairy
Salted Butter
Unsalted Butter
Organic Valley ⓘ
Cultured Unsalted Butter
European Cultured Butter
Pasture Cultured Butter
Salted Butter
Whipped Salted Butter
Our Family
Butter Quarters AA (Salted, Unsalted)
Butter, Solid AA
Prairie Farms
Butter
Price Chopper
Salted Organic Butter
Unsalted Organic Butter
Private Selection (Kroger)
Organic Unsalted Butter
Publix
Organic Butter Salted

Organic Butter Unsalted
Salted Butter
Sweet Cream Butter
Unsalted Butter
Whipped Salted Butter
Whipped Unsalted Butter
Purity Dairies
Butter
Schnucks
Butter (Salted, Unsalted)
Butter Quarters
Whipped Butter (Salted, Unsalted)
Shaw's
Butter Stick Box
Butter Stick Box No Salt
Cream Butter Stick
Grade AA Soft Whipped Butter
Soft Whipped Butter No Salt
Stop & Shop
Salted Sweet Cream Butter Stick
Unsalted Sweet Cream Butter Stick
Straus Family Creamery
Butter (All)
Tillamook
Butter ⛾
Trader Joe's
Butter (All)
Fig Butter
Valu Time (Brookshire)
Butter
Vermont Butter & Cheese Creamery
Vermont Butter & Cheese Creamery (All)
Wegmans
Bearnaise Finishing Butter
Chipotle Lime Finishing Butter
Garlic Cheese Finishing Butter
Lemon Dill Finishing Butter
Solid Butter
Sweet Cream Butter Sticks - Salted
Sweet Cream Butter Sticks - Unsalted
Whipped Butter Tub - Salted
Whipped Butter Tub - Unsalted
Wild Harvest (ACME)
Salted Organic Butter
Unsalted Organic Butter

Wild Harvest (Albertsons)
Organic Salted Butter
Organic Unsalted Butter
Wild Harvest (Cub Foods)
Organic Salted Butter
Organic Unsalted Butter
Wild Harvest (Jewel-Osco)
Organic Salted Butter
Organic Unsalted Butter
Winn-Dixie
Butter (Salted, Unsalted)
Whipped Butter

BUTTERMILK

Albertsons
Buttermilk
Buttermilk Low Fat
Axelrod
Buttermilk
Barber's
Buttermilk
Berkeley Farms
Bulgarian Cultured Buttermilk
Cultured Lowfat Buttermilk
Best Choice
Low Fat Buttermilk
Broughton
1% Lowfat Buttermilk
3.25% Buttermilk
Bakers Blend Buttermilk
Darigold
Darigold (All)
Friendship Dairies
Buttermilk (All)
Gandy's (i)
Buttermilk
Garelick Farms
Buttermilk
Giant
Low Fat Buttermilk
Hiland Dairy
Bulgarian Buttermilk
Low Fat Buttermilk
Hood
Buttermilk

Kalona Organics
Buttermilk (All)
Lehigh Valley Dairy Farms
Buttermilk
Louis Trauth Dairy
Buttermilk
Lucerne (Safeway) ↩
Buttermilk Reduced Fat 1 1/2%
Marsh
2% Buttermilk
Mayfield Dairy
Buttermilk
McArthur Dairy
Cultured Buttermilk
Meadow Brook Dairy
Buttermilk
Meadow Gold
Buttermilk (All)
Meijer
1.5% Buttermilk
Oak Farms Dairy
Buttermilk
Organic Valley (i)
Buttermilk
PET Milk
Buttermilk
Prairie Farms
Buttermilk
Price's Creameries
Buttermilk
Purity Dairies
Lowfat Buttermilk
Whole Buttermilk
Reiter Dairy
Buttermilk
Robinson Dairy
Buttermilk (All)
Saco
Cultured Buttermilk (All)
T.G. Lee Dairy
Cultured Buttermilk

CHEESE & CHEESE SPREADS

4C
100% Imported Cheese (All)

ACME

2% Milk White Cheese Singles
2% String Mozzarella Cheese
American Cheese Singles
American Deluxe Cheese
American Slice Cheese
American White Cheese Singles
Baby Swiss Cheese
Cheese Singles
Colby Jack Cheese
Deluxe American White Cheese
Extra Sharp Cheddar Cheese
Extra Sharp White Cheddar Cheese
Fancy Italian Shredded Cheese
Fancy Mild Shredded Cheese
Fancy Shredded Mexican Cheese
Fancy Shredded Parmesan Cheese
Fancy Shredded Pizza Cheese
Fancy Shredded Sharp Cheese
Fat-Free White Cheese Singles
Mild Cheddar Cheese
Mild White Cheddar Cheese
Monterey Jack Cheese
Mozzarella Cheese Slices
Mozzarella N' Cheddar Cheese String
Mozzarella String Cheese
Muenster Cheese
NY Extra Sharp Cheddar Cheese
NY Sharp Cheddar Cheese
NY Sharp Yellow Cheese
NY White Extra Sharp Cheddar Cheese
NY Yellow Extra Sharp Cheddar Cheese
Pepper Jack Cheese
Pepper Jack Cheese Slices
Provolone Cheese Slices
Sharp Cheddar Cheese
Sharp White Cheddar Cheese
Shredded Colby Jack Cheese
Shredded Colby Monti Jack
Shredded Fancy Mexican Cheese
Shredded Italian Cheese
Shredded Mild Cheddar Cheese
Shredded Mild Cheese
Shredded Mozzarella Cheese
Shredded Reduced Fat 2% Mozzarella
Shredded Sharp Cheese
Singles American Cheese
Swiss Cheese Singles
Swiss Chunk Cheese
Vermont White Sharp Cheese
White American Cheese Singles
White Cheese Singles
White Sharp Cheddar Cheese

Alouette

Baby Brie, Herb
Baby Brie, Plain
Blue Cheese Crumbles
Brie Log
Brie Wedge, Garlic & Herbs
Brie Wedge, Plain
Brie Wedge, Smoked
Crème de Brie, Garlic & Herbs
Crème de Brie, Original
Feta Crumbles
Feta Garlic & Herb Crumbles
Feta Mediterranean Crumbles
Goat Cheese Crumbles
Goat Cheese Provencal Crumbles
Gorgonzola Cheese Crumbles
Gourmet Spreadable Log, Garlic & Herbs
Gourmet Spreadable Log, Sundried Tomato & Garlic
Petite Brie, Plain
Spreadable Cheese, Berries & Cream
Spreadable Cheese, Garlic & Herbs
Spreadable Cheese, Light Garlic & Herbs
Spreadable Cheese, Light Spinach Artichoke
Spreadable Cheese, Limited Edition Cheesecake
Spreadable Cheese, Savory Vegetable
Spreadable Cheese, Spinach Artichoke
Spreadable Cheese, Sundried Tomato
Spreadable Cheese, Sweet & Spicy Pepper Medley

Alta Dena

Goat Milk Cheese
Kefir Cheese
Mild Cheddar Cheese
Monterey Jack Cheese
Pepper Jack Cheese
Sharp Cheddar Cheese

Always Save
Grated Parmesan Cheese

Always Save (Price Chopper)
Imitation Slices
Shredded Imitation Cheddar

Andrew & Everett
Cheese Products (All)

Athenos
Blue Crumbled
Feta Chunk, Black Peppercorn
Feta Chunk, Garlic & Herb
Feta Chunk, Mild
Feta Chunk, Tomato & Basil
Feta Crumbled, Black Peppercorn
Feta Crumbled, Garlic & Herb
Feta Crumbled, Mild
Feta Crumbled, Reduced Fat
Feta Crumbled, Reduced Fat with
Tomato & Basil
Feta Crumbled, Roasted Bell Pepper &
Garlic
Feta Crumbled, Tomato & Basil
Feta Crumbled, Traditional
Feta Crumbled, with Basil & Tomato
Feta Crumbled, with Garlic & Herb
Feta Crumbled, with Lemon, Garlic, &
Oregano
Feta Traditional, Chunk Packed In Brine
Gorgonzola Crumbled

BelGioioso Cheese
BelGioioso Cheese (All)

Best Choice
Grated Parmesan
Grated Parmesan/Romano
Grated Parmesan/Romano/Asiago
Party Cheese American Flavor
Party Cheese Cheddar Flavor
Party Cheese Sharp Cheddar Flavor

Bett's
Bett's (All)

Black Creek
Cheddar

Black Diamond
1 Year White Cheddar
2 Year White Cheddar
2 Year Yellow Cheddar
3 Year White Cheddar

5 Year White Cheddar
Chardonnay & Sharp Cheddar Cold
Pack Spread
Extra Sharp Cheddar Cold Pack Spread
Merlot & Sharp Cheddar Cold Pack
Spread

Black River
Blue
Gorgonzola

Blythedale Vermont Cheese
Blythedale Vermont Cheese (All BUT
Blue Cheese)

Boar's Head
Cheese (All)

Bongards
Cheese (All)

Cabot
Cabot Products (All)

**Central Market Classics
(Price Chopper)**
Asiago Cheese Spread
Baby Swiss Brick Cheese
Blue Cheese Wedge
Crumbled Blue Cheese
Crumbled Feta Cheese
Feta Cheese Chunk
Garlic Herb Spread
New York Cheddar
New York Extra Sharp Cheddar Cheese
Vermont Cheddar
Vermont Extra Sharp Cheddar Cheese

Chavrie
Chavrie Log
Chavrie Log, Herb
Chavrie with Basil & Roasted Garlic
Original Chavrie

County Line
American
Baby Swiss
Brick Cheese
Colby
Colby Jack
Extra Sharp Cheddar
Farmer's Cheese
Hickory Smoked Cheddar
Mild Cheddar
Monterey Jack

Mozzarella
Muenster
Pepper Jack
Provolone
Ricotta
Sharp Cheddar
Smoked Provolone
String Cheese
Swiss

Cracker Barrel ๑

Cheese, Emmentaler Swiss
Cheese, Extra Sharp
Cheese, Extra Sharp Cheddar
Cheese, Extra Sharp Cheddar 2% Milk Reduced Fat
Cheese, Extra Sharp Cheddar 2% Milk Reduced Fat Shredded
Cheese, Extra Sharp Cheddar Cheese Cuts
Cheese, Extra Sharp Cheddar Reduced Fat Cheese Cuts with 2% Milk
Cheese, Extra Sharp White
Cheese, Extra Sharp-White Cheddar
Cheese, Fontina
Cheese, Havarti
Cheese, Natural Baby Swiss
Cheese, Natural Cheddar Vermont Sharp-White
Cheese, Natural Extra Sharp Cheddar
Cheese, Natural Extra Sharp Cheddar 2% Milk Reduced Fat
Cheese, Natural Extra Sharp Cheddar White
Cheese, Natural Extra Sharp White Cheddar Reduced Fat
Cheese, Natural Sharp Cheddar
Cheese, Natural Sharp Cheddar 2% Milk Reduced Fat
Cheese, Natural Sharp Cheddar Slices
Cheese, Natural Sharp White Cheddar Reduced Fat
Cheese, Natural Vermont's Sharp White Cheddar 2% Milk Reduced Fat
Cheese, Sharp Cheddar Shredded
Cheese, Sharp-White Cheddar
Cheese, White Colby

Cracker Cuts ๑

Cheese Cuts, Natural Baby Swiss

DCI Cheese Company ♀

Natural Cheese (All)

DeLallo

50/50 Shredded Blend
American, Sliced
Baby Swiss
Cheddar with Horseradish, Sliced
Ciliegine (with Basil Leaves, with Cherry Tomato)
Ciliegine Piccante
Colby Jack, Sliced
Colby, Sliced
Creamy Havarti with Dill
Domestic Feta
Fresh Marinated Mozzarella
Hot Pepper Cheese
Imported Romano Deli Cup
Monterey Jack, Sliced
Mozzarella, Sliced
Muenster, Sliced
Parmesan Deli Cup
Part Skim Ricotta
Processed Cheddar, Extra Sharp
Provolone, Private Stock
Provolone, Sliced
Swiss, Sliced
Whole Milk Ricotta

Deli Fresh ๑

Cheese, Colby Jack Slices
Cheese, Mild Cheddar Slices
Cheese, Mozzarella Slices Low Moisture
Cheese, Natural Swiss Slices
Cheese, Pepper Jack Spicy Slices
Cheese, Provolone Slices
Cheese, Sharp Cheddar Slices
Cheese, Swiss 2% Milk Reduced Fat Slices
Cheese, Swiss Slices

Delice de France

Black Truffle Brie
Original Brie
Di Lusso Cheese

Dietz & Watson ✓

Aalsbruk Edam
Aalsbruk Gouda

Aalsbruk Smoked Gouda
Aged Aalsbruk Gouda
Aged Cheddar with Habanero &
  Jalapeno
Baby Swiss
Buffalo Wing Hot Sauce Cheddar
Buffalo Wing Wheel
Champagne Cheddar Wheel
Cheddar with Jalapeno & Cayenne
  Pepper
Colby Jack, Mini Horn
Colby Jalapeno, Mini Horn
Colby, Mini Horn
Danish Blue
Danish Havarti
Danish Style Fontina
Double Cream New York State Cheddar
Feta
Gorgonzola
Habanero & Jalapeno Wheel
Havarti with Dill
Horseradish & Bacon Cheddar
Horseradish Cheddar
Horseradish Wheel
Hot Pepper Buffalo Wing Cheddar
Hot Pepper Jack
Jalapeno & Cayenne Pepper Cheddar
Jarlsberg
Lacy Swiss
Monterey Jack
Mozzarella
Muenster
New York State Champagne Cheddar
New York State Sharp White Cheddar
New York State Sharp Yellow Cheddar
NY State Cheddar with Horseradish
NY State Cheddar with Toasted Onion
Peppadew Cheddar
Peppadew New York State Cheddar
Peppadew Wheel
Pepper Jack
Pepperoni Cheddar
Port Salut
Port Wine Cheddar
Provolone
Provolone Cheese
Roasted Garlic

Roasted Garlic Cheddar
Roasted Garlic Wheel
Sharp Cheddar-Red Wax
Sharp Italian Table with Picante Olives
Sharp Italian Table with Tomato & Basil
Sharp White Cheddar
Sharp Yellow Cheddar
Smoked Cheddar Cheese
Smoked Gouda
Smoked Gouda Wheel
Swiss 4X4
Swiss 4X6
Swiss Cheese
Swiss Gruyere
Triple Cream Bergenost Cheese
Triple Cream Bergenost Wheel
White American Cheese
Xtra Sharp NY State Aged Cheddar
XXXtra Sharp Cheddar
Yellow American

Dragone
Mozzarella
Ricotta

Dutch Farms
Cheese (All)

Easy Cheese ✍
Easy Cheese, American
Easy Cheese, Cheddar
Easy Cheese, Sharp Cheddar

Fastco (Fareway)
American Cheese Slices
Cheese Spread
Colby Jack
Colby Jack Chunk
Colby Jack Deli
Deluxe American Slices
Extra Sharp Cheddar
Fancy Shredded Cheddar
Fancy Shredded Colby Jack
Fancy Shredded Mozzarella
Fancy Shredded Taco
Farm Cheese
Medium Cheddar
Medium Cheddar Chunk
Mexican Shredded Cheese
Mild Cheddar
Mild Cheddar Chunk

Moon Colby
Mozzarella
Mozzarella Slices
Natural Cheddar Chunk
Natural Colby Chunk
Natural Mozzarella Chunk
Parmesan Cheese
Pepper Jack
Pepper Jack Chunk
Pepper Jack Deli
Provolone Deli
Sharp Cheddar
Sharp Cheddar Chunk
Sharp Shredded Cheddar
Shredded Cheddar
Shredded Cheddar Chunk
Shredded Cheese
Shredded Colby Jack
Shredded Mozzarella
Shredded Pizza
String Cheese
Swiss
Swiss Chunk
Swiss Deli
Swiss Slices
Finlandia Cheese
Finlandia (All)

Food Club (Brookshire)

2% Four Cheese Mexican Blend
   (Finely Shred)
2% Low Moisture Part Skim Mozzarella
   (Finely Shred)
2% Mild Cheddar (Finely Shred)
2% Pasteurized Processed Sharp Sliced
   Cheese
2% Pasteurized Processed Sliced Cheese
2% Pasteurized Processed Swiss Sliced
   Cheese
Aerosol Cheese (American, Cheddar,
   Sharp Cheddar)
Cheddar Jack (Finely Shred)
Colby Cheese
Colby Jack Cheese
Colby Jack Shred
Colby/Monterey Cheese
Fat Free Individually Wrapped Sliced
   Processed Cheese

Low Moisture Part Skim Mozzerella Bar
Low Moisture Part Skim Mozzerella
   Chunks
Low Moisture Part Skim Shredded
   Mozzarella
Medium Cheddar Bar
Medium Cheddar, Chunks
Mild Cheddar Bar
Mild Cheddar Shred
Mild Cheddar, Chunk
Monterey Jack (Finely Shred)
Monterey Jack, Bar
Monterey Jack, Chunk
Mozzarella (Finely Shred)
Parmesan (Finely Shred)
Pepper Jack, Chunk
Sharp Cheddar Bar
Sharp Cheddar Chunk
Sharp Cheddar Shred
Shredded Cheddar Cheese
Shredded Colby Jack
Shredded Mozzarella Cheese
Shredded Parmesan Cheese

Food Club (Marsh)

Cheddar New York Sharp Bar (Colored)
Cheddar Sliced Shingles
Cheese Food, 2% Individually Wrapped
   Slices
Cheese Product with Calcium,
   Individually Wrapped Slices
Colby Chunk
Colby Jack Bar
Colby Jack Chunk
Colby Jack Longhorn Half Moon
Colby Jack Slices Shingle
Colby Longhorn Half Moon
Extra Sharp Cheddar - Chunk
Extra Sharp Cheddar Bar
Finely Shredded 2% Mexican Blend
Finely Shredded 2% Mozzarella
Finely Shredded Colby Jack
Finely Shredded Italian Blend
   (6 Cheese)
Finely Shredded Jack Cheddar
Finely Shredded Mexican Blend
   (4 Cheese)
Finely Shredded Mild Cheddar

Finely Shredded Mozzarella
Finely Shredded Nacho/Taco
Finely Shredded Pizza 4 Cheese Blend
Finely Shredded Sharp Cheddar
Low Moisture Part Skim Mozzarella Bar
Low Moisture Part Skim Mozzarella
  Shredded
Medium Cheddar Bar
Medium Cheddar Chunk
Mild Cheddar Bar
Mild Cheddar, Chunk
Mild Cheddar, Shredded 2%
Monterey Jack Bar
Mozzarella Shingle Slice
Muenster Slice Shingle
Parmesan Finely Shredded
Pepperjack Chunk
Pepperjack Slices Shingle
Processed Cheese, Fat Free Individually
  Wrapped Slices
Provolone Slices Shingle
Sharp Cheddar Bar
Sharp Cheddar Chunk
Sharp Cheddar, Shredded
Sharp Cheese Food, 2% Individually
  Wrapped Slices
Shredded Cheddar
Shredded Mild Cheddar
Swiss Cheese Food, 2% Individually
  Wrapped Slices
Swiss Chunk
Swiss Finely Shredded
Swiss Slice Shingle

Friendship Dairies
Cheese (All)
Frigo
Blue Crumbled Classic
Gorgonzola Crumbled Classic
Mozzarella
Ricotta
Frigo Cheese Heads
String Cheese
Full Circle (Schnucks)
Organic Greek Feta
Garcia Baquero
Spanish Cheeses (All)

Genuardi's
100% Grated Parmesan and Romano
Giant
1/3 Less Fat Neufchatel Cheese
2% Milk Reduced Fat Yellow American
  Cheese Singles
Big Chunk Mild Cheddar Cheese
Big Chunk Yellow Sharp Cheddar Cheese
Chunk Mild Cheddar Cheese
Chunk Swiss Cheese
Colby Jack Chunk
Crumbled Blue Cheese
Crumbled Feta Cheese (Deli)
Fancy Shredded Mild Cheddar Cheese
Fancy Shredded Mozzarella
Fancy Shredded Parmesan Cheese
Fancy Shredded Reduced Fat Mexican
  Blend
Fancy Shredded Sharp Cheddar Cheese
Fancy Shredded Three Cheese Mexican
  Blend
Grated Parmesan & Romano
Grated Parmesan Cheese
Individually Wrapped Yellow American
  Cheese Slices
Longhorn Colby Chunk
Low Moisture Part Skim Mozzarella
  String Cheese
Monterey Jack Chunk
Monterey Jack with Peppers Chunk
Muenster Cheese Slices
Natural Swiss Cheese Slices
No Fat Ricotta Cheese
Part Skim Mozzarella Chunk
Part Skim Ricotta Cheese
Pepper Jack Chunk
Reduced Fat Mozzarella String Cheese
Reduced Fat Shredded Cheddar Cheese
Regular Sliced Provolone Smoked
  Cheese
Sharp Cheddar Chunk
Shredded Cheddar Cheese
Shredded Mild Cheddar Cheese
Shredded Mozzarella Cheese
Shredded Reduced Fat Mozzarella
Shredded Sharp Cheddar
Sliced Medium Cheddar Cheese

Sliced Mozzarella Cheese
Sliced Provolone
String Cheese
Whole Milk Mozzarella Chunk
Whole Milk Ricotta Cheese
Yellow American Cheese Singles

Giant Eagle
American Cheese, Individually Wrapped
Blue Crumbled Cheese
Colby Jack Cheese Chunk
Colby, High Moisture
Deluxe Sliced American
Easy Melt
Extra-Sharp Cheddar Cheese Chunk
Fancy Shred Colby Jack
Fancy Shred Mild Cheddar
Fancy Shred Parmesan
Fancy Shred RBST Free 2% Mexican
Fancy Shred Sharp Cheddar
Fancy Shred Swiss
Fancy Shred Taco Cheese
Fat Free American Cheese, Individually
  Wrapped
Feta Crumbled Cheese
Gorgonzola Crumbled Cheese
Grated Parmesan & Romano Cheese
Grated Parmesan Cheese
Individually Wrapped 2% American
  Cheese
Lite String Cheese
Low-Moisture Part-Skim Mozzarella
  Chunk
Mild Cheddar Cheese Chunk
Monterey Jack Chunk
Mozzarella Ball
NY Extra Sharp Cheddar Cheese Chunk
NY Sharp Cheddar Cheese Chunk
NY White Cheddar Chunk
Pepper Jack Cheese Chunk
Pepper Jack Cheese, Individually
  Wrapped Slices
Pizza Blend
Reduced Fat Blue Crumbled Cheese
Reduced Fat Feta Crumbled Cheese
Sharp 2% Cheese, Individually Wrapped
  Slices
Sharp Cheddar Cheese Chunk

Sharp Fat Free Cheese, Individually
  Wrapped Slices
Shredded 4 Cheese Italian
Shredded 4 Cheese Mexican
Shredded Fancy Colby Jack Cheese
Shredded Low Fat Mozzarella
Shredded Mexican Blend
Shredded Mild Cheddar
Shredded Mozzarella
Shredded RBST Free 2% Mild Cheddar
Shredded RBST Free 2% Mozzarella
Shredded Sharp Cheddar
Shredded Whole Milk Mozzarella
Sliced Colby Jack Cheese
Sliced Muenster
Sliced Pepper Jack Cheese
Sliced Provolone Cheese
Sliced Sharp Cheddar
Sliced Swiss Cheese
String Cheese
Swiss Cheese Chunk

GoPicnic
Asiago Cheese Spread

Goya
Baby Gouda
Nela Queso de Papa
Queso Blanco
Queso de Freir

Grafton Village Cheese
Grafton Village Cheese (All BUT
  Grafton Duet)

Grass Point Farms
Cheese (All)

Great Hill Blue Cheese
Great Hill Blue Cheese

Great Value (Wal-Mart)
100% Parmesan Grated Cheese
2% Milk American Deluxe Reduced
  Fat Pasteurized Process Cheese with
  Added Calcium
2% Milk Reduced Fat Mild Cheddar
  Cheese Chunk
2% Milk Reduced Fat Sharp Cheddar
  Cheese Chunk
American Pasteurized Prepared Cheese
  Product Singles

American Reduced Fat Pasteurized Process Cheese Food Singles
Cheddar Cheese Chunk, Mild
Cheddar Cheese Cubes, Mild
Cheddar Chunk, Sharp
Cheese Wow American Cheese
Cheese Wow Cheddar Cheese
Cheese Wow Pepper Jack Cheese
Colby And Monterey Jack Cheese Chunk
Colby And Monterey Jack Cheese Cubes
Deluxe American Pasteurized Process Cheese Singles
Deluxe White American Pasteurized Process Cheese Singles
Extra Sharp Cheddar Cheese Chunk
Fancy Shredded Colby & Monterey Jack Cheese
Fancy Shredded Fiesta Blend Cheese
Fancy Shredded Italian Blend Cheese
Fancy Shredded Low-Moisture Part-Skim Mozzarella Cheese
Fancy Shredded Mild Cheddar Cheese
Fancy Shredded Mozzarella Cheese
Fancy Shredded Parmesan Blend
Fancy Shredded Parmesan Cheese
Fancy Shredded Pizza Blend Cheese
Fancy Shredded Sharp Cheddar Cheese
Fancy Shredded Swiss Cheese
Fancy Shredded Taco Blend Cheese
Fat Free Pasteurized Process Cheese Product Singles
Feather Shredded Colby & Monterey Jack Cheese
Feather Shredded Mild Cheddar Cheese
Feather Shredded Mozzarella Cheese
Longhorn Style Colby Cheese Chunk
Longhorn Style Mild Cheddar Cheese Chunk
Medium Cheddar Cheese Chunk
Medium Cheddar Chunk
Melt 'n Dip Pasteurized Processed Cheese Spread
Monterey Jack Cheese Chunk
Mozzarella Cheese Chunk
Muenster Cheese Chunk
Natural Colby Cheese Chunk

Pepper Jack Cheese Chunk
Pepper Jack Cheese Cubes
Sharp Cheddar Cheese Chunk
Shredded Mild Cheddar Cheese
Shredded Mozzarella Cheese
Shredded White Sharp Cheddar Cheese
Sliced Cheddar Cheese, Mild
Sliced Mozzarella Cheese
Sliced Pepper Jack Cheese
Sliced Provolone Cheese
Sliced Swiss Cheese
Swiss Cheese Chunk
White American Pasteurized Prepared Cheese Product Singles
White Mild Cheddar Cheese Chunk
White Sharp Cheddar Cheese Chunk

Haggen

Cheddar, Extra Sharp
Cheddar, Medium
Cheddar, Mild
Cheddar, Sharp
Colby Jack
Colby Jack Bar
Colby Jack Loaf
Colby Jack Shredded
Colby Longhorn
Individually Wrapped Sliced American Cheese
Individually Wrapped Sliced Fat Free American Cheese
Mexican Blend
Monterey Jack
Mozzarella
Parmesan
Pepperjack
Pizza Blend
Ricotta (Low Fat, Part Skim)
String Cheese
Swiss

H-E-B

Cranberry Cinnamon Goat Cheese Log
Crumbled Blue Cheese
Crumbled Goat Cheese
Fresh Mozzarella Bocconcini
Fresh Mozzarella Ciliegine
Garlic and Herb Goat Cheese Log
Havarti with Peppers

Herb & Onion Feta Spread
Honey Goat Cheese Log
Horseradish Cheddar
Peppadew Goat Cheese Log
Plain Goat Cheese Log
Simply Cheesy American
Simply Cheesy Cheddar
Spicy Tomato Feta Spread

Heini's
Cheese (All)

Heluva Good
Cheese Products (All)

Hill Country Fare (H-E-B)
Muenster
Part Skim Mozzarella
Quesadilla with Peppers
Swiss Cheese

Hilmar Cheese
Cheese Products (All)

Horizon Organic
Cheese (All)

Hy-Vee
American Singles
American Singles 2% Milk
Colby Cheese
Colby Jack Cheese
Colby Jack Longhorn Style
Colby Jack Slices
Colby Longhorn Cheese
Colby Slice Singles
Extra Sharp Cheddar Cheese
Fat Free Singles
Fat Free Swiss Cheese Slices
Finely Shredded Cheddar Jack Cheese
Finely Shredded Colby Jack Cheese
Finely Shredded Italian Cheese
Finely Shredded Low Moisture Part
    Skim Mozzarella Natural Cheese
Finely Shredded Mexican Blend Cheese
Finely Shredded Mild Cheddar 2%
    Cheese
Finely Shredded Mild Cheddar Cheese
Finely Shredded Mozzarella 2% Milk
Finely Shredded Mozzarella Cheese
Finely Shredded Parmesan Cheese
Finely Shredded Swiss Cheese
Grated Parmesan Cheese

Grated Parmesan Romano Cheese
Lil' Hunk Colby Jack Cheese
Lil' Hunk Mild Cheddar Cheese
Lil' Hunk Pepper Jack Cheese Cubes
Low Moisture Part Skim Mozzarella
    Cheese
Low Moisture Part Skim Mozzarella
    Slices
Medium Cheddar Cheese
Medium Cheddar Longhorn Cheese
Mild Cheddar Cheese
Mild Cheddar Slices
Monterey Jack Cheese
Muenster Cheese Slices
Orange Rind Muenster Cheese
Pepper Jack Cheese
Pepper Jack Singles
Pepper Jack Slices
Provolone Cheese Slices
Sharp Cheddar Cheese
Sharp Cheddar Longhorn Cheese
Shredded Colby Jack Cheese
Shredded Low Fat Part Skim Mozzarella
    Cheese
Shredded Mild Cheddar Cheese
Shredded Mozzarella Cheese
Shredded Parmesan Cheese
Shredded Pizza Cheese
Shredded Sharp Cheddar Cheese
Shredded Taco Cheese
Sliced Low Moisture Part Skim
    Mozzarella
Smoke Flavored Provolone Cheese
Swiss Cheese
Swiss Singles
Swiss Slices

Ilchester
English Cheeses (All)

Isola
Baked Lemon Ricotta

Jardine's ⓘ
Mi Queso Su Queso

Jarlsberg
Norwegian Cheeses (All)

Jewel-Osco
2% Milk American Cheese Singles
2% Milk Cheese Single

2% Sharp Cheddar Cheese
2% String Mozzarella Cheese
American Cheese Singles
American Deluxe Cheese
Brick Cheese
Cheese Dip
Colby Jack Cheese
Colby Jack Cheese Sticks
Colby Jack Sliced Cheese
Deluxe American Cheese Slices
Extra Sharp Cheddar Cheese
Fancy Shredded Cheddar Jack Cheese
Fancy Shredded Italian Blend Cheese
Fancy Shredded Mexican Cheese
Fancy Shredded Mild Cheddar Cheese
Fancy Shredded Mild Cheese
Fancy Shredded Nacho Blend Cheese
Fancy Shredded Parmesan Cheese
Fancy Shredded Pizza Blend Cheese
Fancy Shredded Sharp Cheddar Cheese
Fancy Shredded Taco Cheese
Fat-Free Cheese Singles
Fat-Free Shredded Mild Cheese

Grated Parmesan Cheese
Grated Romano/Parmesan Cheese
Longhorn Colby Jack Cheese
Medium Cheddar Cheese
Mild Cheddar Cheese Slices
Monterey Jack Cheese
Mozzarella Cheese
Mozzarella Cheese Slices
Mozzarella String Cheese
Muenster Cheese
Pepper Jack Cheese
Provolone Cheese Slices
Sharp Cheddar Cheese
Shredded 2% Colby Jack Cheese
Shredded 2% Mexican Cheese
Shredded 2% Mild Cheddar Cheese
Shredded Colby Jack Cheese
Shredded Mexican Cheddar Jack Cheese
Shredded Mild Cheddar Cheese
Shredded Monterey Jack Cheese
Shredded Mozzarella
Shredded Reduced Fat 2% Mozzarella

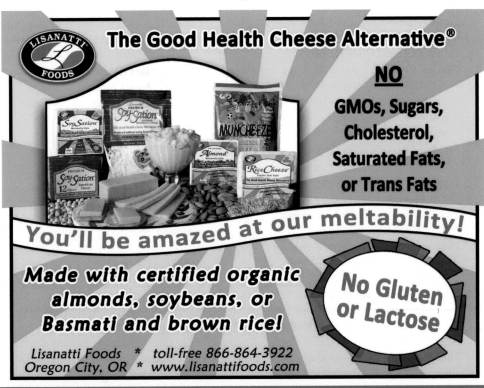

Shredded Reduced Fat 2% Sharp
Cheddar
String Cheese
Swiss Cheese
Swiss Cheese Singles
Swiss Cheese Slices

Joseph Farms
Natural Cheeses (All)

Kalona Organics
Cheese Curds (All)

Kerrygold
Cheese (All BUT Kerrygold Dubliner
with Irish Stout)

Kraft Grated Cheese ᑯ
Grated Cheese, 100% Real Parmesan &
Romano
Grated Cheese, 100% Real Romano
Grated Cheese, Parmesan 100% Grated
Grated Cheese, Parmesan Original
Grated Cheese, Parmesan Reduced Fat
Grated Cheese, Parmesan Shredded
Grated Cheese, Parmesan, Romano &
Asiago Shredded

Kraft Natural Cheese ᑯ
Natural Cheese, Cheddar & Monterey
Jack Marbled
Natural Cheese, Cheddar Extra Sharp
Natural Cheese, Cheddar Medium
Natural Cheese, Cheddar Mild
Natural Cheese, Cheddar Sharp
Natural Cheese, Colby
Natural Cheese, Colby & Monterey Jack
Natural Cheese, Colby & Monterey Jack
Marbled
Natural Cheese, Colby Longhorn Style
Natural Cheese, Extra Sharp Cheddar
Natural Cheese, Medium Cheddar
Natural Cheese, Mild Cheddar
Natural Cheese, Monterey Jack
Natural Cheese, Mozzarella Low-
Moisture Part-Skim
Natural Cheese, Sharp Cheddar

Kraft Natural Cheese Sticks ᑯ
Natural Cheese Sticks, Extra Sharp
Cheddar
Natural Cheese Sticks, Mild Cheddar

Natural Cheese Sticks, Sharp Cheddar
2% Milk Reduced Fat

Kraft Natural Crumbles ᑯ
Natural Cheese Crumbles, Cheddar
Aged Wisconsin

Kraft Natural Shredded Cheese ᑯ
Natural Shredded Cheese, Cheddar &
Monterey Jack
Natural Shredded Cheese, Cheddar Mild
Natural Shredded Cheese, Cheddar
Pepper Jack Finely Shredded
Natural Shredded Cheese, Colby &
Monterey Jack
Natural Shredded Cheese, Colby &
Monterey Jack Finely Shredded
Natural Shredded Cheese, Italian Classic
Finely Shredded
Natural Shredded Cheese, Italian Five
Cheese
Natural Shredded Cheese, Mexican Style
Cheddar Jack Finely Shredded
Natural Shredded Cheese, Mexican Style
Four Cheese
Natural Shredded Cheese, Mexican Style
Taco
Natural Shredded Cheese, Mild Cheddar
Finely Shredded
Natural Shredded Cheese, Monterey
Jack
Natural Shredded Cheese, Mozzarella
Natural Shredded Cheese, Mozzarella
Low Moisture Part-Skim
Natural Shredded Cheese, Pizza Four
Cheese
Natural Shredded Cheese, Pizza
Mozzarella & Cheddar
Natural Shredded Cheese, Sharp
Cheddar Aged Wisconsin
Natural Shredded Cheese, Sharp
Cheddar Finely Shredded Aged
Wisconsin

Kraft Singles ᑯ
Single Cheese Slices, Aged Swiss
Single Cheese Slices, American
Single Cheese Slices, American Fat Free
Single Cheese Slices, American Made
with 2% Milk

Single Cheese Slices, American Slices
Single Cheese Slices, American Slices
Twin Pack
Single Cheese Slices, Cheddar Sharp
Single Cheese Slices, Cheddar Sharp 2%
Milk
Single Cheese Slices, Pepperjack 2%
Milk
Single Cheese Slices, Sharp Cheddar Fat
Free
Single Cheese Slices, Swiss 2% Milk
Single Cheese Slices, Swiss Fat Free
Single Cheese Slices, White American
Single Cheese Slices, White American
2% Milk
Single Cheese Slices, White American
Fat Free

Kraft String-Ums ᧟
String Cheese, Mozzarella

Kraft Twist-Ums & String-Ums ᧟
String Cheese, Mozzarella & Cheddar
String Cheese, Mozzarella & Cheddar
Super Long

Land O'Lakes
Natural Cheeses
Process Cheese
Laughing Cow, The hj33
Laughing Cow Cheese Wedges (All)
Mini Babybel (All)

Lifeway
Lifeway (All)

Lucerne (Safeway) ᧟
Cheese Ball - Mozzarella Part Skim Low
Moisture
Cheese Ball - Mozzarella Whole Milk
Cheese Stick - Colby Jack
Cheese Stick - Pepper Jack
Cheese Sticks - Colby Jack and Pepper
Jack
Cheese Sticks - Mild Cheddar
Cheese Sticks - Sharp Cheddar Reduced
Fat 2%
Feta Cheese, Crumbled
Finely Shredded Asiago Cheese
Finely Shredded Cheddar Jack
Finely Shredded Mexican Four Cheese
Blend

Finely Shredded Mexican Four Cheese
Blend- Reduced Fat 2%
Finely Shredded Mild Cheddar
Finely Shredded Mozzarella
Finely Shredded Parmesan
Finely Shredded Southwest Two Cheese
Blend
Goat Cheese Crumbled
Natural Colby Cheese
Natural Colby Jack Cheese
Natural Colby Jack Cheese- 2%
Reduced Fat
Natural Extra Sharp Cheddar
Natural Longhorn Half Moon Cheese
Natural Medium Cheddar
Natural Medium Cheddar- 2%
Reduced Fat
Natural Mild Cheddar
Natural Monterey Jack
Natural Monterey Jack- 2% Reduced Fat
Natural Mozzarella Low Moisture Part
Skim
Natural Muenster
Natural New York Extra Sharp Aged
Cheddar
Natural Party Pleasers Variety Cheese
Natural Pepper Jack
Natural Ricotta Part Skim
Natural Sharp Cheddar Cheese
Natural Sharp Cheddar- Reduced Fat 2%
Natural Sliced Aged Swiss Cheese
Natural Sliced Colby Jack Cheese
Natural Sliced Havarti Cheese
Natural Sliced Medium Cheddar Cheese
Natural Sliced Medium Cheddar-
Reduced Fat 2%
Natural Sliced Monterey Jack
Natural Sliced Mozzarella
Natural Sliced Muenster
Natural Sliced Pepper Jack
Natural Sliced Provolone
Natural Sliced Provolone- Reduced Fat 2%
Natural Sliced Sharp Cheddar
Natural Sliced Smoked Gouda
Natural Sliced Swiss
Natural Sliced Swiss- Reduced Fat 2%
Natural Swiss

Shredded Cheddar Jack Cheese - Reduced Fat 2%
Shredded Colby Jack
Shredded Medium Cheddar
Shredded Mild Cheddar
Shredded Monterey Jack
Shredded Mozzarella Low Moisture Part Skim
Shredded Mozzarella Provolone
Shredded Mozzarella Reduced Fat 2%
Shredded Sharp Cheddar
Shredded Sharp Cheddar- Reduced Fat 2%
Snacker Cuts - Colby Jack
Snacker Cuts - Mild Cheddar
Snacker Cuts - Sharp Cheddar
String Cheese - Mozzarella Light Low Moisture Part Skim
String Cheese - Mozzarella Low Moisture Part Skim

Lucini Italia
Cheese (All)

Maggio
Mozzarella
Ricotta

Maplebrook Farm
Maplebrook Farm (All)

Market Day
American Cheese
Colby Jack Snack Sticks
String Cheese, 30 Count

Market District (Giant Eagle)
Cheddar Horseradish Spread
Gorgonzola Spread
Jarlsberg Spread
Mediterranean Gorgonzola Spread

Marsh
Cheddar Extra Sharp Bar (Colored)
Cheddar Medium Bar (Colored)
Cheddar Sharp Bar (Colored)
Colby Jack Cheese Cube
Low Moisture Part Skim Mozzarella Bar
Monterey Jack Bar
Pepper Jack Cheese Cube

Meijer
1/3 Less Fat Parmesan Cheese
2% Individually Wrapped Sharp

American Aerosol Cheese
Cheddar Aerosol Cheese
Cheddar Jack Fancy Shred
Cheddar Medium Bar
Cheddar Midget Horn
Cheddar Monterey Jack Bar
Cheddar Sliced Longhorn Half Moon
Cheezy Does It Jalapeno Cheese
Cheezy Does It Processed Spread Loaf
Colby
Colby Bar
Colby Chunk
Colby Jack Bar
Colby Jack Longhorn Half Moon
Colby Jack Sliced Shingle
Colby Longhorn Full Moon
Colby Longhorn Half Moon Sliced
Colby Midget Horn
Extra Sharp Cheddar Bar
Fancy Shredded Cheddar
Fancy Shredded Colby
Fancy Shredded Colby Jack
Fancy Shredded Italian Blend
Fancy Shredded Mexican Blend
Fancy Shredded Mild Cheddar
Fancy Shredded Mozzarella
Fancy Shredded Nacho and Taco Cheese
Fancy Shredded Sharp Cheddar
Grated Parmesan
Grated Romano
Hot Pepper Jack Chunk
Individually Wrapped Cheese
Individually Wrapped Swiss Cheese
Low Moisture Part Skim Mozzarella Chunk
Low Moisture Part Skim Mozzarella Square
Low Moisture Part Skim Shredded Mozzarella
Low Moisture Part Skim Sliced Mozzarella Chunk
Low Moisture Part Skim String Cheese
Marble Cheddar (C&W Cheddar)
Mexican Blend Shredded Cheese
Mild Cheddar Bar
Mild Cheddar Chunk
Monterey Jack Chunk

Mozzarella Sliced Shingle
Muenster Sliced Shingle
Pepper Jack Bar
Pepperjack Sliced
Pizza Shredded Mozzarella and Cheddar
Processed American Cheese
Processed Fat Free Individually
  Wrapped Sharp
Provolone Stacked Slice
Sandwich Cut Sliced Swiss
Sharp Cheddar Aerosol Cheese
Sharp Cheddar Bar
Sharp Cheddar Chunk
Sharp Cheddar, Shredded
Shredded Cheddar
Shredded Cheddar, Zip Pouch
Shredded Mexican
Shredded Mozzarella
Shredded Sharp Cheddar, Zip Pouch
Skim Mozzarella Bars
Sliced Pepper Cheese (Individually
  Wrapped)
Spread Loaf (Cheezy Does It)
String Cheese
Swiss Chunk
Swiss Slice Shingle

Meyenberg
Cheese (All)

Midwest Country Fare (Hy-Vee)
Imitation Shredded Cheddar Cheese
Imitation Shredded Mozzarella Cheese

Montchevre ⓘ
Montchevre (All)

Naturally Good Kosher Cheese
Cheese Products (All)

Nature's Promise (Giant)
Organic Shredded Mexican Blend
  Cheese
Organic Shredded Mild Cheddar Cheese
Organic Shredded Mozzarella Cheese
Organic Shredded Sharp Cheddar
  Cheese

Nature's Promise (Stop & Shop)
Organic Shredded Mexican Blend
  Cheese
Organic Shredded Mozzarella Cheese

Organic Shredded Sharp Cheddar
  Cheese

Nikos Robust Mediterranean 🏅
Feta (All)

O Organics ∼
Kids Cheese Sticks, Colby
Organic Mild Cheddar Cheese
Organic Monterey Jack Cheese
Organic Sharp Cheddar Cheese

Oberweis Dairy
Colby Cheese
Colby Jack Cheese
Mild Cheddar
Pepper Cheddar
Sharp Cheddar

Old Amsterdam
Aged Gouda (All)

Old Chatham Sheepherding Company
Camembert Cheeses (All)

Organic Creamery 🏅
Organic American
Organic American (Processed)
Organic Asiago
Organic Blue
Organic Colby
Organic Feta
Organic Goat Cheese
Organic Gorgonzola
Organic Mild Cheddar
Organic Monterey Jack
Organic Mozzarella
Organic Muenster
Organic Parmesan
Organic Pepper Jack
Organic Sharp Cheddar
Organic String Cheese

Organic Valley ⓘ
Baby Swiss
Cheddar, Mild
Cheddar, Mild Shredded
Cheddar, Raw Mild
Cheddar, Raw Sharp
Cheddar, Reduced Fat and Sodium
Cheddar, Sharp
Cheddar, Vermont Extra Sharp
Cheddar, Vermont Medium
Cheddar, Vermont Sharp

Colby
Feta
Italian Blend, Shredded
Mexican Blend, Shredded
Monterey Jack
Monterey Jack, Reduced Fat
Mozzarella
Mozzarella, Shredded Low Moisture
  Part Skim
Muenster
Parmesan, Shredded
Pepper Jack
Provolone
Ricotta
Stringles, Cheddar
Stringles, Colby-Jack
Stringles, Mozzarella
Wisconsin Raw Milk Jack-Style

Our Family
American Food Singles
Cheddar 2% Bar (Mild, Sharp)
Cheddar Cheese 2%, Shredded
Cheddar with Taco Seasoning
Cheese Food Singles
Colby & Monterey Jack, Shredded
Colby Jack Stick Cheese
Colby Jack, Chunk
Colby Jack, Sliced
Colby, Chunk
Double Cheddar Cheese, Chunk
Fancy Shredded Cheddar
Fancy Shredded Colby Jack
Fancy Shredded Mexican Blend
Fancy Shredded Mild Cheddar
Fancy Shredded Mozzarella
Fancy Shredded Parmesan
Medium Cheddar, Chunk
Mexican Four Cheeses, Shredded
Mild Cheddar, Chunk
Monterey Jack Bar
Mozzarella 2%, Shredded
Muenster Cheese, Chunk
Muenster Shingles
Natural Colby & Monterey Jack 2% Milk
  Shredded Cheese
Natural Swiss, Sliced

Parmesan & Romano Cheese, Grated
  (Canister)
Parmesan Cheese, Fresh Grated (Cup)
Parmesan Cheese, Grated
Pepper Jack Shingles
Pepper Jack, Chunk
Provolone Cheese, Sliced
Sharp Cheddar 2%, Shredded
String Cheese
Swiss Cheese, Shredded

Pastene
Parmesan Cheese, Grated
Romano Cheese, Grated

Polly-O Cheese
Cheese, Mozzarella Parmesan Finely
  Shredded
Cheese, Mozzarella Shredded Whole
  Milk
Cheese, Mozzarella Whole Milk
Cheese, Parmesan Grated
Cheese, Pizza Mozzarella, Provolone
  Romano Parmesan Shredded
Cheese, Ricotta Original
Mozzarella, Fat Free
Mozzarella, Part Skim
Mozzarella, Shredded Fat Free
Mozzarella, Shredded Lite
Mozzarella, Shredded Part Skim
Ricotta Cheese, Fat Free
Ricotta Cheese, Lite
Ricotta Cheese, Original
Ricotta Cheese, Part Skim

Price Chopper
2% White Singles
2% Yellow Singles
Brick Mild Cheddar
Brick Monterey Jack
Brick Sharp Cheddar
Cheese Twister Natural
Colby Cheese
Colby Chunk
Deluxe White American Slices
Deluxe Yellow American Slices
Fancy Shredded Swiss
Fat Free White Singles
Fat Free Yellow Singles
Lite String Cheese

Mild Cheddar Chunk
Monterey Jack & Jalapeno Brick
Monterey Jack
Monterey Jack Chunk
Muenster Chunk
Muenster Slices
Muenster Stick
New York Extra Sharp Cheddar Brick
New York Extra Sharp Cheddar Chunk
Parmesan Grated Cheese
Parmesan Romano Cheese
Pepper Jack Chunk
Primo Parmesan/Pecorino/Romano
Provolone Slices
Sharp Cheddar Cheese
Sharp Cheddar Single Pack Slice
Shredded 2% Reduced Fat Mild
   Cheddar
Shredded 2% Reduced Fat Mozzarella
Shredded 6-Cheese Blend
Shredded Cheddar
Shredded Fat Free Mozzarella
Shredded Mexican Blend
Shredded Mild Cheddar
Shredded Monterey Jack
Shredded Monterey Jack with Jalapeno
Shredded Mozzarella
Shredded Mozzarella Part Skim
Shredded Pizza Blend
Shredded Provolone
Shredded Sharp Cheddar
Shredded Whole Milk Mozzarella
Soft Cream Cheese Tub
String Cheese
Swiss Chunk
Swiss Slices
Swiss Stick
Vermont Sharp Cheddar
Vermont Sharp Cheddar Chunk
White Single Slice
Wisconsin Sharp Cheddar NY
Yellow Single Slice

Primo Taglio (Safeway)
   Brie Wheels
   Provolone Cheese Deli Vacuum Pack
Publix
   Asiago Wedge

Blue Crumbled
Cheddar - Extra Sharp (All Forms:
   Block, Chunk & Shreds)
Cheddar - Medium (All Forms: Block,
   Chunk & Shreds)
Cheddar - Mild (All Forms: Block,
   Chunk & Shreds)
Cheddar - Sharp (All Forms: Block,
   Chunk & Shreds)
Cheese Spread - Processed Cheese
Colby (All Forms: Block, Chunk &
   Shreds)
Colby Jack
Crumbled Feta
Crumbled Goat Cheese
Crumbled Reduced Fat Feta
Feta Chunk
Gorgonzola Crumbled
Italian 6-Cheese Blend - Shredded
Mexican 4-Cheese Blend - Shredded
Monterey Jack & Cheddar - Shredded
Monterey Jack (All Forms: Block, Chunk
   & Shreds)
Monterey Jack with Jalapeño Peppers
   (All Forms: Block, Chunk & Shreds)
Mozzarella (All Forms: Block, Chunk &
   Shreds)
Muenster (All Forms: Block, Chunk &
   Shreds)
Parmesan Wedge
Parmesan, Grated
Provolone (All Forms: Block, Chunk &
   Shreds)
Reduced Fat Feta Chunk
Ricotta
Shredded Parmesan
Singles - Pasteurized Process American
   Cheese Food - Thick Slice
Singles - Pasteurized Process American
   Cheese Food
Singles - Pasteurized Process Swiss
   Cheese Food
Swiss (All Forms: Block, Chunk &
   Shreds)
Redwood Hill Farm
   Cheese (All)

Salemville �
- Amish Blue
- Amish Gorgonzola
- Smokehouse Blue

Saputo Cheese USA Inc.
- Blue Cheese
- Cheddar
- Colby
- Colby Jack
- Edam
- Feta
- Gorgonzola
- Gouda
- Monterey Jack
- Mozzarella
- Muenster
- Provolone
- Queso Rico
- Ricotta
- String Cheese

Sargento
- Natural Cheese (All BUT Blue Cheese)

Sartori ⓘ
- Cheese Products (All BUT Raspberry Bellavitano)

Schneider
- Cheddar
- Colby Jack
- Natural String Cheese

Schnucks
- 6 Cheese Italian, Finely Shredded
- American Cheese (Individually Wrapped Slices)
- Cheddar (Extra Sharp, Sharp)
- Cheddar Bar (Mild, Sharp)
- Cheddar Midget
- Cheddar Slices
- Cheddar, Finely Shredded (Mild, Sharp)
- Cheddar, Shredded
- Colby Chunk
- Colby Jack
- Colby Jack Bar
- Colby Jack, Shredded
- Colby Midget
- Colby Slices
- Colby, Finely Shredded
- Fancy Nacho/Taco Shredded Cheese
- Hot Pepper Cheese
- Medium Cheddar
- Medium Cheddar Slices
- Mexican 2% Blend, Shredded
- Mexican 4 Cheese Blend
- Mexican Blend Shredded Cheese
- Mild Cheddar 2%, Finely Shredded
- Monterey Jack
- Monterey Jack Bar
- Monterey Jack Slices
- Monterey Jack, Finally Shredded
- Mozzarella
- Mozzarella 2%, Finely Shredded
- Mozzarella, Shredded
- Mozzarella, Sliced
- Muenster Chunk
- Muenster Slices
- Parmesan Cheese
- Parmesan, Finely Shredded
- Parmesan, Romano & Asiago
- Parmesano-Romano
- Pepperjack
- Processed Cheese
- Processed Cheese (Individually Wrapped Slices)
- Processed Cheese (WIC)
- Processed Cheese, 2% (Individually Wrapped Slices)
- Processed Cheese, Fat Free
- Provolone Slices
- Ricotta
- Sharp Cheddar Slices
- Sharp Cheddar, Shredded
- Shredded Pizza Cheese
- String Cheese
- Swiss Chunk
- Swiss Slices
- Swiss, Finely Shredded

Shaw's
- American Pasteurized Sliced Cheese
- American Sliced Cheese Box
- Cheese Dip/Spread
- Colby Jack Cheese Bar
- Colby Jack Twisted Cheese Stick
- Extra Sharp Cheddar Cheese Bar
- Fancy Sharp White Cheddar Cheese
- Lite String Cheese

Marble Cheddar Cheese Bar
Mexican 2% Cheese Chunk
Mild Chunk Cheddar Cheese
Mild Yellow Cheddar Cheese
Mild Yellow Cheddar Cheese Bar
Monterey Jack Cheese Bar
Monterey Jack Cheese Chunk
Mozzarella Cheddar String Cheese
Muenster Cheese Bar
New York Sharp Cheddar Cheese Bar
Parmesan Grated Cheese
Pasteurized Cultured Sliced American
  Cheese
Pasteurized Sliced American Cheese
Pasteurized Sliced Wrap White
  American Cheese
Pepper Jack Cheese Bar
Sharp Cheddar Cheese
Sharp Cheddar Cheese Chunk
Sharp Cheddar Cheese Stick
Sharp White Cheddar Cheese Bar
Sharp Yellow Bar Cheese
Shredded 2% Mild Cheddar Cheese
Shredded Cheddar & Monterey Jack
  Cheese
Shredded Cheese
Shredded Fancy Yellow Cheddar Cheese
Shredded Low Fat Muenster Mozzarella
  Cheese
Shredded Monterey Jack Cheddar
  Cheese
Shredded Mozzarella Cheese
Shredded Mozzarella Yellow Cheddar
  Cheese
Shredded Reduced Fat Cheddar
Shredded Reduced Fat Mozzarella
Shredded Wisconsin Parmesan Cheese
Shredded Yellow Cheddar Cheese
Shredded Yellow Monterey Jack
  Pasteurized Cheese
Shredded Yellow Sharp Cheddar Cheese
Sliced American Pasteurized Cheese
Sliced Mild Cheddar Cheese
Sliced Mozzarella Cheese
Sliced Muenster Cheese
Sliced Pasteurized American Cheese Bag
Sliced Pepper Jack Cheese

Sliced Provolone Cheese
Sliced Swiss Cheese
Sliced Wrap American Cheese
Sliced Wrap Pasteurized White
  American Cheese
String Cheese
Vermont White Cheddar Cheese Bar
White Cheddar Cheese
White Cheddar Cheese Chunk
Wrap Cheddar Cheese Bar
Yellow Cheddar Cheese
Yellow Cheddar Cheese Bar
Yellow Cheddar Cheese Stick
Yellow Sharp Cheddar Cheese

Simply Enjoy (Stop & Shop)
  Deli Cheese, Brie Wedge
  Deli Cheese, Triple Crème Brie

Stella
  Blue Cheese
  Feta
  Gorgonzola

Stop & Shop
  Extra Sharp Vermont Cheddar Cheese
    Chunk
  Extra Sharp White New York Cheddar
    Cheese Chunk
  Extra Sharp Yellow New York Cheddar
    Cheese Chunk
  Fancy Shredded Mexican Blend Cheese
  Fancy Shredded Mild Cheddar Cheese
  Fancy Shredded Mozzarella Cheese
  Fancy Shredded Sharp Cheddar Cheese
  Grated Parmesan Cheese
  Grated Pecorino Romano Cheese
  Low Moisture Part Skim Mozzarella
    String Cheese
  Monterey Jack Cheese Board Chunk
  Muenster Cheese Slices
  Part Skim Mozzarella Cheese Chunk
  Pepper Jack Cheese
  Reduced Fat Mozzarella String Cheese
  Regular Sliced Premium Domestic Swiss
    Cheese
  Regular Sliced White American Cheese
  Regular Sliced Yellow American Cheese
  Sharp Wisconsin Yellow Cheddar
    Cheese Chunk

Shredded Mild Cheddar Cheese
Shredded Mozzarella Cheese
Shredded Parmesan Cheese
Shredded Pecorino Romano Cheese
Shredded Taco Blend Cheese
Sliced Provolone Cheese
Sliced Swiss Cheese
Sliced Yellow American Cheese Food
Swiss Cheese Chunk
Thin Sliced Premium Domestic Swiss
   Cheese
Thin Sliced White American Cheese
Thin Sliced Yellow American Cheese
White Vermont Sharp Cheddar Cheese
   Board Chunk
Whole Milk Mozzarella Cheese Chunk

Tillamook
Cheese (All)

Trader Joe's
Cheese (All Shredded, Blocks, and
   Wedges EXCEPT For Blue Cheeses
   and Cheeses Containing Beer)
Cream Cheese (All)
Parmesan And Romano Cheese Blend

Treasure Cave
Blue Cheese
Feta

Trempherbe
Trempherbe Cheeses (All)

Tropical Cheese
American Cheese Food
Cheddar Shreds
El Moli Gouda Wedge
El Molino Rojo Edam
Extra Sharp Cheddar
Gouda Slice
Imitation American
Imitation American Single
Imitation Mexican Topping
Imitation Pizza Topping
Imitation Taco Topping
Medium Cheddar
Mexican Shreds
Mild Cheddar
Monterey Jack
Monterey Pepper Jack
Mozzarella Shreds

Muenster
Muenster Slice Shingle
Muenster Slice Single
Pepper Jack Slice
PepperJack Slice Single
Queso Blanco
Queso Columbiano
Queso Cotija
Queso Crema
Queso De Hoja
Queso de Papa
Queso Duro Blando
Queso Edam
Queso Freir
Queso Fresco
Queso GEO
Queso Gouda
Queso Mild Cheddar Shred
Queso Oaxaca
Queso Pupusas Mozzarella Shred
Queso Quesadilla Shred
Sharp Cheddar
Swiss
Swiss Slice Shingle
Swiss Slice Single
Taco Shreds

V & V Supremo
Cheese Products (All)

Valio
Imported Cheeses (All)

Valu Time (Brookshire)
Cheddar Cheese Imitation
Mozzarella Shred Imitation
Sandwich Sliced Imitation Cheese

Valu Time (Marsh)
Cheese Product, Individually Wrapped
Imitation Cheddar Shredded
Imitation Cheese, Individually Wrapped
Imitation Mozzarella Shredded

Velveeta
Cheese, 2% Milk
Cheese, Mexican Mild
Cheese, Pepper Jack
Cheese, Regular
Cheese, Slices
Cheese, Slices Extra Thick

Vermont Butter & Cheese Creamery
- Vermont Butter & Cheese Creamery (All)

Vons ✍
- Grated Parmesan Cheese

Wegmans
- 2% Colby Jack Cheese - Shredded
- 2% Milk Low-Moisture Part-Skim Mozzarella Cheese - Shredded
- 2% Milk Mexican Blend - Fancy Shredded
- 2% Milk Mild Cheddar Cheese - Shredded
- 2% Milk Sharp Cheddar Cheese - Shredded
- American 2% Milk Reduced Fat - White Slices
- American 2% Milk Reduced Fat - Yellow Slices
- American Fat Free - White Slices
- American Fat Free - Yellow Slices
- American Singles - White Slices
- American Singles - Yellow Slices
- Cheese Spread
- Colby - Sliced
- Colby Jack Cheese - Shredded
- Colby Jack Cheese - Thin Sliced
- Colby Jack Cheese
- Deluxe American - White Slices
- Deluxe American - Yellow Slices
- Extra Sharp White Cheddar Cheese
- Extra Sharp Yellow Cheddar Cheese
- Heart O' Swiss Cheese - Sliced
- Longhorn Style Colby Cheese
- Mexican Cheese - Fancy Shredded
- Mild Cheddar Cheese - Fancy Shredded
- Mild Cheddar Cheese - Shredded
- Mild White Cheddar Cheese
- Mild White Cheddar Cheese - Shredded
- Mild Yellow Cheddar Cheese
- Monterey Jack Cheese
- Muenster Cheese - Thin Sliced
- Muenster Cheese
- Parmesan & Romano Cheese - Grated
- Parmesan Cheese - Finely Shredded
- Parmesan Cheese - Grated
- Part Skim Mozzarella Cheese - Shredded, Low Moisture
- Pepper Jack Cheese
- Pizza Cheese - Fancy Shredded
- Provolone Cheese - Thin Sliced
- Romano Cheese - Grated
- Sharp Cheddar 2% Milk Reduced Fat - Slices
- Sharp Cheddar Cheese - Shredded
- Sharp Cheddar Cheese - Thin Sliced
- Sharp Cheddar Fat Free - Yellow Slices
- Sharp Vermont Cheddar Cheese
- Sharp White Cheddar Cheese
- Sharp Yellow Cheddar Cheese
- Shredded Low Moisture Part Skim Mozzarella
- Shredded Whole Milk Mozzarella
- Swiss 2% Milk Reduced Fat - Slices
- Swiss Cheese - Chunk
- Swiss Cheese - Thin Sliced
- Swiss Fat Free - White Slices
- Taco Cheese - Fancy Shredded
- Thin Sliced Low Moisture Part Skim Mozzarella Cheese
- Whole Milk Mozzarella Cheese - Shredded

Winn-Dixie
- American Pasteurized Process Cheese Product
- Blue Cheese
- Cheddar Jack
- Cheddar, Extra Sharp
- Cheddar, Medium
- Cheddar, Mild
- Cheddar, NY Extra Sharp
- Cheddar, NY Sharp
- Cheddar, Sharp
- Colby
- Colby Jack
- Deluxe American Pasteurized Process Cheese Food
- Feta
- Gorgonzola
- Grated Parmesan
- Grated Parmesan & Romano
- Italian Blend, Shredded
- Mexican Blend

Monterey Jack
Monterey Jack with Jalapeno Peppers
Mozzarella
Muenster
Pasteurized Process Swiss Cheese
    Product
Pimiento Cheese (Chunky, Regular, with
    Jalapenos)
Provolone
Reduced Fat American Pasteurized
    Process Cheese Product
Ricotta (All Types)
String Cheese
Swiss
White Cheddar
Woolwich Dairy Inc.
Goat Cheeses (All)

CHEESE, ALTERNATIVES

Follow Your Heart
Vegan Gourmet Cheddar Cheese
    Alternative
Vegan Gourmet Cream Cheese
    Alternative
Vegan Gourmet Monterey Jack Cheese
    Alternative
Vegan Gourmet Mozzarella Cheese
    Alternative
Vegan Gourmet Nacho Cheese
    Alternative
Vegan Gourmet Sour Cream Alternative
Food Club (Brookshire)
Individually Wrapped Sliced Cheese
    Product
Galaxy Nutritional Foods
Rice American Flavor Slice
Rice Cheddar Flavor Block
Rice Cheddar Flavor Shred
Rice Cheddar Flavor Slice
Rice Mozzarella Flavor
Rice Mozzarella Flavor Block
Rice Mozzarella Flavor Shred
Rice Parmesan Flavor Grated Topping
Rice Pepper Jack Flavor Slice
Rice Swiss Flavor Slice
Rice Vegan American Flavor Slice

Rice Vegan Cheddar Flavor Block
Rice Vegan Mozzarella Flavor Block
Rice Vegan Pepper Jack Flavor Slice
Vegan American Flavor Slice
Vegan Cheddar Flavor Block
Vegan Chive & Garlic Cream Cheese
    Alternative
Vegan Classic Plain Cream Cheese
    Alternative
Vegan Mozzarella Flavor Block
Vegan Mozzarella Flavor Slice
Vegan Parmesan Flavor Grated Topping
Veggie Cheddar Flavor Block
Veggie Chive & Garlic Cream Cheese
    Alternative
Veggie Classic Plain Cream Cheese
    Alternative
Veggie Mozzarella Flavor Block
Veggie Parmesan Flavor Grated Topping
Veggie Pepper Jack Flavor Block
Veggie Shreds Cheddar & Pepper Jack
    Flavor
Veggie Shreds Cheddar Flavor
Veggie Shreds Monterey Jack & Cheddar
    Flavor
Veggie Shreds Mozzarella Flavor
Veggie Shreds Parmesan, Mozzarella &
    Romano Flavor
Veggie Slices American Flavor
Veggie Slices Cheddar Flavor
Veggie Slices Cheddar Flavor with
    Jalapenos
Veggie Slices Mozzarella Flavor
Veggie Slices Pepper Jack Flavor
Veggie Slices Smoked Provolone Flavor
Veggie Slices Swiss Flavor
Veggy American Flavor Slice
Veggy Cheddar Flavor Slice
Veggy Mozzarella Flavor Slice
Veggy Pepper Jack Flavor Slice
Wholesome Valley Organic American
    Flavor Slice
Wholesome Valley Organic Mozzarella
    Flavor Slice
Lisanatti ⓘ ✓
3-Cheeze Blend Vegan Cheeze
Cheddar Vegan Cheeze

Mozzarella Vegan Cheeze
RiceCheeze Cheddar Style Chunks
RiceCheeze Mozzarella Style Chunks
RiceCheeze Pepper Jack Style Chunks
RiceCheeze Snack Sticks American Style
RiceCheeze Snack Sticks Mozzarella
   Style
SoySation 3 Cheese Blend Shreds
SoySation Cheddar Style Chunks
SoySation Cheddar Style Shreds
SoySation Cheddar Style Slices
SoySation Mozzarella Style Chunks
SoySation Mozzarella Style Shreds
SoySation Parmesan Style Shreds
SoySation Pepper Jack Style Slices
SoySation Swiss Style Slices
THE ORIGINAL Almond Cheddar
   Style Chunks
THE ORIGINAL Almond Cheddar
   Style Shreds
THE ORIGINAL Almond Garlic &
   Herb Style Chunks
THE ORIGINAL Almond Jalapeno Jack
   Style Chunks
THE ORIGINAL Almond Mozzarella
   Style Chunks
THE ORIGINAL Almond Mozzarella
   Style Shreds

Lucerne (Safeway)
Cheese Food Slices, American
Cheese Food Slices, American Deluxe
Cheese Food Slices, Sharp Cheddar
Cheese Spread Slices, American 2%
Cheese Spread Slices, American Smooth
   Melting

Publix
Singles - Pasteurized Process American
   Deluxe Cheese Food

Shoppers Value (ACME)
Imitation Shredded Cheddar Cheese
Imitation Shredded Mozzarella
Individually Wrapped Slices Cheese
   Substitute

Shoppers Value (Albertsons)
Imitation Shredded Mozzarella
Individually Wrapped Slices Cheese
   Substitute

Shredded Imitation Cheddar Cheese
Shoppers Value (Cub Foods)
Imitation Shredded Cheddar Cheese
Imitation Shredded Mozzarella
Individually Wrapped Slices Cheese
   Substitute
Shoppers Value (Jewel-Osco)
Imitation Shredded Cheddar Cheese
Imitation Shredded Mozzarella
Individually Wrapped Single Cheese
   Substitute
Sol Cuisine ✓
Veggie Crumbles
Trader Joe's
Soy Cheese Slices
Vegan Gourmet
Cheddar Cheese Alternative
Monterey Jack Cheese Alternative
Mozzarella Cheese Alternative
Nacho Cheese Alternative

COTTAGE CHEESE

Albertsons
2% Cottage Cheese Pasteurized
4% Cottage Cheese Pasteurized
Cottage Cheese Pasteurized
Nonfat Cottage Cheese Regular
Alta Dena
Cottage Cheese with Pineapple
Lowfat Cottage Cheese
Nonfat Cottage Cheese
Small Curd Cottage Cheese
Axelrod
Cottage Cheese
Barber's
Cottage Cheese
Berkeley Farms
Low Fat Cottage Cheese
Low Fat Pineapple Cottage Cheese
Nonfat Cottage Cheese
Small Curd Cottage Cheese
Best Choice
Cottage Cheese
Cottage Cheese 1%
Nonfat Cottage Cheese

Breakstone's
Cottage Cheese, Small Curd 2% Milkfat Lowfat
Cottage Cheese, Small Curd 4% Milkfat Min
Cottage Cheese, Small Curd Fat Free
Cottage Cheese, Small Curd Lowfat 2% Milkfat

Broughton
Large Curd Cottage Cheese
Large Curd Light Cottage Cheese
Light Cottage Cheese
Small Curd Cottage Cheese
Small Curd Light Cottage Cheese

Cabot
Cabot Products (All)

Country Fresh
Cottage Cheese

Creamland Dairies
Cottage Cheese (All)

Crowley Foods
Crowley Foods (All)

Daisy Brand
Daisy Brand (All)

Darigold
Darigold (All)

Dean's
Cottage Cheese (All)

Farmers' All Natural Creamery
Cottage Cheese

Fastco (Fareway)
Cottage Cheese
Cottage Cheese, 1%

Food Club (Brookshire)
1% Low Fat Cottage Cheese
Cottage Cheese
Non Fat Cottage Cheese

Food Club (Marsh)
Cottage Cheese, 1% Lowfat
Cottage Cheese, Large Curd
Cottage Cheese, Small Curd

Friendship Dairies
Cottage Cheese (All)

Gandy's ⓘ
Cottage Cheese

Gay Lea
Gay Lea (All)

Giant
1% Low Fat Small Curd Cottage Cheese
1% Low Fat Small Curd Cottage Cheese No Salt
4% Large Curd Cottage Cheese
4% Small Curd Cottage Cheese
Fat Free Small Curd Cottage Cheese

Great Value (Wal-Mart) 25
1% Lowfat Small Curd Cottage Cheese
2% Lowfat Small Curd Cottage Cheese
2% Small Curd Cottage Cheese
4% Large Curd Cottage Cheese
4% Small Curd Cottage Cheese
Fat Free Small Curd Cottage Cheese

Haggen
Cottage Cheese (2% Low Fat, 4% Small Curd, Fat Free, Large)

Hiland Dairy
Fat Free Cottage Cheese
Large Curd Cottage Cheese
Low Fat 2% Cottage Cheese
Small Curd Cottage Cheese

Hood
Cottage Cheese (All)

Horizon Organic
Cottage Cheese (All)

Hy-Vee
1% Low Fat Small Curd Cottage Cheese
4% Large Curd Cottage Cheese
4% Small Curd Cottage Cheese

Kalona Organics
Cottage Cheese (All)

Kemps ⓘ
Cottage Cheese

Knudsen
Cottage Cheese On the Go, Free Nonfat
Cottage Cheese On the Go, Single Serve Lowfat
Cottage Cheese, Free Nonfat
Cottage Cheese, Pineapple Small Curd 2% Milkfat Lowfat
Cottage Cheese, Small Curd
Cottage Cheese, Small Curd 4% Milkfat Min
Cottage Cheese, Small Curd Lowfat
Cottage Cheese, Small Curd Lowfat 2% Milkfat

Lactaid
  Cottage Cheese
Light N Lively
  Cottage Cheese, Fat Free
  Cottage Cheese, Lowfat
  Cottage Cheese, Lowfat Snack Size
Louis Trauth Dairy
  Cottage Cheese
Lucerne (Safeway)
  1% Low Fat Cottage Cheese
  1% Low Fat Cottage Cheese- No Salt
    Added
  2% Cottage Cheese- Lowfat Calcium
    Fortified
  2% Cottage Cheese- Lowfat Calcium
    Fortified with Chives
  2% Cottage Cheese- Lowfat Calcium
    Fortified with Pineapple
  Cottage Cheese - Large Curd 4%
  Cottage Cheese, Small Curd 4%
  Fat Free Cottage Cheese
Mayfield Dairy
  Cottage Cheese
  Lowfat Cottage Cheese
Meadow Brook Dairy
  Cottage Cheese
Meadow Gold
  Cottage Cheese (All)
Midwest Country Fare (Hy-Vee)
  1% Small Curd Cottage Cheese
  4% Small Curd Cottage Cheese
Nancy's
  Nancy's (All)
Oak Farms Dairy
  Cottage Cheese
Oberweis Dairy
  1% Cottage Cheese
  4% Cottage Cheese
Our Family
  1% Lowfat Cottage Cheese
  2% Lowfat Cottage Cheese
  Cottage Cheese 4% Milkfat
  Small Curd Cottage Cheese 4%
Penn Maid
  Cottage Cheese

Prairie Farms
  Cottage Cheese (Dry Curd, Fat Free,
    Large Curd, Lowfat, Small Curd)
Price Chopper
  Cottage Cheese
  Cottage Cheese, Pineapple
  Non Fat Cottage Cheese
Price's Creameries
  Cottage Cheese
Publix
  Fat Free (All)
  Large Curd, 4% Milkfat (All Styles &
    Flavors)
  Low Fat (All Styles & Flavors)
  Low Fat with Pineapple
  Small Curd, 4% Milkfat (All Styles &
    Flavors)
Purity Dairies
  Cottage Cheese
  Lowfat Cottage Cheese
  No Fat Cottage Cheese
Reiter Dairy
  Cottage Cheese (All)
Robinson Dairy
  Cottage Cheese (All)
Stop & Shop
  Fat Free Small Curd Cottage Cheese
  Low Fat Small Curd Cottage Cheese
  Small Curd Cottage Cheese
Wegmans
  1% Large Curd Cottage Cheese
  1% Small Curd Cottage Cheese
  4% Small Curd Cottage Cheese
  Nonfat Cottage Cheese
  Pineapple Cottage Cheese
  Pineapple Fat Free Cottage Cheese
Winn-Dixie
  Cottage Cheese (Fat Free, Lowfat)
  Large Curd Cottage Cheese, 4% Milkfat
  Small Curd Cottage Cheese, 4% Milkfat

CREAM

Albertsons
  Heavy Whipping Cream
Alta Dena
  Heavy Whipping Cream

Axelrod
Cream

Barber's
Whipping Cream

Berkeley Farms
Gourmet Manufacturing Cream
Heavy Whipping Cream

Best Choice
Heavy Whipping Cream

Broughton
Whipping Cream
Whipping Cream 36%

Country Fresh
Cream

Creamland Dairies
Whipping Cream

Crowley Foods
Crowley Foods (All)

Darigold
Darigold (All)

Dean's
Cream (All)

Food Club (Marsh)
Ultra Pasteurized Processed Heavy
Cream
Ultra Pasteurized Processed Whipping
Cream

Garelick Farms
Fresh Light Cream
Heavy Cream
Light Cream
Whipping Cream

Giant
Table Cream

Giant Eagle
Heavy Cream 36%
Light Whipping Cream 30%

GranoVita
Organic CremoVita

Great Value (Wal-Mart) 25
Heavy Whipping Cream
Light Cream

Hiland Dairy
Heavy Whipping Cream

Hood
Cream (All)

Horizon Organic
Cream (All)

Kalona Organics
Whipping Cream (All)

Lehigh Valley Dairy Farms
Heavy Cream
Light Cream

Louis Trauth Dairy
40% Whipping Cream
Single Cream
UHT Whipping Cream

Lucerne (Safeway) ᗯ
Whipping Cream Heavy Ultra
Pasteurized
Whipping Cream, Ultra Pasteurized

Mayfield Dairy
Whipping Cream

Meadow Brook Dairy
Heavy Whipping Cream
Light Cream

Meadow Gold
Whipping Cream

Meijer
Ultra Pasteurized Heavy Whipping
Cream

O Organics ᗯ
Heavy Whipping Cream

Oak Farms Dairy
Whipping Cream

Oberweis Dairy
Heavy Whipping Cream

Organic Valley ⓘ
Heavy Whipping Cream

Penn Maid
Cream

PET Milk
Heavy Whipping Cream
Whipping Cream

Prairie Farms
Whipping Cream

Price Chopper
Cream

Price's Creameries
Heavy Whipping Cream

Publix
Heavy Whipping Cream
Whipping Cream

Reiter Dairy
Heavy Whipping Cream
Robinson Dairy
Whipping Cream (All)
Rosenberger's Dairies
Cream
Stop & Shop
Light Cream
T.G. Lee Dairy
Heavy Whipping Cream
Tuscan Dairy Farms
Heavy Cream
Light Cream
Vermont Butter & Cheese Creamery
Vermont Butter & Cheese Creamery (All)
Wegmans
Ultra Heavy Cream
Winn-Dixie
Heavy Whipping Cream
Whipping Cream

CREAM CHEESE

Alta Dena
Whipped Cream Cheese
Breakstone's ᗡ
Cream Cheese, Temp Tee Whipped
Fastco (Fareway)
Cream Cheese
Lite Cream Cheese
Lite Soft Cream Cheese
Soft Cream Cheese
Whip Cream Cheese
Food Club (Brookshire)
Cream Cheese Bar
Cream Cheese, 1/3 Less Fat
Cream Cheese, Fat Free
Giant
Cream Cheese Brick
Soft Cream Cheese
Whipped Cream Cheese
Giant Eagle
Cream Cheese Brick
Lite Cream Cheese Brick
Lite Soft Cream Cheese
Soft Cream Cheese

Soft Cream Cheese, Chive and Onion
Soft Cream Cheese, Strawberry
Whipped Soft Cream Cheese
Great Value (Wal-Mart) 🔲25
Chive & Onion Cream Cheese Spread
Cream Cheese Brick
Cream Cheese Spread
Fat Free Cream Cheese Brick
Light Cream Cheese
Neufchatel Cheese
Strawberry Cream Cheese Spread
Whipped Cream Cheese Spread
Horizon Organic
Cream Cheese (All)
Hy-Vee
1/3 Less Than Fat Cream Cheese
Blueberry Cream Cheese
Cream Cheese
Fat Free Cream Cheese
Fat Free Soft Cream Cheese
Garden Vegetable Cream Cheese
Honey Nut Cream Cheese
Onion/Chive Cream Cheese
Soft Cream Cheese
Soft Light Cream Cheese
Strawberry Cream Cheese
Whipped Cream Cheese Spread
Lucerne (Safeway) ᗡ
Cream Cheese
Cream Cheese Spread
Cream Cheese with Chives and Onions
Cream Cheese with Garden Vegetables
Cream Cheese with Strawberry
Fat Free Cream Cheese
Light Cream Cheese
Soft Cream Cheese
Whipped Cream Cheese Spread
Whipped Cream Cheese Spread- Mixed Berry Flavor
Whipped Cream Cheese Spread- With Chives
Nancy's
Nancy's (All)
Organic Valley ⓘ
Cream Cheese
Neufchatel

Philadelphia Cream Cheese ✍

- Cream Cheese Spread, Cheesecake
- Cream Cheese Spread, Regular Chive & Onion
- Cream Cheese, 1/3 Less Fat
- Cream Cheese, 1/3 Less Fat Chive & Onion
- Cream Cheese, 1/3 Less Fat Garden Vegetable
- Cream Cheese, 1/3 Less Fat Neufchatel
- Cream Cheese, 1/3 Less Fat Strawberry
- Cream Cheese, Fat Free
- Cream Cheese, Fat Free Strawberry
- Cream Cheese, Light
- Cream Cheese, Original
- Cream Cheese, Regular
- Cream Cheese, Regular Blueberry
- Cream Cheese, Regular Garden Vegetable
- Cream Cheese, Regular Honey Nut
- Cream Cheese, Regular Pineapple
- Cream Cheese, Regular Salmon
- Cream Cheese, Regular Strawberry
- Cream Cheese, Regular Whipped
- Cream Cheese, The Twin Pack Light
- Cream Cheese, Whipped
- Cream Cheese, Whipped Cinnamon 'N Brown Sugar
- Cream Cheese, Whipped Garlic 'N Herb
- Cream Cheese, Whipped Mixed Berry
- Cream Cheese, Whipped Ranch
- Cream Cheese, Whipped With Chives

Price Chopper

- Cream Cheese Loaf
- Soft Cream Cheese

Publix

- Fat Free Cream Cheese (All Styles)
- Light Soft (All Styles, All Flavors)
- Neufchatel (All Styles, All Flavors)
- Regular (All Styles, All Flavors)
- Regular Soft (All Styles, All Flavors)

Schnucks

- Cream Cheese
- Cream Cheese, Less Fat

Stop & Shop

- Cream Cheese Brick
- Neufchatel Cheese Brick
- Soft Cream Cheese

Vegan Gourmet

- Cream Cheese Alternative

Vita Foods ⓘ

- Vita Cream Cheese with Smoked Salmon

Winn-Dixie

- Cream Cheese (Lite, Soft, Regular)

EGG SUBSTITUTES

ACME

- Egg Substitutes

Albertsons

- Egg Substitute
- Egg White Substitute

All Whites

- Eggs (All)

Better'n Eggs

- Better'n Eggs (All)

Cub Foods

- Eggs 2 Go
- Liquid Eggs

Deb-El

- Deb-El (All)

Egg Beaters

- Egg Beaters (All)

Eggology

- Eggology (All)

Ener-G

- Egg Replacer

Food You Feel Good About (Wegmans)

- Egg Busters

Giant

- Eggs Made Simple

Hy-Vee

- Egg Substitute, Refrigerated

Jewel-Osco

- Egg Substitutes
- Egg White Substitute
- Pasteurized Egg Substitutes

Lucerne (Safeway) ✍

- Best of the Egg
- Best of the Egg Whites

Meijer

- Egg Substitute

Orgran ⓘ ⛨
  No Egg
Price Chopper
  Egg Mates
  Egg Whites
Publix
  Egg Stirs
ReddiEgg
  ReddiEgg Real Egg Product (No Fat No Cholesterol)
Schnucks
  Egg Substitute
Shaw's
  Egg Substitute
Trader Joe's
  Quick Scrambled Egg Whites
Wegmans
  Egg Busters
Wild Harvest (ACME)
  Organic Egg Whites
Wild Harvest (Albertsons)
  Organic Egg Whites
Wild Harvest (Cub Foods)
  Organic Egg Whites
Wild Harvest (Jewel-Osco)
  Organic Egg Whites

EGGNOG & OTHER NOGS

Alta Dena
  Holiday Eggnog
  Holiday Lite Eggnog
  Honey Sweetened Eggnog
  Pumpkin Spice Eggnog
Barber's
  Egg Nog
Berkeley Farms
  Holiday Eggnog
  Light Eggnog
Broughton
  Egg Nog
  Holiday Nog
Bud's of San Francisco
  Famous Eggnog
Creamland Dairies
  Eggnog (All)

Darigold
  Darigold (All)
Hood
  Cinnamon Eggnog
  Gingerbread Eggnog
  Golden Eggnog
  Light Eggnog
  Pumpkin Eggnog
  Sugar Cookie Eggnog
  Vanilla Eggnog
Louis Trauth Dairy
  Eggnog
Mayfield Dairy
  Egg Nog
Meadow Gold
  Eggnog (All)
Oak Farms Dairy
  Eggnog
Oberweis Dairy
  Egg Nog
Organic Valley ⓘ
  Eggnog
PET Milk
  Eggnog
  Pumpkin Spice Nog
Prairie Farms
  Eggnog
  Holiday Nog
Price's Creameries
  Egg Nog
Publix
  Low Fat Egg Nog
  Original Egg Nog
Reiter Dairy
  Eggnog (All)
Robinson Dairy
  Egg Nog (All)
T.G. Lee Dairy
  Eggnog
  Pumpkin Spice Eggnog
Trader Joe's
  Egg Nog (Seasonal)
Turkey Hill
  Eggnog
  Light Vanilla Nog

HALF & HALF

Albertsons
Half And Half
Alta Dena
Half & Half
Axelrod
Half & Half
Barber's
Half & Half
Berkeley Farms
Half & Half
Best Choice
Half & Half
Broughton
Coldstar Half & Half
Half & Half
Creamland Dairies
Half and Half
Crowley Foods
Half & Half
Darigold
Darigold (All)
Fastco (Fareway)
Half & Half Cream
Food Club (Brookshire)
Half & Half
Garelick Farms
Fresh Half & Half
Half & Half (All)
Giant
Fat Free Half & Half
Ultra Half & Half
Giant Eagle
Fat Free Half & Half
Half & Half 10.5%
Great Value (Wal-Mart) 🔲25
Half & Half
GreenWise Market (Publix)
Half & Half
H-E-B
Fat Free Half & Half
Half & Half
Hiland Dairy
Half and Half
Hy-Vee
Fat Free Half & Half

Half & Half
Lehigh Valley Dairy Farms
Half & Half (All)
Louis Trauth Dairy
Half & Half
Sterile Half & Half
Lucerne (Safeway) ᧁ
Half and Half
Half and Half Ultra Pasteurized
Half and Half Ultra Pasteurized Fat Free
Mayfield Dairy
Half & Half
Meadow Brook Dairy
Half & Half
Meadow Gold
Half & Half (All)
Meijer
Ultra Pasteurized Heavy Half and Half
Nature's Promise (Giant)
Organic Half & Half
Nature's Promise (Stop & Shop)
Organic Half & Half
O Organics ᧁ
Half and Half
Half and Half Creamer
Oak Farms Dairy
Half & Half
Oberweis Dairy
Half and Half
Organic Cow of Vermont, The
Organic Cow of Vermont, The (All)
Organic Valley ⓘ
French Vanilla Half and Half
Half and Half
Hazelnut Half and Half
Penn Maid
Half & Half
PET Milk
Half & Half
Prairie Farms
Half & Half
Price's Creameries
Half & Half
Publix
Fat Free Half & Half
Half & Half

Reiter Dairy
Half & Half

Rosenberger's Dairies
Half & Half

Stop & Shop
Fat Free Half & Half
Half & Half

T.G. Lee Dairy
Half & Half

Tuscan Dairy Farms
Fat Free Half & Half
Half & Half

Wegmans
Fresh Half & Half
Half & Half
Ultra Half & Half Pint

Wild Harvest (ACME)
Organic Half & Half

Wild Harvest (Albertsons)
Half & Half

Wild Harvest (Cub Foods)
Organic Half & Half

Wild Harvest (Jewel-Osco)
Organic Half & Half

Winn-Dixie
Half & Half (Fat Free, Regular)

MARGARINE & SPREADS

ACME
65% Margarine Spread Quarters
Soy Oil Soft Spread Margarine
Unbelieve Better Spread Vegetable Oil
Vegetable Oil Soft Spread Margarine

Always Save
52% Spread
Margarine Quarters
Margarine Tub

Benecol
Light Spread
Regular Spread

Berkeley Farms
Margarine

Best Choice
Soft Margarine
Spread Tub
Tastes Like Butter

Vegetable Oil Margarine Quarters

BestLife
Baking Sticks
Spray
Spread
Spread with Extra Virgin Olive Oil

Blue Bonnet
Blue Bonnet Spread

Canoleo
Canoleo

Cub Foods
70% Vegetable Oil Margarine Stick
Soft Spread Margarine Tub

Earth Balance
Earth Balance (All)

Fastco (Fareway)
Could Be Butter
Margarine
Soft Bowl Margarine
Spread Margarine

Flavorite (Cub Foods)
Margarine Quarters

Fleischmann's
Fleischmann's Spread

Food Club (Brookshire)
48% Margarine Spread
60% Margarine Spread
65% Margarine Spread
No Ifs Ands Or Butter
Soft Margarine Tub

Food Club (Marsh)
No Ifs Ands Or Butter
Spread Quarters 65%

Giant
Margarine Stick

Giant Eagle
48% Vegetable Oil Spread
80% Margarine Quarters
Better N' Butter Tub
Soft Margarine Tub

Gold 'n Soft
Gold 'n Soft (All)

Great Value (Wal-Mart) 25
48% Vegetable Oil Soft Spread
Margarine Quarters

Haggen
Margarine, Soft

Vegetable Spread

H-E-B
You'd Think It's Butter

Hy-Vee
100% Corn Oil Margarine
Best Thing Since Butter
Rich & Creamy Soft Margarine
Soft Margarine
Soft Spread
Soft Spread Crock
Vegetable Margarine

Jewel-Osco
65% Original Spread
Kosher Soy Oil Margarine Stick
Soy Oil Soft Spread Margarine
Vegetable Oil Soft Spread Margarine
Whipped Soft Spread Butter Tub

Kroger
Churn Gold Spread
Value Spread

Meijer
48% Crock Spread
70% Quarter Spread
Margarine (Soft Tube, Sleeve)
Margarine, Corn Oil
No Ifs Ands or Butter Spread
Tub Spread

Move Over Butter
Move Over Butter Spread

Nature's Promise (Stop & Shop)
Organic Margarine

Our Family
Best Thing Since Butter
Soft Margarine 80%
Soft Spread 48%
Vegetable Oil Margarine 80% (Quarters)

Parkay
Parkay Spread

Publix
Homestyle Spread - 48% Vegetable Oil
Original Spread Quarters - 70%
   Vegetable Oil

Richfood (ACME)
Family Margarine Spread

Schnucks
Margarine

Shaw's
Margarine and Spread
Soft Salted Soy Oil Margarine
Soft Spread Margarine
Soy Oil Margarine
Spreadable
Sweet Cream Vegetable Oil Spread

Smart Balance
Smart Balance (All)

Valu Time (Brookshire)
40% Margarine Spread
52% Margarine Spread

Value (Kroger)
Spread

Wegmans
48% Vegetable Oil Spread
80% Vegetable Oil Quarters

MILK, CHOCOLATE & FLAVORED

Albertsons
1% Chocolate Milk Low Fat
Chocolate Milk Low Fat
Chocolate Milk Reduced Fat

Alta Dena
Chocolate Lowfat Milk
Chocolate Whole Milk

Always Save
Filled Milk

Barber's
Chocolate Milk (All)

Berkeley Farms
Chocolate Whole Milk
Lowfat Chocolate Milk

Broughton
Coldstar Homogenized
Dairy Fresh Kitchen Guild

Calorie Countdown
Dairy Beverages (All Flavors and Fat
   Levels)

Country Fresh
Milk

Creamland Dairies
Chocolate Milk (All)

Darigold
Darigold (All)

Dean's
Milk

Fastco (Fareway)
Chocolate Milk

Gandy's ⓘ
Chocolate Milk (1%, Skim, Whole)
Strawberry Milk, Skim

Giant
1% Low Fat Chocolate Milk
2% Reduced Fat Chocolate Milk

Grass Point Farms
Milk (All)

Great Value (Wal-Mart) 25
1% Lowfat Chocolate Milk
1/2% Lowfat Chocolate Milk
2% Chocolate Milk

Hiland Dairy
Chocolate Milk
Fat Free Chocolate Milk
Fat Free Vanilla Shake Flavored Milk
Low Fat Chocolate Milk
Low Fat Orange Crème Milk
Low Fat Strawberry Milk
Reduced Fat Chocolate Milk
Reduced Fat Strawberry Milk

Hood
Hood Flavored Milks (All)
Hood Milks (All)

Horizon Organic
Flavored Milk (All)

Kalona Organics
Chocolate Milk (All)

Louis Trauth Dairy
Chocolate Drink
Milk (All)

Lucerne (Safeway) ⌒
2% Reduced Fat Chocolate Milk
Fat Free Chocolate Milk
Mocha Cappuccino Low Fat 1% Milk
Very Berry Strawberry Milk

Marsh
Low Fat Chocolate Milk

Mayfield Dairy
Lowfat Chocolate Milk
Whole Chocolate Milk

McArthur Dairy
Chocolate Milk

Meadow Brook Dairy
Milk (All)

Meadow Gold
Milk (All)

Meijer
1% Chocolate Milk Lowfat
Chocolate Milk
Strawberry Milk

Nesquik
Ready-to-Drink Milk (All Flavors)

O Organics ⌒
Reduced Fat Chocolate Milk

Oak Farms Dairy
Milk (All)

Oberweis Dairy
No Sugar Added Fat Free Vanilla Milk
No Sugar Added Lowfat Chocolate Milk
No Sugar Added Strawberry Milk
Reduced Fat Chocolate Milk
Reduced Fat Strawberry Milk
Reduced Fat Vanilla Milk

Organic Cow of Vermont, The
Organic Cow of Vermont, The (All)

Organic Valley ⓘ
Chocolate 2%
Chocolate 8 oz. Single Serves
Strawberry 8 oz. Single Serves
Vanilla 8 oz. Single Serves

Over the Moon
Milk (All)

Prairie Farms
Candy Cane Milk
Chocolate Cherry Milk
Chocolate Milk (Fat Free, Lowfat,
   Reduced Fat, Regular)
Chocolate Mint Milk
Cookies & Cream Milk
Irish Crème Milk
Pumpkin Spice Milk
Strawberry Milk
Vanilla Milk

Price's Creameries
Milk (All)

Publix
Chocolate Milk
Low Fat Chocolate Milk

Purity Dairies
  1% Lowfat Chocolate Milk
  1% Lowfat Strawberry Milk
  Whole Chocolate Milk
Robinson Dairy
  Milk (All)
Rosenberger's Dairies
  Milk (All)
Simply Smart
  Fat Free Chocolate Milk
Straus Family Creamery
  Milk (All)
T.G. Lee Dairy
  1% Chocolate Lowfat Milk
  1% Strawberry Lowfat Milk
  Chocolate Milk
  Choc-O-Lee
TruMoo
  Chocolate Fat Free Milk
  Coffee Lowfat Milk
  Strawberry Fat Free Milk
Turkey Hill
  Chocolate Cool Moo's
  Premium 1% Lowfat Chocolate Milk
Tuscan Dairy Farms
  Chocolate Milkshake Chug
  Strawberry Lowfat Milk Chug
  Vanilla Milkshake Chug
Wegmans
  Low Fat Chocolate Milk

MILK, LACTOSE-FREE

Best Choice
  2% Lactose Milk
  Lactose Fat Free Milk
  Lactose Whole Milk
Broughton
  100% Lactaid
Food Club (Brookshire)
  100% Lactose Free 2% Milk
  100% Lactose Free Non Fat Milk
  100% Lactose Free Whole Milk
Gay Lea
  Gay Lea (All)
Giant
  2% Reduced Fat Lactose Free Milk

Lactaid
  Milk (All)
Lucerne (Safeway) ✍
  Lactose Free Fat Free Calcium Enriched
    Milk
  Lactose Free Fat Free Milk
  Lactose Free Reduced Fat 2% Calcium
    Enriched Milk
  Lactose Free Reduced Fat 2% Milk
  Lactose Free Whole Vitamin D Milk
McArthur Dairy
  Easy Lactose Free Milk
Meijer
  Lactose Free Milk (Fat Free with
    Calcium, 2% with Calcium)
Meyenberg
  Goat Milk (Lowfat, Whole)
Organic Valley ⓘ
  Lactose Free Milk
Purity Dairies
  0% Acidophilus & Bifudum Milk
  1% Sweet Acidophilus Milk
Smart Balance
  Smart Balance (All)
Trader Joe's
  Dairy Ease Lactose Free Milk

SOUR CREAM

Albertsons
  Grade A Sour Cream Pasteurized
  Light Sour Cream
  Non-Fat Sour Cream Pasteurized
Alta Dena
  Crème Fraiche
  Light Sour Cream
  Sour Cream
Always Save
  Cultured Sour Cream
Axelrod
  Sour Cream (Nonfat, Light, Regular)
Barber's
  Sour Cream
Berkeley Farms
  Fat Free Sour Cream
  Sour Cream

Best Choice
  Fat Free Sour Cream
  Lite Sour Cream
  Sour Cream
Breakstone's ⌒
  Sour Cream, All Natural
  Sour Cream, Fat Free
  Sour Cream, Reduced Fat
Broughton
  Morningstar Sour Cream
  Sour Cream
Cabot
  Cabot Products (All)
Cascade Fresh ⓘ ✓
  Cascade Fresh (All)
Country Fresh
  Sour Cream
Creamland Dairies
  Sour Cream (All)
Crowley Foods
  Crowley Foods (All)
Daisy Brand
  Daisy Brand (All)
Darigold
  Darigold (All)
Dean's
  Sour Cream (All)
Dutch Farms
  Sour Cream (All)
Farmers' All Natural Creamery
  Sour Cream
Food Club (Brookshire)
  Sour Cream, Light
  Sour Cream, Non Fat
Food Club (Marsh)
  Light Sour Cream
  Non Fat Sour Cream
  Sour Cream
Food You Feel Good About (Wegmans)
  Light Sour Cream
Friendship Dairies
  Sour Cream (All)
Gandy's ⓘ
  Sour Cream
Gay Lea
  Gay Lea (All)

Giant
  Lite Sour Cream
  Sour Cream
Great Value (Wal-Mart) 25
  Fat Free Sour Cream
  Light Sour Cream
  Sour Cream
Haggen
  Sour Cream (Fat Free, Light, Regular)
Heluva Good
  Sour Cream (All)
Hiland Dairy
  Light Sour Cream
  Regular Sour Cream
Hood
  Sour Cream (All)
Hy-Vee
  Light Sour Cream
  Sour Cream
Kalona Organics
  Sour Cream (All)
Kemps ⓘ
  Sour Cream
Knudsen ⌒
  Sour Cream, Fat Free
  Sour Cream, Hampshire
  Sour Cream, Hampshire 100% Natural
  Sour Cream, Light
Lakeview Farms
  Sour Cream (All)
Louis Trauth Dairy
  Sour Cream
Lucerne (Safeway) ⌒
  Light Sour Cream
  Sour Cream
Mayfield Dairy
  Sour Cream
Meadow Brook Dairy
  Sour Cream
Meadow Gold
  Sour Cream (All)
Nancy's
  Nancy's (All)
Oak Farms Dairy
  Sour Cream
Oberweis Dairy
  Lite Sour Cream

Sour Cream
Organic Valley ⓘ
Sour Cream (Lowfat, Regular)
Our Family
Sour Cream
Penn Maid
Sour Cream
Prairie Farms
Sour Cream (Fat Free, Light, Regular)
Price Chopper
Lite Sour Cream
Sour Cream
Price's Creameries
Sour Cream
Publix
Fat Free Sour Cream (All Styles)
Light Sour Cream (All Styles)
Regular Sour Cream (All Styles)
Purity Dairies
Sour Cream
Reiter Dairy
Sour Cream (All)
Robinson Dairy
Sour Cream (All)
Senor Rico
Crema Mexicana
Crema Salvadorena
Stop & Shop
Fat Free Sour Cream
Lite Sour Cream
Sour Cream
Straus Family Creamery
Sour Cream (All)
Tillamook
Sour Cream (All) ⚥
Trader Joe's
Sour Cream (All)
Tropical Cheese
Crema CA Dairy Spread
Crema Central American
Crema Mexicana
V & V Supremo
Sour Cream Products (All)
Vegan Gourmet
Sour Cream Alternative
Wegmans
Fat Free Sour Cream

Sour Cream
Wild Harvest (ACME)
Organic Sour Cream
Wild Harvest (Albertsons)
Organic Sour Cream
Wild Harvest (Cub Foods)
Organic Sour Cream
Wild Harvest (Jewel-Osco)
Organic Sour Cream
Winn-Dixie
Sour Cream (Fat Free, Light, Regular)

SOYMILK & MILK ALTERNATIVES

8th Continent ⓘ
Soymilk (All)
Almond Breeze ⚥
Almond Breeze (All)
Almond Dream
Original
Unsweetened Original
Alpro Soya
Soymilk (All)
Best Choice
Chocolate Soymilk
Lite Organic Soymilk
Lite Vanilla Soymilk
Organic Soymilk
Vanilla Soymilk
Central Market (H-E-B)
Organic Original Almond Milk
Organic Original Ancient Grains Milk
Organic Original Rice Milk
Organic Vanilla Almond Milk
Organic Vanilla Rice Milk
Coconut Dream
Coconut Drink
DariFree ⓘ
DariFree Non Dairy Milk Alternative
(Chocolate, Original)
Earth Balance
Earth Balance (All)
Eden Foods
Organic EdenBlend
Organic Edensoy, Unsweetened

Food You Feel Good About (Wegmans)
- Organic Original Rice Beverage
- Organic Original Soymilk
- Organic Rice Beverage, Original
- Organic Rice Beverage, Vanilla
- Organic Vanilla Rice Beverage
- Organic Vanilla Soymilk

Full Circle (Marsh)
- Organic Chocolate Soymilk, Refrigerated (UHT)
- Organic Original Soymilk (UHT)
- Organic Vanilla Soymilk (UHT)

Full Circle (Schnucks)
- Organic Chocolate Soymilk
- Organic Original Soymilk
- Organic Plain Soymilk
- Organic Vanilla Soymilk
- Original Ricemilk
- Vanilla Ricemilk

GranoVita
- Calcium Enriched Soya Drink
- Organic Sugar Free Soya Drink

Great Value (Wal-Mart) 🗓25
- Chocolate Soymilk
- Original Soymilk
- Vanilla Soymilk

GreenWise Market (Publix)
- Chocolate Soymilk
- Plain Soymilk
- Vanilla Soymilk

H-E-B
- Almond Milk, Chocolate
- Almond Milk, Original
- Almond Milk, Unsweetened Vanilla
- Almond Milk, Vanilla
- Chocolate Soymilk
- Light Plain Soymilk
- Light Vanilla Soymilk
- Plain Soymilk
- Vanilla Soymilk

Hy-Vee
- Chocolate Soymilk
- Original Soymilk
- Refrigerated Organic Vanilla Soymilk
- Refrigerated Original Soymilk
- Vanilla Soymilk

Living Harvest ⓘ ✓
- Tempt Hempmilk

Meijer
- Chocolate Soymilk
- Organic Ricemilk
- Organic Soymilk
- Vanilla Rice Milk
- Vanilla Soymilk

MimicCreme ⓘ
- MimicCreme (All)

Nancy's
- Nancy's (All)

Nature's Promise (Giant)
- Chocolate Soymilk
- Chocolate Soymilk (Refrigerated)
- Organic Enriched Original Rice Milk
- Organic Enriched Vanilla Rice Milk
- Organic Original Soymilk
- Organic Plain Soymilk (Refrigerated)
- Organic Vanilla Soymilk (Non-Refrigerated)
- Organic Vanilla Soymilk (Refrigerated)

Nature's Promise (Stop & Shop)
- Chocolate Soymilk
- Chocolate Soymilk (Refrigerated)
- Organic Enriched Original Rice Milk
- Organic Enriched Vanilla Rice Milk
- Organic Original Soymilk
- Organic Plain Soymilk (Refrigerated)
- Organic Vanilla Soymilk (Non-Refrigerated)
- Organic Vanilla Soymilk (Refrigerated)

O Organics ⌒
- Chocolate Soymilk
- Light Vanilla Soy Milk
- Non Dairy Drink Aseptic Original Almond Milk
- Non Dairy Drink Aseptic Vanilla Almond Milk
- Organic Plain Soy Beverage
- Organic Plain Soymilk
- Organic Vanilla Soy Beverage
- Plain Light Soymilk
- Vanilla Soymilk
- Whole Grain Rice Milk Plain
- Whole Grain Rice Vanilla Milk

Organic Valley ⓘ
- Chocolate Soymilk
- Original Soymilk
- Unsweetened Soymilk
- Vanilla Soymilk

Our Family
- Organic Chocolate Soymilk (Refrigerated)
- Organic Original Soymilk
- Organic Vanilla Soymilk (Refrigerated)

Pacific Natural Foods ⓘ
- Hazelnut, Chocolate
- Hazelnut, Original
- Hemp, Chocolate
- Hemp, Original
- Hemp, Vanilla
- Low Fat Rice, Plain
- Low Fat Rice, Vanilla
- Organic Almond Chocolate
- Organic Low-Fat Almond, Original
- Organic Low-Fat Almond, Vanilla
- Organic Soy, Unsweetened
- Organic Unsweetened Almond Original
- Organic Unsweetened Almond Vanilla
- Select Soy, Low Fat Plain
- Select Soy, Low Fat Vanilla
- Ultra Soy, Plain
- Ultra Soy, Vanilla

PEARL Soymilk ()
- Chocolate Organic Soymilk
- Coffee Organic Soymilk
- Creamy Vanilla Organic Soymilk
- Green Tea Organic Soymilk
- Unsweetened Organic Soymilk

Price Chopper
- Chocolate Soymilk
- Original Soymilk

Publix
- Soymilk (Light, Plain and Vanilla)

Pulmuone Wildwood 🏅
- Soymilk (All)

Rice Dream
- Carob Rice Drink
- Enriched Original Rice Drink
- Enriched Vanilla Rice Drink
- Heartwise Original Rice Drink
- Heartwise Vanilla Rice Drink
- Horchata
- Original Rice Drink
- Supreme Chocolate Chai Rice Drink
- Supreme Vanilla Hazelnut Rice Drink
- Vanilla Rice Drink

Silk
- Silk Soymilk (All)

So Delicious Dairy Free
- Coconut Milk Beverage, Chocolate (Refrigerated, Shelf Stable)
- Coconut Milk Beverage, Original (Refrigerated, Shelf Stable)
- Coconut Milk Beverage, Original Sugar Free (Refrigerated, Shelf Stable)
- Coconut Milk Beverage, Unsweetened
- Coconut Milk Beverage, Vanilla (Refrigerated, Shelf Stable)
- Coconut Milk Beverage, Vanilla Sugar Free
- Coconut Milk Creamer, French Vanilla
- Coconut Milk Creamer, Hazelnut
- Coconut Milk Creamer, Original
- Cultured Coconut Milk, Chocolate
- Cultured Coconut Milk, Original
- Cultured Coconut Milk, Strawberry
- Cultured Coconut Milk, Vanilla

So Good
- Chocolate Soya
- Light Soya
- Original Soya
- Soya Life Low Fat
- Unsweetened Soya

Soy Dream
- Chocolate Enriched Soymilk
- Classic Original Soymilk
- Classic Vanilla Soymilk
- Original Enriched Soymilk
- Original Enriched Soymilk (Refrigerated)
- Vanilla Enriched (Refrigerated)
- Vanilla Enriched Soymilk

Trader Joe's
- Almond Smooth Non-Dairy Beverages (Chocolate, Original, Vanilla, Unsweetened Vanilla)
- Coconut Milk Beverage (Unsweetened, Vanilla)

Hemp Drink (Original, Vanilla)
Kefir
Organic Whole Grain Drinks (Regular,
   Unsweetened)
Rice Milk
Soy Beverages (All)
Soymilk (All)

Winn-Dixie
Chocolate Soymilk
Plain Soymilk
Unsweetened Soymilk
Vanilla Soymilk

ZenSoy
ZenSoy Products (All)

WHIPPED TOPPINGS

Alta Dena
Light Whipped Cream

Axelrod
Aerosol Topping

Berkeley Farms
Light Whipped Cream

Best Choice
Extra Creamy Whipped Topping
Light Cream Whipped Topping
Whipped Topping

Broughton
Dairy Fresh Real Cream Whip Cream

Cabot
Cabot Products (All)

Cool Whip ∽
Whipped Topping , Original Regular
Whipped Topping , Season's Delight
   Sweet Cinnamon Regular
Whipped Topping, Extra Creamy
Whipped Topping, Extra Creamy
   Regular
Whipped Topping, Free
Whipped Topping, Lite
Whipped Topping, Original
Whipped Topping, Season's Delight
   French Vanilla Regular
Whipped Topping, Sugar Free

Crowley Foods
Aerosol Topping

Dr. Oetker
Whip It

Dream Whip ∽
Whipped Topping Mix

Dutch Farms
Whipped Cream

Food Club (Brookshire)
Ultra Pasteurized Processed Whipped
   Cream
Whipping Cream

Food Club (Marsh)
Ultra Pasteurized Processed Whipped
   Cream Aerosol

Gay Lea
Gay Lea (All)

Genuardi's ∽
Lite Whipped Topping

Giant
Extra Creamy Whipped Cream
   (Refrigerated) (Aerosol)
Heavy Whipping Cream
Light Whipped Cream (Refrigerated)
   (Aerosol)

Great Value (Wal-Mart)
Aerosol Extra Creamy Sweetened
   Whipped Cream
Aerosol Sweetened Whipped Light
   Cream

Haggen
Aero Whipped Cream

Hood
Instant Whipped Cream
Sugar Free Light Whipped Cream

Lucerne (Safeway) ∽
Whipped Cream - Extra Creamy in
   Aerosol Can
Whipped Cream - Light in Aerosol Can

Meadow Gold
Light Whipped Cream

Meijer
Ultra Pasteurized Whipped Cream
   (Aerosol)

MimicCreme ⓘ
MimicCreme (All)

Our Family
24% Aerosol Whipped Topping

Extra Creamy Whipped Topping with
   Real Cream
Fat Free Whipped Topping
Sugar Free Whipped Topping
Penn Maid
Aerosol Topping
Price Chopper
Extra Creamy Whip Cream
Instant Lite Whip Cream
Xtra Whip Heavy Cream
Publix
Whipped Heavy Cream (Aerosol Can)
Whipped Light Cream (Aerosol Can)
Whipped Topping - Fat Free (Aerosol
   Can)
Reddi-wip
Reddi-wip (All Varieties)
Schnucks
Extra Creamy Whipped Cream
   (Aerosol)
Non-Dairy Whipped Cream
Whipped Cream (Aerosol)
Stop & Shop
Heavy Whipping Cream
Wegmans
Whipped Heavy Cream - Extra Creamy
Whipped Light Cream
Whipped Topping - Extra Creamy
Whipped Topping - Fat Free

YOGURT

Alpro Soya
Yogurt (All)
Alta Dena
All Natural Black Cherry Yogurt
All Natural Peach Yogurt
All Natural Raspberry Yogurt
All Natural Strawberry Banana Yogurt
All Natural Strawberry Yogurt
Low Fat Plain Yogurt
Nonfat Black Cherry Yogurt
Nonfat Lemon Yogurt
Nonfat Peach Yogurt
Nonfat Plain Yogurt
Nonfat Raspberry Yogurt
Nonfat Strawberry Yogurt

Nonfat Vanilla Yogurt
Nonfat Wildberries Yogurt
Axelrod
Yogurt (All)
Berkeley Farms
Fruit on the Bottom Low Fat Blueberry
   Yogurt
Fruit on the Bottom Low Fat
   Boysenberry Yogurt
Fruit on the Bottom Low Fat Cherry
   Yogurt
Fruit on the Bottom Low Fat Peach
   Yogurt
Fruit on the Bottom Low Fat Raspberry
   Yogurt
Fruit on the Bottom Low Fat Strawberry
   Yogurt
Lowfat Blueberry Yogurt
Lowfat Boysenberry Yogurt
Lowfat Cherry Yogurt
Lowfat Lemon Yogurt
Lowfat Peach Yogurt
Lowfat Plain Yogurt
Lowfat Raspberry Yogurt
Lowfat Strawberry Banana Yogurt
Lowfat Strawberry Yogurt
Lowfat Vanilla Yogurt
Nonfat Blueberry Yogurt
Nonfat Cherry Yogurt
Nonfat Peach Yogurt
Nonfat Plain Yogurt
Nonfat Raspberry Yogurt
Nonfat Strawberry Yogurt
Best Choice
Low Fat Blackberry Yogurt
Low Fat Blueberry Yogurt
Low Fat Boston Cream Yogurt
Low Fat Cherry Vanilla Yogurt
Low Fat Lemon Yogurt
Low Fat Peach Yogurt
Low Fat Pina Colada Yogurt
Low Fat Raspberry Yogurt
Low Fat Strawberry Banana Yogurt
Low Fat Strawberry Cheesecake Yogurt
Low Fat Strawberry Yogurt
Low Fat Vanilla Yogurt
Nonfat Blackberry Yogurt

Nonfat Blueberry Yogurt
Nonfat Boston Cream Yogurt
Nonfat Cherry Vanilla Yogurt
Nonfat Key Lime Yogurt
Nonfat Lemon Yogurt
Nonfat Peach Yogurt
Nonfat Plain Yogurt
Nonfat Raspberry Yogurt
Nonfat Strawberry Banana Yogurt
Nonfat Strawberry Cheesecake Yogurt
Nonfat Strawberry Yogurt
Nonfat Vanilla Yogurt

Broughton
Caramel Pecan Yogurt
Dairy Fresh Blueberry Yogurt
Dairy Fresh Cherry Yogurt
Dairy Fresh Mixed Berry Yogurt
Dairy Fresh Peach Yogurt
Dairy Fresh Plain Yogurt
Dairy Fresh Raspberry Yogurt
Dairy Fresh Strawberry Banana Yogurt
Dairy Fresh Strawberry Yogurt
Dairy Fresh Vanilla Yogurt
Peach Yogurt

Brown Cow
Brown Cow Products (All)

Cabot
Cabot Products (All)

Cascade Fresh ⓘ ✔
Cascade Fresh (All)

Chobani
Chobani (All)

Country Fresh
Yogurt

Crowley Foods
Crowley Foods (All)

Dannon
Plain Activia (24 oz. container)
Plain Lowfat Yogurt
Plain Nonfat Yogurt
Plain Oikos Greek Yogurt
Plain Yogurt

Darigold
Darigold (All)

Eating Right ⌒
Light Peach Yogurt
Light Strawberry Yogurt

Light Vanilla Yogurt

Eden
Black Cherry Soya Dessert
Peach & Passion Fruit Soya Dessert
Plain Soya Dessert
Strawberry Soya Dessert

Food Club (Marsh)
Blended Blueberry Yogurt
Blended Cherry Yogurt
Blended Peach Yogurt
Blended Pineapple Orange Banana
  Yogurt
Blended Raspberry Yogurt
Blended Strawberry Banana Yogurt
Blended Strawberry Rhubarb Yogurt
Blended Strawberry Yogurt
Drinkable Mixed Berry Yogurt
Drinkable Strawberry Yogurt
Lite Banana Cream Yogurt
Lite Blackberry Yogurt
Lite Blueberry Yogurt
Lite Cherry Vanilla Yogurt
Lite Cherry Yogurt
Lite Key Lime Yogurt
Lite Lemon Chiffon Yogurt
Lite Peach Yogurt
Lite Raspberry Yogurt
Lite Strawberry Banana Yogurt
Lite Strawberry Kiwi Yogurt
Lite Strawberry Yogurt
Lite Vanilla Yogurt
Lowfat Blended Strawberry Yogurt
Lowfat Blended Vanilla Yogurt
Nonfat Plain Yogurt

**Food You Feel Good About
(Wegmans)**
Blended Lowfat Blueberry Yogurt with
  Pre & Probiotic
Blended Lowfat Peach Yogurt with Pre
  & Probiotic
Blended Lowfat Plain Yogurt with Pre &
  Probiotic
Blended Lowfat Raspberry Yogurt with
  Pre & Probiotic
Blended Lowfat Strawberry Yogurt with
  Pre & Probiotic

Blended Lowfat Vanilla Yogurt with Pre & Probiotic

Friendship Dairies

Yogurt (All)

Full Circle (Schnucks)

Mixed Berry Drinkable Yogurt
Organic Black Cherry Yogurt
Organic Blueberry Yogurt
Organic Peach Yogurt
Organic Raspberry Yogurt
Organic Strawberry Yogurt
Organic Vanilla Yogurt
Peach Drinkable Yogurt
Strawberry Drinkable Yogurt

Giant

Fruit on the Bottom Low Fat Blueberry Yogurt
Fruit on the Bottom Low Fat Boysenberry Yogurt
Fruit on the Bottom Low Fat Cherry Yogurt
Fruit on the Bottom Low Fat Dutch Apple Yogurt
Fruit on the Bottom Low Fat Mixed Berry Yogurt
Fruit on the Bottom Low Fat Peach Yogurt
Fruit on the Bottom Low Fat Pineapple Yogurt
Fruit on the Bottom Low Fat Raspberry Yogurt
Fruit on the Bottom Low Fat Strawberry Banana Yogurt
Fruit on the Bottom Low Fat Strawberry Yogurt
Light Non Fat Banana Cream Yogurt
Light Non Fat Blueberry Yogurt
Light Non Fat Cherry Vanilla Yogurt
Light Non Fat Cherry Yogurt
Light Non Fat Coffee Yogurt
Light Non Fat Lemon Chiffon Yogurt
Light Non Fat Peach Yogurt
Light Non Fat Raspberry Yogurt
Light Non Fat Strawberry Banana Yogurt
Light Non Fat Strawberry Yogurt
Light Non Fat Vanilla Yogurt

Low Fat Plain Yogurt
Low Fat Vanilla Yogurt
Natural Low Fat Vanilla Yogurt
Non Fat Plain Yogurt
Non Fat Vanilla Yogurt

Giant Eagle

Blended Lowfat Blackberry Yogurt
Blended Lowfat Blueberry Yogurt
Blended Lowfat Mixed Berry Yogurt
Blended Lowfat Peach Yogurt
Blended Lowfat Raspberry Yogurt
Blended Lowfat Red Cherry Yogurt
Blended Lowfat Strawberry Yogurt
Blended Lowfat Strawberry/Banana Yogurt
Blended Lowfat Vanilla Yogurt
Light Apple Crumble Yogurt
Light Banana Crème Yogurt
Light Blackberry Yogurt
Light Blueberry Yogurt
Light Key Lime Yogurt
Light Lemon Chiffon Yogurt
Light Mixed Berry Yogurt
Light Orange Crème Yogurt
Light Peach Yogurt
Light Pumpkin Spice Yogurt
Light Raspberry Lemonade Yogurt
Light Raspberry Yogurt
Light Strawberry Yogurt
Light Strawberry/Banana Yogurt
Light Vanilla Yogurt
Lowfat Plain Yogurt
Nonfat Plain Yogurt

Glenoaks Yogurt

Yogurts (All Flavors)

GranoVita

Banana Deluxe Soyage
Black Cherry Deluxe Soyage
Mango Deluxe Soyage
Peach & Apricot Deluxe Soyage
Plain Deluxe Soyage
Raspberry Deluxe Soyage
Strawberry Deluxe Soyage
Tropical Deluxe Soyage

Great Value (Wal-Mart) 25

Benefit Blueberry Probiotic Light Nonfat Yogurt

Benefit Peach Probiotic Light Nonfat Yogurt

Benefit Raspberry Probiotic Light Nonfat Yogurt

Benefit Strawberry Probiotic Light Nonfat Yogurt

Benefit Vanilla Probiotic Light Nonfat Yogurt

Blended Banana Yogurt

Blended Lowfat Black Cherry Yogurt

Blended Lowfat Blueberry Yogurt

Blended Lowfat Cherry Vanilla Yogurt

Blended Lowfat Key Lime Yogurt

Blended Lowfat Mango Yogurt

Blended Lowfat Mixed Berry Yogurt

Blended Lowfat Peach Yogurt

Blended Lowfat Pina Colada Yogurt

Blended Lowfat Raspberry Yogurt

Blended Lowfat Strawberry Banana Yogurt

Blended Lowfat Strawberry Yogurt

Blended Lowfat Vanilla Yogurt

Fat Free Nonfat Plain Yogurt

Light Nonfat Banana Cream Pie Yogurt

Light Nonfat Banana Cream Yogurt

Light Nonfat Black Cherry Yogurt

Light Nonfat Blueberry Yogurt

Light Nonfat Lemon Chiffon Yogurt

Light Nonfat Mixed Berry Yogurt

Light Nonfat Peach Yogurt

Light Nonfat Raspberry Yogurt

Light Nonfat Strawberry Banana Yogurt

Light Nonfat Strawberry Yogurt

Light Nonfat Vanilla Yogurt

Haggen

Light Blueberry Yogurt

Light Cherry Yogurt

Light Keylime Yogurt

Light Mixed Berry Yogurt

Light Orange Yogurt

Light Peach Yogurt

Light Strawberry Yogurt

Light Vanilla Yogurt

Lowfat Blueberry Yogurt

Lowfat Cherry Yogurt

Lowfat Keylime Yogurt

Lowfat Mixed Berry Yogurt

Lowfat Orange Yogurt

Lowfat Peach Yogurt

Lowfat Raspberry Yogurt

Lowfat Strawberry Yogurt

Lowfat Vanilla Yogurt

Hiland Dairy

Low Fat Yogurt (All Flavor Varieties)

Nonfat No Sugar Added Yogurt (All Flavor Varieties)

Horizon Organic

Yogurt (All)

Hy-Vee

Fat Free Key Lime Pie Yogurt

Fat Free Plain Yogurt

Low Fat Black Cherry Yogurt

Low Fat Blueberry Yogurt

Low Fat Cherry-Vanilla Yogurt

Low Fat Lemon Yogurt

Low Fat Mixed Berry Yogurt

Low Fat Plain Yogurt

Low Fat Raspberry Yogurt

Low Fat Strawberry Banana Yogurt

Low Fat Strawberry Yogurt

Nonfat Banana Cream Yogurt

Nonfat Blueberry Yogurt

Nonfat Cherry Yogurt

Nonfat Lemon Chiffon Yogurt

Nonfat Peach Yogurt

Nonfat Raspberry Yogurt

Nonfat Strawberry Banana Yogurt

Nonfat Strawberry Yogurt

Nonfat Vanilla Yogurt

Peach Yogurt

Yogurt To Go - Strawberry

Yogurt To Go Strawberry & Blueberry

Yogurt To Go Strawberry/Banana & Cherry

Kalona Organics

Yogurt (All)

Kemps ⓘ

Yogurt (All)

La Crème

La Crème (All)

Lucerne (Safeway) ✑

Fat Free Light Blackberry Yogurt

Fat Free Plain Yogurt

Greek Nonfat Blueberry Yogurt

Greek Nonfat Plain Yogurt
Greek Nonfat Vanilla Yogurt
Greek Nonfat Yogurt Honey
Greek Nonfat Yogurt Strawberry
Light Banana Cream Yogurt
Light Black Cherry Yogurt
Light Blueberry Yogurt
Light Key Lime Yogurt
Light Lemon Chiffon Yogurt
Light Mix Berry Yogurt
Light Peach Yogurt
Light Raspberry Yogurt
Light Strawberry Banana Yogurt
Light Strawberry Yogurt
Light Vanilla Yogurt
Low Fat Blueberry Yogurt
Low Fat Cherry Yogurt
Low Fat Peach Yogurt
Low Fat Plain Yogurt
Low Fat Raspberry Yogurt
Low Fat Strawberry Yogurt
Low Fat Vanilla Yogurt

Meadow Gold
Yogurt (All)

Meijer
Banana Yogurt Tube
Blended Boysenberry Yogurt
Blended Low Fat Blueberry Yogurt
Blended Lowfat Cherry Yogurt
Blended Lowfat Mixed Berry Yogurt
Blended Lowfat Peach Yogurt
Blended Lowfat Pina Colada Yogurt
Blended Lowfat Raspberry Yogurt
Blended Strawberry Banana Yogurt
Blended Strawberry Yogurt
Blended Tropical Fruit Yogurt
Blueberry Yogurt Tube
Fruit at the Bottom Blueberry Yogurt
Fruit at the Bottom Peach Yogurt
Fruit at the Bottom Raspberry Yogurt
Fruit at the Bottom Strawberry Yogurt
Lite Banana Crème Yogurt
Lite Black Cherry Yogurt
Lite Blueberry Yogurt
Lite Cherry Vanilla Yogurt
Lite Coconut Crème Yogurt

Lite Lemon Chiffon Yogurt
Lite Mint Chocolate Yogurt
Lite Peach Yogurt
Lite Raspberry Yogurt
Lite Strawberry Banana Yogurt
Lite Strawberry Yogurt
Lite Vanilla Yogurt
Lowfat Vanilla Yogurt
Raspberry Yogurt Tube
Strawberry Banana Yogurt Tube
Strawberry Yogurt Tube
Tropical Punch Yogurt Tube
Watermelon Yogurt Tube

Mountain High Yoghurt
Yogurt Products (All)

Nancy's
Nancy's (All)

Nature's Basket (Giant Eagle)
Organic Lowfat Blueberry Yogurt
Organic Lowfat Peach Yogurt
Organic Lowfat Raspberry Yogurt
Organic Lowfat Strawberry Yogurt
Organic Lowfat Vanilla Yogurt

O Organics Ꮗ
Organic Plain Yogurt
Organic Vanilla Yogurt

Oberweis Dairy
100- Calorie Yogurt (All Flavors)
Nonfat Plain Yogurt
Yogurt (All Flavors)

Old Chatham Sheepherding Company
Sheep's Milk Yogurts (All)

Organic Valley ⓘ
Berry Yogurt
Plain Yogurt
Vanilla Yogurt

Our Family
Blueberry Yogurt
Light Blueberry Yogurt
Light Cherry Vanilla Yogurt
Light Lemon Yogurt
Light Peach Yogurt
Light Raspberry Yogurt
Light Strawberry Banana Yogurt
Light Strawberry Yogurt
Plain Yogurt

Strawberry Banana Yogurt
Strawberry Yogurt
Vanilla Yogurt

Penn Maid
Yogurt

Prairie Farms
Fat Free Yogurt (All Flavors)
Lowfat Yogurt (All Flavors)

Price Chopper
Light Nonfat Black Cherry
Light Nonfat Strawberry
Non Fat Cultured Plain Yogurt
Pineapple Cultured Yogurt

Publix
Black Cherry with Chocolate, Limited
Edition
Creamy Blend Black Cherry Yogurt
Creamy Blend Blueberry Yogurt
Creamy Blend Peach Yogurt
Creamy Blend Strawberry Yogurt
Creamy Blend Vanilla Yogurt
Creamy Blends Black Cherry & Mixed
Berry - Multi Pack
Creamy Blends Blueberry & Strawberry
Banana - Multi Pack
Creamy Blends Peach and Strawberry -
Multi Pack
Egg Nog Yogurt, Limited Edition
Fat Free Light "Active" Peach Yogurt
Fat Free Light "Active" Strawberry
Yogurt
Fat Free Light "Active" Vanilla Yogurt
Fat Free Light Apple Pie Yogurt
Fat Free Light Banana Crème Pie Yogurt
Fat Free Light Blueberry Yogurt
Fat Free Light Cappuccino Yogurt
Fat Free Light Caramel Crème Yogurt
Fat Free Light Cherry Vanilla Yogurt
Fat Free Light Cherry Yogurt
Fat Free Light Coconut Crème Pie
Yogurt
Fat Free Light Honey Almond Yogurt
Fat Free Light Key Lime Pie Yogurt
Fat Free Light Lemon Chiffon Yogurt
Fat Free Light Mandarin Orange Yogurt
Fat Free Light Peach Yogurt

Fat Free Light Raspberry Yogurt
Fat Free Light Strawberry Banana
Yogurt
Fat Free Light Strawberry Yogurt
Fat Free Light Vanilla Yogurt
Fat Free Plain Yogurt
Fruit On The Bottom Banana Yogurt
Fruit On The Bottom Black Cherry
Yogurt
Fruit On The Bottom Blackberry Yogurt
Fruit on the Bottom Blueberry Yogurt
Fruit On The Bottom Cherry Yogurt
Fruit On The Bottom Guava Yogurt
Fruit On The Bottom Mango Yogurt
Fruit On The Bottom Mixed Berry
Yogurt
Fruit On The Bottom Peach Yogurt
Fruit On The Bottom Pineapple Yogurt
Fruit On The Bottom Raspberry Yogurt
Fruit On The Bottom Strawberry
Banana Yogurt
Fruit On The Bottom Strawberry Yogurt
Fruit On The Bottom Tropical Blend
Yogurt
Kids Blue Raspberry & Cotton Candy -
Multi Pack
Kids Grape Bubblegum & Watermelon -
Multi Pack
Kids Strawberry & Blueberry - Multi
Pack
Kids Strawberry Banana & Cherry -
Multi Pack
No Sugar Added Blueberry Yogurt
No Sugar Added Cranberry Raspberry
Yogurt
No Sugar Added Peach Yogurt
No Sugar Added Strawberry Yogurt
No Sugar Added Vanilla Yogurt
Original Creamy Blend Yogurt
Strawberry with Chocolate, Limited
Edition

Pulmuone Wildwood ⚕
Soyogurts (All)

Rachel's Yogurt
Organic Yogurt's (All BUT Low Fat
Vanilla Breakfast and Vanilla Yogurt
with Granola)

Redwood Hill Farm ☃
Yogurt (All)

Safeway Select ᨀ
Peach and Blueberry Panna Cotta

Schnucks
Blended Blueberry Yogurt
Blended Cherry Yogurt
Blended Peach Yogurt
Blended Raspberry Yogurt
Blended Strawberry Banana Yogurt
Blended Strawberry Yogurt
Light Banana Cream Yogurt
Light Blueberry Yogurt
Light Cherry Vanilla Yogurt
Light Cherry Yogurt
Light Key Lime Yogurt
Light Lemon Chiffon Yogurt
Light Peach Yogurt
Light Raspberry Yogurt
Light Strawberry Banana Yogurt
Light Strawberry Kiwi Yogurt
Light Strawberry Yogurt
Light Vanilla Yogurt
Low Fat Vanilla Yogurt
Mixed Berry Smoothie Yogurt
Non Fat Plain Yogurt
Peach Smoothie Yogurt
Raspberry Smoothie Yogurt
Strawberry Banana Smoothie Yogurt
Strawberry Kiwi Smoothie Yogurt
Strawberry Smoothie Yogurt
Strawberry Yogurt

Seven Stars Farm
Lemon Yogurt
Low Fat Maple Yogurt
Low Fat Plain Yogurt
Maple Yogurt
Plain Yogurt
Vanilla Yogurt

Shaw's
Summer Berry Yogurt

Silk
Silk Live! Soy Yogurt (All)

Skyr.is ⓘ
Blueberry
Plain
Vanilla

So Delicious Dairy Free
Coconut Milk Blueberry Yogurt
Coconut Milk Chocolate Yogurt
Coconut Milk Greek Blueberry Yogurt
Coconut Milk Greek Chocolate Yogurt
Coconut Milk Greek Plain Yogurt
Coconut Milk Greek Raspberry Yogurt
Coconut Milk Greek Strawberry Yogurt
Coconut Milk Greek Vanilla Yogurt
Coconut Milk Passionate Mango Yogurt
Coconut Milk Pina Colada Yogurt
Coconut Milk Plain Yogurt
Coconut Milk Raspberry Yogurt
Coconut Milk Strawberry Banana
Yogurt
Coconut Milk Strawberry Yogurt
Coconut Milk Vanilla Yogurt

Stonyfield Farm ⓘ
Stonyfield Farm (All BUT YoToddler,
Frozen Yogurt & Ice Cream)

Straus Family Creamery
Plain Yogurts (All)

Tillamook
Yogurt (All) ☃

Trader Joe's
Soy Yogurt (All)
Yogurt (All)

Tropical Cheese
Creme Parfait

Voskos Greek Yogurt
Greek Yogurt (All BUT Voskos and
Granola)

Wallaby Yogurt Company ✓
Yogurt (All)

Wegmans
Blended Lowfat Blueberry Yogurt
Blended Lowfat Cherry Yogurt
Blended Lowfat Coffee Yogurt
Blended Lowfat Key Lime Yogurt
Blended Lowfat Lemon Yogurt

Blended Lowfat Mixed Berry Yogurt
Blended Lowfat Orange Cream Yogurt
Blended Lowfat Peach Yogurt
Blended Lowfat Raspberry Yogurt
Blended Lowfat Strawberry Banana Yogurt
Blended Lowfat Strawberry Yogurt
Blended Lowfat Vanilla Yogurt
Blended Nonfat Light Blueberry Yogurt
Blended Nonfat Light Key Lime Yogurt
Blended Nonfat Light Mixed Berry Yogurt
Blended Nonfat Light Orange Cream Yogurt
Blended Nonfat Light Peach Yogurt
Blended Nonfat Light Raspberry Yogurt
Blended Nonfat Light Strawberry Banana Yogurt
Blended Nonfat Light Strawberry Yogurt
Blended Nonfat Light Vanilla Yogurt
Fruit on the Bottom Fat Free Black Cherry Yogurt
Fruit on the Bottom Fat Free Blueberry Yogurt
Fruit on the Bottom Fat Free Lemon Yogurt
Fruit on the Bottom Fat Free Mixed Berry Yogurt
Fruit on the Bottom Fat Free Peach Yogurt
Fruit on the Bottom Fat Free Raspberry Yogurt
Fruit on the Bottom Fat Free Strawberry Banana Yogurt
Fruit on the Bottom Fat Free Strawberry Yogurt
Fruit on the Bottom Lowfat Apricot Mango Yogurt
Fruit on the Bottom Lowfat Blueberry Yogurt
Fruit on the Bottom Lowfat Cherry Vanilla Yogurt
Fruit on the Bottom Lowfat Cherry Yogurt

Fruit on the Bottom Lowfat Lemon Yogurt
Fruit on the Bottom Lowfat Mixed Berry Yogurt
Fruit on the Bottom Lowfat Peach Yogurt
Fruit on the Bottom Lowfat Pina Colada Yogurt
Fruit on the Bottom Lowfat Pineapple Yogurt
Fruit on the Bottom Lowfat Raspberry Yogurt
Fruit on the Bottom Lowfat Strawberry Banana Yogurt
Fruit on the Bottom Lowfat Strawberry Kiwi Yogurt
Fruit on the Bottom Lowfat Strawberry Yogurt
Lowfat Plain Yogurt
Lowfat Vanilla Yogurt
Nonfat Plain Yogurt

Winn-Dixie
Fat Free Banana Cream Pie Yogurt
Fat Free Black Cherry Yogurt
Fat Free Blueberry Yogurt
Fat Free Key Lime Pie Yogurt
Fat Free Mixed Berry Yogurt
Fat Free Peach Yogurt
Fat Free Pina Colada Yogurt
Fat Free Raspberry Yogurt
Fat Free Strawberry Banana Yogurt
Fat Free Strawberry Yogurt
Fat Free Vanilla Yogurt
Lowfat Blueberry Yogurt
Lowfat Peach Yogurt
Lowfat Pineapple Cherry Yogurt
Lowfat Pineapple Yogurt
Lowfat Plain Yogurt
Lowfat Raspberry Yogurt
Lowfat Strawberry Yogurt
Lowfat Vanilla Yogurt
No Sugar Added Strawberry Yogurt

MISCELLANEOUS

Alouette
  Crème Fraiche
Goya
  Media Crema
  Media Crema Ligera
Lifeway
  Lifeway (All)
Meijer
  Ultra Pasteurized Non Dairy (Aerosol)
  Ultra Pasteurized Non Dairy Creamer
Nancy's
  Kefir (All)
Redwood Hill Farm ♀
  Kefir (All)
Trader Joe's
  Lassi (Alfonso Mango & Plain)
Vita Foods ⓘ
  Sauza Chipotle Cheese Sauce

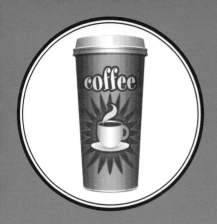

BEVERAGES

Beer

Bard's Tale Beer ⓘ ✓
Bard's Gold
Billabong Brewing
Gluten Free Apple Beer
Gluten Free Blonde Beer
Gluten Free Ginger Beer
Goya
Ginger Beer

Green's
Green's Gluten-Free Beer (All)
Lakefront Brewery
New Grist
New Planet Beer Company ✓
3R Raspberry Ale
Off Grid Pale Ale
Tread Lightly Ale

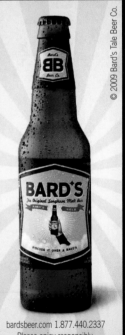

A GLUTEN-FREE BEER. BECAUSE WE'RE PRETTY SURE THE CONSTITUTION INCLUDES SOMETHING ABOUT YOUR RIGHT TO DRINK A COLD ONE.

As beer fans and celiacs, we made it our mission to give beer back to the over two million people who are intolerant to gluten. The result is Bard's Beer, America's first gluten-free sorghum beer and the only beer brewed with 100% malted sorghum. That's right, we even malt the sorghum to give it the traditional taste and aroma that beer lovers demand.

Discuss it over a Bard's

© 2009 Bard's Tale Beer Co.

bardsbeer.com 1.877.440.2337
Please enjoy responsibly.

O'Brien Brewing
- Brown Ale
- Natural Light
- Pale Ale
- Premium Lager

Redbridge
- Redbridge Beer

St. Peter's Brewery ⓘ
- G-Free Sorghum Beer

CARBONATED DRINKS

7Up
- 7Up (All)

A&W
- A&W (All)

Adirondack Beverages
- Naturals (All)

Always Save
- Cherry Cola
- Cola
- Grape Soda
- Lemon Lime Soda
- Orange Soda
- Root Beer
- Strawberry Soda

Barq's
- Caffeine Free Root Beer
- Diet Red Crème Soda
- Diet Root Beer
- Root Beer

Best Choice
- Cherry Cola
- Club Soda
- Cola
- Country Mist Soda
- Crème Soda
- Diet Cola
- Diet Dr. Choice
- Diet Orange Soda
- Diet Root Beer
- Dr. Choice
- Fruit Punch
- Ginger Ale
- Grape Soda
- Grapefruit Soda
- Key Lime Sparkling Water

- Kiwi Strawberry Soda
- Lemon Lime Soda
- Orange Soda
- Peach Soda
- Pineapple Soda
- Red Crème Soda
- Root Beer
- Seltzer Water
- Strawberry Soda
- Strawberry Sparkling Water
- Tonic Water

Big Shot
- Big Shot (All)

Chaser ⓘ
- Chaser

Cheerwine
- Cheerwine Beverage

China Cola ⓘ
- China Cola (All)

Clear 'N' Natural
- Clear 'N' Natural (All)

Clearly Prestige (Winn-Dixie)
- Country Strawberry Sparkling Water Beverage
- Key Lime Sparkling Water Beverage
- Mandarin Orange Sparkling Water Beverage
- Mellow Peach Sparkling Water Beverage
- White Grape Sparkling Water Beverage
- Wild Cherry Sparkling Water Beverage

Coca-Cola Company, The
- Caffeine Free Coca-Cola Classic
- Caffeine Free Diet Coke
- Cherry Coke
- Cherry Coke Zero
- Coca-Cola Classic
- Coca-Cola Zero
- Diet Cherry Coke
- Diet Coke
- Diet Coke Plus
- Diet Coke Sweetened with Splenda
- Diet Coke with Lime
- Vanilla Coke
- Vanilla Coke Zero

Crush
- Crush (All)

Double-Cola ⓘ
  Diet Double-Cola
  Double-Cola
Dr. Pepper
  Dr. Pepper (All)
Fanta
  Fanta Grape
  Fanta Orange
  Fanta Orange Zero
Faygo
  Faygo (All)
Food Club (Brookshire)
  Cherry Cola
  Club Soda
  Cola
  Diet Black Cherry Sparkling Water
  Diet Blackberry Apple Sparkling Water
  Diet Cola
  Diet Dr. Wow
  Diet Key Lime Sparkling Water
  Diet Lemon Lime Soda
  Diet Peach Sparkling Water
  Diet Root Beer
  Diet Strawberry Kiwi Sparkling Water
  Diet Strawberry Sparkling Water
  Diet Tropical Sparkling Water
  Diet White Grape Sparkling Water
  Dr. Wow Soda
  Fruit Punch Soda
  Ginger Ale
  Grape Soda
  Lemon Lime Soda
  Orange Soda
  Peach Soda
  Pineapple Soda
  Punch Soda
  Red Cream Soda
  Root Beer
  Strawberry Soda
  Tonic Soda
  Wild Mountain Soda
Food You Feel Good About (Wegmans)
  Club Soda
  Lemon Sparkling Water
  Lime Sparkling Water
  Mandarin Orange Sparkling Water

  Mixed Berry Sparkling Water
Fresca
  Fresca
Giant
  Black Cherry Seltzer Water
  Club Soda
  Cola
  Cream Soda
  Diet Cola
  Diet Cream Soda
  Diet Ginger Ale
  Diet Grape Soda
  Diet Lemon Lime Soda
  Diet Orange Soda
  Diet Root Beer
  Ginger Ale
  Grape Soda
  Lemon Lime Seltzer Water
  Lemon Lime Soda
  Lemon Seltzer Water
  Lime Seltzer Water
  Mandarin Orange Seltzer Water
  Orange Soda
  Raspberry Seltzer Water
  Root Beer
  Tonic Water
Ginger People, The ()
  Ginger Beer
  Lemon Ginger Beer
Goya
  2 Liter Soda Cola Champagne
  Apple Soda
  Coconut Soda
  El Dorado
  El Dorado Golden Soda
  Fruit Punch Soda
  Grape Soda
  Grapefruit Soda
  Guarana Soda
  Guava Soda
  Jamaica Soda
  Lemon-Lime Soda
  Lime Soda
  Mandarin Soda
  Mango Soda
  Pineapple Soda
  Sangria Soda

Strawberry Soda
Tamarind Soda
Tropical Soda Coconut
Tropical Soda Cola Champagne
Tropical Soda Fruit Punch
Tropical Soda Ginger Beer
Tropical Soda Guava
Tropical Soda Lemon Lime
Tropical Soda Mandarin Orange
Tropical Soda Pineapple
Tropical Soda Strawberry
Tropical Soda Tamarind
Tropicola Soda Diet
Watermelon Soda

GranoVita
NAO Sparkling See Thru Can - Aloe Vera
NAO Sparkling See Thru Can - Apple
NAO Sparkling See Thru Can - Grape
NAO Sparkling See Thru Can - Guava
NAO Sparkling See Thru Can - Lemon
NAO Sparkling See Thru Can - Mango
NAO Sparkling See Thru Can - Peach
NAO Sparkling See Thru Can - Strawberry

Great Value (Wal-Mart) 25
Limeade

GuS Grown-Up Soda
GuS Grown-Up Soda (All Flavors)

Hansen's
Soda (All)

Henry Weinhards
Henry Weinhard's Soda (All)

Hy-Vee
Cherry Cola
Club Soda
Cola
Diet Cola
Diet Dr. Hy-Vee
Diet Orange
Diet Tonic Water
Dr. Hy-Vee
Fruit Punch
Gingerale
Grape
Heee Haw
Lemon Lime

Orange
Root Beer
Seltzer Water
Sour
Strawberry
Tonic Water

Izze
Izze Beverages (All)

Jarritos
Jarritos (All)

Jones
Jones Soda (All)

Kristian Regale
Sparkling Apple Juice
Sparkling Apple Lite Juice
Sparkling Black Currant Juice
Sparkling Lingonberry-Apple Juice
Sparkling Peach Juice
Sparkling Pear Juice
Sparkling Pear Lite Juice
Sparkling Pomegranate-Apple Juice

LaCROIX
LaCROIX (All)

Meijer
Caffeine Free Diet Red Encore
Cherry Cola
Cola
Cranberry Diet
Cranberry Lemonade
Cranberry Soda
Cream Soda
Diet Blue Encore
Diet Cherry Encore
Diet Cola
Diet Cream Soda
Diet Dr. M
Diet Grape
Diet Lemon Lime
Diet Orange
Diet Red Encore
Diet Rocky Mist
Diet Root Beer
Dr. M
Dr. M Cherry Vanilla
Dr. M Diet Cherry Vanilla
Encore Blue
Encore Cherry Cola

Encore Cherry Red
Encore Cola
Encore Diet
Encore Diet Cherry Cola
Encore Red
Encore Red Zero
Fruit Punch
Ginger Ale
Grape Soda
Grapefruit
Lemon Lime
Lemonade
Orange Soda
Organic Cream Lemon Lime Soda
Organic Cream Soda
Organic Orange Cream Soda
Organic Root Beer
Red Pop
Rocky Mist
Root Beer

Mr. Pure
Soda (All)

Natural Springs (Schnucks)
Black Cherry
Diet Black Cherry
Diet Peach
Diet Raspberry
Diet White Grape
Mixed Berry
Peach
Raspberry
Strawberry
Tropical
White Grape

O Organics ✑
Blood Orange Italian Soda
Cranberry Acai Italian Soda
Pink Grapefruit Italian Soda
Pomegranate Italian Soda
Tropical Blend Italian Soda

Our Family
Black Cherry Soda
Black Cherry Sparkling Water
Cola
Root Beer

Pepsi
Pepsi-Cola Products (All)

Price Chopper
Black Cherry
Citrus Dew
Club Soda
Cola
Cream Soda
Diet Cola
Diet Ginger Ale
Diet Lemon/Lime
Diet Orange
Diet Raspberry Ginger Ale
Diet Root Beer
Dr. Sparkle
Ginger Ale
Grape
Lemon/Lime
Lemon/Lime Seltzer
Orange Seltzer
Plain Seltzer
Raspberry Ginger Ale
Raspberry Lime Seltzer
Root Beer
Seltzer
Sparking Pink Grapefruit
Sparkling White Grape
Tropical Punch

Publix
Black Cherry Soda
Cherry Cola
Citrus Hit Soda
Club Soda
Cola
Cream Soda
Diet Cola
Diet Ginger Ale
Diet Tonic Water
Ginger Ale
Grape Soda
Lemon Lime Seltzer
Lemon Lime Soda
Orange Soda
Raspberry Seltzer
Root Beer
Tonic Water

Reed's
China Cola
Energy Elixir

Ginger Brews
Reed's Rx
Sonoma Sparkler
Virgil's

Ritz (Beverage)
Ritz Soda (All)

Safeway Select ⟿
French L Orange
French Lemonade
French Pink Lemonade

Sangria Señorial
Sangria Señorial (All)

Schnucks
Black Cherry Soda
Caffeine Free Diet Cola
Cola
Cream Soda
Diet Cola
Diet Lemon Lime Soda
Diet Mountain Drop
Dr. Phizz
Grape Soda
Lemon Lime Soda
Mountain Drop
Orange Soda
Root Beer
Super Up

Shasta
Shasta (All Flavors)

Sidral Mundet
Sidral Mundet (All)

Simply Enjoy (Giant)
Sparkling Lemonade

Ski Soda ⓘ
Caffeine-Free Diet Ski
Diet Ski
Ski
Ski InfraRED

Sonoma Sparkler
Sonoma Sparkler (All)

Sprite
Sprite
Sprite Zero

St. Nick's
St. Nicks (All)

Stop & Shop
Black Cherry Seltzer Water

Caffeine Free Diet Cola
Club Soda
Cranberry Lime Seltzer Water
Diet Cola
Diet Ginger Ale
Diet Lemon Lime Soda
Diet Orange Soda
Diet Root Beer
Ginger Ale
Lemon Lime Seltzer Water
Lemon Seltzer Water
Lime Seltzer Water
Orange Soda
Peaches & Cream Seltzer Water
Raspberry Lime Seltzer Water
Raspberry Seltzer Water
Root Beer
Wild Berry Seltzer Water

Topo Chico
Topo Chico (All)

Trader Joe's
Organic Sparkling Beverages (Lemon & Grapefruit)
Refreshers (Blueberry, Pomegranate, Tangerine)
Sparkling Juice Beverages (Apple Cider, Blueberry, Cranberry, Pomegranate)

Valu Time (Brookshire)
Cola
Orange Soda
Pineapple Soda
Punch Soda
Red Crème Soda
Root Beer
Strawberry Soda

Wegmans
Aqua Italian Sparkling Mineral Water
Aqua Lemon Flavored Italian Mineral Water
Aqua Lemongrass Flavored Italian Mineral Water
Aqua Lime Flavored Italian Mineral Water
Black Cherry Soda
Black Cherry Sparkling Beverage
Caffeine Free Cola
Caffeine Free Diet Cola

Cherry Cola
Club Soda
Cola
Cranberry Raspberry Sparkling
  Beverage
Cranberry Sparkling Juice Blend
Cream Soda
Diet Cola
Diet Dr. W
Diet Fountain Root Beer
Diet Ginger Ale
Diet Lemon Cola
Diet Lime Cola
Diet Orange Soda
Diet Tonic Water
Diet Vanilla Cola
Diet W-UP
Dr. W
Fountain Root Beet
Frizzante - Blood Orange
Frizzante - Blueberry Lemon
Frizzante - Sicilian Lemon
Frizzante - Sour Cherry Lemon
Ginger Ale
Grape Soda
Green Apple Sparkling Soda
Key Lime Sparkling Beverage
Kiwi Strawberry Sparkling Beverage
Lemon Sparkling Water
Lime Sparkling Water
Merge Cola
Mixed Berry Sparkling Beverage
Mixed Berry Sparkling Water
Mt. W
Orange Soda
Orange Sparkling Water
Peach Grapefruit Sparkling Beverage
Peach Sparkling Beverage
Pink Sparkling Grape Juice
Raspberry Sparkling Water
Red Sparkling Grape Juice
Sparkling Lemonade
Tangerine Lime Sparkling Beverage with
  Sweeteners
Tangerine Lime Sparkling Water
Tonic Water
Vanilla Cola

W RED (Naturally Flavored Citrus
  Cherry Soda)
Wedge Diet Cherry Grapefruit Flavored
  Soda
Wedge Diet Grapefruit Soda
Wedge Diet Peach Grapefruit Flavored
  Soda
White Grape Sparkling Beverage with
  Sweeteners
White Sparkling Grape Juice
W-UP

Welch's
Welch's (All)

Winn-Dixie (Chek)
Black Cherry Soda
Caffeine Free Cola
Cherry Cola
Club Soda
Cola
Cream Soda
Diet Kountry Mist Soda
Diet Lemon-Lime Soda
Diet Orange Soda
Diet Root Beer
Diet Strawberry Soda
Diet Vanilla Cola
Dr. Chek
Ginger Ale
Grape Soda
Green Apple Soda
Kountry Mist Soda
Lemon-Lime Soda
Orange Pineapple Soda
Orange Soda
Peach Soda
Premium Draft Style Root Beer
Punch
Red Alert Soda
Red Cream Soda
Root Beer
Seltzer Water
Strawberry Soda
Vanilla Cola

Zevia
Natural Diet Soda (All Flavors)

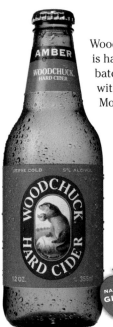

Woodchuck Hard Cider is handcrafted in small batches at our cidery within the Green Mountains of Vermont.

Made with some of nature's best ingredients, Woodchuck Hard Cider is easy to drink with a variety of styles from sweet to dry.

www.woodchuck.com

CHOCOLATE DRINKS

Always Save
Chocolate Drink Mix
Best Choice
Chocolate Drink Mix
Food Club (Brookshire)
Chocolate Flavored Drink Mix
Food Club (Marsh)
Chocolate Flavor Drink Mix
Goya
Chocolate Cortes
Chocolate Cortes Embajador
Chocolate Cortes Molido
Chocolisto
Pinolillo
Sweet Corona Chocolate
Honest CocoaNova
Honest CocoaNova (All)
Hy-Vee
Instant Chocolate Flavored Drink Mix
Meijer
Chocolate Flavored Drink Mix

Midwest Country Fare (Hy-Vee)
Instant Chocolate Flavored Drink Mix
Mocafe ⓘ
Mocafe (All)
Our Family
Chocolate Drink Mix
Trader Joe's
Sipping Chocolate (Seasonal)

CIDER (ALCOHOLIC)

Ace Cider
Ace Cider (All)
Crispin Cider
Apple Cider (All)
Fox Barrel
Cider
Green Mountain Beverage ✓
Woodchuck Hard Ciders (All)
Woodpecker
Wyder's Cider (All)
J.K. Scrumpy's Orchard Gate Gold
Ciders (All)
Magners Irish Cider
Magners Irish Cider (All)
Original Sin Hard Cider
Hard Apple Cider
Hard Pear Cider
Woodchuck Draft Cider
Woodchuck Hard Ciders (All Styles)
Wyder's Cider
Wyder's Hard Cider (All Varieties)

COFFEE DRINKS & MIXES

Always Save
Brick Automatic Drip Coffee
Decaf Coffee
Fully Automatic Coffee Machine Coffee
Instant Coffee
Ambassador Organics
Coffee (All)
Audubon Coffee
Coffee (All)
Autocrat
Coffee

Best Choice
- Breakfast Blend Coffee
- Brick Coffee
- Colombian Brick Coffee
- Colombian Coffee
- Decaf Coffee
- Espresso Roast Ground Coffee
- French Roast Coffee
- Hazelnut Ground Coffee
- Instant Coffee
- Instant Decaf Coffee
- Supreme Coffee

Black Mountain Gold Coffee
- Coffee (All)

Café Jerusalem Kosher Coffee 〇
- Café Jerusalem Kosher Coffee (All)

Caffe Sanora
- Coffee (All)

Caribou Coffee
- Iced Coffee

Chock Full O' Nuts
- Coffee Products (All)

Clearly Organic (Best Choice)
- Colombian Coffee
- Decaf Coffee
- House Blend Coffee
- Peruvian Bag Coffee

Coffee Bean & Tea Leaf
- Coffee (All BUT Cookies & Cream Ice Blended) 〇
- Powders (All) ()

Community Coffee
- Community Coffee (All)

DeLallo
- Café Espresso ⓘ
- Café Espresso Decaf ⓘ

Don Francisco's Coffee
- Coffee (All)

Eight O'Clock Coffee
- Coffee (All)

Equal Exchange ⓘ
- Coffee (All)

Faerie's Finest 〇
- Faerie's Finest (All)

Fairwinds Coffee Company
- Coffee (All)

Food Club (Brookshire)
- Classic Roast Brick Coffee
- Classic Roast Coffee
- Columbian Coffee
- Decaf Coffee
- French Roast Coffee
- Instant Clasico
- Instant Coffee
- Instant Coffee Crystal
- Instant Decaf Coffee Crystal
- Master Roast Coffee

Food Club (Marsh)
- Coffee Instant (Red)
- Coffee, Classic Roast (Red)
- Coffee, Decaf (Green)
- Coffee, French Roast
- Coffee, Instant Decaf (Green)
- Coffee, Lite, 50/50 Blend (Light Blue)

French Market Coffee
- Coffee & Chicory City Roast
- Coffee & Chicory Creole Roast
- Coffee & Chicory Decaf
- Pure Chicory
- Pure Dark Roast
- Pure French Roast
- Restaurant Blend
- Union Coffee & Chicory Roast

Full Circle (Price Chopper)
- Espresso Coffee
- Highland Reserve Coffee

Full Circle (Schnucks)
- Ground Coffee

Giant
- 1/2 the Caffeine Lite Roast Medium Ground Coffee
- 100% Colombian Ground Coffee
- Decaffeinated Instant Coffee
- Instant Coffee

Giant Eagle
- Coffee Singles
- Colombian Coffee
- Decaf Coffee Singles
- Decaf Colombian Coffee
- Decaf Instant Original Blend Coffee
- Decaf Original Blend Coffee
- French Roast Coffee
- French Vanilla Coffee

Hazelnut Coffee
Instant Original Blend Coffee
Lite Coffee
Original Blend Coffee

Goya
Café de Olla
Clasico
Clasico Decaffeinated
Clasico Suave
Coffee Brick Pak
Coffee Can
Coffee Decaf Brick
Coffee Decaffeinated
Nescafe Clasico

Great Value (Wal-Mart) 25
100% Arabica Instant Coffee
100% Arabica Premium Ground Coffee
100% Colombian Naturally
  Decaffeinated Premium Ground
  Coffee
100% Colombian Premium Ground
  Coffee
French Roast 100% Arabica Coffee
Naturally Decaffeinated Instant Coffee

Green Mountain Coffee ()
Café Escapes (All)
Coffees (All)

Harmony Bay
Harmony Bay (All)

Hy-Vee
100% Colombian Coffee
Breakfast Blend Coffee
Classic Coffee
Classic Decaf Coffee
Coffee
Colombian Coffee
Decaf Coffee
Decaffeinated French Roast Coffee
Decaffeinated Hazelnut Coffee (Ground
  and Whole Bean)
French Roast Coffee
Hazelnut Ground Coffee
House Blend (Ground and Whole Bean)
Instant Coffee
Instant Decaf Coffee

Illy
Coffee (All)

Intelligentsia
Coffee (All)

JFG Coffee & Tea
Bonus Blend
Bonus Blend Decaf
Decaf Instant Coffee
Gourmet/Restaurant Blend
Instant Coffee
JFG Decaf
JFG Lite
Rich French Roast
Special

Kalona Organics
Coffee Creamer (All)

Luzianne
Bonus Blend Dark Roast
Bonus Blend Decaf
Bonus Blend Medium Roast
Coffee & Chicory
Coffee & Chicory Decaf
Coffee Partner Chicory
Dark Roast Coffee
Dark Roast Pure
Decaf Coffee
Decaf Coffee & Chicory
Instant Coffee & Chicory
Medium Roast Coffee
Medium Roast Coffee & Chicory
Premium Blend Coffee & Chicory
Red Label Coffee & Chicory
RT Dark Roast Coffee & Chicory
White Label Coffee & Chicory

Market Day
Ice Coffee Mix, Caramel Latte

Market District (Giant Eagle)
Ground Breakfast Coffee
Ground Colombian Coffee
Ground Decaf Coffee
Ground French Roast Coffee
Ground French Vanilla Coffee
Ground Hazelnut Coffee
Ground House Coffee
Ground Jamaican Coffee
Ground Kenya Coffee
Ground Kona Bean Coffee
Ground Sumatran Coffee
Whole Bean Breakfast

Whole Bean Colombian
Whole Bean Decaf Colombian
Whole Bean French Vanilla

Maxwell House 🌀

Coffee Singles, Decaffeinated Instant
  Bags
Coffee Singles, Original Singles
Coffee, Cafe Collection Decaffeinated
Coffee, Cafe Collection French Roast
Coffee, Cafe Collection Hazelnut
Coffee, Cafe Collection House Blend
Coffee, House Blend Medium
Coffee, Instant Original
Coffee, Instant Original Decaffeinated
Coffee, Master Blend Ground
Coffee, Maxwell House Filter Packs
  Original
Coffee, Maxwell House Filter Packs
  Original Decaffeinated
Coffee, Original Decaffeinated Ground

Meijer

Coffee (Decaf, Regular)
Coffee, FACM (Can)
Coffee, Ground Colombian
Coffee, Ground Decaf Lite 50%
Coffee, Ground French Roast
Coffee, Ground Lite 50%

Melitta

Coffee (All)

Millstone ♟

Ground Coffee (All BUT Flavored
  Coffee Products)
Roast Coffee (All BUT Flavored Coffee
  Products)

Mocafe ⓘ

Mocafe (All)

Mountain Blend

Instant Coffee

Mrs. Bryant's

Estate Fresh Gourmet™ L'essence de
  VIRGINIA Colonial Roasted Chestnut
  Organic Coffee Beans
Estate Fresh Gourmet™ L'essence de
  VIRGINIA Revolutionary Roast
  Organic Coffee

Nescafé

Classic Instant Coffee

Taster's Choice Instant Coffee (Flavored
  & Non-Flavored)

New England Coffee

Flavored Coffee (All)

Newman's Own Organics ⓘ

Coffees (All)

O Organics 🌀

Dark French Roast Ground Coffee
Mountain Reserve Blend Medium Light
  Roast Coffee
Wilderness Retreat Blend Medium Dark
  Roast Ground Coffee

Organic Coffee Company, The

Coffee (All)

Our Family

100% Columbian Coffee
Classic Roast Decaf
Coffee Singles (Decaf, Regular)
Decaffeinated Ground Coffee
French Roasted Coffee
French Vanilla Coffee
Ground Coffee (Breakfast Blend, French
  Roast)
Ground Coffee (Can)
Half Caffeine Coffee
Hazelnut Coffee
Instant Coffee
Instant Coffee (Decaffeinated, Regular)
Instant Coffee Clasico Regular
Instant Coffee Crystals (Decaf, Regular)

PapaNicholas

Ground Coffee (All)
Whole Coffee Beans (All)

Price Chopper

Caffeinated Coffee
Colombian Coffee
Decaffeinated Coffee
French Roast
French Vanilla Coffee
Hazelnut Coffee
Instant Coffee
Instant Decaf Coffee
Regular Can Coffee

Publix

Coffee (All Varieties)

Red Diamond

Coffee (All)

Rogers Family Coffee Company, The
  Coffees (All)
RT Coffee
  Coffee (All)
Safeway ⌇
  Café Casero
  Classic Roast Medium Ground Coffee
  Colombian Coffee
  Decaffeinated Coffee
  Half the Caffeine Ground Coffee
  Instant Coffee Crystals
Safeway Select ⌇
  Breakfast Blend Ground Coffee
  Breakfast Blend Whole Bean Coffee
  Café Roast Caramel Coffee
  Café Roast Decaf Creamy Hazelnut
    Flavored Coffee
  Café Roast Double Dutch Chocolate
    Coffee
  Café Roast French Vanilla Coffee
  Colombian Ground Coffee
  Colombian Supremo Cofee
  Costa Rica Ground Coffee
  Creamy Hazelnut Coffee
  Decaf House Blend Ground Coffee
  Decaffeinated Colombian Coffee
  Decaffeinated Colombian Ground
    Coffee
  Decaffeinated Creamy Hazelnut Coffee
  Double Dutch Chocolate Coffee
  Espresso Roast Coffee
  French Roast Coffee
  French Roast Ground Coffee
  Hazelnut Cream Ground Coffee
  House Blend Ground Coffee
  House Blend Whole Bean Coffee
  Kona Blend Coffee Blend
  Kona Blend Whole Bean Coffee
  Sumatra Ground Coffee
  Vanilla Nut and Cream Coffee
  Vanilla Nut Cream Ground Coffee
  Whole Bean Decaf House Blend Coffee
San Francisco Bay Coffee Company
  Coffee (All)
Sanka ⌇
  Coffee, Decaffeinated

Sarkisian Coffee
  Coffee (All)
Singing Dog Vanilla
  Organic Vanilla Coffee
Stewarts
  Coffee
Stop & Shop
  1/2 the Caffeine Ground Lite Coffee
  Colombian Supreme Ground Coffee
Taylors of Harrogate
  Coffee (All)
Trader Joe's
  Coffee (All)
  Coffee Rio's
Ugly Mug Coffee
  Ugly Mug Coffee (All BUT Flavored
    Coffee)
Vons ⌇
  Classic Roast Ground Coffee
  Coffee Singles
  Colombian Coffee
  Decaffeinated Instant Coffee
  French Roast Coffee
  Instant Coffee Crystals
Wegmans
  100% Colombian Decaf Medium Roast
    Whole Bean Coffee
  100% Colombian Ground Coffee
  100% Colombian Medium Roast Whole
    Bean Coffee
  100% Medium Roast Ground
    Colombian Coffee
  Caffeine Lite Ground Coffee
  Dark Espresso Roast Decaf Whole Bean
    Coffee
  Decaf Ground Coffee
  Espresso Dark Roast Decaf Whole Bean
    Coffee
  French Roast Coffee
  French Roast Ground Coffee
  Ground Dark Roast Espresso Coffee
  Instant Coffee
  Traditional Coffee Singles
  Traditional Ground Coffee
  Traditional Light Roast Ground Coffee

Yuban

- 100% Columbian Coffee, 100% Arabica Hazelnut Single Serve
- 100% Columbian Coffee, Dark Roast
- 100% Columbian Coffee, Decaffeinated Single Serve
- 100% Columbian Coffee, Instant
- 100% Columbian Coffee, Organic Rich Medium Roast
- 100% Columbian Coffee, Original
- 100% Columbian Coffee, Single Serve

CREAMERS & FLAVORINGS

Berkeley Farms
- Mocha Mix Creamer

Broughton
- Morning Star Coffee Whitener
- Morning Star Non Dairy Coffee Creamers
- Morning Star Sokreem

Capella Flavor Drops
- Capella Flavor Drops (All)

Coffee-Mate
- Coffee-Mate Liquid (Flavored & Non-Flavored)
- Coffee-Mate Powder (Flavored & Non-Flavored)

Community Coffee
- Creamer

Fastco (Fareway)
- Amaretto Creamer
- French Vanilla Creamer
- Hazelnut Creamer
- Irish Creamer
- Non-Dairy Creamer

Food Club (Brookshire)
- Powdered Creamer
- Powdered Creamer Hazelnut
- Powdered Creamer Lite
- Powdered Creamer, Amaretto
- Powdered Creamer, Chocolate
- Powdered Creamer, Dulce De Leche
- Powdered Creamer, Fat Free
- Powdered Creamer, French Vanilla
- Powdered Creamer, Irish Cream

Food Club (Marsh)
- Fat Free French Vanilla Non Dairy Creamer
- Fat Free Hazelnut Non Dairy Creamer
- Fat Free Powdered Creamer
- French Vanilla Non Dairy Creamer
- Hazelnut Non Dairy Coffee Creamer
- Powdered Creamer
- Ultra Pasteurized Processed Non Dairy Creamer

Giant
- Lite Non Dairy Original Coffee Creamer Powder
- Non Dairy Original Coffee Creamer (Refrigerated)

Giant Eagle
- Coffee Cream 18%
- Non Dairy Creamer

Great Value (Wal-Mart) 25
- Coffee Creamer
- French Vanilla Coffee Creamer

Haggen
- Coffee Creamer
- Powdered Non-Dairy Coffee Creamer

H-E-B
- French Vanilla Creamer
- Hazelnut Creamer
- Plain Creamer

Hood
- Country Creamer
- Fat Free Country Creamer (All)

Hy-Vee
- Chocolate Coffee Creamer
- Fat Free Coffee Creamer
- Fat Free French Vanilla Coffee Creamer - Refrigerated
- Fat Free Hazelnut Coffee Creamer - Refrigerated
- French Vanilla Coffee Creamer
- Hazelnut Coffee Creamer
- Hazelnut Coffee Creamer - Refrigerated
- Original Coffee Creamer
- Sugar Free French Vanilla Coffee Creamer
- Sugar Free Hazelnut Coffee Creamer
- Vanilla Caramel Coffee Cremer

International Delight
International Delight (All)

Kroger
Crème Brulee Coffee Creamer
Sugar Free Hazelnut Non-Dairy
Creamer
Vanilla Caramel Creamer

La Crème
Coffee Creamer (All)

Lucerne (Safeway)
Belgian Chocolate Toffee Non Dairy
Creamer
Coffee Creamer - Caramel Macchiatto
Coffee Creamer - Crème Brulee
Coffee Creamer - French Vanilla
Coffee Creamer - French Vanilla Fat
Free
Coffee Creamer - French Vanilla Sugar
Free
Coffee Creamer - Hazelnut
Coffee Creamer - Hazelnut Fat Free
Coffee Creamer - Hazelnut Sugar Free
Coffee Creamer - Irish Cream
Coffee Creamer - Vanilla Caramel
Coffee Creamer - Vanilla Cinnamon
Macchiatto Caramel Non Dairy
Creamer

Meijer
French Vanilla Creamer
Hazelnut Creamer
Organic Creamer

MimicCreme
MimicCreme (All)

Organic Valley
French Vanilla Soy Creamer
Soy Creamer

Our Family
Coffee Creamer
Fat Free Coffee Creamer
French Vanilla Coffee Creamer, Fat Free
French Vanilla Coffee Creamer, Sugar
Free
French Vanilla Creamer
French Vanilla Creamer, Sugar Free
Hazelnut Coffee Creamer
Hazelnut Creamer
Hazelnut Creamer, Sugar Free

Non Dairy Coffee Creamer
Original Coffee Creamer
Vanilla Caramel Creamer

Price Chopper
Coffee Creamer
Fat Free Creamer
Fat Free Hazelnut Creamer
Fat Free Vanilla Creamer
French Vanilla Creamer
Hazelut Café Creamer
Light Coffee Creamer

Publix
Coffee Creamer
Fat Free Non-Dairy Creamer
Non-Dairy Creamer (Powder)
Non-Dairy French Vanilla Flavored
Creamer (Powder)
Non-Dairy Lite Creamer (Powder)

Pulmuone Wildwood
Soy Creamer

Reiter Dairy
Flavor Charm Non-Dairy Creamer

Robinson Dairy
Creamers (All)

Safeway
Creamer Non Dairy French Vanilla
Non Dairy Creamer
Non Dairy Creamer Value Pack
Non Dairy Hazelnut Creamer
Non Dairy Lite Creamer

Schnucks
Fat Free French Vanilla Coffee Creamer
Fat Free Hazelnut Coffee Creamer
French Vanilla Coffee Creamer
Hazelnut Coffee Creamer
Original Coffee Creamer

Silk
Silk Creamer (All)

Trader Joe's
Non-Dairy Coffee Creamers (Original,
Hazelnut, Vanilla)

Valu Time (Brookshire)
Powdered Creamer

Valu Time (Marsh)
Powdered Creamer

Handwritten margin note (left): Contamination

Handwritten margin note (left): Gatorade has no gluten ingredients but has not been tested for gluten

Winn-Dixie
  Non-Dairy Coffee Creamer (Fat Free, Original)

DIET & NUTRITIONAL DRINKS

Elations
  Elations (All)
FUZE
  FUZE (All Flavors)
Ginger People, The ()
  Ginger Soother
Hy-Vee
  Chocolate Nutritional Supplement
  Chocolate Nutritional Supplement Plus
  Strawberry Nutritional Supplement
  Vanilla Nutritional Supplement
  Vanilla Nutritional Supplement Plus
Meijer
  Diet Quick, Extra Thin (Chocolate, Strawberry, Vanilla)
Metamucil
  Metamucil Powders
Nutiva
  Hempshakes ⓘ
Pedialyte
  Pedialyte (All)
POM Wonderful
  POM Wonderful (All)
Publix
  Balanced Nutritional Drink Supplement - Chocolate
  Balanced Nutritional Drink Supplement - Chocolate Plus
  Balanced Nutritional Drink Supplement - Strawberry
  Balanced Nutritional Drink Supplement - Strawberry Plus
  Balanced Nutritional Drink Supplement - Vanilla
  Balanced Nutritional Drink Supplement - Vanilla Plus
Right Size
  Diet Drinks (All)
Tahiti Trader
  Superfruit Juices (All)

ENERGY DRINKS

4C
  Totally Light Drink Mix Energy Rush (All Flavors)
FUZE
  FUZE (All Flavors)
Ginger People, The ()
  Ginger Energizer
Guayaki Yerba Mate ✓
  Guayaki Yerba Mate (All)
GURU Energy Drink
  GURU Energy Drink
Minute Maid
  Kiwi-Strawberry Energy
Monster Energy
  Monster Beverage Products (All)
NOS
  Energy Drinks (All)
Red Bull
  Red Bull Cola
  Red Bull Energy Drink
  Red Bull Sugarfree
Red Rain Energy Drinks
  Red Rain Energy Drinks & Shots (All)
Rehab Energy Drink
  Rehab Energy Drink
Rip It
  Rip It
Safeway ⤳
  Shake N Run Sugar Free Peach Iced Tea Drink Mix
Sambazon
  Sambazon (All)

FLAVORED OR ENHANCED WATER

Adirondack Beverages
  Flavored Waters (All)
Best Choice
  Black Cherry Water
  Mixed Berry Water
  Peach Flavored Water
  Raspberry Water
  Strawberry/Kiwi Sparkling Water
  White Grape Flavored Water

Cascadia Sparkling Clear
Cascadia Sparkling Clear (All)
ClearFruit
ClearFruit (All)
Crystal Bay
Crystal Bay (All)
Dasani
Dasani Essence
Dasani Lemon
Dasani Plus Cleanse + Restore
Dasani Plus Refresh + Revive
Fastco (Fareway)
Cherry Chiller
Key Lime Chiller
Peach Chiller
Raspberry Chiller
Strawberry Chiller
White Grape Chiller
Hy-Vee
Black Cherry Water Cooler
Black Cherry Water Refreshers
Key Lime Water Cooler
Kiwi Strawberry Water Cooler
Mixed Berry Water Cooler
Peach Melba Water Cooler
Peach Water Cooler
Raspberry Water Cooler
Strawberry Water Cooler
White Grape Water Cooler
Meijer
Fit 20 (Berry, Black Cherry, Grape, Kiwi Strawberry, Lemon)
Flavored Water (Lemon, Orange, Raspberry, Strawberry)
Quencher Black Cherry
Quencher Key Lime
Quencher Kiwi Strawberry
Quencher Mandarin Orange
Quencher Mango Passion Fruit
Quencher Pink Grapefruit
Quencher Pomegranate Cherry
Quencher Raspberry
Quencher Tangerine Lime
Quencher Tropical Island
Quencher White Grape
Price Chopper
Grape Spring Water

Lemon Spring Water
Mango/Orange Seltzer
Raspberry Spring Water
Raspberry Water
Strawberry Water
Propel
Propel
Safeway ᧦
Shake N Run Sugar Free Drink Mix Raspberry Lemonade
Shake N Run Sugar Free Fruit Punch Drink Mix
Shake N Run Sugar Free Lemonade Drink Mix
Shake N Run Sugar Free Raspberry Drink Mix
VIO
Vibrancy Drinks (All)
Wegmans
Aqua V Acai Blueberry Pomegranate Flavored Vitamin Infused Beverage
Aqua V Dragon Fruit Flavored Vitamin Infused Beverage
Aqua V Fruit Punch Flavored Vitamin Infused Beverage
Aqua V Lemonade Flavored Vitamin Infused Beverage
Aqua V Raspberry Apple Flavored Vitamin Infused Beverage

HOT COCOA & CHOCOLATE MIXES

Always Save
Hot Cocoa Mix
Best Choice
Hot Cocoa, Can
Hot Cocoa, Mix
Mini Marshmallows Hot Cocoa
Sugar Free Hot Cocoa
Cub Foods
Fat-Free Hot Cocoa Mix
Hot Cocoa Mix
Faerie's Finest ᔦ
Faerie's Finest (All)
Flavorite (Cub Foods)
Chocolate Drink
Sugar-Free Hot Cocoa Mix

Food Club (Brookshire)
　　Hot Cocoa
　　Hot Cocoa with Mashmallows
Food Club (Marsh)
　　Hot Cocoa
　　Hot Cocoa with Marshmallows
Great Value (Wal-Mart) 25
　　Milk Chocolate Hot Cocoa Mix
　　Milk Chocolate Hot Cocoa Mix with
　　　　Marshmallows
Green Mountain Coffee ()
　　Cocoa (All)
Holy Chocolate ()
　　Holy Chocolate (All)
Hy-Vee
　　Instant Hot Cocoa Mix
　　No Sugar Added Instant Hot Cocoa Mix
Ibarra
　　Ibarra (All)
InJoy Organics
　　Cocoa (All)
Kroger
　　Dutch Cocoa
　　Dutch Cocoa with Marshmallows
Land O'Lakes
　　Cocoa Classics Hot Cocoa Mixes (All)
Market Day
　　Hot Cocoa, Flavored
Meijer
　　Hot Cocoa Mix
　　Hot Cocoa Mix with Marshmallows
　　No Sugar Added Hot Cocoa Mix
　　Sugar Free Hot Cocoa Mix
Meijer Organics
　　Organic Hot Cocoa Regular
Midwest Country Fare (Hy-Vee)
　　Instant Hot Cocoa Mix
Mocafe (i)
　　Mocafe (All)
Our Family
　　Hot Cocoa Mix
　　Hot Cocoa Mix with Marshmallows
　　Hot Cocoa Mix with Mini
　　　　Marshmallows
　　Hot Cocoa Mix, Milk Chocolate
　　No Sugar Added Hot Chocolate

Publix
　　Hot Cocoa
　　Mini Marshmallow Hot Cocoa
　　No Sugar Added Hot Chocolate
Rademaker
　　Cocoa Box
Safeway ✎
　　No Sugar Added Hot Cocoa Mix
　　Rich Chocolate Flavor Fat Free Hot
　　　　Cocoa Mix
　　Rich Chocolate Flavor Hot Cocoa Mix
　　Rich Chocolate Flavor with
　　　　Marshmallows Hot Cocoa Mix
Safeway Select ✎
　　White Chocolate Cocoa
Sally's ⚎
　　Sally's (All)
Schnucks
　　Hot Cocoa Mix
　　Sugar Free Hot Cocoa Mix
Shoppers Value (Cub Foods)
　　Hot Cocoa
Stephen's Gourmet
　　Cocoa (All BUT Ones Containing
　　　　Candy)
Swiss Miss
　　Cocoa (All Varieties)
Taza Chocolate
　　Chocolate Mexicano Discs (All)
Theo Chocolate ()
　　Chipotle Spice
　　Dark Chocolate
Valu Time (Schnucks)
　　Cocoa

INSTANT BREAKFAST DRINKS

Our Family
　　Orange Breakfast Drink Mix

JUICE DRINK MIXES

4C
　　Instant Drink Mixes Sweetened with
　　　　Sugar (All)
　　Totally Light Drink Mixes Sweetened
　　　　with Splenda (All)

Alpine ()
Alpine Apple Cider
Country Time 〜
Drink Mix, Lemonade
Drink Mix, Lemonade Iced Tea Classic
Drink Mix, On The Go Lemonade
Drink Mix, Pink Lemonade
Drink Mix, Raspberry Lemonade
Drink Mix, Strawberry Lemonade
Crystal Light 〜
Drink Mix, Appletini
Drink Mix, Immunity Natural Cherry
Pomegranate
Drink Mix, Margarita
Drink Mix, Metabolism+ Peach Mango
Green Tea
Drink Mix, Mojito
Drink Mix, On The Go Hunger
Satisfaction Natural Strawberry
Banana
Drink Mix, On The Go Skin Essentials
White Peach Tea
Drink Mix, Pink Lemonade
Drink Mix, Pure Fitness Lemon Lime
Drink Mix, Pure Grape
Drink Mix, Pure Lemonade
Drink Mix, Pure Mixed Berry
Drink Mix, Pure Strawberry Kiwi
Drink Mix, Pure Tropical Blend
Drink Mix, Raspberry Ice
Drink Mix, Skin Essentials Pomegranate
Lemonade
Cub Foods
Lemonade
Eating Right 〜
Kids Strawberry Banana 100% Fruit and
Veggie Juice
Fastco (Fareway)
Black Cherry Powdered Drink Mix
Cherry Powdered Drink Mix
Fruit Punch Powdered Drink Mix
Grape Powdered Drink Mix
Lemonade Powdered Drink Mix
Orange Powdered Drink Mix
Pink Lemonade Powdered Drink Mix
Sugar Free Black Cherry Powdered
Drink Mix

Sugar Free Cherry Powdered Drink Mix
Sugar Free Fruit Punch Powdered Drink
Mix
Sugar Free Grape Powdered Drink Mix
Sugar Free Lemon Powdered Drink Mix
Sugar Free Orange Powdered Drink Mix
Sugar Free Pink Lemonade Powdered
Drink Mix
Flavorite (Cub Foods)
Grape Drink Mix
Food Club (Brookshire)
Drink Mix, 50% Less Sugar Lemonade
Drink Mix, 50% Less Sugar Pink
Lemonade
Drink Mix, Cherry
Drink Mix, Fruit Punch
Drink Mix, Grape
Drink Mix, Ice Raspberry
Drink Mix, Ice Tea
Drink Mix, Lemonade
Drink Mix, Orange
Drink Mix, Punch
Drink Mix, Strawberry
Drink Mix, Sunrise Orange
Drink Stix, Grape
Drink Stix, Ice Raspberry
Drink Stix, Iced Tea
Drink Stix, Lemonade
Drink Stix, Peach Tea
Drink Stix, Raspberry Lemonade
Fruit Mixed, Extreme Cherry
Thirst Quencher, Berry (Rain Type)
Thirst Quencher, Fruit Punch
Thirst Quencher, Glacial Chill
Thirst Quencher, Lemon Lime
Thirst Quencher, Orange
Food Club (Marsh)
Drink Mix, Cherry
Drink Mix, Fruit Punch Sugar Free
Drink Mix, Grape
Drink Mix, Lemonade Canister
Drink Mix, Lemonade Sugar Free
Drink Mix, Orange
Drink Mix, Pink Lemonade Sugar Free
Drink Mix, Punch
Drink Mix, Raspberry Ice Sugar Free
Drink Stix, Iced Tea Sugar Free

Drink Stix, Lemonade Sugar Free
Drink Stix, Raspberry Ice Sugar Free

Goya
Nectar Concentrates Guanabana
Nectar Concentrates Guava
Nectar Concentrates Mango Nectar
Nectar Concentrates Passion Fruit/
Parcha/Maracuya
Nectar Concentrates Tamarind

Hy-Vee
Splash Cherry Drink Mix
Splash Grape Drink Mix
Splash Lemonade Drink Mix
Splash Orange Drink Mix
Splash Tropical Fruit Punch Drink Mix
Thirst Splashers Fruit Punch

Juanitas
Champurrado

Kool-Aid Mad Scientwists ✍
Soft Drink Mix, Raspberry Reaction
Invisible Unsweetened
Soft Drink Mix, Wild Watermelon Kiwi
Invisible Unsweetened

Kool-Aid Powdered ✍
Soft Drink Mix, Black Cherry
Unsweetened
Soft Drink Mix, Cherry
Soft Drink Mix, Cherry Sugar Free
Soft Drink Mix, Cherry Sugar-
Sweetened
Soft Drink Mix, Cherry Unsweetened
Soft Drink Mix, Grape
Soft Drink Mix, Grape Sugar Free
Soft Drink Mix, Grape Sugar-Sweetened
Soft Drink Mix, Grape Unsweetened
Soft Drink Mix, Invisible Changin'
Cherry Sugar Sweetened
Soft Drink Mix, Invisible Changin'
Cherry Unsweetened
Soft Drink Mix, Invisible Grape Illusion
Sugar Sweetened
Soft Drink Mix, Invisible Grape Illusion
Unsweetened
Soft Drink Mix, Lemonade
Soft Drink Mix, Lemonade
Unsweetened

Soft Drink Mix, Lemon-Lime
Unsweetened
Soft Drink Mix, On The Go Cherry
Soft Drink Mix, On The Go Tropical
Punch
Soft Drink Mix, On The Go Tropical
Punch Sugar Free
Soft Drink Mix, Orange
Soft Drink Mix, Orange Unsweetened
Soft Drink Mix, Pink Lemonade
Unsweetened
Soft Drink Mix, Singles Cherry
Soft Drink Mix, Singles Grape
Unsweetened
Soft Drink Mix, Singles Orange
Soft Drink Mix, Singles Tropical Punch
Soft Drink Mix, Soarin' Strawberry
Lemonade Unsweetened
Soft Drink Mix, Strawberry Sugar
Sweetened
Soft Drink Mix, Strawberry
Unsweetened
Soft Drink Mix, Tropical Punch
Soft Drink Mix, Tropical Punch Sugar
Free
Soft Drink Mix, Tropical Punch Sugar-
Sweetened
Soft Drink Mix, Tropical Punch
Unsweetened

Kool-Aid Twists ✍
Soft Drink Mix, Berry Blue
Unsweetened
Soft Drink Mix, Blastin' Berry Cherry
Unsweetened
Soft Drink Mix, Ice Blue Raspberry
Lemonade Unsweetened
Soft Drink Mix, Slammin' Strawberry
Kiwi Unsweetened
Soft Drink Mix, Twists Ice Blue
Raspberry Lemonade
Soft Drink Mix, Watermelon Cherry
Unsweetened

Lakewood
Concentrate Organic Juices (All)
Concentrate Premium Juices (All)

Marsh
Drink Mix Orange

Meijer
Breakfast Orange Drink Mix
Cherry Drink Mix
Free and Light Orange Drink Mix
Grape Drink Mix
Lemonade Drink Mix
Lemonade Mix Stix
Orange Drink Mix
Pink Lemonade Drink Mix
Punch Drink Mix
Raspberry Mix Stix
Strawberry Drink Mix
Strawberry Flavored Drink Mix
Strawberry Orange Banana Drink Mix
Sugar Free Lemon Drink Mix
Sugar Free Pink Lemonade Drink Mix
Sugar Free Raspberry Drink Mix

Old Orchard
Old Orchard (All)

Our Family
Iced Tea Sugar Free Drink Mix
Lemonade Sugar Free Drink Mix
Lemonade Sugar Free Drink Mix To Go
Orange Juice Concentrate, Chilled
Orange Sugar Free Drink Mix
Peach Tea Sugar Free Drink Mix To Go
Pink Lemonade Sugar Free Drink Mix
Raspberry Lemonade Sugar Free Drink
  Mix
Raspberry Sugar Free Drink Mix To Go

Price Chopper
Go Fruit Punch Dark
Go Glacial Drink
Go Grape Drink
Go Lemon/Lime Drink
Go Orange Drink

Richfood (ACME)
Unsweetened Cherry Drink Mix

Schnucks
Cherry Drink Mix
Grape Drink Mix
Lemon Drink Mix
Orange Drink Mix
Punch Drink Mix

Trader Joe's
Concentrates (Lemon And Orange)

True Lemon
True Lemon (All)

Valu Time (Brookshire)
Drink Mix- Cherry
Drink Mix- Fruit Punch
Drink Mix- Lemonade

Valu Time (Schnucks)
Cherry Mix
Fruit Punch Mix
Lemonade Mix

Wegmans
Lemonade Flavor Drink Mix
Pink Lemonade Flavor Drink Mix

Welch's
Welch's (All)

JUICES & FRUIT DRINKS

ACME
Country Style Orange Juice Concentrate
Orange Juice Drink Concentrate
Vegetable Juice Cocktail
White Lemonade Drink Concentrate

Albertsons
Apple Juice Concentrate
Apple Raspberry Juice Blend
  Concentrate
Calcium Orange Juice Concentrate
Cranberry Cocktail Juice Concentrate
Cranberry Raspberry Juice Cocktail
  Concentrate
Fruit Punch Drink Concentrate
Limeade Juice / Drink Concentrate
Orange Juice Concentrate
Orange Juice No Pulp Concentrate
Pink Lemonade Drink Concentrate
Purple Grape Juice Cocktail
Raspberry Lemonade Juice Concentrate
Strawberry/Lemonade Fruit Punch
  Concentrate
White Grape Juice Concentrate
White Lemonade Drink Concentrate
Wild Berry Fruit Punch Concentrate

Alta Dena
Apple Juice
Fruit Punch
Orange Juice

Always Save
- Fruit Punch
- Refrigerated Orange Drink
- Refrigerated Orange Juice
- Tomato Juice (Can)

Amy & Brian
- Coconut Waters (All)
- Mangosteen Drinks (All)

Apple & Eve ☷
- 100% Juices (All)
- Juice Beverages (All)

Arctic Splash
- Juice (All)

AriZona
- Juice Products (All)

Axelrod
- Orange Juice

Barber's
- Lemonade
- Orange Juice
- Party Punch

Berkeley Farms
- Fruit Punch
- Grape Drink
- Orange Drink
- Orange Juice

Best Choice
- Apricot Nectar
- Fruit Punch Juice
- Lemonade
- Low Sodium Vegetable Juice (in Plastic Bottle)
- Spicy Vegetable Juice (in Plastic Bottle)
- Strawberry Kiwi
- Tomato Juice (in Plastic Bottle)
- Tropical Punch
- Vegetable Juice (in Plastic Bottle)
- Wild Cherry

Bionaturae
- Nectars (All) ⓘ

Bolthouse Farms ⓘ ✓
- Bolthouse Farms Juices (All BUT Protein Plus Strawberry Parfait Smoothie)

Bom Dia ⓘ
- Bom Dia Juices (All)

Bragg
- Apple Cider Vinegar Drinks (All)

Broughton
- Ardmor Farms Apple Juice
- Ardmor Farms Grape Juice
- Blue Raspberry
- Citrus Drink
- Fruit Drink
- Fruit Punch
- Ice Tea
- Orange Drink
- Orange Juice

Campbell's
- Tomato Juice

Capri Sun ⌇
- Juice Drink, Coastal Cooler/Strawberry Banana Blend
- Juice Drink, Coolers Variety Pack
- Juice Drink, Grape
- Juice Drink, Mountain Cooler Mixed Fruit
- Juice Drink, Orange
- Juice Drink, Pacific Cooler Mixed Fruit Blend
- Juice Drink, Red Berry/Strawberry Raspberry Blend
- Juice Drink, Splash Cooler Mixed Fruit Blend
- Juice Drink, Strawberry
- Juice Drink, Sunrise Berry Strawberry Tangerine Morning
- Juice Drink, Sunrise Orange Wake Up
- Juice Drink, Sunrise Tropical Morning
- Juice Drink, Surfer Cooler Mixed Fruit Blend
- Juice Drink, Tropical Punch Blend
- Juice Drink, Variety Pack
- Juice Drink, Wild Cherry Blend

Central Market Classics (Price Chopper)
- Premium Apple Juice

Ceres
- Juices (All)

Cheribundi ☷
- Cheribundi (All)

Clearly Organic (Best Choice)
- Tomato Juice

Country Fresh
Juice
Creamland Dairies
Orange Juice
Crystal Light ᕫ
Fruit Drink, Fusion Fruit Punch
Fruit Drink, Raspberry Ice Sugar Free
Fruit Drink, Strawberry Kiwi Sugar Free
Lemonade, Energy Peach Mango
Lemonade, On The Go Raspberry
Lemonade
Lemonade, Pink Lemonade Sugar Free
Lemonade, Raspberry Lemonade
Lemonade, Raspberry Lemonade Sugar
Free
Lemonade, Strawberry Orange Banana
Sugar Free
Lemonade, Sugar Free
Lemonade, Value Pack Sugar Free
On the Go, Antioxidant Natural Cherry
Pomegranate
On the Go, Energy Wild Strawberry
On the Go, Fruit Punch Sugar Free
On the Go, Green Tea Honey Lemon
On the Go, Green Tea Raspberry
On the Go, Iced Tea Natural Lemon
On the Go, Lemonade Sugar Free
On the Go, Raspberry Ice
On the Go, Sunrise Classic Orange
Cub Foods
100% Orange Juice
100% Tomato Juice
100% Vegetable Juice
15% Lemonade
16% Pink Lemonade
Vegetable Juice
Dean's
Juice
Dei Fratelli ⓘ
Dei Fratelli (All)
DeLallo
Lemon Juice Plus
Dole ✔
Dole Juices (All)
Dream Foods
Italian Volcano Blood Orange Juice
Italian Volcano Lemon Juice

Italian Volcano Lemonade
Italian Volcano Limeade
Italian Volcano Tangerine Juice
Volcano Lemon Burst
Volcano Lime Burst
Dutch Farms
Orange Juice
Eating Right ᕫ
Kids Raspberry Orange 100% Fruit and
Veggie Juice
Peach Mango Fruit and Vegetable Juice
Pomegranate Blue Fruit and Vegetable
Juice
Eden
Organic Beetroot Juice
Organic Carrot Juice
Organic Red Grape Juice
Organic Vegetable Juice
Prune Juice
Eden Foods
Organic Apple Juice
Organic Cherry Juice Concentrate
Organic Concord Grape Juice
Faerie's Finest ⸙
Flavored Lemonades (All)
Fastco (Fareway)
100% Orange Juice
Flavorite (Cub Foods)
10% Fruit Punch
100% Apple Juice
100% Calcium Fortified Juice
100% Country Blend Orange Juice
100% Grapefruit Juice
100% Pulp Free Orange Juice
15% Grape Juice
Lemonade Drink Mix
Limeade
Tomato Juice
Tropical Drink
Vegetable Juice
Food Club (Brookshire)
10% Fruit Punch Juice
10% Strawberry Kiwi Juice
10% Tropical Punch Juice
10% Wild Cherry
100% All Natural Pomegranate Juice
100% Apple Juice

100% Apple Juice from Concentrate with Vitamin C
100% Cranberry Juice
100% Grape Juice
100% Pink Grapefruit Juice
100% Premium CranGrape Juice
100% Unsweetened Orange Juice
100% Unsweetened Pineapple Juice
100% Unsweetened Pineapple Orange Juice
Apple Cider
Concentrated Apple Juice
Cranberry Apple Juice
Cranberry Blend Juice
Cranberry Cocktail
Cranberry Grape Juice
Cranberry Grape Lite Juice
Cranberry Light
Cranberry Raspberry Juice
Cranberry White Strawberry Juice
Fruit Punch Juice
Orange Peach Mango Juice Blend (Refrigerated)
Orange Strawberry Banana Juice Blend (Refrigerated)
Organic 100% Grape Juice
Pear Juice
Pineapple Juice
Pineapple Orange Banana Blend (Refrigerated)
Pineapple Orange Blend (Refrigerated)
Premium Orange Juice (Refrigerated)
Premium Orange Juice, Pulp Added (Refrigerated)
Premium Orange Juice, With Calcium (Refrigerated)
Prune Juice from Concentrate
Regular Apple Juice 100% from Concentrate
Regular Apple Juice from Concentrate
Ruby Red Grapefruit Juice
Strawberry Kiwi Juice
Sugar Free Pink Lemonade Drink Mix
Tomato Juice
Unsweetened Apple Juice
Unsweetened Orange Juice
Unsweetened Orange Pineapple Juice

Unsweetened Pink Grapefruit Juice
Vegetables Cocktail Juice
White Grape Juice

Food Club (Marsh)

100% Cranberry Blend Juice (Rectangle Bottle)
100% Pomegranate Blend Juice
100% Pomegranate Blueberry Blend Juice
100% Premium Cranberry Grape Juice
Apple Juice Not From Concentrate
Cranberry Apple (Rectangular Bottle)
Cranberry Cocktail Juice (Rectangle Bottle)
Cranberry Grape (Rectangular Bottle)
Cranberry Grape Lite (Rectangular Bottle)
Cranberry Lite Juice (Rectangle Bottle)
Cranberry Raspberry (Rectangular Bottle)
Cranberry Raspberry Lite
Cranberry White Strawberry Juice
Grape Juice (Rectangle Bottle)
Grape White Juice (Rectangle Bottle)
Grapefruit Juice (Rectangle Bottle)
Pineapple Juice
Premium Groves Best Refrigerated Orange Juice
Premium Refrigerated Orange Juice
Premium with Calcium Refrigerated Orange Juice
Prune Juice, Not From Concentrate
Reconstituted Original Refrigerated Orange Juice
Reconstituted Pulp Added Refrigerated Orange Juice
Ruby Red Grapefruit Juice (Rectangular Bottle)
Ruby Red Tangerine Juice (Rectangle Bottle)
Tomato Juice
Vegetable Juice
Vegetable Juice Cocktail

Food You Feel Good About (Wegmans)

100% Cranberry Juice Blend
100% Cranberry Raspberry Juice

100% Premium Orange Juice Extra Pulp (Not From Concentrate)
100% Premium Orange Juice No Pulp (Not From Concentrate)
100% Premium Orange Juice Some Pulp (Not From Concentrate)
100% Premium Orange Juice with Calcium (Not From Concentrate)
100% Premium Orange Juice with Calcium and Vitamins (Not From Concentrate)
100% Ruby Red Grapefruit Juice
100% Tomato Juice
100% Vegetable Juice
100% Vegetable Juice No Salt Added
Apple Juice
Apple Juice Calcium Fortified
Blueberry Flavor Juice Blend
Cherry Flavor Juice Blend
Concord Grape Cranberry Flavor Juice Blend
Cranberry
Cranberry Apple Flavor Juice Blend
Cranberry Flavor Juice Blend
Cranberry Peach
Cranberry Raspberry
Fruit Punch
Grape Juice
Orange Juice (From Concentrate)
Orange Juice Calcium Enriched (From Concentrate)
Orange Juice Concentrate Pulp Free
Pomegranate Flavor Juice Blend
Prune Juice
Ruby Red Grapefruit Juice Blend
White Grape Cranberry Juice Blend
White Grape Peach Blend
White Grape Raspberry Blend

Fruit d'Or
Cranberry Juice Cocktail
Pure Cranberry Juice

Fruit2Day
Juices (All)

Full Circle (Price Chopper)
Blueberry Juice Blend
Cranberry Cocktail
Cranberry Juice

Grape Juice
Lemonade
Natural Apple Juice
Pear Juice

Full Circle (Schnucks)
Apple Juice
Blueberry Acai Juice
Mango Pineapple Juice
Organic Blueberry Juice
Organic Cranberry Raspberry Juice
Organic Grape Juice
Organic Orange Juice
Organic Vegetable Juice
Tomato Juice

Gandy's ⓘ
Fruit Punch Drink
Orange Drink
Pink Lemon Drink

Garelick Farms
Apple Juice
Calcium Rich Orange Juice
Fruit Punch
Lemonade
Not from Concentrate Orange Juice
Orange Juice
Orange Juice from Concentrate

Genuardi's ᴗ
Lite Sugar Free Lemonade Drink

Giant
100% Grape Juice
100% Prune Juice
100% Unsweetened Apple Juice
100% Unsweetened Apple Juice with Added Calcium
100% Unsweetened White Grapefruit Juice
Cranberry Juice Blend
Cranberry Raspberry Juice Blend
Lemon Juice from Concentrate
Premium Orange Juice Pulp Free
Premium Orange Juice with Pulp
Premium Original Orange Juice
Ruby Red Grapefruit Juice
Sunrise Valley Premium Original Orange Juice
White Grape Juice

Giant Eagle
- Low Sodium Tomato Juice
- Spicy Vegetable Juice
- Tomato Juice
- Vegetable Juice

Ginger People, The ()
- Organic Ginger Juice

Goya
- Acai Pulp
- Acai with Guarana Pulp
- Acerola Beverage
- Acerola Pulp
- Apple Nectar
- Apricot Nectar
- Banana Nectar
- Cajuil/Maranon Pulp
- Cana de Azucar
- Coconut Water
- Guanabana Beverage
- Guanabana Nectar
- Guava Beverage
- Guava Nectar
- Guayaba Nectar
- Jocote Corona
- Lemon Beverage
- Mango Beverage
- Mango Nectar
- Mango Verde
- Maranon
- Orange Juice
- Papaya Beverage
- Papaya Nectar
- Passion Fruit Beverage
- Passion Fruit Juice Cocktail
- Passion, Pineapple Beverage
- Peach Nectar
- Pear Nectar
- Pear/Passion Nectar
- Pineapple/Guava Nectar
- Strawberry Banana Nectar
- Strawberry Nectar
- Sugar Cane Juice
- Tamarind Beverage
- Tamarind Nectar

Great Value (Wal-Mart) 25
- 100% Apple Juice
- 100% Cranberry Juice

- 100% Florida Grapefruit Juice
- 100% Grape Juice
- 100% Grape Peach Juice
- 100% Juice Apple Juice Punch Blend
- 100% Juice Fruit Punch
- 100% Juice Unsweetened Apple Juice
- 100% Orange Country Style Juice
- 100% Orange Juice
- 100% Orange Juice From Concentrate
- 100% Pure Orange Juice
- 100% Pure Orange Juice with Calcium
- 100% Tomato Juice
- 100% Vegetable Juice
- 100% White Grape Juice
- Acai Mixed Berry 100% Vegetable & Fruit Juice
- Apple Juice
- Country Style Orange Juice
- Cranberry Apple
- Cranberry Apple Juice Cocktail
- Cranberry Juice Cocktail
- Fruit Punch
- Grape Cranberry
- Grape Cranberry Juice Cocktail
- Grape Drink
- Grape Punch
- Guava Nectar with Calcium
- Kiwi Strawberry Punch
- Lemon Berry Punch
- Lemon Juice
- Lemonade
- Light Apple Juice Cocktail
- Light Apple Juice Cocktail with Splenda
- Light Pomegranate Blueberry Vegetable & Fruit Juice
- Light Strawberry Banana Vegetable & Fruit Juice
- Orange Juice
- Orange Juice with Calcium
- Orange Punch
- Pineapple Juice
- Pineapple Orange Juice
- Pink Grapefruit Juice
- Pink Lemonade
- Pomegranate Blueberry 100% Vegetable & Fruit Juice
- Prune Juice

Strawberry Banana 100% Vegetable & Fruit Juice
Strawberry Banana Nectar
Strawberry Banana Nectar with Calcium
Tomato Juice
Unsweetened Pink Grapefruit Juice
Unsweetened White Grapefruit Juice
Vegetable Juice
Vegetable Juice with Vitamins A&C

Green Mountain Coffee ()
Hot Cider (All)

GreenWise Market (Publix)
100% Organic Apple Juice
Organic Cranberry Juice
Organic Grape Juice
Organic Lemonade
Organic Tomato Juice

Guaranteed Value (Stop & Shop)
Apple Juice Cocktail

Haggen
100% Cranberry Juice
100% Cranraspberry Juice
100% Grape Juice
100% White Grape Juice
Apple Cider
Apple Juice
Cran-Apple Juice
Cranberry Juice Cocktail
Cran-Grape Juice
Lemon Juice
Light Cranberry Juice
Light Cranraspberry Juice
Orange Juice (Premium, Regular, with Calcium) Refrigerated
Pineapple Juice
Prune Juice
Ruby Grapefruit Juice
Ruby Red Grapefruit-Tangerine Juice
Tomato Juice
Vegetable Juice
White Grapefruit Juice

Hiland Dairy
Orange Juice

Honest Ade
Honest Ade (All)

Honest Kids
Honest Kids (All)

Hood
Juices

Hy-Vee
100% Apple Juice From Concentrate
100% Apple Juice from Concentrate with Added Vitamin C
100% Blueberry Pomegranate Juice
100% Cherry Pomegranate Juice
Calcium Fortified Apple Juice From Concentrate
Cranberry Apple Flavored Juice Blend
Cranberry Apple Juice Drink
Cranberry Flavored Juice Blend
Cranberry Juice Cocktail From Concentrate
Cranberry Raspberry Juice Drink
Fruit Punch Coolers
Grape Cranberry Juice Drink
Grape Juice From Concentrate
Grapefruit Juice from Concentrate
Lemonade
Light Apple Cherry Juice Cocktail From Concentrate
Light Apple Juice Cocktail From Concentrate
Light Apple Kiwi Strawberry Juice Cocktail From Concentrate
Light Apple Raspberry Juice Cocktail From Concentrate
Light Cranberry Grape Juice Drink from Concentrate
Light Cranberry Juice Cocktail from Concentrate
Light Cranberry Raspberry Juice Drink
Light Grape Juice Cocktail From Concentrate
Lite Cranberry Juice
Low Sodium Tomato Juice from Concentrate
No Concentrate Country Style Orange Juice
No Concentrate Orange Juice
No Concentrate Orange Juice with Calcium

Not From Concentrate Ruby Red
    Grapefruit Juice
Not from Concentrate Ruby Red
    Grapefruit Juice All Natural No Pulp
Pineapple Juice from Concentrate
Prune Juice
Prune Juice with Added Pulp
Reconstituted Lemon Juice
Ruby Red Grapefruit Juice Drink from
    Concentrate
Splash Apple Cranberry
Splash Cherry
Splash Fruit Punch
Splash Grape
Splash Lemonade
Splash Light Fruit Punch
Splash Light Grape Punch
Splash Light Orange Punch
Splash Orange
Splash Orange Pineapple
Splash Raspberry
Splash Strawberry
Splash Strawberry Kiwi Punch
Splash Tropical Punch
Tomato Juice From Concentrate
Tropical Punch Coolers
Vegetable Juice From Concentrate
White Grape Juice from Concentrate

Jewel-Osco
Apple Juice Concentrate
Calcium Orange Juice Concentrate
Country Style Orange Juice Concentrate
Fruit Punch Drink Concentrate
Limeade Concentrate
No Pulp Orange Juice Concentrate
Orange Juice Concentrate
Quality Pink Lemonade Concentrate
Raspberry Kiwi Punch Concentrate
Raspberry Lemonade Concentrate
Tomato Juice
White Lemonade Drink Concentrate

Juicy Juice
Juicy Juice (All Flavors)

Kern's ⓘ
Nectars (All)

Kool-Aid Jammers ᗥ
Juice Drink, Blue Raspberry

Juice Drink, Cherry
Juice Drink, Grape
Juice Drink, Green Apple
Juice Drink, Jammers Blue Raspberry
Juice Drink, Jammers Cherry
Juice Drink, Jammers Grape
Juice Drink, Jammers Kiwi-Strawberry
Juice Drink, Jammers Orange
Juice Drink, Jammers Tropical Punch
Juice Drink, Kiwi Strawberry
Juice Drink, Orange
Juice Drink, Tropical Punch

Lakewood
Culinary Juices (All)
Light Organic Juices (All)
Organic Juices (All)
Premium Juices (All)
Supplement Juices (All)

Langer Juice Company ⚇
Juice (All)

Lehigh Valley Dairy Farms
Alex's Lemonade
Orange Juice

Little Hugs
Fruit Drinks (All)

Louis Trauth Dairy
Fruit Punch
Lemonade
Orange Drink

Manischewitz
Grape Juice

Mayfield Dairy
Blue Raspberry Juice
Fruit Punch
Lemonade
Orange Juice

McArthur Dairy
Orange Juice

Meadow Brook Dairy
100% Pure Orange Juice
Calcium Added Orange Juice

Meadow Gold
Guava Nectar
Guava Orange Nectar
Juices (All)
Mango Orange Nectar
Orange Juice (All)

Passion Orange Nectar

Pass-O-Guava Nectar

Power POG

Tea (All)

Meijer

Acai and Blueberry Juice Blend (Shelf Stable)

Acai and Grape Juice Blend (Shelf Stable)

Apple

Apple Juice

Apple Juice from Concentrate

Berry 100% (Shelf Stable)

Berry Blend Splash (Shelf Stable)

Cherry 100% (Shelf Stable)

Cherry Juice (Shelf Stable)

CranApple Juice Cocktail (Shelf Stable)

Cranberry Apple Juice Cocktail (Shelf Stable)

Cranberry Flavored with Two Fruit Juices (Shelf Stable)

Cranberry Grape (Shelf Stable)

Cranberry Grape Flavored with Two Juices (Shelf Stable)

Cranberry Grape Juice Cocktail (Shelf Stable)

Cranberry Juice Cocktail (Shelf Stable)

Cranberry Juice Cocktail Light (Shelf Stable)

Cranberry Raspberry (Shelf Stable)

Cranberry Raspberry 100% (Shelf Stable)

Cranberry Raspberry Juice Cocktail (Shelf Stable)

Cranberry Raspberry Juice with Three Fruit Juices (Shelf Stable)

Cranberry Strawberry (Shelf Stable)

Cranberry Strawberry Juice Cocktail (Shelf Stable)

Fruit Punch (Drink Thirst Quencher) (Shelf Stable)

Fruit Punch (Shelf Stable)

Fruit Punch Genuine (Shelf Stable)

Genuine Grape 100% (Shelf Stable)

Genuine Punch 100% (Shelf Stable)

Grape Juice (Shelf Stable)

Grape Juice from Concentrate (Shelf Stable)

Grapefruit (Carafe)

Grapefruit Juice (Shelf Stable)

High Pulp Premium Orange Juice (Carafe)

Lemon Juice (Shelf Stable)

Lemon Juice (Squeeze Bottle) (Shelf Stable)

Lemon Lime (Drink Thirst Quencher) (Shelf Stable)

Lemonade (Carafe)

Light Cranberry Grape Juice (Shelf Stable)

Light Fruit Punch (Shelf Stable)

Light Grape Cranberry Juice Cocktail (Shelf Stable)

Light Grape Juice Cocktail with Splenda (Shelf Stable)

Lime Juice (Shelf Stable)

Limeade (Carafe)

Omega3 Premium Orange Juice

Orange (Drink Thirst Quencher) (Shelf Stable)

Orange Juice

Orange Juice (Shelf Stable)

Orange Juice with Calcium

Orange Peach Mango

Orange Strawberry Banana

Organic Apple Juice (Shelf Stable)

Organic Concord Grape Juice (Shelf Stable)

Organic Cranberry Juice (Shelf Stable)

Organic Lemonade (Shelf Stable)

Pineapple

Pineapple Orange

Pineapple Orange Banana

Pink Grapefruit Juice (Shelf Stable)

Pomegranate and Blueberry Blend (Shelf Stable)

Pomegranate and Cranberry Blend (Shelf Stable)

Premium Orange Juice

Premium Orange Juice with Calcium (Carafe)

Premium Orange Juice with Pulp

Prune Juice (Shelf Stable)

Raspberry Cranberry Juice Cocktail Light (Shelf Stable)
Raspberry Lemonade (Carafe)
Reconstituted Orange Juice (With Calcium, With Pulp)
Ruby Red Grapefruit
Ruby Red Grapefruit Cocktail
Ruby Red Grapefruit Cocktail Light (Shelf Stable)
Ruby Red Grapefruit Cocktail Light 22% (Shelf Stable)
Ruby Red Grapefruit Juice (Shelf Stable)
Strawberry Kiwi Splash (Shelf Stable)
Tangerine
Tangerine and Ruby Red (Shelf Stable)
Tropical Blend Splash (Shelf Stable)
Valencia Orange Juice (Carafe)
Valencia Orange with Pulp (Carafe)
White Cranberry Cocktail Juice (Shelf Stable)
White Cranberry Flavored Juice Blend (Shelf Stable)
White Cranberry Juice Cocktail (Shef Stable)
White Cranberry Peach Juice (Shelf Stable)
White Cranberry Peach Juice Cocktail (Shelf Stable)
White Cranberry Strawberry Juice Cocktail (Shelf Stable)
White Grape Juice (Shelf Stable)
White Grape Juice from Concentrate (Shelf Stable)
White Grape Peach Juice Blend (Shelf Stable)
White Grape Raspberry Juice Blend (Shelf Stable)
White Grapefruit Juice (Shelf Stable)
White Grapefruit Juice Cocktail (Shelf Stable)

Midwest Country Fare (Hy-Vee)
100% Concentrated Orange Juice
100% Unsweeetened Apple Juice from Concentrate
100% Unsweetened Apple Cider from Concentrate
Cranberry Apple Juice Cocktail

Cranberry Juice Cocktail
Cranberry Raspberry Juice
Crushed Pineapple in Natural Juice, No Sugar Added
Grape Juice from Concentrate
Tomato Juice from Concentrate

Minute Maid
Kids + Apple
Lemonade
Light Lemonade
Pomegranate Blueberry Juice
Pomegranate Lemonade

Naked Juice
Naked Juice Products (All BUT Green Machine and Fruit Juice Oat Smoothies)

Nantucket Nectars
Nantucket Nectars (All)

Nature Factor ✓
Organic Coconut Water

Nature's Promise (Giant)
Black Cherry Juice
Cranberry Juice
Organic Apple Juice
Organic Cranberry Juice
Organic Fruit Punch
Organic Lemonade
Organic White Grape Juice
Organic White Tea with Raspberry
Pomegranate Blueberry Juice Blend
Pomegranate Juice Blend

Nature's Promise (Stop & Shop)
Black Cherry Juice
Cranberry Juice
Organic Apple Juice
Organic Concord Grape Juice
Organic Cranberry Juice
Organic Fruit Punch
Organic Lemonade
Pomegranate Blueberry Juice Blend
Pomegranate Cranberry Juice Blend
Pomegranate Juice
Pomegranate Juice Blend

New Leaf
Lemonades (All)

Northland
Juices (All)

O Organics ✍

Orange Juice No Pulp with Calcium
Organic 100% Pure Country Style
Orange Juice
Organic 100% Pure No Pulp Orange
Juice
Organic Apple Juice from Concentrate
Organic Blueberry Flavored Juice Blend
Organic Cranberry Cocktail from
Concentrate
Organic Grape Juice from Concentrate
Organic Lemonade from Concentrate

Oberweis Dairy

Fruit Punch
Lemonade

Ocean Spray

Beverages (All)

Odwalla ⓘ

Apple Juice
Berries Go Mega
Blueberry B Superfood
Citrus C Monster
Mobeta
Orange Juice
Pomegranate Limeade
Red Rhapsody
Strawberry Banana
Strawberry C Monster
Strawberry Lemonade
Summertime Lime
Tangerine
Wellness

Ohana

Ohana

Old Orchard

Old Orchard (All)

Organic Valley ⓘ

Orange Juice, Pulp-Added
Orange Juice, Pulp-Free
Orange Juice, with Calcium

Our Family

100% Apple Juice
100% Berry Juice Blend
100% Cherry Juice Blend
100% Fresh Pressed Apple Cider
100% Fresh Pressed Apple Juice
100% Fruit Punch Juice Blend
100% Grape Juice Blend
100% Orange Tangerine Juice Blend
100% Pomegranate Blueberry Juice
Blend
100% Pomegranate Cranberry Juice
Blend
100% Tangerine Juice Blend
Apple Cherry Cocktail
Apple Cider
Apple Juice
Apple Kiwi Strawberry Cocktail
Apple Raspberry Cocktail
Citrus Punch
Concentrated Tomato Juice
Cranberry Grape Juice Cocktail
Cranberry Juice Cocktail
Fresh Tomato Juice
Fruit Punch
Grape Juice
Grapefruit Juice, Unsweetened
Lemonade
Light Cranberry Grape Juice Cocktail
Light Cranberry Juice Cocktail
Orange Juice
Orange Juice Frozen Concentrate
Orange Juice Pulp Free
Orange Juice with Calcium
Orange Juice with More Pulp
Orange Juice, Chilled
Orange Juice, Unsweetened
Pink Lemonade
Premium Chilled Orange Juice
Prune Juice
Pure Premium Orange Juice with
Calcium from Concentrate
Ruby Red Grapefruit Juice
Tomato Juice
Vegetable Juice
White Cranberry Juice Cocktail
White Cranberry Peach Juice Cocktail
White Grape Juice
White Grapfruit Juice

PET Milk

Blue Raspberry
Fruit Punch
Lemon-Lime
Orange Juice

Pint Coolies, Blue Raspberry
Pint Coolies, Fruit Punch
Pint Coolies, Lemonade
Pint Coolies, Orange

POM Wonderful
POM Wonderful (All)

Prairie Farms
Apple Juice
Blue Raspberry Drink
Fruit Punch Drink
Grape Drink
Grape Juice
Lemon Drink
Lemon Lime Drink
Lemonade
Orange Drink
Orange Juice
Pink Lemonade Drink

Price Chopper
Apple Juice
Calcium Apple Juice
Cranberry Juice Blend
Fruit Punch
Grapefruit Juice
Natural Apple Juice
Organic Apple Juice
Organic Cranberry Juice
Organic Grape Juice
Pineapple Juice
Prune Juice
White Grape Juice

Price's Creameries
Juices (All)

Publix
Apple Juice
Cranberry Apple Juice Cocktail
Cranberry Juice Cocktail
Deli Old Fashion Lemonade
Grape Juice
Grape-Cranberry Juice Cocktail
Orange Juice from Concentrate
Orange with Calcium Juice from
    Concentrate
Pinapple Juice
Premium Orange Juice - Calcium Plus
Premium Orange Juice - Grove Pure
Premium Orange Juice - Old Fashioned

Premium Orange Juice - Original
Premium Ruby Red Grapefruit
Raspberry Cranberry Juice Cocktail
Reduced Calorie Cranberry Juice
    Cocktail
Ruby Red Grapefruit Juice
Tomato Juice
White Grape Juice

Purity Dairies
Fruit Punch
Lemonade
Orange Drink
Orange Juice From Concentrate
Pink Lemonade

Purity Organic
Purity Organic Juices (All)

R.W. Knudsen ⓘ ✓
R.W. Knudsen (All)

Red Gold
Tomato Products (All)

Reiter Dairy
Orange Juice

Right Size
Juices (All)

Robinson Dairy
Fruit Drinks (All)
Orange Juice (All)

Sacramento
Tomato Products (All)

Safeway ✑
Apple Juice
Berry Punch
Calcium Enriched Orange Juice
Concord Grape Juice
Country Style Orange Juice
Cranberry Cocktail Juice
Cranberry Cocktail Juice Blend
Cranberry Raspberry Juice
Cranberry/Pormegranate Juice
Fruit Punch
Grape Cocktail Juice
Grapefruit Ruby Red Prepacked
Light Cranberry Juice Cocktail
Lime Juice
Limeade
Low Sodium Vegetable Juice
Orange Juice

Orange Juice with Calcium
Pink Lemonade
Pink Lemonade Lite Drink Mix
Prune Juice
Pulp Free Orange Juice
Reconstituted Lemon Juice
Ruby Red Grapefruit Cocktail Juice
Spiced Apple Cider
Tomato Juice
White Grape Juice

Safeway Select
Sparkling Apple Cider
Sparkling Apple Pomegranate Cider

Sambazon
Sambazon (All)

Schnucks
Apple Juice
Cranberry Apple Juice Cocktail
Cranberry Grape Juice Cocktail
Cranberry Juice Cocktail
Cranberry Raspberry Juice Cocktail
Grapefruit Juice, Unsweetened
Juice-A-Lot Berry
Juice-A-Lot Cherry
Juice-A-Lot Fruit Punch
Juice-A-Lot Grape
Lite Cranberry Grape Juice Cocktail
Lite Cranberry Juice Cocktail
Lite Grape Juice Cocktail
Orange Juice
Pineapple Juice
Pink Grapefruit Juice, Unsweetened
Prune Juice
Purple Grape Juice
Ruby Red Grapefruit Juice Cocktail
Sugar Free Fruit Punch To Go
Sugar Free Lemonade To Go
Sugar Free Raspberry To Go
Thirst Quencher Cherry
Thirst Quencher Fruit Punch
Thirst Quencher Glacier Chill
Thirst Quencher Grape
Thirst Quencher Lemon Lime
Thirst Quencher Lemonade
Thirst Quencher Orange
Thirst Splasher Lemonade
Thirst Splasher Pink Lemonade

Thirst Splasher Raspberry
Tomato Juice (Bottle)
Vegetable Juice
Vegetable Juice Cocktail
White Grape Juice (Plastic Container)
White Grapefruit Juice

Schnucks Select
Cranberry 100% Juice
Cranberry Grape 100% Juice
Cranberry Raspberry 100% Juice
Premium Apple Juice

Shaw's
100% Grape Juice
Vegetable Juice

Shoppers Value (Cub Foods)
Tagless Tea Bags
Tomato Juice

Shoppers Value (Jewel-Osco)
Tomato Juice

Simply Apple
Simply Apple

Simply Grapefruit
Simply Grapefruit

Simply Lemonade
Simply Lemonade
Simply Lemonade with Raspberry

Simply Limeade
Simply Limeade

Simply Orange
Orange Juice Country Stand Medium
  Pulp with Calcium
Simply Orange with Mango
Simply Orange with Pineapple

Slush Puppie
Slush Puppie (All)

Snapple
Snapple (All)

Stop & Shop
100% Cranberry Juice Blend
100% Low Sodium Vegetable Juice
100% Unsweetened Apple Juice with
  Added Calcium
Cranberry Apple Juice Cocktail
Cranberry Juice Cocktail
Grape Cranberry Juice Cocktail
Grape Juice
Light Apple Juice Cocktail

Reconstituted Lemon Juice
Ruby Red Grapefruit Juice Cocktail
Unsweetened From Concentrate 100%
    Apple Juice
Unsweetened Not From Concentrate
    100% Apple Juice
Unsweetened White Grape Juice
White Cranberry Juice Cocktail

Sunny D
Sunny D (All)

Sunsweet
Sunsweet (All BUT Chocolate Covered
    PlumSweets)

T.G. Lee Dairy
Orange Juice

Tampico
Juices (All)

Trader Joe's
Juices (All BUT Green Juice Blend
    (Fresh) and Green Plant (Shelf Stable))
Organic Mango Lemonade

Tropical Cheese
Energia Drinkable
Lite Drinkable
Low Fat Drinkable

Tropicana
100% Juice Products (All)

Turkey Hill
Fruit Punch
Lemonade
Light Raspberry Lemonade
Limonade
Orangeade
Pink Lemonade
Pomegranate Lemonade
Strawberry Kiwi Lemonade

V8
100% Vegetable Juice
Essential Antioxidants Vegetable Juice
High Fiber Vegetable Juice
Low Sodium Spicy Hot Vegetable Juice
Low Sodium Vegetable Juice
Spicy Hot Vegetable Juice
Splash Berry Blend
Splash Diet Berry Blend
Splash Diet Tropical Blend
Splash Fruit Medley

Splash Mango Peach
Splash Strawberry Kiwi Blend
Splash Tropical Blend
V-Fusion Açai Mixed Berry
V-Fusion Cranberry Blackberry
V-Fusion Goji Raspberry
V-Fusion Light Açai Mixed Berry
V-Fusion Light Cranberry Blackberry
V-Fusion Light Peach Mango
V-Fusion Light Pomegranate Blueberry
V-Fusion Light Strawberry Banana
V-Fusion Peach Mango
V-Fusion Pineapple Mango with Green
    Tea
V-Fusion Pomegranate Blueberry
V-Fusion Pomegranate with Green Tea
V-Fusion Raspberry Green Tea
V-Fusion Strawberry Banana

Valu Time (Brookshire)
Apple Cocktail
Cranberry Cocktail
Cranberry Grape Cocktail
Fruit Punch (Hawaiian Punch)
Fruit Squeeze- Berry (50% Less Sugar)
Fruit Squeeze- Cherry (50% Less Sugar)
Fruit Squeeze- Grape (50% Less Sugar)
Fruit Squeeze- Punch (50% Less Sugar)
Grape Juice
Orange Juice Concentrate

Valu Time (Marsh)
Apple Juice
Apple Juice Cocktail
Tomato Juice

Valu Time (Schnucks)
Apple Juice
Cranberry Cocktail

Vita Coco
100% Pure Coconut Water
Acai & Pomegranate Coconut Water
Peach & Mango Coconut Water
Pineapple Coconut Water
Tangerine Coconut Water
Tropical Fruit Coconut Water

Vons
100% Cranberry Grape Juice
Apple Juice
Cranberry Apple Juice

Cranberry Grape Cocktail Juice
Cranberry Raspberry Juice
Grapefruit Juice
Homestyle Orange Juice with Pulp
Orange Juice
Orange Juice No Pulp with Calcium
Prune Juice
Rich Calcium Orange Juice

Vruit ⓘ
Vruit Juices (Apple Carrot, Berry
Veggie, Orange Veggie, Tropical)

Wacky Apple ♀
Apple Juice

Wegmans
100% Orange Juice (From Concentrate)
100% Tomato Juice
Apple Natural
Berry Flavored Juice Blend
Berry Punch
Cranberry Grape Light
Cranberry Juice Cocktail
Cranberry Light
Cranberry Raspberry Juice Cocktail
Cranberry Raspberry Light
Fruit Punch
Grapefruit
Lemonade
Limeade
Orange Juice Calcium Enriched
Orange Peach Mango Flavor Juice Blend
Organic Apple Juice Concentrate
Organic Apricot Nectar Concentrate
Organic Cranberry Juice Concentrate
Organic Mango Nectar Concentrate
Organic Orange Juice Concentrate
Pineapple Orange Juice
White Grape

Welch's
Welch's (All)

White House
White House (All)

Whole Earth
Organic Cranberry Drink
Organic Elderflower Drink
Organic Ginger Drink
Organic Lemonade Drink

Winn & Lovette (Winn-Dixie)
Black Cherry Juice
Cranberry Juice
Pomegranate Juice

Winn-Dixie
Apple Cider from Concentrate
Apple Juice from Concentrate
Apple Juice, Premium Not from
Concentrate
Cranberry Apple Juice Cocktail
Cranberry Juice Cocktail
Cranberry Raspberry Juice Cocktail
Grape Juice from Concentrate
Grapefruit Juice from Concentrate
Lemon Juice, Reconstituted
Light Cranberry Grape Juice Cocktail
Light Cranberry Juice Cocktail
Light Grape Juice Cocktail
Orange Juice From Concentrate
Orange Juice From Concentrate with
Calcium
Orange Juice, Premium Not From
Concentrate
Organic Apple Juice
Organic Grape Juice
Organic Lemonade
Organic Mango Acai Berry Juice Blend
Organic Orange Mango Juice Blend
Organic Tomato Juice
Pomegranate Blueberry Juice Blend
Pomegranate Cranberry Juice Blend
Pomegranate Juice Blend
Prune Juice from Concentrate
Prune Juice with Pulp from Concentrate
Ruby Red Grapefruit Juice
Ruby Red Grapefruit Juice Cocktail
Tomato Juice
Vegetable Juice Cocktail
White Grape Juice from Concentrate

Winn-Dixie (Chek)
Lemonade

Wyman's
Wyman's (All)

Zico
Zico (All)

Zola Acai ⓘ
Acai Juice with Blueberry

Acai Juice with Pomegranate
Original Acai Juice

Mixers

ACME
Strawberry Daiquiri Fruit Cocktail Mixer

Albertsons
Margarita Fruit Cocktail Mixer
Strawberry Daiquiri Fruit Cocktail Mixer

Baja Bob's
Sugar-Free Cocktail Mixes (All)

Big Bucket ⓘ
Big Bucket (All)

Coco Lopez
Pina Colada Mix

Coco Real ⓘ
Coco Real (All)

Davis & Davis
Frozen Drink Mixes (All)

Demitri's Bloody Mary Seasoning
Demitri's Bloody Mary Seasoning (All)

Faerie's Finest ⚥
Cocktail Rimmers (All)

Finest Call ⓘ
Finest Call (All BUT Bloody Mary Mixes)

Goya
Piña Colada

Jardine's ⓘ
Pomegranate Margarita Mix
Texarita Margarita Mix
Texas Red Snapper Bloody Mary Mix

Jewel-Osco
Margarita Fruit Cocktail Mixer
Strawberry Daiquiri Fruit Cocktail Mixer

Little Hugs
Cocktail Mixers (All)

Martini Gold ⓘ
Martini Gold (All)

Master of Mixes ⓘ
Master of Mixes (All)

Old Orchard
Old Orchard (All)

Sacramento
Tomato Products (All)

Smoothies & Shakes

Bolthouse Farms ⓘ ✓
Bolthouse Farms Smoothies (All BUT Protein Plus Strawberry Parfait Smoothie)

Cascade Fresh ⓘ ✓
Cascade Fresh (All)

Concord Foods
Smoothie Mixes

Full Circle (Schnucks)
Mango Green Smoothie
Mango Smoothie
Strawberry Banana Smoothie

Garelick Farms
Chocolate Milkshake
Vanilla Milkshake

Goya
Smoothies Blackberry
Smoothies Mango
Smoothies Peach
Smoothies Strawberry

Hiland Dairy
Low Fat Shake Base
Shake Mixes (Chocolate, Vanilla)

Lucerne (Safeway) ⌒
Smoothie - Peach Passion
Smoothie - Strawberry
Smoothie - Strawberry Banana
Smoothie - Strawberry Banana Light

Meadow Brook Dairy
Chocolate Chug Milkshake
Vanilla Chug Milkshake

Mocafe ⓘ
Mocafe (All)

Odwalla ⓘ
Protein Monster Chocolate
Protein Monster Strawberry
Protein Monster Vanilla
Super Protein Original
Super Protein Pumpkin

Old Orchard
Old Orchard (All)

Our Family
Mixed Berry Light Smoothie
Peach Smoothie
Strawberry Banana Light Smoothie
Strawberry Smoothie
Prairie Farms
Chocolate Shake Mix
Vanilla Shake Mix
Price Chopper
Light Smoothie Mix Berry
Light Smoothie Strawberry
Low Fat Smoothie Blueberry
Low Fat Smoothie Peach
Low Fat Smoothie Strawberry
Right Size
Smoothies and Shakes (All)
Stonyfield Farm ⓘ
Stonyfield Farm (All BUT YoToddler, Frozen Yogurt & Ice Cream)
V8
Splash Smoothie, Strawberry Banana
Splash Smoothie, Tropical Colada

SPORTS DRINKS

Hy-Vee
Berry Thunder Sports Drink
Fruit Punch Thunder Sports Drink
Glacial Ice Thunder Sports Drink
Lemon Lime Thunder Sports Drink
Orange Thunder Sports Drink
POWERADE
POWERADE ION4 (All Flavors)
Schnucks
MVP Sport Blue Freeze
MVP Sport Fruit Punch
MVP Sport Lemon Lime
MVP Sport Light Fruit Punch
MVP Sport Light Grape
MVP Sport Light Orange
MVP Sport Orange
Wegmans
MVP Blue Freeze Sport Drink
MVP Fruit Punch Sport Drink
MVP Grape Sport Drink
MVP Lemon Lime Sport Drink
MVP Orange Sport Drink

MVP Raspberry Lemonade Sport Drink
Velocity Fitness Water - Berry
Velocity Fitness Water - Black Cherry
Velocity Fitness Water - Grape
Velocity Fitness Water - Kiwi Strawberry
Velocity Fitness Water - Lemon

TEA & TEA MIXES

4C
Instant Iced Tea Mixes Sweetened with Sugar (All)
Light Instant Iced Tea Mixes Sweetened with Splenda (All)
Totally Light Iced Tea Mixes Sweetened with Splenda (All)
ACME
Iced Tea Mix
Square Tea Bags
Tea Bags
Adagio Teas
Teas (All)
Aimee's Livin' Magic
Bone Tea
Red Tea
Yerba Mate
Albertsons
Decaffeinated Tea Bags
Instant Tea Powder
Pekoe Black Tea
Square Tea Bags
Always Save
Ice Tea Mix
Instant Tea
Tagless Tea Bags
Always Save (Price Chopper)
Tea Bags
Ambassador Organics
Tea (All)
Autocrat
Tea
Barry's Tea
Tea (All)
Bentley's
Tea (All)

Best Choice
- Decaffeinated Tea Bags
- Instant Tea Mix (Glass Bottle)
- Instant Tea Mix, Lemon
- Instant Tea Mix, Raspberry
- Tea Bags

Bigelow Tea ✓
- Bigelow Teas (All BUT Blueberry Harvest Herb Tea, Chamomile Mango Herb Tea, & Cinnamon Spice Herb Tea)

Blue Lotus Chai ♨
- Traditional Masala Chai

Boston Tea
- Tea (All)

Bromley Tea Company, The
- Bromley Products (All)

Carrington
- Tea (All)

Central Market Classics (Price Chopper)
- Chamomile Tea
- Decaf Green Tea
- Earl Grey Tea
- English Breakfast Tea
- Green Tea
- Lemon Tea
- Peppermint Tea
- Quiet Time Tea

Chartreuse Organic Tea
- Chartreuse Organic Tea (All)

China Mist
- Tea (All)

Choice Organic Teas
- Tea (All)

Coffee Bean & Tea Leaf
- Tea (All) ♨

Cub Foods
- Black Tea Bags
- Instant Tea

Culinary Circle (Albertsons)
- Chai Black Tea Bags
- Chamomile Tea Bags
- Earl Grey Tea Bags
- English Breakfast Teabags
- Hibiscus Tea Bags, Raspberry
- Lemon Tea Bags, Green
- Mint Green Tea Bags
- Peppermint Tea Bags
- Pomegranate Tea Bags, Green

Culinary Circle (Cub Foods)
- Black Earl Grey Tea Bags
- Black English Breakfast Tea Bags
- Chai Black Tea Bags
- Chamomile Tea Bags
- Lemon Green Tea Bags
- Mint Green Tea Bags
- Peppermint Tea Bags
- Pomegranate Green Tea Bags
- Raspberry Hibiscus Tea Bags

Culinary Circle (Jewel-Osco)
- Black Earl Grey Tea Bags
- Black English Breakfast Tea Bags
- Chai Black Tea Bags
- Chamomile Tea Bags
- Lemon Green Tea Bags
- Mint Green Tea Bags
- Peppermint Tea Bags
- Pomegranate Tea Bags Green
- Raspberry Hibiscus Tea Bags

David Rio
- Chai (All) ◇

Eden Foods
- Lotus Root Tea
- Mu 16 Herb Tea
- Organic Chamomile Herb Tea
- Organic Hojicha Chai Roasted Green Tea
- Organic Hojicha Tea
- Organic Kukicha Twig Tea
- Organic Matcha Tea Refill
- Organic Sencha Ginger Green Tea
- Organic Sencha Green Tea
- Organic Sencha Mint Green Tea
- Organic Sencha Rose Green Tea

Equal Exchange ⓘ
- Tea (All)

Faerie's Finest ♨
- Faerie's Finest (All)

Flavorite (Cub Foods)
- Green Tea Bags with Tags
- Instant Tea
- Tea Bags

Food Club (Brookshire)
Cold Brew Tea Bags
Decaf Tea Bags
Green Tea Bags
Iced Tea Mix
Instant Tea
Tea Bags

Food Club (Marsh)
Instant Tea
Tea Bags
Tea Bags Green
Tea Bags Green Decaf

Full Circle (Marsh)
Organic Earl Grey Tea Bags
Organic English Breakfast Tea Bags
Organic Green Tea Bags
Organic Peppermint Tea Bags

Full Circle (Schnucks)
Organic Breakfast Tea
Organic Chai Tea
Organic Chamomile
Organic Earl Grey
Organic Green Tea
Organic Night Time Tea

Giant
Green Tea Bags

Goya
Cruz de Malta Yerba Mate
Dulce Sueños
Manzanilla
Te de Tila
Te Laxante
Te Manzanilla Anis
Te Negro
Te Verde
Yerba Mate
Yerba Mate Limon
Yerba Mate Naranja

Great Value (Wal-Mart) 25
Decaffeinated Tea 100% Natural
Family Size Decaffeinated Tea 100% Natural
Family Size Tea 100% Natural
Green Tea with Ginseng And Honey

Green Mountain Coffee ()
Teas (All)

Guayaki Yerba Mate ✓
Guayaki Yerba Mate (All)

Hy-Vee
Chai Black Tea
Chamomile Herbal Tea
Cinnamon Apple Herbal Tea
Decaffeinated Green Tea
Decaffeinated Tea Bags
Dream Easy Herbal Tea
Earl Gray Black Tea
English Breakfast Black Tea
Family Size Tea Bags
Green Tea Bags
Instant Tea
Jasmine Green Tea
Orange & Spice Specialty Tea
Peppermint Herbal Tea
Pomegranate White Tea Bags
Rooibos Red Herbal Tea
Strawberry Herbal Tea Bags
Tea Bags

InJoy Organics
Tea (All)

Jewel-Osco
Square Tea Bags
Tagless Tea Bags
Tea Bags

JFG Coffee & Tea
Family Tea Bags
Tea Bags

Luzianne
Decaf Tea Bags
Tea Bags

Meijer
Berry Green Tea
Chai Tea
Chamomile Herbal Tea
Chamomile Mint Herbal Tea
Cinnamon Apple Herbal Tea
Diet Green with Citrus Tea
Diet White with Raspberry Tea
Earl Grey Decaf Tea
Earl Grey Tea
English Breakfast Tea
Green with Citrus Tea
Honey Lemon Ginseng Green Tea
Iced Tea Mix

Instant Tea Mix
Jasmine Green Tea
Orange Spice Black Tea
Peppermint Herbal Tea
Tea Bags (Decaffeinated, Green, Green
  Decaffeinated)
White with Raspberry Tea

Meijer Naturals
Decaf Green Tea
Decaf Tea
Green Tea
Tea

Meijer Organics
Organic Chai Tea
Organic Chamomile Tea
Organic Earl Grey Tea
Organic English Breakfast Tea
Organic Green Tea
Organic Peppermint Tea

Midwest Country Fare (Hy-Vee)
Black Tea

Mighty Leaf Tea ()
Mighty Leaf Tea (All)

Mocafe ⓘ
Mocafe (All)

Mrs. Bryant's
Estate Fresh Gourmet™ L'essence of the
  South Colonial Southern Organic
  Fruit Tea
Estate Fresh Gourmet™ L'essence of the
  South Colonial Southern Organic
  Peach Tea

Nestea (Nestlé)
Nestea Iced Tea Mix Unsweetened
Nestea Iced Tea Mix Unsweetened
  Decaffeinated
Nestea Stick Packs (All Flavors)

Newman's Own Organics ⓘ
Teas (All)

O Organics ⌒
Organic Earl Grey Tea
Organic Green Tea
Organic Peppermint Herb Tea

Original Ceylon Tea Company, The
Teas and Tea Bags (All)

Our Family
Cold Brew Tea Bags (Family Size)

Decaffeinated Tea Bags
Green Tea (Envelope)
Green Tea, Decaffeinated (Envelope)
Instant Tea 100%
Tea Bags
Tea Bags (Family Size)

Pacific Chai
Chai Teas (All)

Price Chopper
Black Tea Bags
Decaf Tea Bags
Iced Tea

Publix
Decaffeinated Tea Bags
Tagless Tea Bags
Tea Bags (All Varieties)

Red Diamond
Tea (All)

Red Rose
Red Rose Teas (All)

Revolution Tea ⚱
Black Tea
Green Tea
Herbal Tea
Oolong Tea
Organic Tea
Red Tea
White Tea

Rishi Tea
Rishi Tea (All)

Safeway ⌒
Black Tea Bags
Shake N Run Sugar Free Iced Tea Drink
  Mix

Salada
Salada (All)

Schnucks
Decaf Tea Bags
Green Tea Bags
Instant Tea
Tea Bags
Tea Bags (Family Size)

Shaw's
Decaf Square Tea Bags
Ice Tea Mix Can
Powdered Iced Tea Mix
Tea Bags

Shoppers Value (ACME)
Tagless Tea Bags
Shoppers Value (Albertsons)
Tagless Tea Bags
St. Dalfour ⓘ
Organic Teas (All)
Stash Tea
Acai Premium Tea
American Classic Iced
Apple Cinnamon Premium Tea
Blackcurrant Iced
Blueberry Herbal Iced
Blueberry Herbal Premium Tea
Blueberry Superfruit Premium Tea
Chai Spice Premium Tea
Chai White Premium Tea
Chamomile Premium Tea
Chanakara Blue Ginger
Chanakara Dragonfruit
Chanakara Guanabana
Chanakara Red Berry Rooibos
Chanakara Vanilla Honeybush
Chocolate Mint Oolong Premium Tea
Christmas Eve Premium Tea
Christmas Morning Premium Tea
Cinnamon Apple Chamomile Premium
  Tea
Cinnamon Vanilla Premium Tea
Coconut Mango Oolong Premium Tea
Cranberry Pomegranate Premium Tea
Decaf Chai Spice Premium Tea
Decaf Chocolate Hazelnut Premium Tea
Decaf Crème Caramel Premium Tea
Decaf Earl Grey Iced
Decaf Earl Grey Premium Tea
Decaf English Breakfast Premium Tea
Decaf Lemon & White Premium Tea
Decaf Premium Green Tea
Decaf Pumpkin Spice Premium Tea
Decaf Raspberry & White Premium Tea
Decaf Vanilla Chai Premium Tea
Decaf Vanilla Nut Crème Premium Tea
Double Bergamot Earl Grey Premium
  Tea
Earl Grey Iced
Earl Grey Premium Tea
English Breakfast Premium Tea

Fusion Breakfast Premium Tea
Fusion Green & White Premium Tea
Fusion Honey Ginseng & White
  Premium Tea
Fusion Red & White Premium Tea
Fusion Red, White & Blueberry
  Premium Tea
Ginger Breakfast Premium Tea
Ginger Peach Green with Matcha
  Premium Tea
Goji Green Premium Tea
Green Chai Premium Tea
Holiday Chai Premium Tea
Jasmine Blossom Premium Tea
Lemon Blossom Herbal Iced
Lemon Blossom Premium Tea
Lemon Ginger Premium Tea
Lemon Iced
Lemon Spice Premium Tea
Licorice Spice Premium Tea
Mango Passionfruit Iced
Mango Passionfruit Premium Tea
Mangosteen Green Premium Tea
Mellow Moments Premium Tea
Meyer Lemon Premium Tea
Mojito Green Premium Tea
Moroccan Mint Iced
Moroccan Mint Premium Tea
Orange Cranberry Iced
Orange Spice on Ice
Orange Spice Premium Tea
Orange Starfruit Premium Tea
Organic Cascade Mint
Organic Chai Spice
Organic Chamomile Herbal
Organic Decaf Premium Green
Organic Earl Grey
Organic Honeybush
Organic Lavender Tulsi
Organic Lemon Ginger Green
Organic MerryMint Premium Tea
Organic Premium Green
Organic Vanilla Honeybush
Organic White Tea with Mint
Peach Black Premium Tea
Peach Herbal Iced
Peppermint Iced

Peppermint Premium Tea
Pomegranate Raspberry with Matcha
    Premium Tea
Premium Green Tea
Premium Green Tea with Matcha
Pyramid Chamomile Citrus
Pyramid Rooibos Blood Orange
Red Tea Premium
Ruby Mist on Ice
Ruby Mist Premium Tea
Strawberry Pomegranate Premium Tea
Teas of India Kashmiri Green Chai
Traditional on Ice
Tropical Fruit Iced
Tropical Iced
White Christmas Premium Tea
White Peach Oolong Premium Tea
Wild Blackcurrant Iced
Wild Raspberry Iced
Wild Raspberry Premium Tea
Yamamotoyama Chrysanthemum
Yamamotoyama Ginger Green
Yamamotoyama Pu-erh
Yumberry Blackcurrant Premium Tea

Steviva
Organic Yerba Mate Green Tea
Stevia Tea Leaves

Stop & Shop
Iced Tea Mix
Sugar Free Iced Tea Mix
Sugar Free Lemonade Drink Mix

Taylors of Harrogate
Tea (All)

Tazo ()
Teas (All BUT Green Ginger,
    Honeybush, Lemon Ginger & Tea
    Lemonade)

Tea Forte
Tea (All)

Teekanne
Herbal Wellness Teas (All BUT
    Lemon Twist, Mandarin Breeze, and
    Passionfruit Mango)

Trader Joe's
Tea (All)

Traditional Medicinals Tea ⓘ
Teas (All BUT PMS Tea and St. John's
    Good Mood Tea)

Triple Leaf Tea ()
Triple Leaf Tea (All)

Twinings
Herbal Infusions (All)
Teas (All)

Uncle Lee's Tea ⚕
Teas (All)

Valu Time (Brookshire)
Tagless Tea Bags

Valu Time (Marsh)
Tea Bags Tagless

Valu Time (Schnucks)
Tea Bags (Family Size)
Tea Bags (Tagless)

Vons 〰
Tea Bags Decaf

Wegmans
Black Tea, Orange Pekoe
Decaf Black Tea Bags
Decaf Earl Grey Black Tea Bags
Decaf Green Tea Bags
Decaf Iced Tea Mix
Earl Grey Black Tea Bags
Earl Grey Green Tea Bags
English Breakfast Black Tea Bags
Genmaimatcha- Loose Green Tea
Green Tea Bags
Iced Tea Mix
Iced Tea Mix with Natural Lemon
    Flavor & Sugar
Lavender Sencha- Loose Green Tea
Organic Chai Tea
Organic Chamomile Tea
Organic Decaffinated Earl Grey Loose
    Black Tea
Organic Decaffinated Lemon Ginger
    Tea
Organic Dragon Well Loose Green Tea
Organic Earl Grey Tea
Organic English Breakfast Loose Black
    Tea
Organic English Breakfast Tea
Organic Jasmine Green Tea

Organic Lapsang Souchong Loose Black Tea

Organic Peppermint Tea

Organic Rooibos Loose Herbal Tea

Organic Rooibos Strawberry Cream Tea

Organic Silver Needle Loose White Tea

Organic Yerba Mate Loose Herbal Tea

Pekoe Cut Black Tea Bags

Regular Tea Bags

Sencha Pure Japanese Tea

Ti Guan Yin- Loose Oolong Tea

Toma Sencha- Loose Green Tea

Windsor

Anise Tea

Coca Tea

Fruit Tea

Mate de Manzanilla

Tea Classic

Tea With Cinnamon and Clove

Trimate

Windsor Classic

Winn-Dixie

Decaffeinated Tea Bags (Family Size, Regular)

Tea Bags (Family Size, Regular)

World Classics (Schnucks)

Black Chai Tea Tin

English Breakfast Tea Tin

Green Berry Tea Tin

Red Chai/Rooibos Tea Tin

Spearmint Tea Tin

White Jasmine Tea Tin

Yogi Tea ⓘ

Tea (All BUT Calming, Healthy Fasting, Kava Stress Relief & Stomach Ease Teas)

TEA DRINKS

ACME

Cold Brew Tea

Diet Decaf Iced Tea

Diet Green Tea With Ginseng/Honey

Diet Lemon Iced Tea

Green Tea With Ginseng/Honey

Lemon Iced Tea Carton

Peach Iced Tea Jug

AriZona

Teas (All)

Best Choice

Sweet Tea

Bolthouse Farms ⓘ ✓

Bolthouse Farms Tea (All BUT Protein Plus Strawberry Parfait Smoothie)

Crystal Light ⌇

Iced Tea, Antioxidant Raspberry Green Tea Sugar Free

Iced Tea, Decaffeinated Iced Tea Natural Lemon

Iced Tea, Decaffeinated Sugar Free

Iced Tea, Lemon Sugar Free

Iced Tea, Natural Lemon

Iced Tea, Raspberry Sugar Free

FUZE

FUZE (All Flavors)

Genuardi's ⌇

Lite Iced Tea Drink Mix

Peach Lite Iced Tea

Gold Peak

Lemon Iced Tea

Golden Star

White Jasmine Sparkling Tea

Good Earth Tea

Teas (All)

Great Value (Wal-Mart) 🔲25

Diet Green Tea with Ginseng And Honey

Ready To Drink Sweetened Tea

Sugar Free Sweet Iced Tea

Sweet Iced Tea

Guayaki Yerba Mate ✓

Guayaki Yerba Mate (All)

Honest Tea

Honest Tea (All)

Hy-Vee

Honey Lemon Ginseng Green Tea

Thirst Splashers Raspberry Tea

Inko's

Inko's (All)

Ito En

Traditional Tea Line (All)

ITO EN Shot

Ito En Shot (All)

Luzianne
Ready to Drink Diet Peach Tea
Ready to Drink Green with Mint Sweet Tea
Ready to Drink Lemon Sweet Tea
Ready to Drink Raspberry Sweet Tea
Ready to Drink Sweet Tea

MaryAnna's Tea
Berry Sweet Tea
Peachy Sweet Tea
Summer Sweet Tea

McArthur Dairy
Southern Style Sweet Tea
Sweetened Iced Tea with Lemon

Milo's Famous Tea
Milo's Sweet Tea (All)
Milo's Sweet Tea Splenda (All)
Milo's Unsweetened Tea (All)

Minute Maid
Pomegranate Flavored Tea

Nature's Promise (Giant)
Organic Black Tea with Lemon
Organic Black Tea with Plum
Organic Green Tea with Spearmint
Organic Red Tea with Mandarin Mango

Nature's Promise (Stop & Shop)
Organic Black Tea with Lemon
Organic Red Tea with Mandarin Mango
Organic White Tea with Raspberry

Nestea (Coca-Cola Company, The)
Citrus Green Tea
Diet Citrus Green Tea
Diet Lemon Tea
Lemon Sweet Tea
Red Tea
Sweetened Lemon Tea

New Leaf
Iced Teas (All)

NOH of Hawaii ◊
Hawaiian Iced Tea

O Organics ⌇
Organic Black Tea with Lemon
Organic Green Tea with Honey
Organic Peach Flavored Oolong Tea
Organic White Tea with Spearmint
Pomegranate White Tea

Oberweis Dairy
Lemon Tea

Oi Ocha ⓘ
Oi Ocha (All)

Our Family
Diet Green Tea with Honey
Green Tea with Honey Ginseng

POM Wonderful
POM Wonderful (All)

Prairie Farms
Iced Tea

Price Chopper
Green Tea

Publix
Deli Iced Tea - Sweetened
Deli Iced Tea - Unsweetened

Purity Dairies
Tea

Reiter Dairy
Iced Tea

Safeway ⌇
Regular Green Tea with Citrus

Schnucks
Sugar Free Iced Tea To Go
Thirst Splasher Tea

Sencha Shot
Sencha Shot

Shaw's
Lemon Iced Tea

Snapple
Snapple (All)

Steaz ⓘ
Steaz Tea Drinks (All)

Swiss Premium
Tea (All)

Teas' Tea
Teas' Tea (All)

Trader Joe's
Kettle Brewed Unsweetened Green & White Tea

Turkey Hill
Cherry Pomegranate Black Tea
Decaf Tea
Diet Blackberry Sweet Tea
Diet Decaf Iced Tea
Diet Decaf Orange Tea
Diet Green Tea

Diet Green Tea Mango
Diet Iced Tea
Green Tea
Green Tea Mango
Iced Tea
Lemonade Tea
Light Wildberry Green Iced Tea
Orange Tea
Peach Tea
Raspberry Tea
Sweet Tea
Unsweetened Iced Tea

Wegmans

Diet Iced Tea
Iced Tea

Winn-Dixie

Organic Sweet Black Tea with Lemon
Organic Sweet Green Tea
Organic Sweet Red Tea with Mango and
  Mandarin Orange
Organic Sweet White Tea with
  Raspberry
Organic Unsweetened Green Tea
Organic Unsweetened Red Tea with
  Pomegranate

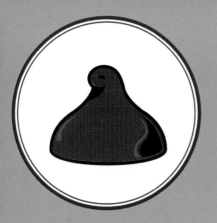

BAKING AISLE

BAKING CHIPS & BARS

Aimee's Livin' Magic
Really Raw Cacao Nibs
Really Raw Coconut Chips
Always Save
Imitation Chocolate Chips
Baker's Chocolate
Baking Chocolate, Bittersweet
Baking Chocolate, Semi-Sweet
Baking Chocolate, Unsweetened

Baking Chocolate, White Chocolate
Chocolate Bar, German's Sweet
Chocolate Chunks, Semi-Sweet
Best Choice
Butterscotch Chips
Chocolate Almond Bark
Milk Chocolate Chips
Mini Chocolate Chips
Semi Sweet Chips
Vanilla Almond Bark

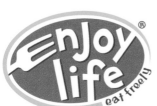
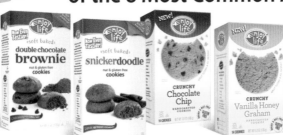
 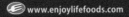

White Chips
Candiquik ⓘ
Candiquik (All)
Enjoy Life Foods ⚕ ✓
Semi-Sweet Chocolate Mega Chunks
Semi-Sweet Chocolate Mini Chips
Fastco (Fareway)
Real Chocolate Chips
Food Club (Brookshire)
Chocolate Flavor Baking Chips
Milk Chocolate Baking Chips
Semi Sweet Chocolate Baking Chips
Food Club (Marsh)
Baking Chips, Milk Chocolate
Baking Chips, Peanut Butter
Baking Chips, Semisweet Chocolate
Baking Chips, Vanilla
Giant
Milk Chocolate Baking Chips
Great Value (Wal-Mart) 🔟25
Semi Sweet Chocolate Chips
Haggen
Chocolate Chips
Hy-Vee
Butterscotch Baking Chips
Milk Chocolate Baking Chips
Mini Semi Sweet Chocolate Chips
Peanut Butter Baking Chips
Semi Sweet Chocolate Chips
Vanilla Flavored White Baking Chips
Kroger
Jumbo Semi-Sweet Chips
Log House
Almond Bark
Manischewitz
Chocolate Morsels
Meijer
Almonds (Natural Sliced, Slivered, Whole)
Almonds, Blanched (Sliced, Slivered)
Butterscotch Baking Chips
Milk Chocolate Chips
Peanut Butter Chips
Pecan Chips
Pecan Halves
Semi Sweet Chocolate Chips
Walnut Halves and Pieces

Walnuts (Black, Chips)
White Baking Chips
Midwest Country Fare (Hy-Vee)
Chocolate Flavored Chips
Nestlé Toll House ⸰
Milk Chocolate & Peanut Butter Swirled Morsels
Milk Chocolate Morsels
Peanut Butter & Milk Chocolate Morsels
Premier White Morsels
Semi-Sweet Chocolate & Premier White Swirled Morsels
Semi-Sweet Chocolate Chunks
Semi-Sweet Chocolate Mini Morsels
Semi-Sweet Morsels
Our Family
Butterscotch Chips
Milk Chocolate Chips
Real Semi Sweet Chocolate Chips
Price Chopper
Chocolate Chips
Milk Chocolate Chips
Publix
Butterscotch Morsels
Milk Chocolate Morsels
Semi-Sweet Chocolate Morsels
Saco
Chocolate Chunks (All)
Safeway ⸰
Baking Chips Butterscotch
Baking Chips Milk Chocolate
Chocolate Chips
Schnucks
Milk Chocolate Chips
Real Chocolate Chips
Taza Chocolate
Baking Chocolate (All)
Trader Joe's
Chocolate Chips (Semi-Sweet, White Chocolate)
Milk Chocolate Peanut Butter Chips
Unsweetened Belgian Baking Chocolate
Tropical Source
Semi-Sweet Chocolate Chips
Valu Time (Brookshire)
Chocolate Chip Baking Chips

Valu Time (Marsh)
Baking Chips, Chocolate
Wegmans
Chocolate Morsels Semi-Sweet
Chocolate Chips

BAKING MIXES

1-2-3 Gluten Free ♟ ✓
Aaron's Favorite Rolls Mix
Allie's Awesome Buckwheat Pancakes
Mix
Chewy Chipless Scrumdelicious Cookie
Mix
Delightfully Gratifying Poundcake Mix
Devilishly Decadent Brownies Mix
Devil's Food Cake Mix
Divinely Decadent Brownies Mix
Lindsay's Lipsmackin' Sugar Cookies
Mix
Meredith's Marvelous Muffin Mix
Micah's Mouthwatering Corn Bread Mix
Peri's Perfect Chocolate Poundcake Mix
Southern Glory Biscuits Mix
Sweet Goodness Pan Bars Mix
Yummy Yellow Cake Mix
Arrowhead Mills
Bake with Me Gluten-Free Chocolate
Cupcake Mix
Bake with Me Gluten-Free Vanilla
Cupcake Mix
Gluten-Free All Purpose Baking Mix
Gluten-Free Brownie Mix
Gluten-Free Chocolate Chip Cookie
Mix
Gluten-Free Pancake & Waffle Mix
Gluten-Free Vanilla Cake Mix
Authentic Foods
Baking Mixes (All)
Bella Gluten-Free
Bella Gluten-Free (All)
Better Batter
Gluten Free Brownie Mix
Gluten Free Chocolate Cake Mix
Gluten Free Pancake/Biscuit Mix
Gluten Free Yellow Cake Mix

Betty Crocker
Gluten-Free Brownie Mix
Gluten-Free Chocolate Chip Cookie
Mix
Gluten-Free Devil's Food Cake Mix
Gluten-Free Yellow Cake Mix
Bi Aglut
Bi Aglut (All)
Biscuiterie de Provence ⓘ
Gluten Free Organic Cakes (All)
Bisquick
Bisquick Gluten Free
Bob's Red Mill
GF Brownie Mix
GF Chocolate Cake Mix
GF Chocolate Chip Cookie Mix
GF Cinnamon Raisin Bread Mix
GF Cornbread Mix
GF Hearty Whole Grain Bread Mix
GF Homemade Bread Mix
GF Pancake Mix
GF Pizza Crust Mix
GF Shortbread Cookie Mix
GF Vanilla Cake Mix
Wheat Free Biscuit Mix
Bodhi's Bakehouse
Fibre Rich Pancake Mix
Breads From Anna
Apple Pancake & Muffin Mix
Banana Bread Mix
Black Bean Brownie Mix
Classic Herb Bread Mix
Cranberry Pancake & Muffin Mix
Gluten Free Bread Mix
Gluten, Corn, Dairy, Soy, Nut & Rice
Free Bread Mix
Maple Pancake & Muffin Mix
Pie Crust Mix
Pizza Crust Mix
Pumpkin Bread Mix
Chebe ♟
All-Purpose Bread Mix
Cinnamon Roll Mix
Focaccia Mix
Garlic-Onion Breadstick Mix
Original Cheese Bread Mix
Pizza Crust Mix

Cherrybrook Kitchen
- Gluten-Free Dreams Chocolate Cake Mix
- Gluten-Free Dreams Chocolate Chip Cookies Mix
- Gluten-Free Dreams Chocolate Chip Pancake Mix
- Gluten-Free Dreams Fudge Brownie Mix
- Gluten-Free Dreams Pancake & Waffle Mix
- Gluten-Free Dreams Sugar Cookie Mix
- Gluten-Free Dreams Yellow Cake Mix

Chi-Chi's
- Fiesta Sweet Corn Cake Mix

Cravings Place, The ⌀
- Chocolate Chunk Cookie Mix
- Cinnamon Crumble Coffee Cake Mix

Dowd & Rogers ✓
- Dark Chocolate Brownie Mix
- Dark Vanilla Cake Mix
- Dutch Chocolate Cake Mix
- Golden Lemon Cake Mix

Eating Gluten Free ✓
- Eating Gluten Free (All)

Farmo ✓
- Farmo (All)

Fast & Fresh ◯
- Low Sodium Microwave Gluten Free Dairy Free White Cake Kit
- Low Sodium Microwave Gluten Free Dairy Free Yellow Cake Kit
- Low Sodium Microwave Gluten Free Double Chocolate Cake Kit
- Low Sodium Microwave Gluten Free Gooey Brownie Decadence Kit
- Low Sodium! Microwave Gluten Free Dairy Free Chocolate Cake Kit
- Low Sodium! Microwave Gluten Free Dairy Free Cinnamon Coffee Cake Mix
- Low Sodium! Microwave Gluten Free Dairy Free Cornbread Kit
- Microwave Gluten Free Dairy Free Pizza Crust Kit
- Microwave Gluten Free Dairy Free Pizza Crust Mix
- Microwave Gluten Free Hamburger Bun Kit
- Microwave Gluten Free Hamburger Bun Refill
- Microwave Gluten Free Waffle Kit
- Microwave Gluten Free Waffle Mix
- Microwave Gluten Free White Bread Kit
- Microwave Gluten Free White Bread Mix
- No Sodium Gluten Free Dairy Free Chocolate Flavored Icing
- No Sodium Gluten Free Dairy Free Vanilla Flavored Icing

Food-Tek ◯
- Gluten-Free Fast & Fresh Line (All)
- Gluten-Free Quick-Bake Kids Line (All)

Gifts of Nature ✓
- Basic Muffin Mix
- Buttermilk Biscuit & Baking Mix
- Buttermilk Cornbread Mix
- Buttermilk Pancake & Waffle Mix
- Cinnamon Spice Muffin Mix
- Cranberry Orange Muffin Mix
- Fancy Cookie Mix
- French Bread & Pizza Crust Mix
- Fudge Brownie Mix
- Sandwich White Bread & Roll Mix
- Triple Treat Cookie Mix
- Vanilla Poppy Seed Muffin Mix
- Yellow Cake Mix

Gillian's Foods ⌀
- Gillian's Foods (All)

Gluten Free Harvest, A
- A Gluten Free Harvest (All)

Gluten Free Mama
- Mama's Cookie Mix
- Mama's Pancake Mix
- Mama's Pie Crust Mix
- Mama's Pizza Crust Mix
- Mama's Scone Mix

Gluten Free Sensations ⌀ ✓
- Chocolate Chip Cookie Mix
- Pancake & Waffle Mix
- Sugar Cookie Cutout Mix

Gluten-Free Naturals ⌀ ✓
- Gluten-Free Naturals (All)

Gluten-Free Pantry, The
Brown Rice Pancake & Waffle Mix
Chocolate Chip Cookie & Cake Mix
Chocolate Truffle Brownie Mix
Decadent Chocolate Cake Mix
Favorite Sandwich Bread Mix
French Bread & Pizza Mix
Muffin & Scone Mix
Old Fashioned Cake & Cookie Mix
Perfect Pie Crust Mix
Yankee Cornbread and Muffin Mix

Gluuteny
Gluuteny (All)

Goya
Arepa Rellenas
Masarica
Pao de Queijo

Grandpa's Kitchen
Grandpa's Kitchen (All)

HGD Foods
Gluten Free Baking Mixes (All)

Hodgson Mill
Gluten Free Sweet Yellow Cornbread Mix
Gluten-Free Apple Cinnamon Muffin Mix
Gluten-Free Bread Mix
Gluten-Free Brownie Mix
Gluten-Free Chocolate Cake Mix
Gluten-Free Cookie Mix
Gluten-Free Multi Purpose Baking Mix
Gluten-Free Pancake & Waffle Mix
Gluten-Free Pizza Crust Mix
Gluten-Free Yellow Cake Mix

Hol-Grain
Chocolate Brownie Mix
Pancake & Waffle Mix

Inspired Cookie, The
Bliss Brownie Mix

Jules Gluten Free
Bread Mix
Cookie Mix
Graham Cracker/Gingersnap Mix

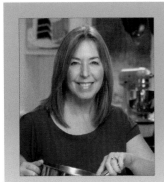

King Arthur
 Gluten-Free Bread Mix
 Gluten-Free Brownie Mix
 Gluten-Free Chocolate Cake Mix
 Gluten-Free Cookie Mix
 Gluten-Free Muffin Mix
 Gluten-Free Pancake Mix
 Gluten-Free Pizza Crust Mix

Kinnikinnick Foods ☗
 Kinnikinnick Foods (All)

Larrowe's
 Buckwheat Pancake Mix

Little Aussie Bakery, The
 The Little Aussie Bakery (All)

Maple Grove Farms
 Gluten-Free Pancake Mix ☗ ✔

Marion's Smart Delights ☗
 Delightfully Delicious Gluten-Free
  Lemon Bar Mix
 Gluten-Free Cookie & Muffin Baking
  Mix

Mom's Place Gluten-Free ☗
 Mom's Place Gluten-Free (All)

Namaste Foods ☗ ✔
 Baking Mixes (All)
 Biscuit Mix
 Waffle/Pancake Mix

Orgran ⓘ ☗
 All Purpose Pastry Mix
 Alternative Grain Wholemeal Bread Mix
 Apple & Cinnamon Pancake Mix
 Buckwheat Pancake Mix
 Chocolate Cake Mix
 Chocolate Mousse Mix
 Chocolate Muffin Mix
 Cornbread & Muffin Mix
 Easy Bake Bread Mix
 Gluten Free Gluten Replace Mix
 Pizza & Pastry Mix
 Vanilla Cake Mix

Pamela's Products ⓘ
 Baking & Pancake Mix
 Chocolate Brownie Mix
 Chocolate Cake Mix
 Chocolate Chunk Cookies Mix
 Classic Vanilla Cake Mix
 Cornbread & Muffin Mix

 Gluten-Free Bread Mix

Purely Elizabeth
 Purely Elizabeth (All)

Quick-Bake ⓘ
 Gluten Free Biscuit Mix
 Gluten Free Brownies
 Gluten Free Chocolate Chip Cookies
 Gluten Free Chocolate Cookie
 Gluten Free Dairy Free Chocolate Cake
 Gluten Free Dairy Free Yellow Cake
 Gluten Free Sugar Cookie
 Low Sodium Gluten Free Chocolate
  Chip Cookie Mix
 Low Sodium Gluten Free Dairy Free
  Sugar Cookie Mix
 Low Sodium Gluten Free Double
  Chocolate Chip Cookie Mix

Really Great Food ☗
 Really Great Food (All)

Schar ☗
 Classic White Bread Mix

Simply Organic
 Banana Bread Mix ✔
 Carrot Cake Mix ✔
 Chai Spice Scone Mix ✔
 Cocoa Brownie Mix ✔
 Cocoa Cayenne Cupcake Mix ✔
 Devil's Food Cake Mix ✔
 Golden Vanilla Cake Mix ✔
 Pancake & Waffle Mix ✔
 Pizza Crust Mix ✔
 Spice Cookie Mix ✔

Sof'ella ⓘ
 All Purpose Baking Mix
 Chocolate Cake Mix

Something Good
 Something Good (All)

Streit's ⓘ
 Gluten Free Chocolate Cake Mix
 Gluten Free Vanilla Cake Mix

Sweet Cake Bake Shop ☗
 Gluten Free Flour Blends and Mixes
  (All)

Sylvan Border Farm
 Chocolate Cake Mix
 Lemon Cake Mix
 Pancake & Waffle Mix

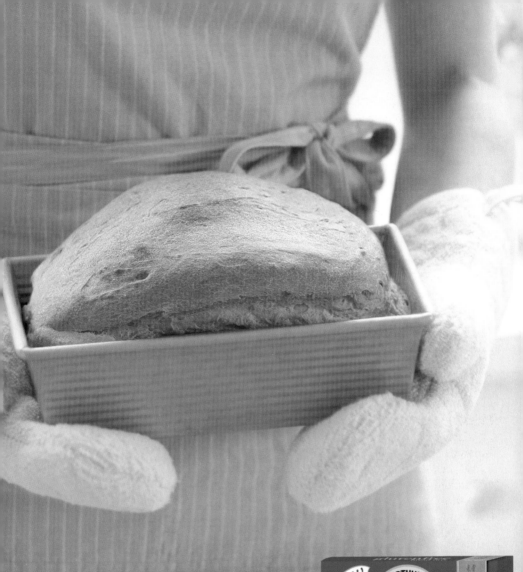

Worth the wait.

The tempting aroma of freshly baked bread fills your kitchen, filling *you* with the anticipation of your first warm, buttery bite. At long last, you can enjoy all the tastes you've been craving, thanks to a new line of certified gluten-free mixes from King Arthur Flour. It's the feast for the senses you've been waiting for.

BREAD • MUFFINS • BROWNIES • CAKE
PIZZA • FLOUR • COOKIES • PANCAKES

Learn more about our complete line of new gluten-free mixes at
kingarthurflour.com/glutenfree

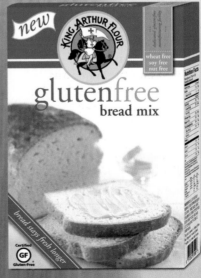

new

KING ARTHUR FLOUR

wheat free
soy free
nut free

glutenfree
bread mix

bread stays fresh longer

Certified
GF
Gluten-Free

Trader Joe's
 Gluten Free Brownie Mix
 Gluten Free Homestyle Pancakes
Vons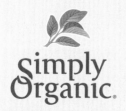
 Corn Starch, Holiday
Well & Good ⚕
 Well & Good (All)
Wholesome Chow ✓
 Gluten Free All-Purpose/Pancake Mix
 Gluten Free Chocolate Cake Mix
 Gluten Free Chocolate Lavender Cake
  Mix
 Gluten Free Vanilla Cake Mix
WOW Baking ⚕
 Cake Mix (All)

BAKING POWDER

Always Save
 Baking Powder
Best Choice
 Baking Powder

Bob's Red Mill
 Baking Powder
Clabber Girl ✓
 Baking Powder
Davis Baking Powder ✓
 Baking Powder
Dr. Oetker
 Baking Powder
Durkee
 Baking Powder
Ener-G
 Baking Powder
Hain Pure Foods
 Gluten-Free Featherweight Baking
  Powder
Hearth Club ✓
 Baking Powder
Hy-Vee
 Double Acting Baking Powder
KC
 Baking Powder

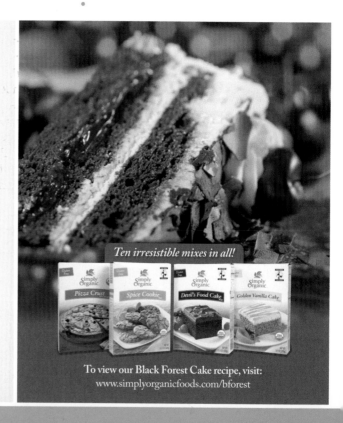

Our Family
Baking Powder
Price Chopper
Baking Powder
Really Great Food ♀
Really Great Food (All)
Royal Baking Powder
Baking Powder
Rumford
Baking Powder
Spice Islands
see also Durkee
Tone's
see also Durkee
Wegmans
Baking Powder, Double Acting

BAKING SODA

Always Save
Baking Soda
Arm & Hammer
Baking Soda
Bob's Red Mill
Baking Soda
Clabber Girl ✓
Baking Soda
Cub Foods
Baking Soda
Durkee
Baking Soda
Ener-G
Baking Soda
Flavorite (Cub Foods)
Baking Soda
Food Club (Brookshire)
Baking Soda
Food Club (Marsh)
Baking Soda
Giant
Baking Soda
Baking Soda (Guaranteed Value)
Haggen
Baking Soda
Hy-Vee
Baking Soda

Meijer
Baking Soda
Price Chopper
Baking Soda
Schnucks
Baking Soda
Spice Islands
see also Durkee
Tone's
see also Durkee

BREAD CRUMBS & OTHER COATINGS

Aleia's ♀ ✓
Italian Bread Crumbs
Plain Bread Crumbs
Bodhi's Bakehouse
Gluten Free Bread Crumbs
Ener-G
Bread Crumbs
Gillian's Foods ♀
Gillian's Foods (All)
Glutino
Breadcrumbs
Hodgson Mill
Gluten-Free Seasoned Coating Mix ♀
Hol-Grain ⓘ ♀
Brown Rice Bread Crumbs
Chicken Coating Mix
Onion Ring Batter Mix
Tempura Batter Mix
I.M. Healthy
Corn Crumbs
Katz Gluten Free
Bread Crumbs
Kinnikinnick Foods ♀
Kinnikinnick Foods (All)
Luzianne
Seafood Coating Mix
Mary's Gone Crackers
Mary's Gone Crackers (All)
Mom's Place Gluten-Free ♀
Mom's Place Gluten-Free (All)
Orgran ⓘ ♀
All Purpose Rice Crumbs
Corn Crispy Crumbs

Oven Fry
Seasoned Coating, Fish Fry For Fish
Schar
Bread Crumbs
Shabtai Gourmet Gluten-Free Bakery
Pread Crumbs - Gluten Free Bread
Crumb Substitute
Shake 'N Bake
Seasoned Coating Mix, BBQ Glaze For
Chicken Or Pork with 2 Packets &
Shaker Bags
Slap Ya Mama
Cajun Fish Fry
Southern Homestyle
Corn Flake Crumbs
Tortilla Crumbs
Sunbird
Tempura Batter

Cocoa Powder

Aimee's Livin' Magic
Really Raw Cacao Powder
Always Save
Baking Cocoa
Foods Alive
Organic Raw Cacao Powder
Goya
Chocolate Menier Cocoa
Hy-Vee
Baking Cocoa
Our Family
Cocoa Powder
Saco
Premium Cocoa (All)
Trader Joe's
Organic Cocoa Powder (Seasonal)
Organic Conacado Cocoa

Hersheys cocoa - gf

Coconut

Aimee's Livin' Magic
Really Raw Shredded Coconut
Baker's Chocolate
Sweetened Coconut, Angel Flake
Best Choice
Flake Coconut

Food Club (Brookshire)
Coconut Flakes
Unsweetened Coconut Flakes
Goya
Grated Coconut
Great Value (Wal-Mart) 25
Sweetened Coconut Flakes
Sweetened Flaked Coconut
Haggen
Coconut Flakes
Hy-Vee
Sweetened Flake Coconut
Let's Do...Organic ✓
Organic Coconut Flakes
Organic Reduced Fat Shredded Coconut
Organic Shredded Coconut
Our Family
Coconut Flakes, Sweetened
Shredded Coconut, Sweetened
Publix
Coconut Flakes
Schnucks
Coconut Flakes
Stop & Shop
Sweetened Tender Coconut Flakes
Valu Time (Brookshire)
Coconut Flake
Vons
Shredded Coconut
Wegmans
Coconut
Sweetened Flaked Coconut

Corn Syrup

Brer Rabbit ⓘ
Syrup - Full
Syrup - Light
Crosby's
Corn Syrup
Food Club (Brookshire)
Lite Corn Syrup
Food Club (Marsh)
Lite Corn Syrup
Golding Farms ⓘ
Light Corn Syrup

Hill Country Fare (H-E-B)
Dark Corn Syrup
Light Corn Syrup
Karo
Karo Syrups (All)
Meijer
Lite Corn Syrup
Valu Time (Brookshire)
Lite Corn Syrup
Wholesome Sweeteners
Organic Light Corn Syrup

CORNMEAL

Arrowhead Mills
Blue Corn Meal
Yellow Corn Meal
Bob's Red Mill
GF Cornmeal
Food Club (Brookshire)
Instant Grits, Butter
Instant Grits, Regular
Quick Grits
Gifts of Nature ✓
Yellow Cornmeal
Goya
Arepa de Choclo
Coarse Corn Meal ()
Fine Corn Meal ()
Harina P.A.N. White ()
Harina P.A.N. Yellow ()
Maiz ()
Masarepa/White ()
Masarepa/Yellow ()
Pinol (Ground Toasted Corn)
Hodgson Mill
Organic Yellow Corn Meal ⓘ
White Corn Meal, Plain ⓘ
Yellow Corn Meal, Plain ⓘ
Kinnikinnick Foods
Kinnikinnick Foods (All)
Publix
Plain Yellow Corn Meal
Really Great Food
Really Great Food (All)
Rice River Farms ⓘ
Cornmeal, Blue

Cornmeal, Red
Sam Mills ✓
Corn Grits
Corn Meal
Valu Time (Brookshire)
Instant Grits- Regular
Vons
Yellow Corn Meal

EXTRACTS AND FLAVORINGS

Aimee's Livin' Magic
Peruvian Mesquite Powder
Really Raw Tahitian Vanilla Powder
Always Save
Imitation Vanilla Extract
Authentic Foods
Natural Flavors (All)
Autocrat
Coffee Extract
Tea Extract
Bakto Flavors
Bakto Flavors (All)
Best Choice
Pure Vanilla
Bombay
Biryani Paste
Curry Pastes (All)
Butter Buds
Butter Buds (All)
Capella Flavor Drops
Capella Flavor Drops (All)
DeLallo
Lime Juice ⓘ
Durkee
Liquid Extracts (All)
Liquid Flavorings (All)
Encore Woodland
Liquid Smoke, Hickory
Liquid Smoke, Mesquite
Faerie's Finest
Faerie's Finest (All)
Flavorganics
Organic Flavor Extracts (All)
Organic Flavor Syrups (All)
Food Club (Brookshire)
Coconut Flavoring Imitation

Orange Flavoring Imitation
Peppermint Flavoring Imitation
Pure Almond Extract
Pure Lemon Extract
Rum Flavoring Imitation
Vanilla Extract
Vanilla Flavor Clear Imitation
Vanilla Flavor Imitation

Giant
Pure Vanilla Extract

Gifts of Nature ✔
Cook Vanilla Powder

Gold Medal Spices ()
Almond Extract, Imitation
Lemon Extract, Artificial Non-Alcoholic
Lemon Extract, Pure
Vanilla Extract, 3 Star Imitation
Vanilla Extract, Imitation
Vanilla Extract, Imitation & Natural
Vanilla Extract, Pure

Goya
Vanilla Extract

Great Value (Wal-Mart) 25
100% Lemon Juice

Griffin Foods
Griffin Foods (All)

H-E-B
Sabor Tradicional Cajeta

Hill Country Fare (H-E-B)
Imitation Vanilla

InJoy Organics
Cinnamon Sweet

King Arthur
Madagascar Bourbon Vanilla Extract
Mexican Vanilla Extract

Molly McButter 🏅
Molly McButter Products (All)

Nielsen-Massey ✔
Nielsen-Massey (All)

Orgran ⓘ 🏅
Custard Powder

Our Family
Imitation Vanilla Extract
Vanilla Extract

Perfect Puree, The ⓘ
Perfect Puree, The (All)

Price Chopper
Pure Vanilla Extract
Squeeze Lemon Juice

Publix
Almond Extract
Lemon Extract
Vanilla Extract

Really Great Food 🏅
Really Great Food (All)

Rice River Farms ⓘ
Bourbon Style Vanilla Extract
Champignon Powder Extract
Madagascar Vanilla Extract
Tamarind Concentrate
Vanilla Beans, Bourbon Madagascar
Vanilla Beans, Tahitian Papua New
Guinea

Rodelle ⓘ
Gourmet Vanilla Extract
Organic Almond Extract
Organic Lemon Extract
Organic Pure Vanilla Extract
Pure Vanilla Extract
Vanilla Beans
Vanilla Flavor (Alcohol Free)

Safeway 〰
Extract Pure Almond
Pure Vanilla Extract

Sauer's ()
Almond Extract, Pure
Anise Extract, Pure
Banana Extract, Imitation
Black Walnut Extract, Imitation
Brandy Flavor, Pure
Butter Flavor
Cinnamon Extract, Pure
Coconut Extract, Imitation
Lemon Extract, Pure
Maple Extract, Imitation
Mint Extract, Pure
Orange Extract, Pure
Peppermint Extract
Pineapple Extract, Imitation
Rum Flavor, Pure
Sherry Flavor, Pure
Strawberry Extract, Imitation
Vanilla Butter & Nut Extract, Imitation

Vanilla Colorless Extract, Imitation
Vanilla Extract, Natural & Imitation
Vanilla Extract, Pure
Schnucks
Imitation Vanilla
Liquid Smoke (Hickory, Mesquite)
Vanilla
Simply Organic
Almond Extract ☷
Lemon Flavor ☷
Orange Flavor ☷
Peppermint Flavor ☷
Vanilla Extract ☷
Vanilla Extract, Ugandan ☷
Singing Dog Vanilla
Pure Vanilla Extract
Vanilla Bean Paste
Spice Islands
see also Durkee
Specialty - Vanilla Bean
Stop & Shop
Almond Extract
Lemon Extract
Pure Vanilla Extract
Supreme Spice ()
Supreme Spice (All)
Taza Chocolate
Chocolate Mexicano Extracts (All)
Tone's
see also Durkee
Trader Joe's
Vanilla Extract (All)
TryMe
Liquid Smoke
Valu Time (Brookshire)
Vanilla, Imitation
Valu Time (Marsh)
Vanilla, Imitation
Wegmans
Lemon Juice From Concentrate
Vanilla Extract
Wright's Liquid Smoke ⓘ
Liquid Smoke - Hickory
Liquid Smoke - Mesquite

FLAX MEAL

Bob's Red Mill
Brown Flaxseed Meal
Golden Flaxseed Meal
Organic Brown Flaxseed Meal
Organic Golden Flaxseed Meal
Hill Country Fare (H-E-B)
Corn Masa Mix
Hodgson Mill
Brown Milled Flax Seed ☷
Milled Flax Seed
Milled Flax Seed "Travel Flax"
Organic Golden Milled Flax Seed
Organic Golden Milled Flax Seed
"Travel Flax"
Organic Milled Flax Seed ☷
Linusit
Premium Vitality Assured Organic
Ground Flaxseed
LinuSprout
Organic Sprouted Flax Powder
Organic Sprouted Flax Powder with
Blueberries
Organic Sprouted Flax Powder with
Cranberries
Organic Sprouted Flax Powder with Goji
Berries
Mom's Place Gluten-Free ☷
Mom's Place Gluten-Free (All)

FLOURS & FLOUR MIXES

1-2-3 Gluten Free ☷ ✓
Olivia's Outstanding Multi-Purpose
Fortified Flour Mix
Ancient Harvest ☷
Quinoa Flour
Arrowhead Mills
Brown Rice Flour
Buckwheat Flour
Long Grain Brown Rice Flour
Millet Flour
Soy Flour
White Rice Flour
Authentic Foods
Baking Flours (All)

Bay State Milling
Gluten-Free All Purpose Flour
Better Batter
Gluten Free All-Purpose Flour
Gluten Free Seasoned Flour
Bi Aglut
Bi Aglut (All)
Bisquick
Bisquick Gluten Free
Bob's Red Mill
Almond Meal/Flour
Black Bean Flour
Brown Rice Flour
Fava Bean Flour
Garbanzo Bean Flour
Garbanzo/Fava Bean Flour
GF All Purpose Baking Flour
GF Corn Flour
GF Masa Harina
GF Oat Flour
Green Pea Flour
Hazelnut Flour/Meal
Millet Flour
Millet Grits/Meal
Organic Amaranth Flour
Organic Brown Rice Flour
Organic Coconut Flour
Organic Quinoa Flour
Organic White Rice Flour
Potato Flour
Sorghum Flour
Sweet White Rice Flour
Tapioca Flour
Teff Flour
White Bean Flour
White Rice Flour
Breads From Anna
Gluten & Yeast Free Bread Mix (All-Purpose Flour Blend)
Coconut Secret ⓘ
Coconut Flour
Dowd & Rogers ✓
California Almond Flour
Italian Chestnut Flour
Eating Gluten Free ✓
Eating Gluten Free (All)

Ener-G
Brown Rice Flour
Corn Mix
Gluten-Free Gourmet Blend
Potato Flour
Potato Mix
Potato Starch Flour
Rice Mix
Sweet Rice Flour
Tapioca Flour
White Rice Flour
Fearn Natural Foods ⓘ
Brown Rice Baking Mix
Natural Soya Powder
Rice Baking Mix
Rice Flour
Foods Alive ⚱
Organic Raw Mesquite Powder/Flour
Gifts of Nature ✓
All Purpose Flour
Baby Lima Bean Flour
Brown Rice Flour
Chick Pea Flour
Montina All Purpose Blend
Sweet Rice Flour
Tapioca Flour
White Rice Flour
Gillian's Foods ⚱
Gillian's Foods (All)
Glutano
Gluten-Free Flour Mix
Gluten Free Mama
Mama's Almond Blend Flour
Mama's Coconut Blend Flour
Gluten-Free Naturals ⚱ ✓
Gluten-Free Naturals (All)
Gluten-Free Pantry, The
All-Purpose Flour Mix
Gluuteny ⚱
Gluuteny (All)
GoGo Quinoa ✓
GoGo Quinoa (All)
Goya
Bacalaitos ⧗
Donarepa Corn Flour/White
Donarepa Corn Flour/Yellow
Extra Fine Corn Flour ⧗

Farinha de Mandioca ()
Harina de Arvejas ()
Harina de Habas ()
Mandioca
Masarepa ()
Rice Flour ()
Trigo ()
Yuca Flour (Tapioca) ()

Grandpa's Kitchen
Grandpa's Kitchen (All)

Hodgson Mill
Brown Rice Flour ⓘ
Buckwheat Flour ⓘ
Gluten-Free All Purpose Flour
Organic Soy Flour ⓘ
Soy Flour ⓘ

Honeyville
Bakers Soy Flour
Blanched Almond Flour
Natural Almond Flour
Potato Flour
White Corn Flour
Yellow Corn Flour

JK Gourmet
Almond Flour

Jules Gluten Free
All Purpose Flour

King Arthur
Ancient Grains Flour Blend
Gluten-Free Brown Rice Flour
Gluten-Free Multi-Purpose Flour
Gluten-Free Sorghum Flour
Gluten-Free Whole Grain Flour Blend

Kinnikinnick Foods
Kinnikinnick Foods (All)

Let's Do…Organic ✓
Organic Coconut Flour

Little Aussie Bakery, The
The Little Aussie Bakery (All)

Living Intentions
Super Flour (All)

Lundberg Family Farms
Eco-Farmed Brown Rice Flour
Organic Brown Rice Flour

Mom's Place Gluten-Free
Mom's Place Gluten-Free (All)

Montana Monster Munchies ⓘ ✓
Gluten Free Whole Grain Oat Flour

Montana
All-Purpose Flour Blend
Brown Rice Flour Blend
Pure Baking Flour Supplement

Namaste Foods ✓
Flour Blend

NutraSprout
Sprouted Broccoli Seed Powder

Nu-World Amaranth
Amaranth Flour (All)
Toasted Amaranth Bran Flour (All)

Orgran ⓘ
All Purpose Plain Flour
Self Raising Flour

Pocono
Buckwheat Flour

Really Great Food
Really Great Food (All)

Rice River Farms ⓘ
Blanched Almond Meal
Buckwheat Flour
Masa Harina
Roasted Chestnut Powder
White Rice Flour
Wild Rice Flour

Ritrovo
Gluten-Free Hazelnut Flour

Sam Mills ✓
Corn Flour

Simpli ⓘ
Gluten Free Whole Oat Flour

Something Good
Something Good (All)

Sylvan Border Farm
General Purpose Flour

Tom Sawyer
All Purpose Gluten-Free Flour (All)

Trader Joe's
Almond Nut Meal

Well & Good
Well & Good (All)

Zocalo Gourmet
Zocalo Gourmet (All)

Food Coloring

Durkee
Food Coloring (All)
Food Club (Brookshire)
Food Color Set
Red Food Color
Yellow Food Color
Gold Medal Spices ()
Red Color
Safeway ⌒
Food Coloring Assorted
Sauer's ()
Green Food Color
Red Food Color
Yellow Food Color
Spice Islands
see also Durkee
Tone's
see also Durkee

Frosting

Betty Crocker
Butter Cream Whipped Frosting
Cherry Rich & Creamy Frosting
Chocolate Rich & Creamy Frosting
Chocolate Whipped Frosting
Coconut Pecan Rich & Creamy Frosting
Cream Cheese Rich & Creamy Frosting
Cream Cheese Whipped Frosting
Dark Chocolate Rich & Creamy Frosting
Fluffy White Whipped Frosting
Lemon Rich & Creamy Frosting
Milk Chocolate Rich & Creamy Frosting
Milk Chocolate Whipped Frosting
Rainbow Chip Rich & Creamy Frosting
Strawberry Mist Whipped Frosting
Triple Chocolate Fudge Chip Rich &
    Creamy Frosting
Vanilla Rich & Creamy Frosting
Vanilla Whipped Frosting
Whipped Cream Whipped Frosting
Dr. Oetker
Cake Glaze - Clear
Chocolate Icing
Vanilla Icing

Food Club (Brookshire)
Coating Chocolate Microwavable Candy
Coating Vanilla Microwaveable Candy
Food-Tek ()
Gluten-Free Quick-Bake Line (All)
Grainless Baker, The ⸸
The Grainless Baker (All)
Namaste Foods ⸸ ✓
Frosting Mix (All)
Pamela's Products ⓘ
Dark Chocolate Frosting Mix
Vanilla Frosting Mix

Honey

BeeMaid
Honey (All)
Burleson's Honey
Burleson's Honey (All)
Capilano
Capilano (All)
**Central Market Classics
(Price Chopper)**
Blueberry Honey
Buckwhite Honey
Organic Blossom Honey
Darbo
Creamy Clover
Creamy Sunflower
Fine Acacia
Fine Blossom
Fine Fir and Spruce
Fine Forest
Fine Highland
Dutch Gold Honey
Dutch Gold Honey (All)
Fischer's Honey
Honey Products (All)
Food Club (Brookshire)
Honey
Food Club (Marsh)
Honey, Inverted Squeeze Bottle
Honey, Squeeze Bear
Full Circle (Schnucks)
Honey Inverted Bottle
Organic Honey Bear

Giant
Pure Clover Honey
Golding Farms ⓘ
Clover Honey
Goya
Honey
Great Value (Wal-Mart) 🔲25
Clover Honey
GreenWise Market (Publix)
Organic Honey
Haggen
Honey
Hawkshead Relish
Honey (All)
Honey Acres
Honey (All)
Hy-Vee
Honey (Squeeze Bear)
Madhava 🎖
Honey (All)
Meijer
Honey (Squeeze Bear, Squeeze Bottle)
Mother's Mountain
Orange Blossom Honey
Star Thistle Honey
Wildflower Honey
Mountain Ridge ⓘ
Pure Raw Honey
Naturally Healthy ⓘ
Pure Honey
Nature's Promise (Giant)
Organic Golden Honey
Nature's Promise (Stop & Shop)
Organic Golden Honey
O Organics 〰
Honey
Our Family
Honey Bear
Price Chopper
Honey
Honey Bears
Publix
Clover Honey
Orange Blossom Honey
Wildflower Honey
Really Raw Honey
Honey (All) ⟲

Rice River Farms ⓘ
Honey, Granulated
Honey, Powdered
Rice's Honey
Rice's Honey (All)
Savannah Bee Company
Savannah Bee Company (All)
Schnucks
Honey
Honey Bear
Silverbow Honey
Silverbow Honey (All)
Stop & Shop
Pure Clover Honey
Sue Bee Honey
Honey (All)
Suzanne's Specialties 🎖
Honey
Tassos
Honey (All)
Trader Joe's
Honey (All)
Valu Time (Brookshire)
Honey
Valu Time (Marsh)
Honey
Valu Time (Schnucks)
Honey
Vita Foods ⓘ
Virginia Brand Pure Honey
Vons 〰
Honey Clover
Honey Clover Squeeze Bear
Wegmans
100% Pure Clover Honey
Clover Honey - Grade A
Clover Honey
Orange Blossom Honey
Squeezeable Bear 100% Pure Clover
Honey
Wholesome Sweeteners
Organic Amber Honey
Organic Raw Honey
Zocalo Gourmet
Organic Mesquite Honey

Marshmallows

Always Save
Marshmallows
Mini Marshmallows

Best Choice
Marshmallows
Mini Marshmallows

Flavorite (Cub Foods)
Mini Marshmallows

Food Club (Brookshire)
Marshmallow Crème
Marshmallow, Mini
Marshmallow, Regular

Food Club (Marsh)
Marshmallow Creme
Marshmallows Mini
Marshmallows Regular

Giant
Marshmallows

Giant Eagle
Marshmallows
Mini Marshmallows

Great Value (Wal-Mart) 25
Marshmallow Creme
Marshmallows
Marshmallows Miniature
Miniature Flavored Marshmallows
Miniature Marshmallows

Haggen
Marshmallow Crème
Marshmallows (Mini, Regular)

Hy-Vee
Colored Miniature Marshmallows
Marshmallows
Miniature Marshmallows

Jet-Puffed
Marshmallow Creme, Marshmallow
   Creme
Marshmallows
Marshmallows, Mini Variety Pack
Marshmallows, Miniature
Marshmallows, Miniature Choco
   Mallows
Marshmallows, Miniature Strawberry
   Mallows
Marshmallows, Starmallows Vanilla
Marshmallows, Strawberrymallows

Marshmallows, Swirl Mallows Caramel
   & Vanilla
Marshmallows, Toasted Coconut
Miniature Marshmallows, Funmallows

Jewel-Osco
Regular Marshmallows
White Mini Marshmallows

Kroger
Big Marshmallows
Mini Marshmallows

Manischewitz
Marshmallow Cups
Marshmallows

Marshmallow Fluff
Marshmallow Fluff

Meijer
Marshmallows
Mini Flavored Marshmallows
Mini Marshmallows

Our Family
Marshmallows (Mini, Fruit Flavored,
   Regular)

Price Chopper
Mini Marshmallow
Pastel Mini Marshmallow
Regular Marshmallow

Publix
Marshmallows

Safeway
Regular Marshmallows

Schnucks
Marshmallow Crème
Marshmallows
Mini Marshmallows

Solo ()
Marshmallow Crème
Toasted Marshmallow Crème

Stop & Shop
Marshmallows
Mini White Marshmallows

Suzanne's Specialties
Marshmallows

Valu Time (Marsh)
Marshmallow Creme

Winn-Dixie
Marshmallows (Mini, Regular)

MARZIPAN

Marzipan House, The
The Marzipan House (All)
Solo ◇
Almond Paste
Marzipan

MILK, CONDENSED

Albertsons
Sweetened Condensed Milk
Best Choice
Sweetened Condensed Milk
Eagle Brand
Sweetened Condensed Milk
Food Club (Brookshire)
Sweetened Condensed Milk
Food Club (Marsh)
Sweetened Condensed Milk
Giant
Sweetened Condensed Milk
Goya
Condensed Milk
Fat Free La Lechera
La Lechera "Christmas"
La Lechera Condensed Milk
La Lechera Mini
La Lechera Squeeze
Nela Condensed Milk
Nestle La Lechera 50% Less Sugar
Great Value (Wal-Mart) 25
Fat Free Sweetened Condensed Milk
Sweetened Condensed Milk
Hy-Vee
Sweetened Condensed Milk
Meijer
Sweetened Condensed Milk
Nestlé Carnation
Sweetened Condensed Milk
Our Family
Sweetened Condensed Milk
Schnucks
Sweetened Condensed Milk
Shaw's
Kosher Condensed Milk
Shoppers Value (Albertsons)
Canned Milk

Shoppers Value (Cub Foods)
Canned Milk
Stop & Shop
Sweetened Condensed Milk
Valu Time (Brookshire)
Sweetened Condensed Milk
Vons ↩
Condensed Milk Sweetened
Wegmans
Sweetened Condensed Milk

MILK, EVAPORATED

Best Choice
Evaporated Milk
Food Club (Brookshire)
Evaporated Fat Free Milk
Evaporated Milk
Food Club (Marsh)
Evaporated Milk
Giant
Evaporated Milk
Evaporated Milk with Vitamin D
Goya
Nela Evaporated Milk
Nestle Nido + Kinder
Great Value (Wal-Mart) 25
Evaporated Fat Free Milk
Evaporated Milk
Fat Free Evaporated Skimmed Milk
Hy-Vee
Fat Free Evaporated Milk
Meijer
Evaporated Milk
Lite Skimmed Evaporated Milk
Meyenberg
Evaporated Goat Milk
Nestlé Carnation
Evaporated Milk
Fat Free Evaporated Milk
Low Fat Evaporated Milk
Our Family
Evaporated Milk
Schnucks
Evaporated Milk
Stop & Shop
Evaporated Milk with Vitamin D

Fat Free Evaporated Milk
Valu Time (Brookshire)
Evaporated Milk
Valu Time (Marsh)
Filled Evaporated Milk
Valu Time (Schnucks)
Evaporated Milk
Vons ↝
Evaporated Milk
Fat Free Evaporated Milk
Wegmans
Evaporated Milk
Fat Free Evaporated Milk

MILK, INSTANT OR POWDERED

Always Save
Instant Milk
Best Choice
Instant Milk
Food Club (Brookshire)
Instant Milk
Giant
Non Fat Instant Dry Milk
Goya
Nido
Meijer
Instant Milk
Meyenberg
Powdered Goat Milk
Nestlé Carnation
Instant Nonfat Dry Milk
Organic Valley ⓘ
Buttermilk Blend Powder
Nonfat Dry Milk Powder
Our Family
Instant Nonfat Dry Milk
Price Chopper
Instant Milk
Publix
Instant Nonfat Dry Milk
Saco
Mix'n Drink (All)
Safeway ↝
Dry Milk, Nonfat
Instant Non Fat Dry Milk

Schnucks
Instant Milk
Stop & Shop
Instant Non Fat Dry Milk
Winn-Dixie
Instant Nonfat Dry Milk

MOLASSES

Brer Rabbit ⓘ
Molasses - Blackstrap
Molasses - Full
Molasses - Mild
Crosby's 🎖
Molasses
Golding Farms ⓘ
Molasses
Grandma's Molasses ⓘ
Original
Robust
Griffin Foods
Griffin Foods (All)
Imperial Sugar
Molasses (All)
Oskri
Molasses (All)
Plantation Molasses
Barbados Molasses
Blackstrap Molasses
Certified Organic Blackstrap
Holiday Blackstrap Molasses
Suzanne's Specialties 🎖
Molasses
Wholesome Sweeteners
Organic Blackstrap Molasses

OIL & OIL SPRAYS

ACME
Canola Cooking Spray
Vegetable Cooking Spray
Albertsons
Cooking Spray Butter Flavor
Extra Virgin Olive Oil Spray
Peanut Oil
Pure Corn Oil
Soybean Vegetable Oil

Vegetable Canola Oil
Vegetable Cooking Spray Can

Always Save
Canola Oil
Corn Oil
Pan Coating
Pure Vegetable Oil
Vegetable Oil

Always Save (Price Chopper)
Corn Oil
Vegetable Oil

Ambassador Organics
Olive Oil (All)

B.R. Cohn
Olive Oils (All)

Best Choice
Blended Vegetable Oil
Butter Pan Coating
Canola Oil
Canola Pan Spray
Corn Oil
Corn Oil Pan Coating
Extra Virgin Olive Oil
Extra-Virgin Lite Olive Oil
Olive Oil
Olive Oil Pan Coating
Peanut Oil
Pure Corn Oil
Pure Vegetable Oil
Pure Vegetable Shortening
Vegetable Oil

Bionaturae
Extra Virgin Olive Oil ⅊

Blue Plate
Oil

Bragg
Bragg (All)

Brookfarm ⓘ
Lemon Myrtle Infused Macadamia Oil
Lime and Chili Infused Macadamia Oil
Premium Natural Macadamia Oil

Cat Cora's Kitchen
Extra Virgin Olive Oil
Kalamata DOP Extra Virgin Olive Oil
Organic Extra Virgin Olive Oil

Sitia, Crete DOP Extra Virgin Olive Oil

**Central Market Classics
(Price Chopper)**
Basil Olive Oil
Extra Virgin Olive Oil
Garlic Herb Basil Olive Oil
Garlic Olive Oil
Grape Seed Oil
Hot Dipping Oil
Italian Dipping Oil
Lemon Olive Oil
Roasted Pepper Olive Oil

China Sun
Pure Sesame Oil

Clearly Organic (Best Choice)
Extra Virgin Olive Oil

Colavita
Oil (All)

Cub Foods
Butter Spray
Olive Oil Spray

Davis & Davis
Cooking & Dipping Oil (All Flavors)

DeLallo
Basil Flavored Dipping Oil ⓘ
Canola Oil ⓘ
Extra Light Olive Oil ⓘ
Extra Virgin Olive Oil ⓘ
Extra Virgin Olive Oil, Unfiltered
   Organic ⓘ
Garlic Flavored Dipping Oil
Grapeseed Oil ⓘ
Lemon Flavored Dipping Oil ⓘ
Pure Olive Oil ⓘ
Red Pepper Flavored Dipping Oil ⓘ
Vegetable Oil ⓘ

Eden Foods
Hot Pepper Sesame Oil
Organic Safflower Oil
Organic Sesame Oil
Organic Soybean Oil
Spanish Olive Oil - Extra Virgin
Toasted Sesame Oil

Edible Haven
- 100% Natural and Organic Virgin Coconut Oil

EMERIL'S ♱
- Cooking Sprays (Canola Oil, Buttery)

Fastco (Fareway)
- Canola Oil
- Corn Oil
- Regular Cooking Spray
- Vegetable Oil

Filippo Berio
- Olive Oil (All)

Flavorite (Cub Foods)
- Butter Cooking Spray
- Olive Oil Cooking Spray
- Vegetable Oil Spread

Food Club (Brookshire)
- Baker's Release Cooking Spray
- Canola Oil
- Cooking Spray, Butter
- Cooking Spray, Canola
- Cooking Spray, Extra Virgin Olive Oil
- Cooking Spray, Vegetable Oil
- Corn Oil
- Extra Virgin Olive Oil
- Olive Oil, Mild
- Peanut Oil
- Pure Olive Oil
- Vegetable Oil

Food Club (Marsh)
- Canola Oil
- Cooking Spray, Butter
- Cooking Spray, Canola
- Cooking Spray, Extra Virgin Olive Oil
- Corn Oil
- Extra Virgin Olive Oil
- Mild Olive Oil
- Pure Olive Oil
- Vegetable Oil

Food You Feel Good About (Wegmans)
- Black Truffle Extra Virgin Olive Oil
- Grapeseed Oil
- Organic High Oleic Sunflower Oil
- Pumpkin Seed Oil

- Pure Walnut Oil
- Sicilian Lemon Extra Virgin Olive Oil

Foods Alive ♱
- Organic Green Gold Hemp Oil
- Organic High Lignan Flax Oil

Full Circle (Price Chopper)
- Extra Virgin Olive Oil
- Olive Oil

Full Circle (Schnucks)
- Canola Oil
- Canola Oil Cooking Spray
- Extra Virgin Olive Oil
- Olive Oil Cooking Spray
- Organic Balsamic Vinegar
- Soybean Oil
- Vegetable Oil Cooking Spray

Gaea ()
- Olive Oil (All)

Giant
- All Natural Non Stick Butter Flavored Cooking Spray
- Canola Oil
- Corn Oil
- Extra Light Olive Oil
- Extra Virgin Olive Oil
- Non Stick Canola Oil Cooking Spray
- Olive Oil Cooking Spray
- Peanut Oil
- Pure Olive Oil
- Vegetable Oil

Giant Eagle
- Extra Light Olive Oil
- Pure Olive Oil

Goya
- Extra Virgin Olive Oil
- Light Olive Oil
- Pure Corn Oil
- Pure Olive Oil
- Vegetable Oil

Grand Selections (Hy-Vee)
- 100% Pure & Natural Olive Oil
- Balsamic Vinegar of Modina
- Extra Virgin Olive Oil
- Olive Oil Lemon

Great Value (Wal-Mart) 25
   100% Extra Virgin Olive Oil
   Blended Canola Oil
   Canola Oil
   Canola Oil Blend
   Corn Oil
   Extra Virgin Olive Oil
   Light Tasting Olive Oil
   Olive Oil
   Pure Canola Oil
   Pure Corn Oil, Bilingual
   Pure Vegetable Oil

Haggen
   Blended Oil
   Canola Oil
   Cooking Spray, Butter
   Cooking Spray, Canola
   Cooking Spray, Olive Oil
   Corn Oil
   Extra Virgin Olive Oil
   Light Olive Oil
   Olive Oil
   Vegetable Cooking Oil
   Vegetable Oil

Hawkshead Relish
   Flavored Oils (All)

Hy-Vee
   100% Pure Canola Oil
   100% Pure Corn Oil
   100% Pure Vegetable Oil
   Natural Blend Oil

Italian Classics (Schnucks)
   Basil Garlic Olive Oil
   Extra Virgin Olive Oil
   Garlic Olive Oil
   Pure Olive Oil

Italian Classics (Wegmans)
   Campania Oil
   Tuscany Oil

Jewel-Osco
   48% Vegetable Oil Spread
   Butter Flavor Cooking Spray
   Canola Cooking Spray
   Olive Oil Cooking Spray
   Vegetable Cooking Spray

Kernel Season's ⓘ
   Popping and Topping Oil

Kevala
   Toasted Sesame Oil

Lapas ()
   Olive Oil

Linusit
   Organic Premium Flax Oil
   Organic Premium Flax Oil with Toasted
    Sesame

Living Harvest ⓘ ✔
   Living Harvest Hemp Oil

Lucini Italia
   Oils (All)

Manischewitz
   Cooking Sprays (All Varieties)
   Vegetable Oil

Market District (Giant Eagle)
   Extra Virgin Olive Oil

Mazola
   Oils & Sprays (All)

Meijer
   100% Pure Italian Classic Olive Oil
   Blended Canola & Vegetable Oil
   Canola Oil
   Cooking Spray, Butter
   Cooking Spray, Extra Virgin Olive Oil
   Cooking Spray, Vegetable Oil
   Corn Oil
   Extra Virgin Italian Classic Olive Oil
   Extra Virgin Olive Oil
   Infused Italian Garlic and Basil Olive Oil
   Infused Italian Roasted Garlic Olive Oil
   Infused Italian Spicy Red Pepper Olive
    Oil
   Italian Select Premium Extra Virgin Oil
   Milder Tasting Olive Oil
   Olive Oil
   Peanut Oil
   Shortening
   Sunflower Oil
   Vegetable Oil

Midwest Country Fare (Hy-Vee)
   100% Pure Vegetable Oil
   Vegetable Oil

Montebello ()
   Olive Oil

Mrs. Bryant's
Estate Fresh Gourmet™ L'essence de Oil Melange (Olive Oil Blend)

Napa Valley Naturals ()
Culinary Oils (All)

Nature's Basket (Giant Eagle)
Virgin Olive Oil

Nature's Promise (Giant)
Organic Canola Oil Cooking Spray (Non Stick)
Organic Olive Oil Cooking Spray (Non Stick)

Nature's Promise (Stop & Shop)
Organic Cooking Spray, Olive Oil (Non-Stick)

Newman's Own Organics ⓘ
Olive Oil

Nunez de Prado ()
Olive Oil

Nutiva
Coconut Oils (All) ♀
Hemp Oil ♀

O Olive Oil ♀
Oils (All)

O Organics ⤶
Canola Oil Cooking Spray
Extra Virgin Olive Oil
Olive Oil Cooking Spray

Olivado
Olivado (All)

Oskri
Oils (All)

Our Family
Butter Flavor Cooking Spray
Canola Oil
Canola Spray
Cooking Spray
Corn Oil
Extra Virgin Olive Oil
Light Olive Oil
Olive Oil
Peanut Oil
Vegetable Oil
Vegetable Shortening

Pastene
Extra Virgin Olive Oil
Garlic Oil

Olive Oil
Organic Olive Oil
Pure Olive Oil

Pinnaroo Hill
Olive Oil (All)

Pompeian
Grapeseed Oil (All)
Olive Oil (All)
OlivExtra Blends (All)

Price Chopper
Butter Cooking Spray
Canola Oil
Canola/Soy Bean Oil
Classic Olive Oil
Corn Oil
Extra-Virgin Olive Oil
Light Olive Oil
Olive Oil Cooking Spray
Organic Olive Oil
Peanut Oil
Pure Classic Olive Oil
Sunflower Oil
Vegetable Oil

Publix
Butter Flavored Cooking Spray
Canola Oil
Corn Oil
Olive Oil
Olive Oil Cooking Spray
Original Canola Cooking Spray
Peanut Oil
Vegetable Oil

Red Island Australia
Olive Oil

Rice River Farms ⓘ
Truffle Oil Spray, Black French
Truffle Oil Spray, White French
Truffle Oil, Black
Truffle Oil, White

Ruth's Hemp Foods ✓
Hemp Oil

Safeway ⤶
Canola Blend Vegetable Oil
Grill Cooking Spray
Peanut Oil, One Time Buy Holiday
Vegetable Oil

Safeway Select 🪶
- Brown Rice with Extra Virgin Olive Oil
- Extra Virgin Olive Oil
- Pure Light Olive Oil
- Verdi Extra Light Olive Oil
- Verdi Extra Virgin Olive Oil
- Verdi Pure Olive Oil

Sam Mills ✓
- Extra Virgin Corn Oil

Santa Barbara Olive Co.
- Santa Barbara Olive Co. (All)

Schnucks
- Canola Blend
- Canola Oil
- Corn Oil
- Extra Virgin Olive Oil
- Modified Oil
- Olive Oil
- Peanut Oil
- Shortening
- Vegetable Oil

Shaw's
- All Natural Canola Cooking Spray
- Cooking Spray
- Natural Cooking Spray

Shoppers Value (ACME)
- Vegetable Oil

Shoppers Value (Albertsons)
- Vegetable Oil

Shoppers Value (Cub Foods)
- Vegetable Oil

Shoppers Value (Jewel-Osco)
- Vegetable Oil

Smart Balance
- Smart Balance (All)

Stop & Shop
- Canola Oil
- Canola Oil Cooking Spray
- Extra Light Olive Oil
- Extra Virgin Olive Oil
- Non Stick Butter Cooking Spray
- Non Stick Vegetable Oil Cooking Spray
- Olive Oil Cooking Spray
- Vegetable Oil

Sun Luck
- Chili Oil (Hot, La Yu)
- Chili Sesame Oil, Hot
- Seasoned Wok Oil
- Sesame Oil, Pure

Tassos
- Olive Oil (All)

Trader Joe's
- Canola Oil Spray (All)
- Oils (All)

Valu Time (Brookshire)
- Canola Oil
- Cooking Spray- Vegetable Oil
- Corn Oil
- Shortening
- Vegatable Oil

Valu Time (Marsh)
- Canola Oil
- Corn Oil
- Vegetable Oil

Valu Time (Schnucks)
- Canola Oil
- Corn Oil
- Vegetable Oil

Villa Flor ()
- Olive Oil

Vons 🪶
- Cooking Spray Olive Oil
- Corn Oil
- Oil, All Natural Vegetable
- Oil, Canola
- Salad Oil

Weber
- Grill 'N Spray

Wegmans
- 100% Pure Olive Oil
- 100% Soybean Vegetable Oil
- Basting Oil
- Campania Style Extra Virgin Olive Oil
- Canola Oil
- Canola Oil Cooking Spray
- Corn Oil Cooking Spray
- Extra Virgin Olive Oil
- Mild Olive Oil
- Natural Butter Flavor Canola Oil Cooking Spray
- Novello Unfiltered Extra Virgin Olive Oil
- Olive Oil Cooking Spray
- Peanut Oil

Puglia Oil
Puglia Style Extra Virgin Olive Oil
Pure Olive Oil
Sicilian Style Extra Virgin Olive Oil
Submarine Sandwich Oil
Tuscany Style Extra Virgin Olive Oil
Vegetable Oil
Wesson
Oils (All)
Wilderness Poets
Wilderness Poets (All)
Winn-Dixie
Canola Oil
Corn Oil
Olive Oil
Peanut Oil
Vegetable Oil

PECTIN

Ball ()
Pectin (All)
MCP ✎
Fruit Pectin, Premium 100% Natural For
Homemade Jams & Jellies
Sure.Jell ✎
Fruit Pectin, Premium
Fruit Pectin, Premium 100% Natural
Taco Bell ✎
Jam Pectin, No Cook
Williams
Jel-Ease Pectin

RICE SYRUP

Lundberg Family Farms ⚇
Eco-Farmed Sweet Dreams Rice Syrup
Organic Sweet Dreams Rice Syrup
Suzanne's Specialties ⚇
Rice Syrup (All BUT Organic Barley
Malt Extract)

SHORTENING & OTHER FATS

Albertsons
Shortening

Always Save
Pre-Creamed Shortening
Always Save (Price Chopper)
Shortening
Fastco (Fareway)
Butter Cooking Spray
Vegetable Shortening
Food Club (Brookshire)
Shortening
Food Club (Marsh)
Shortening
Goya
Lard
Great Value (Wal-Mart) 25
All Vegetable Shortening
Animal Vegetable Shortening
Haggen
Vegetable Shortening
Hy-Vee
Vegetable Oil Shortening
Vegetable Shortening, Butter Flavor
Midwest Country Fare (Hy-Vee)
Pre-Creamed Shortening
Price Chopper
Vegetable Shortening
Publix
Vegetable Shortening
Shoppers Value (Albertsons)
Shortening
Valu Time (Marsh)
Shortening
Spread, 40% Crock
Valu Time (Schnucks)
Shortening
Wegmans
Vegetable Shortening

SPICES & SPICE PACKETS

Ac'cent ⓘ
Flavor Enhancers (All Varieties)
Aimee's Livin' Magic
Himalayan Crystal Salt
Alamo ⚇
All Purpose Seasoning (All)
Always Save
Black Pepper

Garlic Powder
Minced Onion

Amazing Taste ()
Beef Seasoning
Burger Seasoning
Cajun Seasoning
Chili Seasoning
Fajita Seasoning
Garlic & Rosemary Seasoning
Honey BBQ Seasoning
Lemon Pepper Seasoning
Lemon, Butter & Dill Seasoning
Malibu Seasoning
Mr. Grill Seasoning
Orange Chipotle Seasoning
Peppercorn, Garlic & Herb Seasoning
Pork Seasoning
Southwest Seasoning
Steak House Seasoning

Andy's Seasoning
Seasoned Salt

Badia
Cajun Seasoning (Check Label - Previously Contained MSG)
Five Spice (Check Label - Previously Contained MSG)
Garam Masala (Check Label - Previously Contained MSG)
Herbs de Provence (Check Label - Previously Contained MSG)
Italian Seasoning (Check Label - Previously Contained MSG)
Jerk Seasoning (Check Label - Previously Contained MSG)
Poultry Seasoning (Check Label - Previously Contained MSG)
Rotisserie Seasoning (Check Label - Previously Contained MSG)
Sazon Tropical (Check Label - Previously Contained MSG)
Seasoned Salt (Check Label - Previously Contained MSG)
Steak Seasoning (Check Label - Previously Contained MSG)
Straight 100% Spices (All)

Ball ()
Spices (All)

Bell's ()
Bell's Seasoning

Best Choice
Alum
Basil
Basil Leaves
Black Pepper
Celery Seed
Chili Powder
Chives
Cinnamon
Cream of Tartar
Crushed Red Pepper
Curry Powder
Dill Seed
Dill Weed
Fennel Seed
Garlic Powder
Ground Allspice
Ground Cinnamon
Ground Cloves
Ground Cumin
Ground Ginger
Ground Mustard
Ground Oregano
Ground Red Pepper
Ground Sage
Ground White Pepper
Minced Garlic
Mustard Seed
Nutmeg
Onion Powder
Onion, Chopped
Oregano Leaves
Paprika
Parsley Flakes
Poppy Seed
Rosemary Leaves
Rubbed Sage
Salt & Pepper Shakers
Sesame Seed
Thyme Leaves
Turmeric
Whole Cloves

Bombay
Curry Powders (All)

Bone Suckin' Sauce
Bone Suckin' Seasonings & Rubs (All) ()

Bragg
Seasonings (All)

Burnt Sacrifice ()
Spice Rubs (All)

Cajun Injector ⓘ
Cajun- Blended Spice Mix
Cajun Herbed Spice Mix
Cajun Shake Canister
Hickory- Grill Shake Canister
Lemon Pepper Shake Canister

Casa Fiesta ⓘ
Burrito Seasoning Mix
Chili Seasoning Mix
Fajita Seasoning Mix
Guacamole Seasoning Mix
Taco Salad Seasoning Mix
Taco Seasoning Mix

Cat Cora's Kitchen
Red Saffron

Cavender's
Greek Seasoning Salt Free

Celtic Sea Salt
Celtic Sea Salt (All)

Chi-Chi's
Fiesta Restaurante Seasoning Mix

Crockery Gourmet
BBQ Seasoning Mix
Chicken Seasoning Mix
Italian Seasoning Mix
Southwest Seasoning Mix

Cugino's ()
SPANK! Dry Rub Seasoning, Butta
  Beatin' Garlic Butter
SPANK! Dry Rub Seasoning, Marvelous
  Mesquite
SPANK! Dry Rub Seasoning,
  Peppercorn A Crackin'

Dave's Gourmet
Chile Powder (All)

DeLallo
Dipping Seasoning Spices
Sea Salt, Natural (Coarse, Fine) ⓘ

Dr. Gonzo's Uncommon Condiments
Dr. Gonzo's Uncommon Condiments
  (All)

Durkee
Allspice
Alum
Anise Seed
Apple Pie Spice
Basil
Bay Leaves
Caraway Seed
Cardamom
Cayenne Pepper
Celery Flakes
Celery Seed
Chicken & Rib Rub
Chicken Seasoning
Chili Powder
Chives
Cilantro
Cinnamon
Cloves
Coriander
Crazy Dave's Lemon Pepper
Crazy Dave's Pepper & Spice
Crazy Dave's Salt & Spice
Cream of Tartar
Crushed Red Pepper
Cumin
Curry Powder
Dill Seed/Weed
Fennel
Garlic Minced
Garlic Pepper
Garlic Powder
Garlic Salt
Ginger
Green Bell Pepper
Hickory Smoke Salt
Italian Seasoning
Jamaican Jerk Seasoning
Lemon & Herb
Lemon Garlic Seasoning
Lemon Pepper
Lime Pepper
Mace
Marjoram
Meat Tenderizer
Mint Leaves
Mr. Pepper

MSG
Mustard
Nutmeg
Onion Powder
Onion Salt
Onion, Minced
Orange Peel
Oregano
Oriental 5-Spice
Paprika
Parsley
Pepper (Black, White)
Pickling Spice
Pizza Seasoning
Poppy Seed
Poultry Seasoning
Pumpkin Pie Spice
Rosemary
Rosemary Garlic Seasoning
Sage
Salt-Free Garden Seasoning
Salt-Free Garlic & Herb
Salt-Free Lemon Pepper
Salt-Free Original All-Purpose
   Seasoning
Salt-Free Vegetable Seasoning
Seasoned Pepper
Sesame Seed
Six Pepper Blend
Smokey Mesquite Seasoning
Spaghetti/Pasta Seasoning
Spicy Spaghetti Seasoning
Steak Seasoning
Tarragon
Thyme
Turmeric

Eden Foods
Eden Shake (Furikake)
Organic Black & Tan Gomasio (Sesame
   Salt)
Organic Black Gomasio (Sesame Salt)
Organic Garlic Gomasio (Sesame Salt)
Organic Gomasio (Sesame Salt)
Organic Seaweed Gomasio (Sesame
   Salt)
Sea Salt - French
Sea Salt - Portuguese

EMERIL'S ☷
Essence (Bayou Blast, Italian, Original,
   Southwest)
Garlic Parmesan Essence for Bread
Rubs (Chicken, Fish, Rib, Turkey, and
   Steak)

Faerie's Finest ☷
Faerie's Finest (All)

Food Club (Brookshire)
Allspice (Ground, Whole)
Alum, Granulated
Apple Pie Spice
Basil Leaves
Bay Leaves
Black Pepper
Cajun Spice
Cayenne Pepper
Celery Salt
Chicken Grilling Seasoning
Chili Powder
Chili Powder Texas Style
Chives, Chopped
Cilantro Leaves
Cinnamon & Sugar
Cinnamon P.E.T
Cinnamon Sticks
Cloves, Whole
Coarse Ground Black Pepper
Cream of Tartar
Crushed Red Pepper
Crushed Thyme
Curry Powder
Dill Weed
Garlic Bread Spice Sprinkle
Garlic Pepper
Garlic Powder
Garlic Powder California Style
Garlic Powder P.E.T
Garlic Salt
Garlic Salt California Style
Garlic Salt P.E.T
Ground Cinnamon
Ground Cloves
Ground Cumin
Ground Mustard
Ground Sage
Ground Thyme

Ground Turmeric
Groung Nutmeg
Iodized Salt
Italian Seasoning
Meat Tenderizer, Non Seasoned
Meat Tenderizer, Seasoned
Minced Garlic
Minced Onions
Minced Onions P.E.T
Mustard Seed
Onion Powder
Onion Powder California Style
Onion Salt P.E.T
Onions, Chopped
Oregano Leaves
Oregano P.E.T
Paprika P.E.T
Parsley Flakes
Parsley P.E.T
Pepper & Lemon Seasoning
Pepper Medley Grinder
Peppercorns
Pickling Spice
Plain Salt
Rosemary Leaf
Salad Seasoning with Cheese
Salt & Pepper Shaker Set
Sea Salt Grinder
Seafood Grilling Seasoning
Seasoned Salt
Seasoning for Poultry
Seasoning Spice for Fried Chicken
Spice for Pumpkin Pie
Steak Grilling Seasoning
Steak Grilling Seasoning, Spicy
Whole Grinder Black Pepper

Food Club (Marsh)
Beef Stew Seasoning Mix
Black Pepper
Cinnamon
Garlic Powder
Garlic Salt
Onion, Minced
Paprika
Rice, Instant Boil In Bag
Roasting Bag Pot Roast
Salt & Pepper Shaker Set

Salt, Iodized
Salt, Plain
Taco Seasoning Mix

Foods Alive ⚕
Himalayan Crystals Mineral Salt
Organic Raw Maca Powder

Full Circle (Schnucks)
Basil
Bay Leaves
Black Pepper, Whole
Cayenne Pepper
Chili Powder
Cinnamon
Cloves, Ground
Coriander, Ground
Cumin, Ground
Curry Powder
Dill Weed
Garlic Powder
Ginger
Italian Seasoning
Nutmeg, Ground
Oregano Leaves
Paprika
Parsley
Poultry Seasoning
Rosemary, Crushed
Sage
Sesame Seed
Thyme Leaves
Turmeric

Fusion Flavors ⚕
Seasoning Blends (All)

Gaea ()
Spices (All)

Gayelord Hauser
Spice Garden Spices (All BUT Seas 'n
  Grill)
Spike 5Herb Magic!
Spike Garlic Magic!
Spike Hot 'n Spicy Magic!
Spike Onion Magic!
Spike Original Magic!
Spike Salt Free Magic!
Spike Vegit Magic!
Swiss Kriss Flake and Tablets

Giant
- Garlic
- Iodized Salt
- Paprika
- Salt & Pepper

GoGo Quinoa ✓
- GoGo Quinoa (All)

Gold Medal Spices ()
- Black Pepper, Ground
- Celery Seed
- Chili Powder
- Cinnamon, Ground
- Garlic Powder
- Garlic Salt
- Italian Seasoning
- Lemon Pepper
- Meat Tenderizer, Seasoned
- Nutmeg, Ground
- Onion, Minced
- Oregano, Whole
- Paprika
- Parsley Flakes
- Poultry Seasoning
- Red Pepper, Ground
- Sage, Rubbed
- Seasoning Salt
- Soul Seasoning
- Spaghetti Sauce Mix

Goodness Gardens
- Fresh Herbs (All)

Goya
- Adobo Con Comino
- Adobo con Limon
- Adobo Con Pimienta
- Adobo Con Pique
- Adobo Goya
- Adobo Naranja Agria
- Adobo Sin Pimienta
- All Spice
- Anise Seed
- Azafran
- Bay Leaf
- Camomile Manzanilla
- Chili Powder
- Cilantro & Tomato Seasoning
- Comino Molino
- Con Azafran
- Con Comino
- Con Limon
- Con Naranja
- Cooking Wine, Golden
- Crushed Red Pepper
- Culantro y Achiote Jumbo
- Culantro y Achiote Low Sodium
- Cumin Seed
- Dominican Sazonador
- Flor de Tilo
- Garlic Powder
- Garlic Salt
- Ground Black pepper
- Ground Cinnamon
- Ground Cumin
- Ground Oregano
- Ground Pepper
- Hojas de Laurel
- Jam Curry Powder
- Onion Powder
- Oregano Leaf
- Oregano Molido
- Paprika
- Pimienta Molida
- Salad & Vegetable Seasoning
- Salt
- Sazon Ajo y Cebolla
- Sazon Azafran
- Sazon Culantro Achiote
- Sazon Natural y Comp
- Sazon Regular Econo
- Sazon Regular Family
- Star Anise
- Stick Cinnamon
- Whole Black Pepper
- Whole Cloves

Grandmas
- Spaghetti Seasoning

Great Value (Wal-Mart) 25
- Iodized Salt
- Salt Iodized Seasoning
- Salt Seasoning

Haddon House
- Jane's Krazy Mixed Up Seasonings (All)
- Tropical Pepper (All)

Haggen
- Salt & Pepper Shaker Set

Salt (Iodized, Plain)

H-E-B
Blackened Seasoning
Borracho Seasoning
Brisket Rub
Cajun Seasoning
Creole Seasoning
Fajita Seasoning, Beef
Fajita Seasoning, Chicken
Seafood Boil
Seafood Seasoning
Steak Seasoning

Hill Country Fare (H-E-B)
Chicken Fajita Spice
Chili Powder
Chopped Onions
Fajita Spice
Garlic Powder
Garlic Salt
Ground Black Pepper
Ground Comino
Lemon Pepper
Meat Tenderizer
Nutmeg
Onion Powder
Onion Salt
Parsley Flakes
Rubbed Sage
Seasoning Salt

Hol-Grain ⓘ ☓
Chili Seasoning Mix
Fajitas Seasoning Mix

Hurst's Brand Soups ()
Seasonings (All BUT Cajun 15 Bean Soup)

Hy-Vee
California Garlic and Sea Salt
California Garlic, Granulated
California Onion, Chopped
Chicken Grill Seasoning
Fish and Seafood Seasoning
Garlic Pepper
Garlic Salt
Iodized Salt
Kosher Sea Salt
Malabar Black Pepper
Mediterranean Sea Salt

Mesquite Grilling Seasoning
Orange & Lemon Pepper
Pepper Supreme
Plain Salt
Steak Grilling Seasoning
Tex-Mex Chipotle Seasoning

InJoy Organics
Cinnamon Herb Sweet
Erythritol
Sea Shakes Sea Salt (All Flavors) (All)

Instant Gourmet
Seasonings (All)

J&D's
Natural Bacon Salt

Jardine's ⓘ
5-Star Ranch Rub
Fajita Seasoning

Jodie's Kitchen
Seasoning Blends (All)

Johnny's Fine Foods ⓘ
Chicken & Pork Seasoning
Dill Ranch
Garlic Salt
Great! Caesar Garlic Spread & Seasoning
Hunter's Blend
Jamaica Me Crazy Lemon Pepper
Jamaica Me Crazy Seasoned Pepper
Johnny's Seasoning Salt (Original ONLY, No Added MSG version CONTAINS GLUTEN)
Lemon Dill Seasoning
Pasta Elegance
Popcorn Salt
Salad Elegance
Salmon Seasoning
Seasoned Tenderizer
Steak Seasoning

Kernel Season's ⓘ
Seasoning Flavors (All)

Kikkoman
Tandoori Chicken Seasoning Mix ()

King Arthur
Cake Enhancer

Konriko ⓘ ☓
Chipotle Seasoning
Creole Seasoning

Greek Seasoning
Gulf Coast Seasoning Blend
Jalapeno Seasoning
Mojo Seasoning

Las Palmas ⓘ
Chiles

Leila Bay Trading Company
Finishing Salts (All)
Sea Salts (All)

Lisa Shively's ⓘ
BBQ & Steak Rub
Fiesta Pork Chops Mix
Firehouse Chili Mix
Jamaican Chicken Mix
Meatloaf Mix
Ranch Chicken Mix
Sloppy Joe Mix
Spaghetti Mix

Louisiana Fish Fry ⓘ
Blackened Fish Seasoning
Cajun Seasoning
Cayenne Papper
Crawfish Crab and Shrimp Boil
(Granulate and Liquid)
Fish Fry All Natural
Fish Fry New Orleans Style with Lemon
Fish Fry Seasoned
Gumbo File

Luzianne
Cajun Seasoning

Lydia's Organics ⚭
Lydia's Organics (All)

Manischewitz
Salt

Mas Guapo
Sazon Mas Guapo

Meijer
Black Pepper
Chili Powder
Cinnamon
Garlic Powder
Garlic Salt
Imitation Vanilla
Mild TacoMinced Onion
Onion Salt
Oregano Leaves
Paprika

Parsley Flakes
Salt (Seasoned, Iodized, Plain)
Spaghetti Mix
Vanilla Extract

Mexene ⓘ
Chili Powder Seasoning

Mom's Place Gluten-Free ⚭
Mom's Place Gluten-Free (All)

Mrs. Bryant's
Estate Fresh Gourmet™ L'essence de 7 SEA SALT FUSION
Estate Fresh Gourmet™ L'essence de Africa
Estate Fresh Gourmet™ L'essence de Cuba
Estate Fresh Gourmet™ L'essence de Dravida
Estate Fresh Gourmet™ L'essence de France
Estate Fresh Gourmet™ L'essence de Germany
Estate Fresh Gourmet™ L'essence de India
Estate Fresh Gourmet™ L'essence de Italy
Estate Fresh Gourmet™ L'essence de Jamaica
Estate Fresh Gourmet™ L'essence de Louisiana
Estate Fresh Gourmet™ L'essence de Mexico
Estate Fresh Gourmet™ L'essence d'England Mulling Spices

Nantucket Off-Shore ⟨⟩
Bayou Rub
Dragon Rub
Garden Rub
Mt. Olympus Rub
Nantucket Rub
Prairie Rub
Pueblo Rub
Rasta Rub
Renaissance Rub
Shellfish Boil
St. Remy Rub

No Salt
No Salt Salt Substitute

NOH of Hawaii ()
- Chinese Lemon Chicken Mix
- Hawaiian Spicy Chicken Mix
- Hawaiian Style Curry Mix
- Korean Kim Chee Mix
- Portuguese Vinha D'Alhos Mix

Nueva Cocina ⓘ
- Picadillo Seasoning
- Taco Fresco Seasoning
- Taco Seasoning with Chipotle

NU-Salt
- NU-Salt (All)

O Organics
- Coriander
- Ground Cumin
- Ground Curry Powder
- Organic Basil Leaves
- Organic Bay Leaves
- Organic Black Pepper
- Organic Garlic Powder
- Organic Oregano
- Organic Parsley
- Organic Rosemary
- Organic Rubbed Sage
- Organic Thyme Leaves
- Paprika

Ortega ⓘ
- 40% Less Sodium Taco Mix
- Chipotle Mix
- Guacamole Mix
- Jalapeno & Onion Mix
- Taco Seasoning - Hot & Spicy
- Taco Seasoning

Oskri
- Spices (All)

Our Family
- Baking Soda
- Black Pepper
- Black Pepper, Pure Ground
- Chicken Grilling Seasoning
- Chicken Season N Bake Roasting Bag
- Chili Powder
- Cinnamon, Ground
- Crushed Red Pepper
- Garlic Powder
- Garlic Salt
- Ginger, Ground
- Iodized Salt
- Italian Seasoning
- Lemon Pepper Seasoning
- Nutmeg, Ground
- Onion Powder
- Onions, Minced
- Oregano Leaves
- Paprika
- Parsley Flakes
- Plain Salt
- Pork Chop Season N Bake Roasting Bag
- Sage, Ground
- Seasoning Salt
- Spaghetti Seasoning
- Steak Grilling Seasoning
- Taco Seasoning

Polaner ⓘ
- Ready To Use Wet Spices - Basil
- Ready To Use Wet Spices - Garlic
- Ready To Use Wet Spices - Jalapenos

Price Chopper
- Arnold's Beef Seasoning
- Arnold's Chicken Seasoning
- Iodized Salt
- Regular Salt

Private Selection (Kroger)
- Living Basil

Publix
- Adobo Seasoning with Pepper
- Adobo Seasoning without Pepper
- Black Pepper
- Chili Powder
- Cinnamon
- Garlic Powder
- Garlic Powder with Parsley
- Garlic Salt
- Ground Ginger
- Ground Red Pepper
- Italian Seasonings
- Lemon & Pepper
- Minced Onion
- Onion Powder
- Paprika
- Parsley Flakes
- Salt
- Seasoned Salt
- Taco Seasoning Mix

Whole Basil Leaves
Whole Bay Leaves
Whole Black Pepper
Whole Oregano

Red Ape Cinnamon
Organic Cinnamon Sticks
Organic Ground Cinnamon

Rice River Farms ⓘ
Adobo Seasoning
Aji Amarillo Powder
Aji Panca Powder
Allspice, Jamaican
Amchur Powder
Ancho Powder
Arrowroot
Artichoke Powder
Bay Leaves, Ground
Bay Leaves, Semi Select
BBQ Seasoning
Beet Powder
Black Sea Salt (Kala Namuk)
Black Truffle Sea Salt
Boletes Mushroom Powder
Cajun Blackened Seasoning
Cajun Blackening Blend
Canadian Steak Blend
Cape Cod Seasoning
Caraway Seed
Caraway Seed, Black (Nigella)
Cardamom, Green Pods
Cardamom, Ground
Cardamom, Whole Black Pods
Carrot Powder
Carrots & Celery Mix
Celery Flakes
Celery Salt
Champignon (White Button)
   Mushroom Powder
Chicken Seasoning
Chile Verde Sea Salt
Chili Blend, Powder
Chipotle BBQ Seasoning
Chipotle Powder, Brown
Chipotle Powder, Morita
Chives, Air Dried
Cici Bean Powder (Garbanzo Bean
   Powder)

Cinnamon Sticks (4", 12")
Cinnamon, Sri Lankan Ground
Cinnamon, Vietnamese Ground
Cloves, Ground
Cloves, Hand Picked
Coriander Seed, Extra Bold
Coriander, Cracked
Coriander, Ground
Cubeb Berry
Cumin, Extra Fancy
Cumin, Ground
Curry, Hot
Curry, Madras Style
De Arbol Powder
Epazote, Crushed
Epazote, Ground
Espresso Brava Sea Salt
Fajita Marinade Seasoning
Fajita Spice
Fennel Pollen
Fenugreek Seed
Five Spice Powder
Fleur de Sel
Garam Masala
Garlic & Pepper Steak Seasoning
Garlic Peppercorn Seasoning
Garlic Powder, Roasted
Garlic Salt
Garlic, Granulated
Ghost Chile Powder
Ginger Galangal, Whole
Grains of Paradise (Melegueta Pepper)
Gray Sea Salt
Greek Sea Salt
Guajillo Powder
Gumbo File
Habanero Pepper Sea Salt
Habanero Powder, Blend
Habanero Powder, Pure
Hawaiian Black Sea Salt
Hawaiian Red Sea Salt, Coarse
Herbes de Provence
Hibiscus Flower
Hibiscus Powder
Hickory BBQ Seasoning
Himalayan Pink Sea Salt
Hot Paprika, Sweet

Hungarian Paprika (Sweet)
Jalapeno Powder
Jamaican Jerk Seasoning
Jerk Seasoning
Juniper Berries, Jumbo
Lavender Flowers, Super Blue
Lemon Peel, Granulated
Lemon Pepper Blend
Lime Fresco Sea Salt
Lime Peel, Granulated
Long Pepper
Maple Apple Seasoning
Mulling Spices
Mustard Seed, Black
Mustard Seed, Yellow
New Mexico/Anaheim Chile Powder
Nutmeg, Ground
Nutmeg, Whole
Onion Powder
Orange Peel, Granulated
Oregano, Mexican
Paella Seasoning
Paprika (All)
Paprika, Smoke (Sweet)Paprika, Smoked (Bittersweet)
Pasilla Negro Chile Powder
Peppercorns (All)
Pickling Spice
Pimente de Espelette (French Chile Powder)
Pineapple, Granulated
Pink Sea Salt
Pizza Blend
Porcini Mushroom Powder
Poultry Seasoning
Pumpkin Powder
Ras El Hanout
Raspberry Powder
Red Bell Pepper Powder
Red Wine Vinegar Powder
Rosemary, Extra Fancy
Saffron Powder
Saffron Threads
Sea Salt
Sea Salt, Coarse
Sea Salt, Mill Grind
Sea Salt, Smoked (Coarse, Fine)

Seasoning Salt
Serrano Smoked Powder
Shiitake Mushroom Powder
Spicy Curry Sea Salt
Spinach Powder
Star Anise
Strawberry Powder
Sumac, Ground
Szechuan Pepper Sea Salt
Tandoori Spice
Thai Ginger Sea Salt
Thyme, Extra Fancy
Tomato Powder
Truffle Powder, Black
Truffle Powder, White
Turmeric, Ground
Vegetable Blend, Dried
Wasabi Powder
Wasabi, Genuine Pure
Wild Mushroom Powder
Zahtar

Rub With Love ⓘ
Rubs (All)

Safeway ✍
Basil Leaves
Bay Leaves
Black Pepper Tin
Cayenne Pepper
Chili Powder
Cinnamon Powder
Coarse Black Pepper
Cream of Tartar
Crushed Red Pepper
Garlic and Herb Salt Free Seasoning
Garlic Powder
Garlic Salt with Parsley
Ground Black Pepper
Ground Cloves
Ground Cumin
Ground Ginger
Ground Mustard
Italian Seasoning
Lemon Pepper Seasoning
Minced Garlic
Nutmeg
Onion Powder
Onions Minced

Oregano Leaves
Paprika
Parsley Flakes
Salt and Pepper Shaker
Whole Black Pepper

Sally's ⚕
Sally's (All)

Sauce Goddess ✓
Spice Rubs (All)

Sauer's ()
7 Pepper Seasoning
Allspice (Ground, Whole)
Alum
Anise Seed
Apple Pie Spice
Barbecue Spice
Basil Leaves
Bay Leaves
Black Peppercorns
Brown Sugar Glazed Veggie Steamer
Buffalo Wings Baking Bag
Buffalo Wings Spicy Baking Bag
Caraway Seed
Cayenne Pepper, Ground
Celery Flakes
Celery Salt
Celery Seed
Cheddar Veggie Steamer Mix
Chicken Seasoning Canadian Style
Chicken Seasoning Canadian Style, Less
  Sodium
Chicken Seasoning Rub
Chicken Seasoning, Fried
Chili Powder
Chili Powder, Hot
Chives, Freeze Dried Chopped
Cinnamon (Ground, Whole Stick)
Cinnamon Sugar
Cloves (Ground, Whole)
Coriander, Ground
Crab Boil
Cream of Tartar
Cumin, Ground
Curry Powder
Dill Seed
Dill Weed
Econo Meat Tenderizer

Econo Meat Tenderizer, Seasoned
Econo Poultry & Pork Brine
Econo Seasoning Salt
Egg White Magic
Fennel Seed
Garlic Herb Grinder
Garlic Herb Veggie Steamer Mix
Garlic Pepper
Garlic Powder
Garlic Salt
Garlic Salt, Parslied
Garlic, Minced
Ginger, Ground
Ground Black Pepper
Hamburger Seasoning
Home Style Potato Steamer Mix
Italian Herb Grinder
Italian Seasoning
Jamaican Jerk Seasoning
Lemon Herb Seasoning
Lemon Pepper Seasoning
Mace, Ground
Marjoram Leaves
Meat Loaf Seasoning Mix
Meat Tenderizer
Meat Tenderizer, Seasoned
Mesquite Grill Seasoning
Monosodium Glutamate
Mustard Seed
Mustard, Ground
Nutmeg (Ground, Whole)
Onion Powder
Onion Salt
Onion, Minced
Oregano (Ground, Whole)
Paprika
Parsley Flakes
Peppercorn Grinder
Peppercorn Medley Grinder
Peppermill Grind Pepper
Pickling Spice
Poppy Seed
Pork Seasoning Rub
Poultry Seasoning
Prime Rib & Roast Rub
Pumpkin Pie Spice
Red Pepper (Crushed, Ground)

Rosemary & Garlic Seasoning
Rosemary Leaves
Sage, Rubbed
Salad Delight
Sea Salt Grinder
Seafood Seasoning, Cajun
Seafood Seasoning, Chesapeake
Seasoning Salt
Seasoning Salt, Garlic
Sesame Seed
Sour Cream & Chive Potato Steamer Mix
Steak Seasoning
Steak Seasoning Canadian Style
Steak Seasoning Canadian Style,
   Less Sodium
Steak Seasoning Canadian Style, Spicy
Steak Seasoning Rub
Steak Seasoning, Blackened
Swiss Steak Baking Bag
Thyme (Ground, Leaves)
Turmeric
White Pepper, Ground

Schnucks

Bay Leaves
Black Pepper
Chili Powder
Cinnamon
Cumin Powder
Garlic Powder
Garlic Salt
Iodized Salt
Nutmeg
Onion, Minced
Oregano
Organic Basil
Organic Chives
Organic Dill
Organic Edible Flowers
Organic Fresh Sage
Organic Mint
Organic Oregano
Organic Rosemary
Organic Tarragon
Organic Thyme
Parsley
Red Pepper, Crushed
Sage, Ground

Sweet Basil
Taco Mix

Shoppers Value (ACME)
Salt

Shoppers Value (Albertsons)
Salt

Shoppers Value (Cub Foods)
Salt

Simply Organic
All-Purpose Seasoning ☿
All-Seasons Salt ☿
Basil Leaf, Sweet ☿
Bay Leaf ☿
BBQ Ground Up ☿
Black Bean Seasoning Mix ✓
Cayenne ☿
Celery Salt ☿
Chicken Seasoning ☿
Chili Powder ☿
Chipotle Pepper ☿
Chophouse Seasoning ☿
Cilantro ☿
Cinnamon Powder ☿
Citrus A'peel ☿
Cloves ☿
Coriander Seed ☿
Crushed Red Pepper ☿
Cumin Seed ☿
Curry Powder ☿
Daily Grind ☿
Dill Weed ☿
Dirty Rice Seasoning Mix ✓
Enchilada Sauce Seasoning ✓
Fajita Seasoning ✓
Fish Taco Seasoning ✓
Garam Masala ☿
Garlic ☿
Garlic N Herb Seasoning ☿
Garlic Salt ☿
Get Crackin' ☿
Ginger ☿
Grind to a Salt ☿
Gumbo Base Seasoning Mix ✓
Herbes de Provence ☿
Italian Seasoning ☿
Jambalaya Seasoning Mix ✓
Lemon Peel ☿

Lemon Pepper ☷
Marjoram Leaf ☷
Mild Chili Seasoning Mix ✓
Mole Sauce Seasoning ✓
Mulling Spice ✓
Mustard Seed, Yellow ☷
Nutmeg ☷
Onion ☷
Oregano ☷
Paprika ☷
Parsley Leaf ☷
Pepper, Black ☷
Peppercorns, Black ☷
Poppy Seed ☷
Poultry Seasoning ☷
Pumpkin Pie Spice ☷
Red Bean Seasoning Mix ✓
Rosemary Leaf ☷
Sage Leaf ☷
Salsa Verde Seasoning ✓
Seafood Seasoning ☷
Sesame Seed, Black ☷
Sesame Seeds ☷
Sloppy Joe Seasoning Mix ✓
Southwest Taco Seasoning ✓
Spicy Chili Seasoning Mix ✓
Spicy Steak Seasoning ☷
Spicy Taco Seasoning ✓
Steak Seasoning ☷
Tarragon Leaf ☷
Thyme Leaf ☷
Turmeric Root ☷
Vegetable Seasoning ☷
Vegetarian Chili Seasoning Mix ✓

Singing Dog Vanilla
Organic Vanilla Beans

Slap Ya Mama
Cajun Seasoning (All)
Seafood Boil

Spice Islands
see also Durkee
Specialty - Beau Monde
Specialty - Chili Powder
Specialty - Crystallized Ginger
Specialty - Fines Herbs
Specialty - Garlic Pepper Seasoning
Specialty - Italian Herb Seasoning

Specialty - Old Hickory Smoked Salt
Specialty - Saffron
Specialty - Summer Savory
Spice Islands Grilling Gourmet & World
   Flavors (All)
Spice Islands Salt-Free (All)

Spice World
Garlic (All)
Speciality Spices (All)

Spicely
Spicely Organic Spices (All)

Stop & Shop
Celery Salt
Garlic Salt
Iodized Salt
Iodized Salt & Pepper
Paprika
Peppercorn (Grinder)
Sea Salt (Grinder)

Stubb's
Bar-B-Q Rub
Chile-Lime Rub
Herbal Mustard Rub
Rosemary Ginger Rub

Sun Luck
Classic Stir Fry Mix
Five Spice Powder
Hot Mustard Powder
Sweet & Sour Mix

Sunbird
Asian Skillet Classics - Sweet & Sour Pork
Beef & Broccoli
Chinese Chicken Salad
Chop Suey
Chow Mein
Fried Rice
General Tso's Chicken
Honey Sesame Chicken
Hot & Spicy Fried Rice
Hot & Spicy Kung Pao
Hot & Spicy Szechwan
Lemon Chicken Stir Fry
Mongolian Beef
Oriental Vegetable Stir Fry
Phad Thai
Spare Rib
Spicy Orange Beef

Stir Fry
Sweet & Sour
Thai Chicken
Thai Fried Rice
Thai Red Curry
Thai Spicy Beef
Thai Stir Fry
Tabasco ⓘ
Crushed Pepper
Dry Flavoring
Pepper Chaff
Processors Blend
Taste of Thai, A
Taste of Thai, A (All)
Tone's
see also Durkee
Trader Joe's
Private Label Spices (All)
Taco Seasoning
TryMe
Tiger Seasoning
Valu Time (Brookshire)
Barbeque Seasoning
Basil Leaves
Bay Leaves
Black Pepper
Cajun Seasoning
Cayenne Pepper
Celery Salt
Chili Powder
Crushed Red Pepper
Garlic Powder
Garlic Salt
Ground Cinnamon
Ground Sage
Italian Seasoning
Lemon Pepper Seasoning
Meat Tenderizer
Minced Onions
Onion Powder
Onion Salt
Oregano Leaf
Paprika
Parsley Flakes
Poultry Seasoning
Seafood Seasoning
Seasoned Salt

Soul Seasoning
Steak Seasoning
Weber
Beer Can Chicken Seasoning
Burgundy Beef Rub
Burgundy Beef Seasoning
Chicago Steak Grinder
Chicago Steak Seasoning
Classic BBQ Rub
Classic BBQ Seasoning
Cracked Black Pepper and Herb Rub
Gourmet Burger Seasoning
Kick 'N Chicken Grinder
Kick 'N Chicken Seasoning
Mango Lime Seasoning
New Orleans Cajun Seasoning
Roasted Garlic & Herb Grinder
Roasted Garlic & Herb Seasoning
Seasoning Salt
Six Pepper Fusion Grinder
Smokey Mesquite Seasoning
Summer Citrus Rub
Sweet and Savory Salmon Rub
Tex Mex Fiesta Rub
Tex Mex Fiesta Seasoning
Twisted Citrus-Garlic Grinder
Veggie Grill Seasoning
Zesty Lemon Grinder
Zesty Lemon Seasoning
Wegmans
Black Pepper
Fine Crystals Sea Salt
Fleur de Sel (Sea Salt)
Iodized Salt
Plain Salt
Sea Salt - Coarse Crystals
Wick Fowler's
Taco Seasoning
Williams
Chili Seasoning (Fancy, Original)
Chili with Onions Seasoning
Chipotle Chili Seasoning
Chipotle Taco Seasoning
Country Store Chili Soup Mix
Country Store Tortilla Soup Mix
Taco Seasoning
Tex-Mex Chili Seasoning

Tex-Mex Taco Seasoning (Hot)
White Chicken Chili Seasoning
Zocalo Gourmet
Zocalo Gourmet (All)

SPRINKLES

Genuardi's 〰
Party Sprinkles
Let's Do… ✔
Carnival Sprinkelz
Chocolatey Sprinkelz
Confetti Sprinkelz
Market Day
Autumn Sprinkles
Safeway 〰
Decorations Pastel Party Sprinkles
Decorations Rainbow Sugar Sprinkles
Stop & Shop
Chocolate Sprinkles
Non Pareils Sprinkles
Rainbow Sprinkles

STARCHES

Argo
Corn Starch
Authentic Foods
Starches (All)
Benson's
Corn Starch
Best Choice
Corn Starch
Bob's Red Mill
Arrowroot Starch
Corn Starch
Potato Starch
Canada
Corn Starch
Clabber Girl ✔
Cornstarch
Durkee
Arrowroot
Eden Foods
Kuzu Root Starch
Food Club (Brookshire)
Corn Starch

Gifts of Nature ✔
Expandex (Modified Tapioca Starch)
Potato Starch
Goya
Pan de Yuca
Hill Country Fare (H-E-B)
Corn Starch
Hol-Grain ⓘ ⸸
Rice Starch
Honeyville
Corn Starch
Potato Starch
Hy-Vee
Cornstarch
King Arthur
Gluten-Free Potato Starch
Gluten-Free Tapioca Starch
Kingsford
Corn Starch
Kinnikinnick Foods ⸸
Kinnikinnick Foods (All)
Let's Do…Organic ✔
Organic Cornstarch
Organic Tapioca Starch
Little Aussie Bakery, The
The Little Aussie Bakery (All)
Manischewitz
Potato Starch
Meijer
Corn Starch
Mom's Place Gluten-Free ⸸
Mom's Place Gluten-Free (All)
Our Family
Corn Starch
Price Chopper
Corn Starch
Really Great Food ⸸
Really Great Food (All)
Streit's ⓘ
Potato Starch

SUGAR & SUGAR SUBSTITUTES

ACME
Light Brown Sugar
Sugar

Albertsons
  Brown Sugar
  Powdered Sugar
Alter Eco Fair Trade ⓘ
  Sugar (All)
Always Save
  Brown Sugar
  Granulated Sugar
  Powdered Sugar
Authentic Foods
  Maple Sugar (All)
Best Choice
  Brown Sugar
  Granulated Sugar
  Powdered Sugar
  Sugar Packets
C&H Sugar
  Sugar (All)
Caring Candies
  Pure Xylitol Crystals
Clearly Organic (Best Choice)
  Pure Cane Sugar

Coconut Secret ⓘ
  Coconut Crystals
  Coconut Nectar
Community Coffee
  Sugar
Crosby's 🍴
  Drink Crystals
Crystal Sugar
  Brown Sugar (Light, Dark)
  Granulated Sugar
  Powdered Sugar
Cub Foods
  Granulated Sugar
Dixie Crystals
  Sugar Products (All)
Domino
  Sugars (All)
Dr. Oetker
  Natural Vanilla Sugar
  Vanilla Sugar
Eden Foods
  Organic Sweet Sorghum

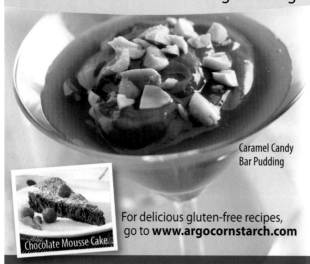
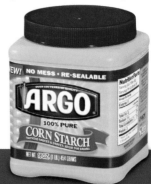

Edible Haven
Natural Coconut Sugar
Emerald Forest
Xylitol Products (All)
Equal
Equal
Faerie's Finest
Flavored Sugars (All)
Sugar & Spice Blends (All)
Fasweet
Fasweet Liquid Sweetener
Flavorite (Cub Foods)
Powdered Sugar
Florida Crystals
Sugar Products (All)
Food Club (Brookshire)
Aspartame Sweetener
Confectioners Sugar
Dark Brown Sugar
Light Brown Sugar
Sucralose, Sugar Substitute
Sugar

Sugar Substitute
Food Club (Marsh)
Aspartame Sweetener
Confectioners Sugar
Light Brown Sugar
Sugar
Sugar Substitute
Fructevia
Fructose Sweeteners (All)
Full Circle (Price Chopper)
Brown Sugar
Demerara Sugar
Sugar Cane
Full Circle (Schnucks)
Demerara Cane Sugar
Light Brown Sugar
Giant
Aspartame Sweetener Packets
Calorie Free Sweetener Packets
Dark Brown Sugar
Granulated Pure Cane Sugar
Light Brown Sugar

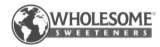
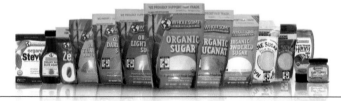

Powdered Confectioners Sugar

Giant Eagle
Granulated Sugar
Sucralose Sugar Substitute

Gifts of Nature ✓
Turbinado Sugar

Goya
Azucar Morena/Sugar

Great Value (Wal-Mart) 25
Altern No Calorie Sweetener
Calorie Free Sweetener
Confectioners Powdered Sugar
Extra Fine Granulated Sugar
Light Brown Sugar
Pure Cane Sugar

Haggen
Brown Sugar (Dark, Light)
Powdered Sugar
Sugar

Hy-Vee
Confectioners Powdered Sugar
Dark Brown Sugar
Delecta Sugar Substitute
Light Brown Sugar

Ideal
Ideal (All)

Imperial Sugar
Sugar Products (All)

Jewel-Osco
Dark Brown Sugar
Granulated Sugar
Light Brown Sugar
Organic Cane Sugar
Organic Light Brown Sugar
Powdered Raw Sugar

Leila Bay Trading Company
All-Natural Flavored Cane Sugars (All)

Madhava 🥇
Agave (All)

Maple Grove Farms 🥇 ✓
Granulated Maple Sugar

Meijer
Confectioners Sugar
Dark Brown Sugar
Light Brown Sugar
Sugar

Midwest Country Fare (Hy-Vee)
Granulated Sugar
Light Brown Sugar
Powdered Sugar

Nevella
Nevella (All)

Nielsen-Massey ✓
Nielsen-Massey (All)

O Organics 🌱
Light Brown Sugar
Organic Granulated Sugar
Powdered Sugar
Raw Agave Sweetener
Turbinado

Organic Nectars
PalmSweet

Our Family
Aspartame
Brown Sugar
Dark Brown Sugar
Granulated Sugar
Sucralose Sweetener

Price Chopper
Brown Sugar
Confectioners Sugar
Golden Brown Sugar
Granulated Sugar

Publix
Dark Brown Sugar
Granulated Sugar
Light Brown Sugar
Powdered Sugar - 10X
Powdered Sugar - 4X

PureVia
PureVia (All)

Rice River Farms ⓘ
Brown Granulated Sugar
Brown Sugar Sticks
Coconut Palm Sugar
Demerara Sugar
Fondant & Icing Powder
Maple Sugar
Turbinado Sugar

Richfood (ACME)
Sugar

Rodelle ⓘ
Vanilla Sugar

Safeway ᔐ
- Aspartame Sweetener
- Dark Brown Sugar
- Fine Granulated Sugar
- Granulated Sucralose No Calorie Sweetener
- Light Brown Sugar
- Powdered Sugar
- Stevia
- Sucralose No Calorie Sweetener

Schnucks
- Aspartame Sweetener
- Brown Sugar (Dark, Light)
- Powdered Sugar
- Sugar
- Sugar Substitute

Smart Sugar
- Smart Sugar (All)

Splenda
- Splenda Sweetener Products (All)

Stevia Extract in the Raw
- Stevia Extract in the Raw

Steviva
- Fructose
- Stevia Sweeteners (All)
- Xylitol

Stop & Shop
- Dark Brown Sugar
- Light Brown Sugar
- Powdered Confectioners Sugar
- Pure Cane Granulated Sugar

Sugar in the Raw
- Sugar In The Raw

Sweet Leaf
- Sweet Leaf (All)

Sweet N' Low
- Sugar (All)

Tate & Lyle
- Sugar Products (All)

Trader Joe's
- Sugar (All)

Truvia
- Truvia

Valu Time (Brookshire)
- Aspartame Sweetener
- Dark Brown Sugar
- Light Brown Sugar

- Powdered Sugar
- Sugar
- Sugar Substitute

Valu Time (Marsh)
- Sugar

Vita Foods ⓘ
- Sauza Agave

Vons ᔐ
- Dark Brown Sugar
- Light Brown Sugar
- Powdered Sugar
- Sugar Granulated

Wegmans
- Dark Brown Sugar
- Granulated Sugar
- Granulated White Sugar
- Light Brown Sugar
- Mandarin Cocktail Sugar
- Sugar Substitute with Saccharin
- Sweetener with Aspartame

Wholesome Sweeteners
- Dark Muscovado Sugar
- Evaporated Cane Juice (Sugar) (All Types)
- Light Muscovado Sugar
- Organic Agave Syrups
- Organic Blue Agave Cinnamon Flavored Syrup
- Organic Blue Agave Maple Flavored Syrup
- Organic Blue Agave Strawberry Flavored Syrup
- Organic Blue Agave Vanilla Flavored Syrup
- Organic Cane Syrups, Inverts, and Blends (All Types)
- Organic Coconut Palm Sugar
- Organic Evaporated Cane Juice (Sugar) (All Types)
- Organic Powdered Sugar
- Organic Stevia
- Organic Sucanat (All Types)
- Organic Sucanat with Honey
- Wholesome Sweeteners Zero (Erythritol)

Wild Harvest (ACME)
- Organic Cane Sugar
- Organic Light Brown Sugar

Wild Harvest (Albertsons)
Organic Light Brown Sugar
Wild Harvest (Cub Foods)
Organic Cane Sugar
Winn-Dixie
Granulated Sugar
Light Brown Sugar
Powdered Sugar, 10X

WHOLE GRAINS

Aimee's Livin' Magic
Really Raw Hempseeds
Alter Eco Fair Trade ⓘ
Quinoa (All)
Ancient Harvest ⚭
Black Quinoa
Inca Red Quinoa
Polenta Quinoa
Quinoa Flakes
Traditional Quinoa
Arrowhead Mills
Amaranth
Buckwheat Groats
Flax Seeds
Hulled Millet
Organic Golden Flax Seeds
Quinoa
Bob's Red Mill
Brown Flaxseeds
GF Rolled Oats
GF Steel Cut Oats
Golden Flaxseed
Grain Teff
Hulled Millet
Organic Amaranth Grain
Organic Brown Flaxseed
Organic Buckwheat Groats
Organic Golden Flaxseeds
Organic Kasha
Organic Quinoa Grain
Bora Bora ✓
Traditional Apricot Quinoa
Cream Hill Estates
Gluten-Free Rolled Oats/Flakes
Gluten-Free Whole Grain Oat Flour

Eden Foods
Organic Buckwheat
Organic Millet
Organic Quinoa
Organic Red Quinoa
Food Merchant Polenta ⚭
Quinoa
Gifts of Nature ✓
Certified GF Old Fashioned Rolled Oats
Certified GF Whole Oat Groats
GoGo Quinoa ✓
GoGo Quinoa (All)
Goya
Semilla de Quinoa ⟨⟩
GranoVita
Linseed Plus
Organic Golden Linseed
Organic Quinoa
Organic Red Quinoa
Hodgson Mill
Whole Grain Flax Seed ⚭
Linusit
Linusit Gold
Mom's Place Gluten-Free ⚭
Mom's Place Gluten-Free (All)
Nu-World Amaranth
Amaranth Grain (All)
Puffed Amaranth (All)
Pocono
Kasha
Whole Buckwheat Groats
Rice River Farms ⓘ
Amaranth
Buckwheat Groats
Chia Seed, Black
Chia Seed, White
Flax Seed, Brown
Flax Seed, Golden
Kañiwa
Kasha
Millet Seed
Quinoa
Quinoa Blend
Quinoa, Black
Quinoa, Golden
Quinoa, Puffed
Quinoa, Red

Gluten-Free RED STAR ☆
Mock Black Russian Bread

Wet Ingredients:	Dry Ingredients:	
1+1/3 cup Water	2+1/4 tsp (1 package)	3 TBSP, packed Dark
2 TBSP Molasses	RED STAR® Active Dry Yeast	Brown Sugar
3 Eggs, large, lightly beaten	2 cup Brown Rice Flour	1 TBSP egg replacer, optional
1 tsp Cider Vinegar	1/2 cup Potato Starch	1/2 cup Non-fat Dry Milk
3 TBSP Olive Oil	1/2 cup Tapioca Starch	1 tsp Instant Coffee
	1/3 cup Rice Bran	4+1/2 tsp Cocoa
THIS RECIPE	1 TBSP Xanthan Gum	2 TBSP Caraway Seeds
MAKES 1 LOAF	1+1/2 tsp Salt	

Traditional Method: All ingredients should be at room temperature (70º - 80ºF). Combine the wet ingredients in a mixing bowl and whisk together. Thoroughly blend all dry ingredients, including the Active Dry Yeast. Add blended dry ingredients on top of the wet ingredients. Using a mixer, beat ingredients about 10 minutes until all ingredients are well-blended. Pour batter into greased bread pan. Allow batter to rise approximately 1 hour. Bake at 375ºF for 45 to 60 minutes; use a toothpick to test for doneness. Remove from pan and cool on wire rack before slicing.

Bread Machine Method: All ingredients should be at room temperature (70º - 80ºF). Combine wet ingredients; pour carefully into baking pan. Measure dry ingredients; mix well to blend. Add to baking pan. Carefully set pan in bread maker. Select NORMAL/WHITE cycle, or GLUTEN FREE CYCLE (if machine has one); start machine. After mixing action begins, help any unmixed ingredients into the dough with a rubber spatula, keeping to edges and top of batter to prevent interference with the paddle. Remove pan from the machine when bake cycle is complete. Invert pan and shake gently to remove bread. Cool upright on a rack before slicing.

Join us 📘 🐦

For more gluten-free recipes, go to www.redstaryeast.com or call 800-445-4746.

CAROL'S COLLECTION

Quinoa, Red & Black Blend
Teff, Brown
Trader Joe's
Organic Polenta
Organic Quinoa
TruRoots
Organic Chia Seeds
Organic Quinoa
Organic Sprouted Quinoa
Wolff's
Kasha
Whole Buckwheat Groats
Zocalo Gourmet
Zocalo Gourmet (All)

YEAST

Bakipan
Fast Rising Instant Yeast
Traditional Baking Active Dry Yeast
Best Choice
Active Yeast
Fast Rise Yeast
Yeast Mix

Bob's Red Mill
Active Dry Yeast
Nutritional Yeast
Bragg
Bragg (All)
Fleischmann's Yeast
Yeast (All)
Foods Alive ⚥
Nutritional Yeast
Gayelord Hauser
Brewers Yeast
Our Family
Active Dry Yeast Envelopes
Rapid Rise Yeast
Really Great Food ⚥
Really Great Food (All)
Red Star Yeast
Active Dry Yeast (ADY)
Bread Machine Yeast
Quick Rise Yeast
SAF
Bread Machine Yeast
Gourmet Perfect Rise Yeast
Traditional Active Dry Perfect Rise Yeast

MISCELLANEOUS

Aimee's Livin' Magic
Really Raw Goji Berries
Really Raw Peruvian Maca Powder
Shilajit, Conqueror of Mountains and Destroyer of Weakness
Wild Vanilla Beans
Authentic Foods
Dough Enhancer
Guar Gum
Xanthan Gum
Bob's Red Mill
Guar Gum
Organic Textured Soy Protein
Rice Bran
Soy Lecithin
Textured Vegetable Protein (TVP)
Xanthan Gum
Ener-G
Xanthan Gum

Fearn Natural Foods ⓘ
  Lecithin Granules
  Liquid Lecithin
  Soya Granules
Fondarific
  Fondant (All)
Gifts of Nature ✓
  Unflavored Gelatin
  Xanthan Gum
Goya
  Api Morado
  Corn Patties, Cheese Arepas
  Guava Paste
  Guava Paste Sugar Free
  Guava Paste with Jelly Center
Hodgson Mill
  Gluten-Free Xanthan Gum ⚕
King Arthur
  Hi-Maize Natural Fiber
Konjac Foods
  Konjac Glucomannan Powder (Konjac
    Root Fiber)
Let's Do…Organic ✓
  Organic Tapioca Granules
  Organic Tapioca Pearls
Little Aussie Bakery, The
  Guar Gum
Mom's Place Gluten-Free ⚕
  Guar Gum
  Xanthan Gum
Our Family
  Unflavored Gelatin
Really Great Food ⚕
  Xantham Gum

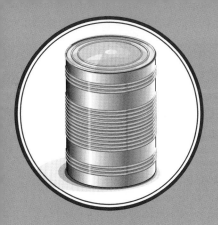

CANNED AND PRE-PACKAGED FOODS

ASIAN SPECIALTY ITEMS

ACME
Whole Water Chestnuts
Albertsons
Whole Water Chestnuts
Culinary Circle (Albertsons)
Chicken Tikka Masala
Eden Foods
Agar Agar Bars
Agar Agar Flakes
Arame
Bonito Flakes
Daikon Radish - Shredded and Dried
Hiziki
Kombu
Lotus Root
Maitake Mushrooms, Dried
Mekabu Wakame
Nori
Organic Shiro Miso
Pickled Daikon Radish
Shiitake Mushrooms, Dried (Whole and
  Sliced)
Shiso Leaf Powder (Pickled Beefsteak
  Leaf)
Sushi Nori
Tekka (Miso Condiment)
Toasted Nori Krinkles
Ume Plum Balls
Ume Plum Concentrate (Bainiku Ekisu)
Umeboshi Paste
Umeboshi Plums
Wakame
Wakame, Instant Flakes
Wasabi Powder

Yansen (Dandelion Root Concentrate)
Pacific Natural Foods ⓘ
Beef Pho Soup Starter
Chicken Pho Soup Starter
Vegetarian Pho Starter
Safeway 〰
Water Chesnuts Sliced
Safeway Select 〰
Shelled Edamame Boiled Soybeans
Snapdragon Pan-Asian Cuisine
Chinese Mushroom Soup
Hong Kong Seafood Rice Noodle Soup
  Bowl
Hunan Sweet & Sour Stir Fry
Indonesian Peanut Stir Fry
Pad Thai Ginger Stir Fry
Singapore Curry Rice Noodle Soup
  Bowl
Sun Luck
Bamboo Shoots (Sliced, Strip)
Bean Sprouts
Phad Thai Rice Sticks, 3mm
Sesame Seeds (Toasted, White)
Shiitake Mushrooms
Stir Fry Vegetables
Straw Mushrooms (Stir Fry, Whole/
  Peeled)
Waterchestnuts (Sliced, Whole)
World Classics (Price Chopper)
Sliced Fancy Water Chestnuts

BEANS, BAKED

ACME
Baked Beans With Smoked Ham

Pork 'n Beans
Vegetarian Baked Beans

Albertsons
Baked Beans
Baked Beans With Onions
Vegetarian Baked Beans

Always Save
Pork & Beans

Amy's Kitchen ✓
Vegetarian Baked Beans

B&M Baked Beans ⓘ
Baked Beans (All)

Best Choice
Baked Beans
Country Style Beans
Homestyle Beans
Onion Baked Beans
Pork & Beans

Bush's Best
Bush's Best Products (All)

Castleberry's Brands, Inc.
Cattle Drive Brown Sugar & Bacon
    Baked Beans

Crest Top
Canned Products (All)

Eden Foods
Organic Baked Beans with Sorghum &
    Mustard

Fastco (Fareway)
Pork & Beans

Flavorite (Cub Foods)
Baked Beans

Food Club (Brookshire)
Baked Beans
Baked Beans with Onions
Baked Beans, Homestyle
Baked Beans, Maple Cured

Food Club (Marsh)
Baked Beans
Baked Beans with Onions
Baked Beans, Homestyle
Baked Beans, Maple Cured
Baked Beans, Vegetarian
Pork And Beans

**Food You Feel Good About
(Wegmans)**
Vegetarian Baked Beans

Full Circle (Schnucks)
Baked Beans
Maple Baked Beans

Great Value (Wal-Mart) 25
Pork & Beans

Haggen
Pork and Beans

Hanover Foods
Beans & Franks
Brown Sugar & Bacon Baked Beans
Homestyle Baked Beans
Pork & Beans
Vegetarian Baked Beans

Heinz
Vegetarian Beans

Hill Country Fare (H-E-B)
Baked Beans with Onions
Homestyle Baked Beans
Original Baked Beans
Pork-n-Beans

Hy-Vee
Country Style Baked Beans
Home Style Baked Beans
Maple Cured Bacon Baked Beans
Onion Baked Beans
Original Baked Beans
Pork and Beans
Pork and Beans in Tomato Sauce

Jewel-Osco
Brown Sugar Baked Beans
Homestyle Whole Baked Beans
Vegetarian Whole Baked Bean

Kroger
Baked Beans

Meijer
Pork and Beans

Country Fare (Hy-Vee)
Pork and Beans in Tomato Sauce

Our Family
Baked Beans (Country Style, Homestyle,
    Onion, Original)
Pork and Beans

Publix
Baked Beans
Pork & Beans

Safeway ᔕ
Baked Beans Original

Schnucks
Baked Beans
Baked Beans with Onion
Homestyle Baked Beans
Pork N Beans
Vegetarian Baked Beans
Valu Time (Schnucks)
Pork & Beans
Wagon Master
Canned Items (All)
Wegmans
Homestyle Baked Beans
Original Baked Beans
Pork & Beans in Tomato Sauce
Whole Earth
Organic Baked Beans
Winn-Dixie
Baked Beans
Baked Beans with Bacon & Onion

BEANS, OTHER

ACME
Black Beans
Blackeyed Peas
Dark Red Kidney Beans
Dried Black Eyed Peas
Dried Split Peas
Dried Whole Beans Navy
Dried Whole Pinto Beans
Garbanzo Beans
Great Northern Beans
Light Red Kidney Beans
Light Red Whole Kidney Beans
Pinto Beans
Whole Cannellini Beans
Whole Dried Great Northern Beans
Whole Large Lima Beans
Aimee's Livin' Magic
Mucuna, The Velvet Bean
Really Raw Peeled Cacao Bean
Albertsons
Baby Lima Beans
Cannellini Beans
Dark Red Kidney Beans
Dried Lima Beans
Dried Pinto Beans

Dried Red Beans
Dried Whole Baby Lima Beans
Garbanzo Beans
Great Northern Beans
Italian Style Cut Green Beans
Navy Beans
Pinto Beans
Red Kidney Beans
Sliced French Style Green Beans
Whole Beans
Whole Black Eyed Peas
Whole Butter Beans
Whole Dried Garbanzo Beans
Whole Dried Pinto Beans
Whole Pink Beans
Allens
Canned Products (All)
Always Save
Black Eyed Peas
Chili Beans
Great Northern Beans
Pinto Beans
Red Kidney Beans
Amy's Kitchen ✓
Refried Black Beans
Arrowhead Mills
Adzuki Beans
Anasazi Beans
Chickpeas (Garbanzos)
Pinto Beans
Soybeans
Aunt Penny's
Beans (All)
Bar Harbor
Vegetarian Soldier Beans
Vegetarian Yellow Eye Beans
Best Choice
Dark Kidney Beans
French Stuffed Green Beans
Garbanzo Beans
Great Northern Beans
Large Lima Beans
Lentils
Light Red Kidney Beans
Mexican Chili Beans
Mexican Style Beans
Navy Beans

Pinto Beans
Red Beans
Red Kidney Beans
Seasoned Black Beans

Bush's Best
Bush's Best Products (All)

Carlita (Jewel-Osco)
Black Beans
Frijoles Pinto Beans

Carmelina
Carmelina Beans (All)

Casa Fiesta ⓘ
Bean and Green Chili Burrito Filling
Jalapeno Pinto Beans
Mexican Style Chili Beans
Pinto Beans

Clearly Organic (Best Choice)
Black Beans
Chili Beans
Dark Red Kidney Beans
Great Northern Beans
Pinto Beans

Cub Foods
Baked Beans
Black Beans
Butter Beans
Chili Beans
Dark Red Kidney Beans
Great Northern Beans
Lentils
Light Kidney Beans
Regular Pinto Beans

DeLallo
Black Beans
Butter Beans
Cannellini Beans
Chick Peas
Chili Beans in Sauce
Gigantes Beans (in Natural Juice, in Tomato Sauce, in Vinaigrette)
Great Northern Beans
Kidney Beans, Light Red
Lentils
Lupini Beans, Imported
Navy Beans
Pinto Beans
Romano Beans

East Texas Fair
Canned Products (All)

Eden Foods
Caribbean Black Beans
Green Lentils
Green Split Peas
Organic Aduki Beans
Organic Black Beans
Organic Black Eyed Peas
Organic Black Soybeans
Organic Butter Beans (Baby Lima)
Organic Cajun Rice & Small Red Beans
Organic Cannellini (White Kidney) Beans
Organic Caribbean Rice & Black Beans
Organic Curried Rice & Lentils
Organic Garbanzo Beans (Chick Peas)
Organic Great Northern Beans
Organic Kidney Beans
Organic Mexican Rice & Black Beans
Organic Moroccan Rice & Garbanzo Beans
Organic Navy Beans
Organic Pinto Beans
Organic Rice & Garbanzo Beans
Organic Rice & Kidney Beans
Organic Rice & Lentils
Organic Rice & Pinto Beans
Organic Small Red Beans
Spanish Rice & Pinto Beans

Fastco (Fareway)
Green Beans, Cut
Green Beans, French
Kidney Beans

Flavorite (Cub Foods)
Baby Lima Beans
Blackeyed Peas
Butter Beans
Great Northern Beans
Lentil Beans
Navy Beans
Pinto Beans

Food Club (Brookshire)
Black Beans
Blackeye Peas with Jalapenos
Chili Beans
Cut Waxed Beans

Dried Blackeye Peas
Garbanzo Beans
Great Northern Beans
Green Beans, Cut
Green Beans, Cut (No Salt)
Green Beans, French Style
Green Beans, Italian Cut
Large Lima Beans
Lentil Beans
Light Red Kidney Beans
Navy Beans
Pinto Beans
Pinto Beans with Jalapeno
Pork and Beans
Red Beans
Texas Style Ranch Beans
White Hominy Beans
Yellow Hominy Beans

Food Club (Marsh)
Black Beans
Butter Beans
Chili Beans
Dark Red Kidney Beans
French Style Green Beans, Veri Green
Garbanzo Beans
Great Northern Beans
Navy Beans
Pinto Beans
Red Beans

Full Circle (Marsh)
Organic Black Beans
Organic Dark Red Kidney Beans
Organic Pinto Beans

Full Circle (Price Chopper)
Black Beans
Dark Kidney Beans
Garbanzo Beans
Great Northern Beans
Green Lentils
Kidney Beans
Pinto Beans

Full Circle (Schnucks)
Black Beans
Dark Red Kidney Beans
Garbanzo Beans
Great Northern Beans
Kidney Beans

Lentil Beans
Navy Beans
Pinto Beans
Spicy Black Beans

Furmano's
Furmano's (All)

Gaea
Beans (All)

Genuardi's
Dark Red Kidney Beans
Pinto Beans

Giant
Black Beans
Black-Eyed Peas
Chick Peas
Dark Red Kidney Beans
Dry Baby Lima Beans
Dry Black Beans
Dry Lentils
Dry Navy Beans
Dry Split Green Peas
Golden Wax Beans, Cut
Light Red Kidney Beans
No Salt Added Sweet Peas
Roman Beans
Small Green Lima Beans
Wax Beans, Cut

Goya
Baby Lima Beans-Dry ()
Bean Soup Mix-Dry ()
Black Beans
Black Beans (Low Sodium)
Black Beans-Dry ()
Black Volteados
Black with Cheese
Blackeye Peas
Blackeye Peas-Dry ()
Bola Roja Beans
Bola Roja Beans-Dry ()
Butter Beans
Canary Beans
Canary Beans-Dry ()
Canary Beans-Frijol Canario-Dry ()
Cannellini Beans
Central American Red Beans-Dry ()
Chick Peas
Chick Peas (Low Sodium)

Chick Peas- Dry ()
Cow Peas-Dry ()
Dark Kidney Beans
Dominican Red Beans-Dry ()
Ducal Red with Chorizo
El Jibarito Pigeon Peas ()
French Style Green Beans
Frijol Black Volteado
Frijol Black Volteado Cobanero
Frijol Black Volteado Jalapeño
Frijol Centroamericano-Dry ()
Frijol de Seda
Frijol Parado
Frijoles Negros (Low Sodium)
Garbanzos (Low Sodium)
Giant White Corn-Dry ()
Great Northern Beans
Great Northern Beans-Dry ()
Green Lima Beans
Green Split Peas-Dry ()
Habichuelas Blancas (Low Sodium)
Habichuelas Coloradas (Low Sodium)
Habichuelas Pintas (Low Sodium)
Habichuelas Rosadas (Low Sodium)
Kirby Black Beans
Large Fava Beans-Dry ()
Large Lima Beans-Dry ()
Lentils
Lentils - Dry ()
Listo Frijol Negro
Maiz Cancha Chulpe-Dry ()
Maiz Trillado Amarillo-Dry ()
Maiz Trillado/White Hominy-Dry ()
Mexican Hominy
Navy Beans
Navy Beans-Dry ()
Organic Black Beans
Organic Black Beans- Dry ()
Organic Chick Peas
Organic Navy Beans
Organic Pinto Beans- Dry ()
Organic Red Kidney Beans
Organic Red Kidney Beans- Dry ()
Pardina Lentils-Dry ()
Peeled Fava Beans-Dry ()
Pigeon Peas ()
Pigeon Peas-Dry ()

Pink Beans
Pink Beans (Low Sodium)
Pink Beans-Dry ()
Pinto Beans
Pinto Beans (Low Sodium)
Pinto Beans-Dry ()
Pintos Frijoles
Red Cargamanto Beans
Red Cargamanto Beans-Dry ()
Red Kidney Beans (Low Sodium)
Red Kidney Beans-Dry ()
Red Lentils-Dry ()
Red Volteados
Roman Beans
Roman Beans-Dry ()
Small Red Beans
Small Red Beans-Dry ()
Small White Beans (Low Sodium)
Small White Beans-Dry ()
Spanish Style Red Kidney Beans
White Beans
White Cargamanto Beans
White Cargamanto Beans-Dry ()
White Kidney/Cannellini Beans-Dry ()
Whole Green Peas-Dry ()
Whole Yellow Peas-Dry ()
Yellow Split Peas-Dry ()

Great Value (Wal-Mart) 25

Baby Lima Beans
Black Beans
Chick Peas (Garbanzos), Bilingual
Great Northern Beans
Large Lima Beans
Lentils
Light Red Kidney Beans
Mayocoba Beans, Bilingual
Navy Beans
Pink Beans, Bilingual
Pinto Beans
Small Red Beans
Southern Ranch Beans

GreenWise Market (Publix)

Organic Black Beans
Organic Garbanzo Beans
Organic Kidney Beans, Dark Red
Organic Pinto Beans
Organic Soy Beans

Haggen
Black Beans
Chili Beans
Dark Red Kidney Beans
Garbanzo Beans
Great Northern Beans
Hominy (Golden, White)
Kidney Beans
Lima Beans, Large
Low Sodium Black Beans
Low Sodium Garbanzo Beans
Low Sodium Kidney Beans
Navy Beans
Pinto Beans
Red Beans, Small
Red Kidney Beans

Hanover Foods
3 Bean Salad
4 Bean Salad
Black Beans
Blackeye Peas
Butter Beans
Cannellini Beans
Chick Peas
Chili Beans
Great Northern Beans
Limagrands
Pink Beans
Pinto Beans
Red Beans
Redskin Kidney Beans (Light & Dark)
Roman/ Shellie/ Cranberry Beans
Seasoned Black Beans
Superfine Diced Green & White Lima
    Beans
Superfine Midget Green Butter Beans
Vegetarian Beans in Tomato Sauce

Hill Country Fare (H-E-B)
Texas Style Beans

Hy-Vee
Black Beans
Black-Eyed Peas
Butter Beans
Chili Style Beans in Chili Gravy
Dark Red Kidney Beans
Garbanzo Beans (Chick Peas)
Great Northern Beans

Large Lima Beans
Lentils
Light Red Kidney Beans
Navy Beans
Pinto Beans
Red Beans
Red Kidney Beans

Italian Classics (Wegmans)
Cannellini Beans
Garbanzo Beans

Jewel-Osco
Blackeyed Peas
Brown Black Beans
Cannellini Beans
Dark Red Kidney Beans
Dried Lentils
Dried Pinto Beans
Dried Whole Navy Beans
Garbanzo Beans
Great Northern Beans
Large Lima Beans
Light Red Beans
Light Red Kidney Beans
Lima Beans
Pinto Beans
Pork & Beans
Whole Beans
Whole Black Beans
Whole Butter Beans

Joan of Arc ⓘ
Black Beans
Butter Beans
Garbanzo Beans
Great Northern Beans
Light & Dark Red Kidney Beans
Pinto Beans
Red Beans

La Costena
Beans (All)

Meijer
Black Beans
Blackeye Peas
Butter Beans
Garbanzo Beans
Great Northern Beans
Green Beans (Cut, Whole)
Green Beans Cut, Blue Lake

Green Beans Cut, No Salt
Green Beans Cut, Veri Green
Green Beans French Style
Green Beans French Style, Blue Lake
Green Beans French Style, No Salt
Green Beans French Style, Veri Green
Green Split Peas
Kidney Beans (Dark Red, Light Red)
Lentils
Lima Beans
Mexican Style Beans
Navy Beans
Organic Baked Beans
Organic Black Beans
Organic Garbanzo Beans
Organic Green Beans French Style
Organic Green Beans, Cut
Organic Kidney Beans, Dark Red
Organic Pinto Beans
Pinto Beans
Red Beans
Wax Beans, Cut

Midwest Country Fare (Hy-Vee)
Chili Style Beans

Nature's Promise (Giant)
Organic Black Beans
Organic Cut Green Beans
Organic Dark Kidney Beans
Organic Garbanzo Beans

Nature's Promise (Stop & Shop)
Lentil
Organic Black Beans
Organic Dark Kidney Beans
Organic Garbanzo Beans
Organic Light Kidney Beans

O Organics
Organic Black Beans
Organic Garbanzo Beans
Organic Pinto Beans
Organic Red Kidney Beans

Our Family
Black Beans
Garbanzo Beans
Great Northern Beans
Green Beans, (Cut, Cut No Salt Added,
    French Style, Whole)
Kidney Beans (Dark Red, Light)

Lentils
Navy Beans
Pinto Beans
Split Peas (Dry Pack)
Wax Beans, Cut

Pastene
Black Beans
Chick Peas
Kidney Beans, Red
Kidney Beans, White
Lupini

Price Chopper
Kidney Beans

Publix
Baby Lima Beans (Dry Beans)
Black Beans (Dry Beans)
Blackeye Peas (Dry Beans)
Garbanzo Beans (Dry Beans)
Great Northern Beans (Dry Beans)
Green Lima Beans
Green Split Peas (Dry Beans)
Kidney Beans - Dark and Light
Large Lima Beans (Dry Beans)
Lentils (Dry Beans)
Light Red Kidney Beans (Dry Beans)
Navy Beans (Dry Beans)
Pinto Beans (Dry Beans)
Small Red Beans (Dry Beans)

Rice River Farms ⓘ
10 Bean Blend
21 Bean Blend
Adzuki Beans
Anasazi Beans
Appaloosa Beans
Black Beans, Fermented
Black Turtle Beans
Calico Soup Blend
Calypso Beans, Black
Cannellini Beans
Christmas Bean Mix
Corona/Runner Beans, Sweet White
Cranberry (Borlotti) Beans
Eight Bean Blend
European Soldier Beans
Exotic Bean Blend
Fava Beans, Extra Large
Flageolet Beans

French Navy Beans
Garbanzo Beans
Garbanzo Beans, Black
Gourmet Bean Blend
Great Northern Beans
Habas (Peeled Fava)
Jacobs Cattle Gold Beans
Jacobs Cattle/Trout Beans
Kidney, Dark Red
Kidney, Light Red
Lentils, Black Beluga
Lentils, Brown (Spanish Pardina)
Lentils, French Green
Lentils, Green
Lentils, Green (Eston)
Lentils, Ivory White
Lentils, Multi-Colored Blend
Lentils, Petite Crimson
Lentils, Petite Golden
Lentils, Red Chief
Lima Beans, Baby Butter
Lima Beans, Christmas
Lima Beans, Giant Peruvian
Lupini Beans, Extra Large
Marrow Beans
Mayocoba Beans/Canary Beans
Mung Beans, Whole
Peas, Blackeye
Peas, Green Split
Peas, Green Whole
Peas, Pigeon
Peas, Red Split
Peas, Yellow Split
Peas, Yellow Whole
Pebble Beans
Pinto Beans
Rattlesnake Beans
Rice Beans
Runner Beans, Scarlet
Small Red Beans
Snow Cap Beans
Swedish Brown Beans
Tongues of Fire
Yellow Eye Stueben Beans

Safeway 𑅐
Baked Beans Vegetarian
Black Beans

Dark Red Kidney Beans
Garbanzo Beans
Lentils
Low Sodium Black Beans
Navy Beans
Pinto Beans

Schnucks
Black Beans
Blackeye Peas
Dark Red Kidney Beans
Great Northern Beans
Green Beans, Cut
Green Beans, Cut Low Sodium
Green Beans, French Style
Green Beans, French Style Low Sodium
Green Beans, Whole
Lentils
Lima Beans
Lima Beans, Baby
Lima Beans, Large
Navy Beans
Pinto Beans
Red Beans
Red Beans, Small
Split Green Peas
Wax Beans, Cut

Shaw's
Dried Blackeyed Peas
Dried Great Northern Beans Bag
Dried Navy Beans Bag
Dried Red Kidney Bean
Dried Split Green Peas Bag
Dried Whole Black Beans
Dried Whole Lentils
Dried Whole Lima Beans
Great Northern Beans
Pinto Beans
Whole Dried Red Beans

Stop & Shop
Black Beans
Dark Red Kidney Beans
Dry Navy Beans
Garbanzo Beans
Green Beans, Cut
White Cannellini Kidney Beans

Teasdale ⓘ ⛌
Beans in Brine (All)

Organic Beans (All)

Trader Joe's
Beans (All)

TruRoots
Organic Sprouted Bean Trio
Organic Sprouted Green Lentils
Organic Sprouted Mung Beans

Valu Time (Brookshire)
Blackeye Peas
Chili Style Beans
Cut Green Beans
Green Beans- Cut
Green Beans- Cut French Style
Green Beans- Short Cut
Hominy White Beans
Lima Beans
Pinto Beans
Pork & Beans
Red Kidney Beans

Valu Time (Marsh)
Blackeye Peas
Pork and Beans
Red Kidney Beans
White Hominy Beans
Yellow Hominy Beans

Valu Time (Schnucks)
Kidney Beans
Pinto Beans

Vons ᐸ
Light Red Kidney Beans
Red Kidney Beans

Wegmans
Black Beans
Butter Beans
Dark Kidney Beans
Dark Red Kidney Beans - No Salt Added
Great Northern Beans
Light Kidney Beans
Lima Beans
Pinto Beans
Seasoned Chili Beans
Wax Beans

Wild Harvest (ACME)
Organic Black Beans
Organic Garbanzo Beans
Organic Pinto Beans

Wild Harvest (Albertsons)
Organic Black Beans
Organic Pinto Beans

Wild Harvest (Cub Foods)
Organic Black Beans
Organic Garbanzo Beans
Organic Pinto Beans

Wild Harvest (Jewel-Osco)
Organic Black Beans
Organic Garbanzo Beans
Organic Pinto Beans

Winn-Dixie
Garbanzo Beans
Green & White Lima Beans
Green Beans (Cut, French Style Sliced, Veggi-Green, Whole)
Green Beans, No Salt Added (Cut, French Style Sliced)
Green Lima Beans
Kidney Beans (Dark Red, Light Red, Red)

Zocalo Gourmet
Zocalo Gourmet (All)

BEANS, REFRIED

ACME
Fat-Free Refried Beans
Traditional Refried Beans
Vegetarian Refried Beans

Albertsons
Spicy Refried Beans
Vegetarian Refried Beans

Always Save
Refried Beans

Amy's Kitchen ✓
Light in Sodium Refried Black Beans
Light in Sodium Traditional Refried Beans
Refried Beans with Green Chiles
Traditional Refried Beans

Bush's Best
Bush's Best Products (All)

Casa Fiesta ⓘ
Refried Beans (No Fat, Original, with Chilies)
Refried Beans with Green Chilies

Refried Black Beans

Eden Foods
Organic Refried Black Beans
Organic Refried Black Soy & Black
Beans
Organic Refried Kidney Beans
Organic Refried Pinto Beans
Organic Spicy Refried Black Beans
Organic Spicy Refried Pinto Beans

Food Club (Brookshire)
Refried Beans
Vegetarian Refried Beans

Food Club (Marsh)
Refried Beans
Refried Beans, Authenic
Refried Beans, Fat Free

Full Circle (Price Chopper)
Fat Free Refried Beans
Refried Black Beans
Vegetarian Refried Beans

Full Circle (Schnucks)
Fat Free Refried Beans
Lime Refried Beans
Refried Beans
Refried Black Beans

Goya
Black-Refried Beans
Chipotle-Refried Beans
Chorizo-Refried Beans
Rancheros-Refried Beans
Refried Beans Mayocoba
Speckled Beans
Traditional-Refried Beans
Volteados Black
Volteados Red

Haggen
Refried Beans (Fat Free, Regular,
Vegetable)

Hill Country Fare (H-E-B)
Refried Beans
Refried Beans with Jalapenos

Hy-Vee
Black Refried Beans
Fat Free Refried Beans
Spicy Refried Beans
Traditional Refried Beans
Vegetarian Refried Beans

Jewel-Osco
Fat-Free Refried Beans
Low-Fat Vegetable Refried Beans
Spicy Refried Beans
Vegetarian Refried Beans

La Costena
Refried Beans (All)

Las Palmas ⓘ
Refried Beans

Meijer
Organic Refried Beans, (Black Bean,
Black Bean & Jalapeno, Roasted Chili
& Lime, Traditional)
Refried Beans (Fat Free, Vegetarian)

Ortega ⓘ
Refried Beans - Fat Free
Refried Beans - Regular

Our Family
Fat Free Refried Beans
Refried Beans
Vegetarian Refried Beans

Safeway ᗡ
Refried Beans

Taco Bell ᗡ
Refried Beans, Fat Free
Refried Beans, Vegetarian Blend

Valu Time (Schnucks)
Refried Beans

Vons ᗡ
Refried Beans No Fat

Wild Harvest (Albertsons)
Organic Garbanzo Beans

BOUILLON

Better than Bouillon
All Natural Reduced Sodium Chicken
Base
Au Jus Base
Beef Base (Organic, Regular)
Chicken Base (Organic, Regular)
Chili Base
Clam Base
Fish Base
Ham Base
Kosher Chicken Base
Kosher Vegetable Base

Lobster Base
No Beef Base
No Chicken Base
Turkey Base (Organic, Regular)
Vegetable Base (Organic, Regular)
Edward & Sons ✓
Garden Veggie Bouillon Cubes
Low Sodium Veggie Bouillon Cubes
Not-Beef Bouillon Cubes
Not-Chick'n Bouillon Cubes
Food Club (Brookshire)
Cube Beef Bouillon
Instant Beef Bouillon
Food Club (Marsh)
Bouillon Cube Beef
Bouillon Instant Beef
Giant
Beef Bouillon Cubes
Chicken Bouillon Cubes
Goya
Bouillon-Beef
Bouillon-Chicken
Ham Flavored Concentrate
Herb-Ox
Beef
Chicken
Garlic Chicken
Vegetable
Hy-Vee
Beef Bouillon Cubes
Beef Instant Bouillon
Chicken Bouillon Cubes
Chicken Instant Bouillon
Mom's Place Gluten-Free ⚕
Mom's Place Gluten-Free (All)
Mrs. Bryant's
Garden Fresh Gourmet™ Vegan
  CHICKEN Flavored Broth Seasoning
  (Powder Concentrate)
Organic Gourmet
Natural Bouillon Cubes
Our Family
Beef Bouillon Cubes
Chicken Bouillon Cubes
Instant Beef Bouillon
Instant Chicken Bouillon Granules

Price Chopper
Chicken Instant Bouillon
Schnucks
Beef Cube Bouillon
Instant Beef Bouillon
Streit's ⓘ
Soup Bases (All Flavors)

BROTH & STOCK

Bar Harbor
Clam Stock
Fish Stock
Lobster Stock
Seafood Stock
Best Choice
Beef Broth Box
Chicken Broth Box
Low Sodium Chicken Broth
Central Market (H-E-B)
Organic Free Range Chicken Broth
Organic Low Sodium Chicken Broth
Organic Vegetable Broth
Organics Beef Broth
Clearly Organic (Best Choice)
Chicken Broth
Vegetable Broth
College Inn Broth ⓘ
Bold Stock Tender Beef Flavor
Garden Vegetable Variety
No MSG Low Sodium Chicken Broth
  (Fat Free, Light)
Organic Beef Broth Variety
White Wine & Herb Culinary Broth
DeLallo
Clam Juice Broth
Colonial Inn Beef Broth
Colonial Inn Chicken Broth
EMERIL'S ⚕
Stocks (Beef & Chicken)
Food Club (Brookshire)
Aseptic Chicken Broth
Fat Free Low Sodium Chicken Broth
Thin Beef Broth
Food Club (Marsh)
Beef Broth Ready to Serve Soup (Thin)
Chicken Broth (Aseptic)

Chicken Broth Fat Free, Low Sodium,
Thin

**Food You Feel Good About
(Wegmans)**
All-Natural Beef Flavored Culinary
Stock
All-Natural Chicken Culinary Stock
All-Natural Thai Culinary Stock
All-Natural Vegetable Culinary Stock

Full Circle (Schnucks)
Chicken Broth
Chicken Broth, Aseptic
Vegetable Broth, Aseptic

G. Washington
G. Washington (All)

Giant Eagle
Beef Broth, Aseptic
Chicken Broth, Aseptic
Low Sodium Chicken Broth

Goya
Cubitos de Pollo
Cubitos en Polvo

Great Value (Wal-Mart) 25
Beef Broth Ready To Serve
Chicken Broth Ready To Serve

Haggen
Chicken Broth (Aseptic)

H-E-B
Beef Broth
Chicken Broth
Reduced Sodium Beef Broth
Reduced Sodium Chicken Broth

Hill Country Fare (H-E-B)
Reduced Sodium Chicken Broth

Imagine
Organic Beef Flavored Broth
Organic Free Range Chicken Broth
Organic Low Sodium Beef Flavored
Broth
Organic Low Sodium Vegetable Broth
Organic No Chicken Broth
Organic Vegetable Broth

Kallo
Organic Beef Stock Cubes
Organic Chicken Stock Cubes
Organic French Onion Stock Cubes
Organic Garlic & Herb Stock Cubes

Organic Low Salt Beef Stock Cubes
Organic Low Salt Chicken Stock Cubes
Organic Low Salt Vegetable Stock Cubes
Organic Mushroom Stock Cubes
Organic Tomato & Herb Stock Cubes
Organic Vegetable Stock Cubes
Yeast Free Vegetable Stock Cubes

Kitchen Basics ✓
Kitchen Basics (All)

Kroger
Beef Broth
Fat Free Low Sodium Chicken Broth

Market District (Giant Eagle)
Beef Stock, Aseptic
Chicken Stock, Aseptic
Vegetable Stock, Aseptic

Meijer
Chicken Broth

Nature's Basket (Giant Eagle)
Organic Broth, Chicken
Organic Broth, Low Sodium Chicken
Organic Broth, Vegetable

Nature's Promise (Giant)
Beef Flavored Broth
Organic Chicken Broth
Organic Chicken Stock
Organic Low Sodium Chicken Broth
Organic Vegetable Broth
Organic Vegetable Stock

Nature's Promise (Stop & Shop)
Flavored Beef Broth
Low Sodium LowFat Beef Broth
Organic Chicken Broth
Organic Chicken Stock
Organic Low Sodium Chicken Broth
Organic Low Sodium Fat Free Chicken
Broth
Organic Vegetable Broth
Organic Vegetable Stock

O Organics
Low Sodium Chicken Broth Aseptic
Organic Chicken Broth
Organic Vegetable Broth

Our Family
Beef Broth
Chicken Broth (Aseptic)
Chicken Broth, Reduced Sodium

Pacific Natural Foods ⓘ
Natural Beef
Natural Free Range Chicken
Organic Beef
Organic Free Range Chicken
Organic Low Sodium Beef Broth
Organic Low Sodium Chicken
Organic Low Sodium Vegetable
Organic Mushroom
Organic Vegetable

Progresso
Beef Flavored Broth
Chicken Broth
Reduced Sodium Chicken Broth

Safeway ᧬
Beef Broth
Beef Broth Aseptic
Beef Stock
Chicken Broth
Chicken Stock

Savory Choice ⓘ ✓
Beef Broth Concentrate
Chicken Broth Concentrate
Reduced Sodium Chicken Broth
   Concentrate
Reduced Sodium Vegetable Broth
   Concentrate
Turkey Broth Concentrate

Shelton's ⓘ
Chicken Broth Fat Free
Chicken Broth Regular

Swanson
Beef Stock (Aseptic)
Chicken Broth (Aseptic & Canned)
Chicken Stock (Aseptic)
Natural Goodness Chicken Broth
   (Aseptic & Canned)
Vegetable Broth (Canned)

Trader Joe's
Organic Free Range Chicken Broth
Organic Hearty Vegetable Broth
Organic Low Sodium Chicken Broth
Reduced Sodium Chicken Broth
   Concentrate

Valu Time (Schnucks)
Chicken Broth

Vogue Cuisine ⓘ 🍴
Soup & Seasoning Bases (All)

Vons ᧬
Broth, Chicken
Low Sodium Fat Free Chicken Broth

CHILI & CHILI MIXES

ACME
Spicy Chili Beans

Albertsons
Chili Beans
Chili with Beans Hot

Amy's Kitchen ✓
Black Bean Chili
Light in Sodium Medium Chili
Light in Sodium Spicy Chili
Medium Chili
Medium Chili with Vegetables
Southwestern Black Bean Chili
Spicy Chili

Bear Creek
Chili

Best Choice
Chili Sauce

Bush's Best
Bush's Best Products (All)

Carroll Shelby Chili
Original Texas Chili Kit
White Chicken Chili

Casa Fiesta ⓘ
Green Chili Burrito Filling

Castleberry's Brands, Inc.
Cattle Drive Chicken Chili
Cattle Drive Chili with Beans
Chili No Beans
Chili with Beans
Hot Dog Chili Sauce
Hot Dog Chili Sauce with Onion

Cub Foods
Chili With Beans

Eden Foods
Black Bean & Quinoa Chili

Fastco (Fareway)
Chili Beans

Flavorite (Cub Foods)
Chili Beans

Food Club (Brookshire)
- Chili with Beans
- Mild Chili with Beans

Food Club (Marsh)
- Chili with Beans, Mild

Food You Feel Good About (Wegmans)
- Spicy Red Lentil Chili

Frontier Soups ⓘ
- California Gold Rush White Bean Chili
- Michigan Ski Country Chili
- Midwest Weekend Cincinatti Chili

Full Circle (Schnucks)
- Chili Beans, Ranchero
- Chili Beans, Seasoned
- Chili with Black Beans
- Mild Vegetarian Chili
- Spicy Vegetarian Chili

Goldwater
- Goldwater (All) ()

Grandmas
- Chili Package

Hormel
- Chili Master - Chipotle Chicken No Bean
- Chili Master - Chipotle Chicken with Beans
- Chili Master - White Chicken Chili with Beans
- Chili with Beans (Beef Only) - Chunky
- Chili with Beans (Beef Only) - Hot
- Chili with Beans (Beef Only) - Regular
- Low Sodium Chili with Beans

Hy-Vee
- Chili with Beans
- Hot Chili with Beans

Jardine's ⓘ
- Cowboy Kettle Chili Original
- Texas Chili Bag O' Fixins
- Texas Chili Works

Jewel-Osco
- Mild Chili Beans
- Spicy Chile Beans

Kunzler ⛉
- Hot Dog Chili Sauce

Meijer
- Chili (No Beans, With Beans)

- Hot Dog Chili Sauce

O Organics ⌇
- Chili Beans in Sauce

Our Family
- Chili Beans
- Chili with Beans

Sauer's ()
- Chili Seasoning, Tex Mex

Schnucks
- Chili Beans, Hot

Shaw's
- Chili Can

Shelton's ⓘ
- Turkey Chili Mild
- Turkey Chili Spicy

Skyline Chili ⓘ
- Canned Chili (All)

Stagg
- Chunkero Chili
- Classic Chili
- Dynamite Hot Chili
- Ranch House Chicken Chili
- Silverado Beef Chili
- Steak House Chili
- Vegetable Garden Chili
- White Chicken Chili

Trader Joe's
- Organic Vegetarian Chili
- Vegetarian 3 Bean Chili

Vietti ⓘ
- Chili No Beans
- Chili with Beans
- Family Style Chili with Beans
- Hot Chili with Bean with Louisiana Hot Sauce
- Keys Chili with Beans
- Rudy's Chili with Beans
- Southgate Chili no Beans
- Southgate Chili with Beans
- Southgate Vegetarian Chili with TVP
- Texas Pete Chili No Beans
- Tony Packo Chicken Chili with Bean
- Tony Packo Chili with Beans
- Varallo Chili with Beans

Whitey's
- Beef with Bean Chili
- Jalapeno Beef No Bean Chili

Wick Fowler's
2-Alarm Chili Kit
Chicken Chili Mix
False Alarm Chili Kit
One Step Wick Fowler Chili
Winn-Dixie
Mexican Style Chili Beans
Zeigler ()
Chili Con Carne

COCONUT MILK

Coco Lopez
Coconut Milk
Cream of Coconut
Reduced Fat Cream of Coconut
Goya
Coconut Milk
Coconut Pulp
Let's Do…Organic ✓
Organic Creamed Coconut
Native Forest ✓
Organic Coconut Milk
Organic Light Coconut Milk
NOH of Hawaii ()
Coconut Milk
Sun Luck
Coconut Milk (Regular, Light)
Taste of Thai, A
Taste of Thai, A (All)
Trader Joe's
Light Coconut Milk

CRANBERRY SAUCE

Food Club (Brookshire)
Cranberry Sauce
Full Circle (Price Chopper)
Cranberry Sauce
Giant
Jellied Cranberry Sauce
Whole Berry Cranberry Sauce
Great Value (Wal-Mart) 25
Jellied Cranberry Sauce
Whole Berry Cranberry Sauce
Haggen
Cranberry Sauce (Jelly, Whole)

Ocean Spray
Sauces (All)
Our Family
Jellied Cranberry Sauce
Whole Cranberry Sauce
Price Chopper
Jellied Cranberry Sauce
Whole Cranberry Sauce
Publix
Whole Cranberry Sauce
Schnucks
Jellied Cranberry Sauce
Whole Cranberry Sauce
Stop & Shop
Jellied Cranberry Sauce
Whole Cranberry Sauce
Tiptree
Cranberry Sauce
Vons 〰
Cranberry Sauce Jellied
Cranberry Sauce Whole
Wegmans
Jellied Cranberry Sauce
Whole Berry Cranberry Sauce
Wild Thymes ⓘ
Original Cranberry Sauce
Winn-Dixie
Jellied Cranberry Sauce

FRUIT

Albertsons
Mandarin Oranges Light Syrup
Pineapple Chunks
Sliced Pineapple Unsweetened
Always Save
Chunk Pineapple
Crushed Pineapple
Fruit Mix
Lite Peach Halves
Mandarin Oranges
Peach Pieces
Peach Slices
Pear Halves
Pears Irregular Sliced in Light Syrup
Sliced Pineapple

Best Choice
- Apricot Halves
- Diced Mixed Fruit
- Diced Peaches
- Fruit Cocktail
- Grapefruit Sections
- Lite Chunk Mixed Fruit
- Lite Fruit Cocktail
- Lite Peach Slices
- Lite Pear Halves
- Mandarin Oranges
- Peach Halves
- Peach Slices
- Pear Halves in Heavy Syrup
- Pear Halves in Light Syrup
- Pineapple Chunks
- Pineapple Crushed
- Pineapple Slices
- Pineapple Tidbits
- Red Grapefruit Sections
- Sliced Pears in Syrup
- Tropical Fruit Salad
- Yellow Cling Peach Halves
- Yellow Cling Peach Slices

Central Market Classics (Price Chopper)
- Macintosh Apple Slices

Del Monte ⓘ
- Canned/Jarred Fruits (All)

DeLallo
- Champion Pitted Prune
- Colonial Inn Cherries

Flavorite (Cub Foods)
- Cherries
- Green Cherries

Food Club (Brookshire)
- Clinged Peach Halves in Light Syrup
- Crushed Pineapple in Juice
- Diced Peach Bowl in Light Syrup
- Diced Peaches in Strawberry Gel
- Diced Peaches with Banana Berry Flavor
- Fruit Cocktail in Heavy Syrup
- Fruit Cocktail in Juice
- Fruit Cocktail with Splenda
- Mandarin Oranges with Lite Syrup
- Mixed Fruit Bowl in Light Syrup
- Peaches with Splenda
- Pear Halves with Splenda
- Pears Bartlett Halves in Juice
- Pears Bartlett Halves, Heavy Syrup
- Pineapple Bites in Juice
- Pineapple Chunks in Juice
- Pitted Prunes
- Red Pitted Cherries, Tart
- Sliced Cling Peaches in Heavy Syrup
- Sliced Peaches Cling in Juice
- Sliced Pears Bartlett in Juice
- Sliced Pears Bartlett, Heavy Syrup
- Sliced Pineapple in Juice

Food Club (Marsh)
- Apricot Halves, Unpeeled In Heavy Syrup
- Fruit Cocktail in Heavy Syrup
- Fruit Cocktail in Juice
- Fruit Cocktail with Splenda
- Imported Pineapple Chunks in Juice
- Imported Pineapple Crushed in Juice
- Imported Pineapple Sliced in Juice
- Mandarin Oranges in Lite Syrup
- Maraschino Cherry, Green
- Maraschino Cherry, Red
- Maraschino Cherry, Red with Stems
- Mixed Fruit Bowl, Cherry in Lite Syrup
- Mixed Fruit, Extreme Cherry
- Peaches Cling Halves Heavy Syrup
- Peaches Cling Sliced In Juice
- Peaches Diced Bowl In Light Syrup
- Peaches Sliced with Splenda
- Peaches, Cling Sliced in Heavy Syrup
- Pears Bartlett Halves Heavy Syrup
- Pears Bartlett Halves Juice
- Red Tart Pitted Cherries

Food You Feel Good About (Wegmans)
- Apricots, Halved Unpeeled
- Chunk Pineapple
- Crushed Pineapple
- Fruit Cocktail
- Fruit Cocktail in Pear Juice
- Halved Peaches
- Halved Yellow Cling Peaches
- Peaches, Sliced in Juice
- Pear Halves
- Pear Halves, Lite

Pineapple Tidbits
Sliced Peaches
Sliced Pears
Sliced Pears, Lite
Sliced Pineapple
Solid Pack Pumpkin

Full Circle (Price Chopper)
Raspberries

Full Circle (Schnucks)
Organic Pear Halves
Organic Pear Slices

Geisha
Mandarin Oranges
Mandarin Oranges in Light Syrup
Mixed Fruits
Peaches Sliced
Pear Halves
Pineapple Chunk
Pineapple Crushed
Pineapple Sliced
Sliced Peaches in Light Syrup
Tropical Fruit Salad

Giant
Blueberries in Heavy Syrup
Crushed Pineapples in Juice
Fruit Cocktail
Mandarin Orange Segments in Syrup
  Fruit Cups
Mandarin Oranges in Syrup
No Sugar Added Pear Halves in Pear
  Juice
Peach Halves in Pear Juice
Pear Halves in Syrup
Pineapple Chunks in Heavy Syrup
Pineapple Tidbits in Juice Fruit Cups
Sliced Pineapple in Juice
Unpeeled Apricot Halves in Pear Juice
Yellow Cling Peaches in Pear Juice,
  Sliced
Yellow Cling Peaches in Syrup, Sliced
Yellow Cling Peaches, Sliced

Goya
Ancel Papaya Chunks
Brevas Almibar
Chirimoya Pulp
Chunks of Pineapple
Coctel de Frutas

Cream of Coconut
Curuba Pulp
Feijoa Pulp
Fruit Cocktail
Grape Preserve
Guanabana Pulp
Guanabana Tubes Fruit Pulp
Guava Coronilla Pulp
Guava Preserve
Guayaba Pulp
Jocote
Limon Pulp
Lucuma Pulp
Lulo Pulp
Mamey Pulp
Mandarin Pulp
Mango Preserve
Mango Pulp
Mango Slices with Pulp
Mango Tubes Fruit Pulp
Maracuya/Parcha
Mora Pulp
Nance
Orange Shells
Papaya Chunks
Papaya Preserve
Papaya Pulp
Papaya Slices
Papaya Tubes Fruit Pulp
Passion Fruit Preserve
Passion Fruit Tubes Pulp
Peach Halves
Peaches, Sliced
Pejivalles/Chontaduro
Pineapple Chunks
Pineapple Preserve
Pineapple, Sliced
Pitahaya Pulp
Ponche Mexicano
Strawberry Preserve
Strawberry Pulp
Tamarind Pulp
Whole Guavas
Whole Jocote-Plum
Whole Mora/Black Raspberry
Whole Nance
Whole Tejocote

Whole Zapote-Mamey

Great Lakes International Trading ⓘ

Pitted Prunes

Great Value (Wal-Mart) 🔲

Bartlett Pear Halves In Heavy Syrup
Bartlett Sliced Pears In Heavy Syrup
Blackberries
Blueberries
Crushed Pineapple
Fruit Cocktail In Heavy Syrup
Fruit Cocktail Sweetened with Splenda
Fruit Selections Crushed Pineapple
Fruit Selections Diced Peaches & Pears In Strawberry & Raspberry Light Syrup
Fruit Selections Diced Peaches In Light Syrup
Fruit Selections Diced Peaches In Strawberry & Banana Light Syrup
Fruit Selections Diced Peaches with Splenda
Fruit Selections Mandarin Oranges In Light Syrup
Fruit Selections Mixed Fruit In Light Syrup
Fruit Selections Mixed Fruit with Splenda
Fruit Selections Pineapple Chunks
Fruit Selections Pineapple Slices
Fruit Selections Pineapple Tidbits In Pineapple Juice
Fruit Selections Tropical Fruit Mix In Light Syrup
Fruit Slices
Maraschino Cherries with Stems
No Sugar Added Bartlett Pear Halves
No Sugar Added Chunky Mixed Fruits
No Sugar Added Fruit Cocktail
No Sugar Added Yellow Cling Peach Halves
No Sugar Added Yellow Cling Sliced Peaches
Peaches & Pears In Cherry Gel
Pineapple Chunks
Pineapple Slices
Red Raspberries
Sliced Peaches

Tidbit Pineapple
Triple Cherry Fruit Mix In Light Syrup
Tropical Fruit Salad
Whole Segment Mandarin Oranges In Light Syrup
Whole Strawberries
Yellow Cling Peach Halves In Heavy Syrup
Yellow Cling Sliced Peaches Sweetened with Splenda

Haggen

Apricot Halves
Fruit Cocktail (in Heavy Syrup, in Juice)
Mixed Fruit with Cherry
Peach Halves (in Heavy Syrup, in Juice)
Peaches, Sliced (in Heavy Syrup, in Juice)
Pear Halves (in Heavy Syrup, in Juice)
Pears, Sliced in Heavy Syrup
Pumpkin

Hawkshead Relish

Fruit Pastes (All)
Pickled Fruits (All)
Preserved Fruits (All)

Hy-Vee

Bartlett Pear Halves
Bartlett Pear Slices
Chunk Pineapple
Crushed Pineapple
Fruit Cocktail
Lite Bartlett Pear Halves
Lite Chunk Mixed Fruit
Lite Fruit Cocktail
Lite Yellow Cling Peach Halves
Lite Yellow Cling Peach Slices
Mandarin Oranges
Purple Plums
Sliced Pineapples
Unpeeled Apricot Halves
Whole Plums in Heavy Syrup
Yellow Cling Peach Halves
Yellow Cling Peach Slices

Kroger

Mandarin Oranges

Libby's

100% Pure Pumpkin

Meijer
Apricot Halves Unpeeled In Pear Juice
Fruit Cocktail In Heavy Syrup
Fruit Cocktail in Juice
Fruit Cocktail in Pear Juice Light
Fruit Mix Juice
Grapefruit Sections in Juice
Grapefruit Sections in Syrup
Lite Cling Sliced Peaches in Pear Juice
Mandarin Oranges Light Syrup
Peaches Cling Sliced In Heavy Syrup
Peaches Cling Sliced In Juice
Peaches, Cling Halves In Heavy Syrup
Peaches, Cling Halves In Light Juice
Peaches, Cling Halves In Pear Light
   Juice
Peaches, Yellow Sliced In Heavy Syrup
Pear Halves in Heavy Syrup
Pear Halves in Juice
Pears Halves in Juice Light
Pears Sliced in Heavy Syrup
Pears Sliced in Juice Light
Pears, Halves Light
Pineapple Chunks in Heavy Syrup
Pineapple Chunks in Juice
Pineapple Crushed in Heavy Syrup
Pineapple Crushed in Juice
Pineapple Juice
Pineapple Sliced in Heavy Syrup
Pineapple Sliced in Juice
Tropical Fruit Salad

Midwest Country Fare (Hy-Vee)
Bartlett Pear Halves in Light Syrup
Fruit Cocktail in Heavy Syrup
Pineapple Chunks in Natural Juice, No
   Sugar Added
Pineapple Slices in Natural Juice, No
   Sugar Added
Pineapple Tidbits in Natural Juice, No
   Sugar Added
Yellow Cling Peach Halves in Light
   Syrup
Yellow Cling Sliced Peaches in Heavy
   Syrup
Yellow Cling Sliced Peaches in Light
   Syrup

Native Forest ✓
Organic Asian Pears, Sliced
Organic Grapefruit Segments
Organic Mandarin Oranges
Organic Mango Chunks
Organic Mangosteen
Organic Papaya Chunks
Organic Peach & Apricot Medley
Organic Peaches, Sliced
Organic Pineapple (Chunks, Crushed,
   Slices)
Organic Rambutan
Organic Tropical Fruit Salad

Nature's Promise (Giant)
Organic Turkish Apricots
Organic Turkish Figs

Nature's Promise (Stop & Shop)
Organic Turkish Apricots
Organic Turkish Figs

Our Family
Apricot Halves, Unpitted
Fruit Cocktail
Fruit Cocktail in Heavy Syrup
Fruit Cocktail in Splenda
Fruit Cocktail, Lite
Grapefruit Sections
Mandarin Oranges
Mandarin Oranges in Light Syrup
Mixed Fruit, Triple Cherry
Peaches, Sliced in Pear Juice
Peaches, Sliced Sweetened with Splenda
Pear Halves
Pear Halves in Heavy Syrup
Pear Halves, Lite
Pear Slices, Lite
Pears, Sliced in Heavy Syrup
Pineapple, Chunks in Juice
Pineapple, Crushed in Juice
Pineapple, Sliced in Juice
Sliced Peaches
Tropical Fruit Salad
Tropical Fruit Salad with Banana
Yellow Cling Peach Halves
Yellow Cling Peach Halves in Heavy
   Syrup
Yellow Cling Peaches, Sliced

Yellow Cling Peaches, Sliced in Heavy Syrup

POM Wonderful
POM Wonderful (All)

Price Chopper
Mandarin Orange

Publix
Apricot Halves - Unpeeled in Heavy Syrup
Bartlett Pears in Heavy Syrup (Halves and Slices)
Chunky Mixed Fruit in Heavy Syrup
Fruit Cocktail in Heavy Syrup
Lite Bartlett Pear Halves in Pear Juice
Lite Chunky Mixed Fruit in Pear Juice
Lite Fruit Cocktail in Pear Juice
Lite Yellow Cling Peaches in Pear Juice (Halves and Slices)
Mandarin Oranges in Light Syrup
Pineapple (All Styles)
Yellow Cling Peaches in Heavy Syrup (Halves and Slices)

S&W Fine Foods ⓘ
Canned/Jarred Fruits (All)

Safeway ⤳
Berries and Cherries
California Apricots
Cherries
Cranberries
Dried Cranberries Organic
Philippine Mango

Schnucks
Apricot Halves, Unpeeled in Heavy Syrup
Apricot Halves, Unpeeled in Juice
Dark Sweet Pitted Cherries
Fruit Bowl with Diced Peaches
Fruit Bowl with Peaches & Berries
Fruit Bowl with Peaches & Pears
Fruit Cocktail
Fruit Cocktail Heavy Syrup
Fruit Cocktail, Juice Pack
Grapefruit Sections
Mandarin Oranges
Mixed Fruit Bowl
Mixed Fruit Chunks
Peach Halves in Juice

Peach Halves, Sliced in Juice
Peaches, Sliced
Pear Halves in Heavy Syrup
Pear Halves in Juice
Pears, Sliced in Heavy Syrup
Pineapple Chunks (in Heavy Syrup, in Juice, Plain)
Pineapple Tidbits
Pineapple, Crushed (in Heavy Syrup, in Juice, Plain)
Pineapple, Sliced (in Heavy Syrup, in Juice, Plain)
Red Tart Pitted Cherries
Sliced Peaches Juice Pack
Tropical Fruit Salad
Yellow Cling Peach Halves in Heavy Syrup
Yellow Cling Sliced Peach No Juice
Yellow Cling Sliced Peaches in Heavy Syrup
Yellow Cling Sliced Peaches in Juice

Stop & Shop
No Sugar Added Fruit Cocktail in Pear Juice
No Sugar Added Pear Slices in Juice
No Sugar Added Sliced Peach Clings in Pear Juice
No Sugar Added Sliced Yellow Cling Peaches in Pear Juice
Pineapple Chunks in Juice
Yellow Cling Peach Slices in Pear Juice

Thrifty Maid (Winn-Dixie)
Bartlett Pears (Halves, Slices)
Yellow Cling Peaches (Halves, Slices)

Trader Joe's
Apple Banana Fruit Sauce Crushers
Chunky Spiced Apples
Mandarin Oranges In Light Syrup
Sweet Pineapple Chunks

Valu Time (Brookshire)
Fruit Cocktail in Light Syrup
Mandarin Orange in Lite Syrup
Peach Halves in Light Syrup
Pear Halves
Sliced Peaches
Sliced Peaches in Light Syrup
Sliced Pears in Light Syrup

Valu Time (Marsh)
Fruit Cocktail Light Syrup
Peaches Cling Halves Light
Peaches Sliced Light Syrup
Pears Halves Light Syrup

Valu Time (Schnucks)
Cling Peaches, Sliced
Pear Halves, Lite

Vons ✍
Apricot Halves in Heavy Syrup
Diced Peaches in Light Syrup Fruit
Fruit Cocktail
Light Sugar Fruit Cocktail
Light Sugar Yellow Cling Peach Halves
Pear Halves in Heavy Syrup
Pear Halves in Light Juice
Pears, Sliced in Light Syrup
Pineapple, Crushed
Pineapple, Sliced in Juice
Triple Cherry Mixed Fruit in Light Syrup
Unpeeled Light Apricot Halves
Yellow Cling Peach Halves in Heavy
Syrup

Wegmans
Fruit Cocktail in Heavy Syrup
Half Pears in Heavy Syrup
Mandarin Oranges
Sliced Peaches in Heavy Syrup
Sliced Pears in Heavy Syrup
Sliced Pineapple in Heavy Syrup
Sliced Yellow Cling Peaches in Heavy
Syrup
Sliced Yellow Cling Peaches, Raspberry
Flavor
Triple Cherry Fruit Mix - Cherry
Flavored, Light Syrup
Tropical Fruit Salad in Light Syrup
Whole Segment Mandarin Oranges

White House
White House (All)

Winn-Dixie
Apricot Halves, Unpeeled
Bartlett Pears (Halves, Slices)
Chunky Mixed Fruit
Fruit Cocktail
Mandarin Orange Segments
Mandarin Oranges Fruit Cup

Mixed Fruit Cup
Peaches Fruit Cup
Pears Fruit Cup
Pineapple (Chunks, Crushed, Sliced,
Tidbits)
Yellow Cling Peaches (Halves, Slices)

Wyman's
Wyman's (All)

MEALS & MEAL STARTERS

ACME
Corned Beef Hash

Albertsons
Corned Beef Hash

Annie's Homegrown
Gluten Free Deluxe Rice Pasta and
Cheddar
Gluten Free Rice Pasta & Cheddar

Asian Helper
Beef Fried Rice Skillet Meal
Chicken Fried Rice Skillet Meal

Best Choice
Beef Tamales

Caesar's Pasta ⓘ ✔
Gluten-Free Cheese Lasagna in
Marinara Sauce
Gluten-Free Gnocchi without Sauce
(Potato, Spinach)
Gluten-Free Manicotti in Marinara
Sauce
Gluten-Free Stuffed Shells in Marinara
Sauce
Gluten-Free Vegetable Lasagna in
Marinara Sauce

Casa Fiesta ⓘ
Taco Dinner

Cat Cora's Kitchen
Sundried Tomato Bruschetta

Chi-Chi's
Fiesta Plates Creamy Chipotle Chicken
Fiesta Plates Salsa Chicken
Fiesta Plates Savory Garlic Chicken

Cub Foods
Corned Beef Hash
Old Fashioned Potato Salad

Culinary Circle (ACME)
Chicken Tikka Masala

Culinary Circle (Cub Foods)
Chicken Tikka Masala

Dave's
Coleslaw

Davis & Davis
Cheeseball Kits (All)

DeBoles
Gluten Free Rice Angel Hair Plus
   Golden Flax
Gluten Free Rice Elbow Style Pasta &
   Cheese
Gluten Free Rice Shells & Cheddar

DeLallo
Artichoke Bruschetta ⓘ
Calabrese Style Mushroom Antipasto
Capers in Brine Antipasto
Caponata
Fresh Garlic & Pepper Antipasto
Genovese Salad
Greek Feta Salad
Green Asparagus Bruschetta
Hot Pepper & Cauliflower Salad
Marinated Artichoke Antipasto
Mexicalo Jalapeno Mushroom Antipasto
Muffalatta Antipasto
Olive Bruschetta ⓘ
Pearl Martini Onion Antipasto
Piquillo Pepper & Artichoke Bruschetta
Prince Omar Stuffed Grape Leaves
Roasted Pepper Bruschetta ⓘ
Roasted Piquillo Bruschetta
Sun Dried Tomato Bruschetta ⓘ
Sweet Martini Onion Antipasto
Whole Roasted Garlic Antipasto

Dietz & Watson ✓
Buffalo Cheese Panino
Pizzaz Panino
Prosciutto Panino
Salame Panino
Toasted Onion Cheese Panino

Dinty Moore
Microwaveable Cups - Beef Stew
Microwaveable Cups - Scalloped
   Potatoes & Ham

Divine Brine ()
Caponata

Dr. McDougall's Right Foods ⓘ
Pad Thai Asian Entrée

Eating Right ↷
Veggie Party Platter

Flavorite (Cub Foods)
Corned Beef Hash

Food Club (Brookshire)
Canned Spanish Rice
Corned Beef Hash
Dinner Taco Kit
Dried Hash Browns

Food Club (Marsh)
Corned Beef Hash

Gaea ()
Dolmas

GalloLea Organics ⓘ
Gluten Free Pizza Kit

Giant
Ready to Eat Amish Potato Salad
Ready to Eat Cole Slaw
Ready to Eat Dixie Cole Slaw
Ready to Eat Potato Salad
Ready to Eat Potato Salad with Egg
Ready to Eat Red Skinned Potato
Ready to Heat Balsamic Chicken
Ready to Heat Broccoli Au Gratin
Ready to Heat Creamed Spinach
Ready to Heat Deli Fresh Organic
   Creamy Tomato Soup
Ready to Heat Garlic Mashed Potatoes
Ready to Heat Homestyle Mashed
   Potatoes
Ready to Heat Lemon Thyme Chicken
Ready to Heat Maryland Crab Soup
Ready to Heat Sweet Potato Casserole

Giant Eagle
Baked Beans
Broccoli Cheese and Rice
Cheddar Mashed White Potato
Chicken Salad
Cinnamon Caramel Apples
Cole Slaw
Deluxe Potato Salad
Egg Salad
Four Bean Salad

Garlic Mashed Potatoes
Ham Off the Bone
Ham Salad
Health Salad
Homestyle Mashed Potatoes
Italian Pasta Salad
Loaded Mashed Potatoes
Macaroni Salad
Mashed Sweet Potatoes
Potato Salad
Rotini Supreme
Seashell Macaroni Salad
Sour Cream and Chive Potatoes
Sour Cream Dill Potato
Sour Cream Macaroni and Cheddar
Southern Potato Salad

Glutenfreeda ⓘ 🏅
Pizza Wraps (All)

GoGo Quinoa ✔
GoGo Quinoa (All)

GoPicnic
Hummus & Crackers
Salmon & Crackers
St. Dalfour Three Beans with Sweetcorn
St. Dalfour Wild Salmon with
Vegetables
Steak Nuggets & Cheese
Sunbutter & Crackers
Tuna & Crackers
Turkey Pepperoni & Cheese
Turkey Stick & Crunch

Goya
Anticucho
Classic Entrees - Picadillo with Rice
Classic Entrees - Stew Rice
Hoppin'John- Blackeye Peas ()
Mediterranean Salad
Paella ()
Papa Criolla
Plantain Turnovers- Blue Crab
Plantain Turnovers- Cheese
Plantain Turnovers- Shrimp
Plantain Turnovers- Tuna
Rice & Black Beans ()
Rice & Pigeon Peas ()
Rice & Pinto Beans ()
Rice & Red Beans ()

Yellow Rice & Corn ()
Yellow Rice & Red Beans ()

Grandmas
Bag N Bake Chicken

GranoVita
Nut Luncheon
Vegetable Hotpot

GreenWise Market (Publix)
Organic Baby Arugula Salad
Organic Baby Lettuce Salad
Organic Baby Romaine Salad
Organic Baby Spinach Blend
Organic Baby Spinach Salad
Organic Fresh Herb Salad
Organic Mix Baby Greens
Organic Romaine Hearts

Hamburger Helper
Cheesy Hashbrowns Skillet Meal

H-E-B
Artisan Capicolla & Pepperoncini
Mozzarollo
Artisan Prosciutto & Basil Mozzarollo
Artisan Wine Salami Mozzarollo

Hormel
Beef Tamales
Compleats Microwave Meals - Chicken
& Rice
Compleats Microwave Meals - Santa Fe
Chicken
Party Trays (Crackers do contain gluten)
Refrigerated Entrées - Beef Roast Au Jus
Refrigerated Entrées - Italian Style Beef
Roast
Refrigerated Entrées - Pork Roast Au Jus
Refrigerated Entrées - Turkey Breast
Roast

Isola
Antipasti (All)

Jewel-Osco
Corned Beef Hash
Dixie Cole Slaw

Juanitas
Refrigerated Entrees, Barbacoa
Refrigerated Entrees, Carnitas

Kroger
Sloppy Joe

Leahey Gardens ⓘ
Gluten Free Red Beans and Rice

Luzianne
Creole Dinner Kit

Market District (Giant Eagle)
Fresh Bruschetta

Mezzetta
Giardiniera (All)
Italian Olive Antipasto

Molly's Tamales
Tamales (All)

Mon Cuisine
MonPassover 2-pack
MonPassover Beef Goulash
MonPassover Braised Veal
MonPassover Dairy Cheese Blintzes
MonPassover Dairy Eggplant Parmesan
MonPassover Fillet Salmon
MonPassover Prime Ribeye
MonPassover Roast Chicken
MonPassover Roast Turkey
MonPassover Salsibury Steak

Nueva Cocina ⓘ
Black Beans and Rice Mix
Chicken Rice Mix
Mexican Rice Mix
Red Beans and Rice Mix
Seafood Rice Mix

Orgran ⓘ ♉
Falafel Mix
Pasta & Sauce Tomato & Basil
Spaghetti in Tomato Sauce
Spaghetti with Tomato and Basil
Spirals in Tomato Sauce

Ortega ⓘ
Chicken Breast Mexican Style Sauce
Chicken Breast Santa Fe Style Sauce
Sponge Bob Dinner Kit
Taco Kit (12-count and 18-count)

Our Family
Corned Beef Hash

Pastariso
Dolphin Rice Macaroni and Yellow
Cheese
Elephant Rice Macaroni & White
Cheese

Orangutan Rice Mini Shells and White
Cheese
Panda Potato Macaroni and Cheese
Phino Rice Mini Shells & Yellow
Cheddar Cheese
Potato Orangutan Macroni and White
Chedder Cheese
White Rice Rabit Macaroni & Cheese

Pastene
Eggplant Caponata
Hot Garden Salad

Peloponnese
Dolmas
Eggplant Meze

Publix
Chicken Tarragon Salad
Classic Blend Salad
Cole Slaw Blend Salad
European Blend Salad
Italian Blend Salad
Packaged Blends Salad
Romaine Lettuce Heart Salad
Spinach Salad

Road's End Organics ✓
GF Alfredo Chreese Mix
GF Cheddar Chreese Mix
Organic GF Alfredo Mac & Chreese
Organic GF Cheddar Penne & Chreese

Sacla
Antipasti in Oil

Safeway Farms 〰
American Blend
Baby Spinach
Caesar Romaine
Hearts of Romaine Prepacked
Italian Blend Prepacked
Spring Mix
Sweet Butter Blend

Simply Potatoes
Simply Potatoes (All BUT Macaroni and
Cheese)

Sof'ella ⓘ
Basmati Rice and Green Lentils
Broccoli & Cheddar Pilaf
Cuban Rice and Beans
Garlic Herb & Risotto

Spaa Natural Foods ⓘ
Curry Spicy Thai Rice Meal
Peanut Satay Noodles Meal
Tasty Thai Pad Thai Noodels Meal

St. Dalfour ⓘ
Gourmet on the Go, Three Beans
Gourmet on the Go, Wild Salmon

Stop & Shop
Heat & Serve Creamed Spinach
Heat & Serve Garlic Mashed Potatoes
Heat & Serve Homestyle Mashed
  Potatoes
Homestyle Cole Slaw Salad

Tassos
Bruschetta (All)

Taste of China, A
Taste of China, A (All)

Taste of Thai, A
Taste of Thai, A (All)

Tasty Bite ⓘ
Agra Peas & Greens
Aloo Palak
Bangkok Beans
Bengal Lentils
Bombay Potatoes
Channa Masala
Chunky Chickpeas
Jaipur Vegetables
Jodhpur Lentils
Kashmir Spinach
Kerala Vegetables
Lentil Magic
Madras Lentils
Mushroom Takatak
Paneer Makhani
Peas Paneer
Punjab Eggplant
Snappy Soya
Spinach Dal
Tofu Corn Masala
Vegetable Korma
Zesty Lentils & Peas

Trader Joe's
Artichoke Antipasto
Baby Spinach Salad
Balela
Bruschetta

Channa Masala
Chef Salad
Chicken Enchiladas In Salsa Verde
Chicken Gorgonzola
Chicken Masala
Chicken Pomodoro
Chicken Salad
Classic Cole Slaw
Classic Greek Salad
Curried Lentils with Basmati Rice
Dolmas
Egg White Salad
Eggplant Caponata Appetizer
Enchilada – Organic Black Bean And
  Corn
Garden Salad
Genova Pesto
Gorgonzola Walnut Salad
Grilled Chicken (Strips, Lemon Pepper,
  Plain, Balsamic & Rosemary Chicken
  Breast)
Grilled Chicken Salad with Orange
  Vinaigrette
Grilled Vegetable Bruschetta
Indian Fare Meals (All)
Mixed Olive Bruschetta
Palak Paneer
Paneer Tikka Masala
Peruvian Style Chimichurri Rice with
  Vegetables
Powerhouse Salad
Rice Pasta & Cheddar
Roasted Chicken
Steamed Beets
Steamed Lentils
Sun-Dried Tomato Bruschetta
True Thai Green Papaya Salad
Vegetable Panang Curry

Urbane Grain
Indian Coconut Curry Quinoa Blend
Miso with Edamame & Scallions
  Quinoa Blend
Southwest Black Bean Quinoa Blend
Sundried Tomato & Basil Quinoa Blend
Thai Red Curry Quinoa Blend
Three Cheese & Mushroom Quinoa
  Blend

Vietti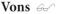
Beef Barbecue
GAF Beans and Franks in Sauce
Pork Barbecue
Southgate Beans and Franks in Sauce
Southgate Corned Beef Hash
Sun Meadow Potatoes and Ham in
Cheese Sauce
Vons
Corned Beef
Williams
Bag-N-Bake Chicken

MEAT

Albertsons
Fat Free Chunk Chicken In Water
Fat Free Chunk White Chicken
Premium Chunk Chicken Breast
Always Save
Vienna Sausage
White/Dark Chunk Chicken
Best Choice
Chunk White Chicken
Corned Beef Hash
Cub Foods
Premium Chunk Chicken
Flavorite (Cub Foods)
Breast Of Chicken
Food Club (Brookshire)
Canned Luncheon Meat
Chicken Chunks, 98% Fat Free
Food Club (Marsh)
Chicken, Chunk White (98% Fat Free)
Giant
Corned Beef Hash
Giant Eagle
Chunk White Chicken
Great Value (Wal-Mart) 🔲25
Luncheon Meat
Potted Meat Product
Vienna Sausage
H-E-B
Canned Chicken
Premium Chicken Breast
Hill Country Fare (H-E-B)
Lite Vienna Sausage

Vienna Sausage
Hormel
Black Label Canned Hams
Breast of Chicken Chunk Meats
Chicken Chunk Meats
Corned Beef
Corned Beef Hash
Dried Beef
Ham Chunk Meats
Turkey Chunk Meats
Hy-Vee
Luncheon Meat
Premium Chunk Chicken Breast with
Rib Meat and Water
Jewel-Osco
Canned Luncheon Meat
Chunk Chicken
Chunk Chicken Breast
White Chicken
Meijer
Chicken, Chunk White
Corned Beef Hash
Plumrose ✓
Plumrose (All)
Safeway
Canned Chicken
Shaw's
Chunk Chicken In Water
Corned Beef Hash Can
Shelton's ⓘ
Canned Chicken Breast Meat
SPAM
Classic
Hot and Spicy
Less Sodium
Lite
Oven Roasted Turkey
Smoke Flavored
SPAM with Bacon
SPAM with Cheese
Thrifty Maid (Winn-Dixie)
Chicken Vienna Sausage
Underwood ⓘ
Deviled Ham Spread
Valley Fresh
Chicken
Turkey

Valu Time (Brookshire)
- Potted Meat Spread
- Vienna Sausage
- White Chicken Chunks in Water

Valu Time (Marsh)
- Chicken Chunk White in Water

PIE FILLINGS

Albertsons
- Instant Pie Filling, Chocolate
- Instant Pie Filling, Vanilla

Baker ()
- Dessert Fillings (All Flavors)
- Pie Fillings (All Flavors)

E.D. Smith
- E.D. Smith (All)

Farmer's Market (i)
- Organic Pumpkin Pie Mix

Fischer & Wieser (i)
- Classic Cherry Pie Filling
- Fredericksburg Golden Peach Pie Filling
- Harvest Apple & Brandy Pie Filling

Flavorite (Cub Foods)
- Apple Pie Filling
- Blueberry Pie Filling

Food Club (Brookshire)
- Pie Filling (Apple, Cherry, Cherry Lite, Peach)
- Pumpkin

Food Club (Marsh)
- Pie Filling Apple
- Pie Filling Blueberry
- Pie Filling Cherry
- Pie Filling Cherry Lite
- Pie Filling Peach

Goya
- Calabaza/Auyama

Grainless Baker, The
- The Grainless Baker (All)

Grandmother's
- Apple Pie Filling
- Blueberry Pie Filling
- Cherry Pie Filling
- Fig Pastry Filling
- Red Raspberry Pie & Pastry Filling
- Rum Flavored Mincemeat
- Traditional Mincemeat

Great Value (Wal-Mart) `25`
- Apple Pie Filling
- Blueberry Pie Filling
- Cherry Pie Filling
- No Sugar Added Apple Pie Filling with Splenda
- No Sugar Added Cherry Pie Filling with Splenda

Hy-Vee
- Cook and Serve Chocolate Pudding & Pie Filling
- Cook and Serve Vanilla Pudding & Pie Filling
- Instant Butterscotch Pudding & Pie Filling
- Instant Chocolate Pudding & Pie Filling
- Instant Lemon Pudding & Pie Filling
- Instant Pistachio Pudding & Pie Filling
- Instant Vanilla Pudding and Pie Filling
- More Fruit Cherry Pie Filling Or Topping

Kroger
- Apple Pie Filling
- Cherry Pie Filling
- Extra Peach Pie Filling
- Light Cherry Pie Filling
- Strawberry Pie Filling

Libby's
- Easy Pumpkin Pie Mix

Meijer
- Pie Filling (Apple, Blueberry, Cherry, Cherry Light, Peach)
- Pumpkin

Midwest Country Fare (Hy-Vee)
- Apple Pie Filling
- Cherry Pie Filling

Our Family
- Apple More Fruit Pie Filling
- Apple Pie Filling
- Blueberry Pie Filling
- Cherry More Fruit Pie Filling
- Cherry Pie Filling
- Pumpkin
- Strawberry Pie Filling

Price Chopper
- Pumpkin Solid Pack

Schnucks
- Apple Pie Filling
- Blueberry Pie Filling
- Cherry Pie Filling
- Light Cherry Pie Filling
- Pumpkin

Shaw's
- Blueberry Pie Fillng
- Cherry Pie Filling

Solo ()
- Cake & Pastry Fillings (All Flavors)

Vons ∿
- Red Tart Pitted Pie Cherries

Winn-Dixie
- Apple Pie Filling
- Blueberry Pie Filling
- Cherry Pie Filling

SEAFOOD, OTHER

Always Save
- Jack Mackerel

Bar Harbor
- Chopped Clams
- Clam Juice
- Whole Cherrystone Clams
- Whole Maine Lobster
- Whole Maine Mussels

Best Choice
- Pink Salmon
- Red Salmon

Chicken of the Sea
- Chicken of The Sea (All BUT Tuna Salad Kit)

Crown Prince ♛
- Canned Seafood Products (All)

DeLallo
- Anchovies, Flat Fillet ⓘ
- Anchovies, Rolled with Capers ⓘ
- San Martino Crabmeat
- Sea Clams (Chopped, Minced)

Ducktrap River of Maine
- Ducktrap River of Maine (All)

Geisha
- Chopped Clams
- Crab Meat
- Jack Mackerel
- Lump Crab Meat
- Minced Clams
- Oyster
- Smoked Oysters
- Tiny Shrimp
- Whole Baby Clams

Goya
- Angulas Surimi
- Bonito en Aceite de Oliva
- Bonito in Tomato Sauce
- Calamares en Tinta
- Calamares Picante
- Filete Calamares en Tinta
- Mejillones Escabeche
- Pulpo a la Marinera
- Pulpo al Ajillo
- Pulpo en Aceite de Oliva
- Pulpo Picante
- Sardinas con Limon
- Sardinas en Aceite
- Sardinas en Tomate
- Sardinas Lata Ovalada/Tomate
- Sardinas Spice
- Sardines
- Sardines in Hot Sauce
- Sardinilla
- Tinapa Sardinas /Picantitas
- Tinapa Sardinas en Tomate

Great Value (Wal-Mart) 25
- Crab Meat
- Lightly Smoked Sardines In Oil
- Naturally Smoked Kipper Snacks
- Smoked Oysters (China)
- Smoked Oysters (South Korea)
- Tiny Shrimp

Hill Country Fare (H-E-B)
- Pink Salmon

Hy-Vee
- Alaska Pink Salmon
- Alaska Red Salmon

Isola
- Anchovies

Kasilof
- Boxed Salmon Items (All)

Meijer
- Salmon (Pink, Sockeye Red)

Our Family
Pink Salmon
Pastene
Anchovy Fillets, Wild Caught
Schnucks
Anchovies, Italian
Spence & Co. Ltd.
Spence & Co. Ltd. (All BUT Lox in a
Box)
Trader Joe's
Skinless & Boneless Sardines in Olive
Oil
Whole Smoked Oysters in Olive Oil
Trans Ocean Products ()
Crab Classic Chunk
Lobster Classic Chunk
Vons ᧞
Salmon Pink
Wild Planet ()
Wild Planet (All)

SEAFOOD, TUNA

ACME
White Chunk Chicken In Water
Always Save
Chunk Lite Tuna in Water
Best Choice
Chunk Lite Tuna in Water
Chicken of the Sea
Chicken of The Sea (All BUT Tuna
Salad Kit)
Food Club (Brookshire)
Light Chunk Tuna in Water
Premium White Tuna
**Food You Feel Good About
(Wegmans)**
Low Sodium Tuna, No HVP
Tuna in Water
Yellowfin Light Tuna in Water
Giant
Light Chunk Tuna in Water
Solid White Albacore Tuna in Water
Goya
Atun con Elote/Maiz ()
Atun con Jalapeño ()
Atun con Vegetales ()

Great Value (Wal-Mart) [25]
Chunk Light Tuna In Water
Premium Chunk Light Tuna In Water
Solid White Albacore Tuna In Water
H-E-B
Albacore in Water
Albacore Tuna Pouch
Chunk Light Tuna in Pouch
Chunk Light Tuna in Spring Water
Chunk Light Tuna in Water
Hill Country Fare (H-E-B)
Chunk Light Tuna in Spring Water
Chunk Light Tuna in Water
Solid White Albacore in Water
Hy-Vee
Chunk Light Tuna in Water
Nature's Promise (Giant)
Albacore Tuna in Water
Light Chunk Tuna in Water
Our Family
Albacore Tuna
Light Chunk Tuna in Water
Pastene
Tonno (Tuna)
Tuna with Fresh Ginger
Tuna with Hot Chili Pepper
Price Chopper
Chunk Light Tuna
Safeway ᧞
Chunk Light Tuna in Water
StarKist Tuna
Starkist Canned & Pouch Tuna (All
BUT Crackers in Lunch To-Go and
Charlie's Lunch Kit)
Starkist Seasations (All BUT Teriyaki
Orange & Ginger and Thai with Basil)
Starkist Tuna Creations (All BUT Herb
& Garlic and Tomato Pesto Albacore)
Trader Joe's
Tuna (All)
Valu Time (Brookshire)
Light Chunks of Tuna in Water
Vons ᧞
Tuna Chunk Light in Water
Wegmans
Albacore Tuna in Water

Wild Planet ()
  Wild Planet (All)

SOUPS & SOUP MIXES

4C
  Dehydrated Onion Soup Mix
ACME
  Ham Flavor 16 Bean Soup Mix
  Onion Soup Mix
Albertsons
  Onion Soup Mix
Amy's Kitchen ✓
  Black Bean Vegetable Soup
  Chunky Tomato Bisque
  Chunky Vegetable Soup
  Cream of Tomato Soup
  Curried Lentil Soup
  Fire Roasted Southwestern Vegetable
    Soup
  Hearty Spanish Rice & Red Bean Soup
  Indian Golden Lentil Soup
  Lentil Soup
  Lentil Vegetable Soup
  Light in Sodium Chunky Tomato Bisque
  Light in Sodium Cream of Tomato Soup
  Light in Sodium Lentil Soup
  Light in Sodium Lentil Vegetable Soup
  Light in Sodium Split Pea Soup
  Organic Hearty French Country
    Vegetable Soup
  Organic Hearty Rustic Italian Vegetable
  Split Pea Soup
  Summer Corn & Vegetable Soup
  Thai Coconut Soup (Tom Kha Phak)
  Tuscan Bean & Rice Soup
Andean Dream
  Tomato Quinoa Noodle Soup
  Vegetarian Quinoa Noodle Soup
Bear Creek
  Cheddar Broccoli
  Cheddar Potato
  Clam Chowder
  Creamy Potato
  Creamy Wild Rice
  Navy Bean
  Split Pea

  Tortilla
Best Choice
  Chunky Broccoli Cheese Soup
  Chunky Chicken Gumbo
Bineshii Wild Rice
  Wild Rice Soup Mix
Casa Fiesta ⓘ
  Gazpacho Soup Mix
Cub Foods
  16 Bean Soup Mix
Dr. McDougall's Right Foods ⓘ
  Black Bean & Lime Soup Cup
  Black Bean Soup
  Chunky Tomato Soup
  Lentil Soup
  Light Sodium Split Pea Soup Cup
  Low Sodium Garden Vegetable Soup
  Low Sodium Lentil Soup
  Pad Thai Noodle Soup Cup
  Roasted Red Pepper Tomato Soup
  Split Pea Soup
  Spring Onion Noodle Soup Cup
  Tamale Soup Cup
  Tortilla Soup Cup
  Vegetable Soup
Eating Right ◡
  Enlighten Potato Leek Soup
Eden Foods
  Organic Genmai (Brown Rice) Miso
Edward & Sons ✓
  Miso-Cup, Japanese Restaurant Style
  Miso-Cup, Original Golden Vegetable
  Miso-Cup, Reduced Sodium
  Miso-Cup, Savory Seaweed
  Miso-Cup, Traditional with Tofu
Flavorite (Cub Foods)
  16 Bean Soup Mix
Food Club (Brookshire)
  Chunky Grilled Chicken Sausage
    Gumbo
  Condensed Chicken Rice Soup
Food Club (Marsh)
  Condensed Chicken Rice Soup
**Food You Feel Good About
(Wegmans)**
  Broccoli & Vermont White Cheddar
    Soup

Caribbean Black Bean Soup
Moroccan Lentil with Chick Pea Soup

Frontier Soups ⓘ
Carolina Springtime Asparagus Almond Soup
Chicago Bistro French Onion Soup
Connecticut Cottage Chicken Noodle Soup
Far East Ginger Beef Bowl
Florida Sunshine Red Pepper Corn Chowder
Holiday Gathering Cranberry Bean Soup
Idaho Outpost Potato Leek Soup
Illinios Prairie Corn Chowder
Indiana Harvest Sausage Lentil Soup
Louisiana Red Bean Gumbo
Minnesota Heartland 11-Bean Soup
Mississippi Delta Tomato Basil Soup
Missouri Homestead Garden Gazpacho Soup
Nebraska Barnraising Green Split Pea Soup
New Mexico Mesa Spicy Fiesta Soup
New Orleans Jambalaya Soup
Oregon Lakes Wild Rice & Mushroom Soup
San Francisco Thai Golden Peanut Soup
South of the Border Tortilla Soup
Texas Wrangler Black Bean Soup
Virginia Blue Ridge Broccoli Cheddar Soup
Wisconsin Lakeshore Wild Rice Soup

Full Flavor Foods ✓
Soup Mixes (All)

Giant
Onion Soup Mix

Giant Eagle
Butternut Squash
Southwestern Black Bean Soup
Tomato Basil Soup

GoGo Quinoa ✓
GoGo Quinoa (All)

Goya
Ajiaco
Black Bean Soup
Caldo de Bola

Consomme de Pollo
Frijol Mixed Pallet
H&S Menudo
Menudo
Pozole
Sancocho

Haggen
16 Bean Soup Mix
Chunky Vegetable Soup
Homestyle Chicken & Rice

H-E-B
Cheesy Chicken Enchilada Soup
Creamy Mushroom Pouch Soup
Fall Harvest Pouch Soup
Loaded Baked Potato Pouch
Poblano Corn Chowder Pouch

Hill Country Fare (H-E-B)
Chicken Rice Soup
Condensed Chicken and Rice Soup

Hormel
Microwaveable Cup Bean & Ham Soup
Microwaveable Cup Chicken with Vegetables & Rice Soup

Imagine
Creamy Portobello Mushroom Soup
Creamy Sweet Corn & Lemongrass Soup
Organic Creamy Acorn Squash & Mango Soup
Organic Creamy Broccoli Soup
Organic Creamy Butternut Squash Soup
Organic Creamy Potato Leek Soup
Organic Creamy Sweet Pea Soup
Organic Creamy Tomato Basil Soup
Organic Creamy Tomato Soup

Jewel-Osco
16 Bean Soup Mix
Onion Soup Mix Powder

Johnny's Fine Foods ⓘ
Potato Soup

Juanitas
Cocido de Res
Pozole
Pozole de Pollo

Leahey Gardens ⓘ
Gluten Free Broccoli Cheese Soup
Gluten Free No Beef Rice Soup

Lipton - Onion Soup Mix

Gluten Free No Chicken Rice Soup
Gluten Free Potato Soup
Lucini Italia
Soups (All BUT Rustic Minestrone)
Manischewitz
Borscht (All)
Meijer
Chicken, Aspectic
Condensed Chicken with Rice Soup
Homestyle Chicken with Rice Soup
Traditional New England Clam
Chowder
Midwest Country Fare (Hy-Vee)
Onion Soup
Mom's ⓘ
Limited Edition Tomato Basil Soup
Mom's Place Gluten-Free ⚇
Mom's Place Gluten-Free (All)
Mrs. Bryant's
Garden Fresh Gourmet™ Bombay Lentil
Dry Soup Mix
Garden Fresh Gourmet™ Moroccan
Black Bean Dry Soup Mix
Nature's Promise (Giant)
Butternut Squash Soup
Cream of Tomato Soup
Nature's Promise (Stop & Shop)
Butternut Squash Soup
Cream of Brocolli Soup
Cream of Tomato
New England Country Soup ◇
Caribbean Black Bean
Chicken Corn Chowder
Lentil
Nana's Chicken Soup
New England Clam Chowder
Sweet Chicken Curry
Yankee White Bean
Nueva Cocina ⓘ
Black Bean Soup with Chipotle
Cuban Black Bean Soup
Latin Lentil Soup
Red Bean Soup
White Bean Soup
O Organics 〰
Black Bean Soup
Lentil Soup

Organic Gourmet
Instant Soup N Stock Concentrates
Organic Oat Miso Pastes ✓
Orgran ⓘ ⚇
Tomato Soup
Our Family
16 Bean Ham Soup Mix
Chicken with Rice Soup (Condensed)
Chunky Grilled Chicken & Sausage
Gumbo, 98% Fat Free 42% Less
Sodium
Pacific Natural Foods ⓘ
All Natural Rosemary Potato Chowder
Cashew Carrot Ginger
Curried Red Lentil
Organic Chicken and Wild Rice Soup
Organic Cream of Celery Condensed
Soup
Organic Cream of Chicken Condensed
Soup
Organic Cream of Mushroom
Condensed Soup
Organic Creamy Butternut Squash
Organic Creamy Roasted Red Pepper &
Tomato
Organic Creamy Tomato
Organic French Onion
Organic Hearty Tomato Bisque
Organic Light Sodium Creamy
Butternut Squash
Organic Light Sodium Creamy Tomato
Organic Light Sodium Roasted Red
Pepper & Tomato
Organic Roasted Red Pepper & Tomato
Bisque
Organic Sante Fe Style Chicken Soup
Spicy Black Bean Soup
Pastene
Minestrone Soup
Tuscan Vegetable Soup
White Bean Soup
Progresso
99% Fat Free New England Clam
Chowder
High Fiber Chicken Tuscany
Reduced Sodium Garden Vegetable
Soup

Rich & Hearty Chicken Corn Chowder
Rich & Hearty New England Clam
  Chowder
Traditional Chicken Cheese Enchilada
Traditional Chicken Rice with Vegetable
Traditional Manhattan Clam Chowder
Traditional New England Clam
  Chowder
Traditional Potato Broccoli Cheese
  Chowder
Traditional Southwestern Style Chicken
Traditional Split Pea with Ham
Vegetable Classics 99% Fat Free Lentil
Vegetable Classics Black Bean & Bacon
Vegetable Classics Creamy Mushroom
Vegetable Classics French Onion
Vegetable Classics Garden Vegetable
Vegetable Classics Lentil

Really Great Food
Really Great Food (All)
Richfood (ACME)
Onion Soup Mix
Safeway
Soup Mix Onion
Schnucks
Chicken Rice Soup
Homestyle Chicken Rice Soup
Shaw's
Bean Dry Soup Mix
Stop & Shop
Onion Recipe Soup Mix
Taste of Thai, A
Taste of Thai, A (All)
Trader Joe's
Butternut Squash Soup
Carrot Ginger Soup
Chicken Chili With Beans
Creamy Corn And Roasted Red Pepper
  Soup
Creamy Polenta with Spinach & Carrots
Instant Rice Noodle Soup (Roasted
  Garlic, Mushroom or Spring Onion)
Latin Black Bean Soup
Lentil Soup With Vegetables (All)
Miso Soup
Organic Black Bean Soup

Organic Creamy Corn & Roasted Red
  Pepper Soup
Organic Creamy Tomato Soup (Regular,
  Low Sodium)
Organic Split Pea Soup
Organic Sweet Potato Bisque
Organic Tomato And Roasted Red
  Pepper Soup (Regular, Low Sodium)
Organic Tomato Bisque Soup
Sweet Potato Bisque
Valu Time (Brookshire)
Dry Onion Soup Mix
Vietti
Sundown Chicken Rice Soup
Value Ready to Eat Beef Soup
Value Ready to Eat Vegetable Soup
Vons
Chicken Rice Soup
Soup, Homestyle Lentil
Wegmans
Gaspacho
Lobster Bisque
World Classics (Price Chopper)
Southwestern Style Chicken Soup

STEWS

Best Choice
Beef Stew
Castleberry's Brands, Inc.
Beef Stew
Brunswick Stew
Cub Foods
Beef Stew
Dinty Moore
Beef Stew
Chicken Stew
Flavorite (Cub Foods)
Beef Stew
Food Club (Brookshire)
Beef Stew
Food Club (Marsh)
Beef Stew
Frontier Soups
Colorado Campfire Chicken Stew
Hungarian Goulash
New England Seaport Fisherman's Stew

Goya
- Bacalao Vizcaina
- Mondongo
- Mondongo Dominicano
- Tropical Stew-Sancocho

Juanitas
- Hot & Spicy Menudo, Picoso
- Menudo Without Hominy
- Menudo, Menudito
- Pico Pica , Hot & Spicy Menudo
- Pico Pica, Menudo
- White Menudo

Our Family
- Beef Stew

Shaw's
- Beef Stew

Vietti ⓘ
- Bristol Beef Stew
- Bristol Meat Ball Stew
- Family Style Beef Stew
- Hatch Green Chili Stew with Pork
- Southgate Beef Stew
- Sun Meadow Chicken Stew
- Sun Meadow Stew

TOMATO PASTE

Best Choice
- Fancy Tomato Paste

Contadina ⓘ
- Flavored Tomato Paste (All BUT Italian Tomato Paste with Italian Seasonings)
- Tomato Paste

Cub Foods
- Tomato Paste
- Tomato Sauce

Del Monte ⓘ
- Tomatoes & Tomato Products (All BUT Spaghetti Sauce Flavored with Meat)

DeLallo
- Tomato Paste ⓘ

Food Club (Brookshire)
- Tomato Paste

Food Club (Marsh)
- Domestic Tomato Paste

Full Circle (Price Chopper)
- Tomato Paste

Full Circle (Schnucks)
- Tomato Paste

Giant
- Tomato Paste

Giant Eagle
- Tomato Paste

Goya
- Tomato Paste

Great Value (Wal-Mart) 🔲25
- Tomato Paste

GreenWise Market (Publix)
- Organic Tomato Paste

Haggen
- Tomato Paste

Hunt's
- Tomato Paste

Hy-Vee
- Tomato Paste

Jewel-Osco
- Tomato Paste

Meijer
- Tomato Paste (Domestic, Organic)
- Tomatoes Crushed in Puree

Nature's Basket (Giant Eagle)
- Organic Tomato Paste

Nature's Promise (Giant)
- Organic Tomato Paste

Nature's Promise (Stop & Shop)
- Organic Tomato Paste

O Organics
- Organic Tomato Paste

Our Family
- Tomato Paste

Pastene
- Tomato Paste

Price Chopper
- Tomato Paste

Publix
- Tomato Paste

S&W Fine Foods ⓘ
- Tomato & Tomato Products

Safeway
- Tomato Paste

Schnucks
- Tomato Paste

Shaw's
- Tomato Paste

Shoppers Value (Albertsons)
Tomato Paste
Shoppers Value (Cub Foods)
Tomato Paste
Shoppers Value (Jewel-Osco)
Tomato Paste
Valu Time (Brookshire)
Tomato Paste
Wegmans
Tomato Paste
Winn-Dixie
Tomato Paste

TOMATOES

ACME
Diced Italian Style Tomatoes
Diced Petite Tomatoes
No Salt Tomato Sauce
Premium Diced Peeled Tomatoes
Premium Tomato Sauce
Sliced Italian Style Stewed Tomatoes
Tomato Juice
Tomato Puree
Whole Peeled Tomatoes
Always Save
Crushed Tomatoes
Diced Tomatoes
Tomato Sauce
Whole Tomatoes
Whole/Peeled Tomatoes
Best Choice
Canned Tomato Juice
Crushed Tomatoes
Diced Tomatoes & Chilis
Diced Tomatoes
Diced Tomatoes with Garlic & Onion
Diced Tomatoes with Onion & Chilis
Diced Tomatoes with Sweet Onion
Fancy Stewed Tomatoes
Fancy Tomato Sauce
Italian Diced Tomatoes
Italian Stewed Tomatoes
Mexican Diced Tomatoes
Mexican Stewed Tomatoes
Petite Diced Tomatoes

Petite Diced Tomatoes with Garlic and
Onion
Tomato Sauce
Tomatoes & Green Chili
Whole Peeled Tomatoes
Bionaturae
Canned Tomatoes ⅋
Bubbies ⅋
Pickled Green Tomatoes (All)
Carlita (Cub Foods)
Diced Tomatos With Green Chilies
Clearly Organic (Best Choice)
Crushed Tomato
Diced Tomatoes
Tomato Sauce
Whole Peeled Tomatoes
Contadina ⓘ
Crushed Tomatoes (All)
Diced Tomatoes (All)
Stewed Tomatoes (All)
Tomato Puree
Tomato Sauces (All)
Whole Tomatoes
Cub Foods
Crushed Tomatoes
Diced Petite Tomatoes
Diced Tomatoes
Diced Tomatoes With Sweet Onion
Italian Style Diced Tomatos
Regular Tomato Paste
Southwest Style Diced Tomatos
Stewed Tomatoes
Tomato Juice
Whole Tomatoes
Dei Fratelli ⓘ
Dei Fratelli (All BUT Tomato Soup)
Del Fuerte
Tomato Sauce
Del Monte ⓘ
Tomatoes & Tomato Products (All BUT
Spaghetti Sauce Flavored with Meat)
DeLallo
Cherry Tomatoes, Imported Sun
Roasted ⓘ
Crushed Tomatoes, Chunky Style ⓘ
Fire Roasted Tomatoes, Diced ⓘ
Imported Italian Crushed Tomatoes

Imported Italian Diced Tomatoes
Italian Organic Crushed Tomatoes
Italian Organic Diced Tomatoes
Italian Organic Whole Peeled Tomatoes
Italian Stewed Tomatoes ⓘ
Italian Whole Peeled Tomatoes,
    Imported ⓘ
Organic Italian Tomatoes (Crushed,
    Diced, Whole Peeled) ⓘ
Organic San Marzano Tomatoes,
    Imported ⓘ
San Marzano Tomatoes, Imported ⓘ
Sun Dried Tomato Sauce, Imported ⓘ
Sun Dried Tomatoes ⓘ
Sun Dried Tomatoes in Olive Oil ⓘ
Sun Roasted Cherry Tomatoes,
    Imported
Sundried Tomatoes, Marinated with
    Garlic
Tomato Puree ⓘ
Tomato Sauce ⓘ
Tomatoes in Juice, Whole ⓘ
Tomatoes, Crushed in Light Puree ⓘ
Tomatoes, Diced in Juice ⓘ

Eden Foods
Organic Crushed Tomatoes
Organic Crushed Tomatoes with Basil
Organic Crushed Tomatoes with Onion
    & Garlic
Organic Diced Tomatoes
Organic Diced Tomatoes with Basil
Organic Diced Tomatoes with Green
    Chilies
Organic Diced Tomatoes with Roasted
    Onion & Garlic
Organic Whole Tomatoes
Organic Whole Tomatoes with Basil

Flavorite (Cub Foods)
Diced Tomatoes
Puree Tomatoes
Tomato Sauce

Food Club (Brookshire)
Crushed Tomatoes
Crushed Tomatoes in Puree
Diced Petite Peeled Tomatoes with
    Green Chilies
Diced Petite Tomatoes

Diced Petite Tomatoes with Roasted
    Garlic & Onions
Diced Petite Tomatoes with Sweet
    Onions
Diced Petite Tomatoes, Smoked
    Chipotle
Diced Petite Tomatoes, Southwestern
Diced Tomatoes
Diced Tomatoes in Juice
Diced Tomatoes in Tomato Juice, No
    Salt Added
Diced Tomatoes with Green Chilies
Diced Tomatoes with Green Chilies-
    Mild
Diced Tomatoes, Italian
Diced Tomatoes, Mexican Style
Stewed Tomatoes
Stewed Tomatoes, Italian
Stewed Tomatoes, Mexican
Stewed Tomatoes, No Salt Added
Tomato Sauce
Tomato Sauce, Hot Mexican
Tomato Sauce, No Salt Added
Whole Peeled Tomatoes (Regular and
    No Salt Added)

Food Club (Marsh)
Tomato Puree
Tomato Sauce
Tomatoes Crushed
Tomatoes Crushed In Puree
Tomatoes Diced & Green Chilies
Tomatoes Diced & Green Chilies,
    Milder
Tomatoes Diced
Tomatoes Diced In Juice
Tomatoes Diced In Juice No Salt Added
Tomatoes Diced Petite
Tomatoes Diced with Onion, Chili
    Ready
Tomatoes Diced with Roasted Garlic &
    Onion
Tomatoes Diced, Chili Ready
Tomatoes Petite Dice Peeled with Green
    Chilies
Tomatoes Stewed
Tomatoes Stewed Italian
Tomatoes Stewed Mexican

Tomatoes Whole Peeled

Food You Feel Good About (Wegmans)
Chili Style Diced Tomatoes
Roasted Garlic & Onion Diced
Tomatoes
Tomato Puree

Full Circle (Price Chopper)
Crushed Tomatoes
Diced Tomato
Tomato Juice
Whole Peeled Tomato

Full Circle (Schnucks)
Diced Italian Tomatoes
Organic Crushed Tomatoes
Organic Diced Tomatoes
Tomato Puree
Tomato Sauce
Whole Peeled Tomatoes

Furmano's
Furmano's (All)

Gaea
Tomatoes (All)

Giant
Crushed & Peeled Tomatoes
Diced Tomatoes
No Salt Added Tomato Sauce
Sliced Stewed Tomatoes
Stewed Tomatoes
Tomato Sauce
Whole Peeled Tomatoes

Giant Eagle
Crushed Tomato in Puree
Diced Tomato
Diced Tomato Garlic and Onion
Diced Tomatoes and Green Chilies
Italian Stew Tomatoes
Stewed Tomatoes
Stewed Tomatoes with Celery and
Pepper
Tomato Sauce
Whole Peeled Tomatoes
Whole Peeled Tomatoes, NSA

Goya
Hot Tomato Sauce
Low Sodium Tomato Sauce
Tomate de Arbol Pulp

Great Lakes International Trading ⓘ
Sun Dried Tomatoes (All)

Great Value (Wal-Mart) 25
Chili Ready Tomatoes
Concentrated Crushed Tomatoes
Crushed Tomatoes In Puree
Diced No Salt Added Tomatoes
Diced Tomatoes In Tomato Juice
Italian Diced Tomatoes
Italian Stewed Tomatoes
Italian Stewed Tomatoes with Basil,
Garlic, & Oregano
Mexican Hot Style Tomato Sauce,
Bilingual
No Salt Added Diced Tomatoes
No Salt Added Tomato Sauce
Pear Tomato Strips
Pear Tomato Strips with Basil In Puree
Petite Diced Tomatoes
Sliced Stewed Tomatoes In Tomato Juice
Tomato Puree
Tomato Sauce
Whole Peeled Pear Tomatoes
Whole Tomatoes
Whole Tomatoes In Tomato Juice

GreenWise Market (Publix)
Organic Crushed Tomatoes
Organic Diced Tomatoes, Basil, Garlic,
and Oregano
Organic Diced Tomatoes, Regular
Organic Tomato Sauce

Haggen
Tomato Sauce
Tomato Sauce, No Salt Added
Tomato Sauce, Roasted
Tomatoes, Diced
Tomatoes, Diced Italian
Tomatoes, Diced Petite
Tomatoes, Diced Roasted
Tomatoes, Diced with Chilies
Tomatoes, Stewed
Tomatoes, Stewed Italian
Tomatoes, Stewed Mexican
Tomatoes, Whole
Tomatoes, Whole No Salt Added

Hanover Foods
Superfine Tomatoes with Okra

Tomato Juice
Tomato Puree
Tomato Sauce

Hunt's
Canned Tomatoes (All Varieties)
Tomato Sauce (NOT Pasta Sauces)

Hy-Vee
Chili Ready Diced Tomatoes
Crushed Italian Style Tomatoes in
  Heavy Puree
Diced Italian Style Tomatoes
Diced Tomatoes
Diced Tomatoes with Green Chilies
Diced Tomatoes with Roasted Garlic &
  Onions
Petite Cut Diced Tomatoes
Petite Cut Diced Tomatoes with Garlic
  & Olive Oil
Petite Cut Diced Tomatoes with Sweet
  Onion
Petite Diced Tomatoes
Stewed Italian Style Tomatoes
Stewed Tomatoes
Tomato Sauce
Tomato Sauce, No Salt Added
Whole Peeled Tomatoes

Italian Classics (Wegmans)
Coarse Ground Tomatoes
Crushed Tomatoes with Herb
Marinated Sun-Dried Tomatoes with
  Capers
Whole Roma Tomatoes

Jewel-Osco
Crushed Tomatoes Puree
Diced Peeled Tomatoes
Diced Petite Tomatoes
Diced Tomatoes With Chiles
Diced Tomatoes With Garlic Onion
Italian Diced Tomatoes
Mexican Stewed Tomatoes
No Salt Add Diced Tomatoes
No Salt Added Diced Peeled Tomatoes
No Salt Tomato Sauce
Peeled Whole Tomatoes
Premium Diced Tomatoes
Premium Sliced Stewed Tomato
Premium Tomato Sauce

Sliced Stewed Tomatoes
Stewed Tomatoes
Tomato Sauce
Whole Peeled Tomatoes

Just Tomatoes
Just Tomatoes (All)

L'Esprit de Campagne
Dried Tomatoes (All)

Lucini Italia
Tomatoes (All)

Meijer
Diced Tomatoes
Diced Tomatoes in Italian
Diced Tomatoes in Juice
Diced Tomatoes, Chili Ready
Organic Diced Tomatoes
Organic Tomato Sauce
Organic Tomatoes with Basil
Organic Tomatoes, Whole Peeled
Stewed Tomatoes
Stewed Tomatoes, Italian
Stewed Tomatoes, Mexican
Tomato Puree
Tomato Sauce
Tomatoes Diced with Green Chilies
Tomatoes Petite Diced
Tomatoes Whole Peeled
Tomatoes Whole Peeled No Salt

Mezzetta
Sundried Tomatoes (All)

Midwest Country Fare (Hy-Vee)
Diced Tomatoes
Stewed Tomatoes
Tomato Sauce
Whole Peeled Tomatoes

Nature's Basket (Giant Eagle)
Organic Diced Tomatoes
Organic Tomato Sauce
Organic Whole Peeled Tomatoes

Nature's Promise (Giant)
Organic Crushed Tomatoes with Basil
Organic Diced Tomatoes
Organic Tomato Sauce
Organic Whole Peeled Tomatoes

Nature's Promise (Stop & Shop)
Organic Crushed Tomatoes with Basil
Organic Tomato Sauce

O Organics ✍

Diced Tomatoes
Diced Tomatoes with Garlic, Basil, and
   Oregano
No Salt Diced Tomatoes
Organic Diced Tomatoes in Tomato
   Juice
Organic Tomato Sauce
Organic Whole Peeled Tomatoes in
   Tomato Juice

Our Family

Crushed Tomatoes
Crushed Tomatoes with Basil
Diced Tomatoes
Diced Tomatoes with Garlic
Diced Tomatoes with Green Chilies
   (Mild, Original, with Cilantro & Lime)
Diced Tomatoes, Mexican Fiesta
Diced Tomatoes, No Salt Added
Petite Diced Tomatoes with Garlic &
   Olive Oil
Petite Diced Tomatoes with Onion,
   Celery, & Green Pepper
Petite Diced Tomatoes with Sweet
   Onion
Stewed Tomatoes
Stewed Tomatoes with Italian
Stewed Tomatoes with Mexican
Tomato Sauce
Whole Tomatoes

Pastene

California Plum Tomatoes with Basil
California Tomatoes, Whole Peeled
Chateau Tomato Sauce
Diced Tomatoes with Green Chilis
Italian Tomatoes
Kitchen Ready (Chunky, No Salt,
   Regular)
Marinara Tomato
San Marzano Tomatoes
Sun Dried Tomato (Halves, Julienne
   Cut)
Sun Dried Tomato Pesto
Tomato Puree
Whole Tomatoes, Small

Price Chopper

Crushed Tomato

Tomato Sauce

Publix

Tomato Puree
Tomato Sauce
Tomatoes - Crushed
Tomatoes - Diced
Tomatoes - Diced with Green Chilies
Tomatoes - Diced with Roasted Garlic
   & Onion
Tomatoes - Diced, Italian Style
Tomatoes - Diced, No Salt Added
Tomatoes - Diced, Petite
Tomatoes - Peeled Whole
Tomatoes - Sliced, Stewed
Tomatoes Sauce, No Salt Added

Red Gold

Tomato Products (All)

Rice River Farms ⓘ

Diced Natural Sun Dried Tomatoes
Diced Super Red Sun Dried Tomatoes
Julienne Natural Sun Dried Tomatoes
Julienne Super Red Sun Dried Tomatoes
Julienne Traditional Sun Dried
   Tomatoes
Sun Dried Tomato Halves, Super Red
Sun Dried Tomatoes Halves, Traditional

S&W Fine Foods ⓘ

Tomato & Tomato Products (All)

Safeway ✍

Diced Petite Tomatoes with Green
   Peppers, Celery, Onions
Fire Roasted Diced Tomatoes
Fire Roasted Diced Tomatoes with
   Garlic
No Salt Stewed Tomatoes
Petite Diced Tomatoes

Schnucks

Crushed Tomatoes in Puree
Diced Italian Tomatoes
Diced Tomatoes
Diced Tomatoes with Chili
Diced Tomatoes with Chili and Onion
Diced Tomatoes with Garlic
Diced Tomatoes with Green Chilis
Diced Tomatoes with Jalapeno
Diced Tomatoes, No Salt Added
Peeled Tomatoes

Petite Diced Tomatoes
Stewed Italian Tomatoes
Stewed Tomatoes
Stewed Tomatoes, No Salt
Tomato Juice
Tomato Sauce
Tomato Sauce, No Salt
Tomatoes with Mild Green Chili
Whole Peeled Tomatoes, No Salt

Shaw's
Crushed Tomatoes
Diced Tomato & Onion & Roasted
  Garlic
Diced Tomato With Green Chile
Diced Tomato With Jalapeno
Diced Tomatoes
Italian Diced Tomatoes
Italian Stewed Tomatoes
Mexican Stewed Tomatoes
No Salt Diced Tomatoes
No Salt Stewed Tomatoes
Petite Diced Tomatoes
Sliced Stewed Tomatoes
Tomato Juice, Canned
Tomato Puree Sauce
Tomato Sauce
Whole Peeled Tomatoes

Shoppers Value (Albertsons)
Stewed Tomatoes
Tomato Juice
Tomato Sauce

Shoppers Value (Cub Foods)
Whole Peeled Tomatoes

Shoppers Value (Jewel-Osco)
Stewed Tomatoes
Tomato Sauce
Whole Peeled Tomatoes

Stop & Shop
Cut & Peeled Diced Tomatoes
Peeled Crushed Tomatoes
Tomato Sauce

Tassos
Sun-Dried Tomatoes (All)

Trader Joe's
Sun-Dried Tomatoes (All)
Whole Peeled Tomatoes With Basil (All)

Tuttorosso
Tomato Products

Valu Time (Brookshire)
Diced Tomatoes
Stewed Tomatoes
Tomato Sauce
Whole Peeled Tomatoes

Valu Time (Marsh)
Tomato Sauce

Valu Time (Schnucks)
Diced Tomatoes
Stewed Tomatoes
Tomato Juice (Canned)
Tomato Sauce
Whole Peeled Tomatoes

Vons ✍
Diced Italian Style Tomatoes
Diced Tomatoes
Diced Tomatoes with Diced Green
  Chiles
No Salt Diced Tomatoes
No Salt Tomato Sauce
Stewed Mexican Tomatoes
Tomato Sauce
Tomatoes, Stewed
Whole Peeled Tomatoes

Wegmans
Crushed Tomatos
Diced Tomatoes
Italian Style Diced Tomatoes
Italian Style Stewed Tomatoes
Italian Style Whole Tomatoes with Basil
Kitchen Cut Tomatoes with Basil
Peeled Whole Tomatoes
Petite Diced Tomatoes
Stewed Tomatoes
Tomato Sauce
Whole Tomatoes
Whole Tomatoes - No Salt

Wild Harvest (ACME)
Organic Diced Tomatoes
Organic Whole Peeled Tomatoes

Wild Harvest (Albertsons)
Organic Diced Tomatoes
Organic Tomato Sauce
Organic Tomatoes with Italian Herbs

Wild Harvest (Cub Foods)
Organic Crushed Tomatoes With Basil
Organic Tomato Sauce
Organic Tomatoes With Italian Herbs

Wild Harvest (Jewel-Osco)
Organic Diced Tomatoes
Organic Tomato Sauce
Organic Tomatoes With Basil Crushed
Organic Tomatoes With Italian Herbs
Organic Whole Peeled Tomatoes

Winn-Dixie
Tomato Puree
Tomato Sauce
Tomatoes, Crushed
Tomatoes, Diced
Tomatoes, Diced with Green Chilies
Tomatoes, Italian Style Stewed
Tomatoes, Mexican Style Stewed
Tomatoes, Petite Diced
Tomatoes, Sliced Stewed
Tomatoes, Whole Peeled

VEGETABLES

ACME
Quartered Artichoke Hearts

Albertsons
Artichoke Hearts Quartered
Chopped Onions
Chopped Turnip Greens
Mushroom Pieces
Small Corn On The Cob
Split Green Peas
Super Sweet White Corn
Whole Green Peas
Whole Kernel Corn
Whole Petite Peas

Allens
Canned Products (All)

Alma
Canned Products

Always Save
Creamed Corn
Golden Hominy
Green Beans, Cut
Mixed Vegetables
Mushroom Pieces & Stems

Sliced Beets
Sliced Carrots
Spinach, Chopped
Sweet Peas
White Hominy
Whole Kernel Corn
Whole White Potatoes

Arrowhead Mills
Green Lentils
Green Split Peas
Red Lentils

Best Choice
Button Mushrooms
Corn, Whole Kernel
Cream-Style Corn
Early Peas
Fancy Mixed Vegetables
Fancy Sliced Beets
Fancy Sliced Carrots
Fancy Whole Beets
Golden Hominy
Green Beans, Cut
Green Beans, French Style
Green Beans, Whole
Green Split Peas
Italian Green Beans
Leaf Spinach, Whole
Lima Beans
Mixed Vegetables
Mushroom Pieces & Stems
Mustard Greens, Chopped
No Salt Cut Green Beans
No Salt French-Style Green Beans
No Salt Mixed Vegetables
No Salt Sweet Peas
No Salt Whole Kernel Corn
Peas & Sliced Carrots
Sliced Button Mushrooms
Sliced White Potatoes
Sweet Peas
Sweet Potatoes
Turnip Greens, Chopped
Wax Beans, Cut
White Hominy
White Potatoes, Whole

Bineshii Wild Rice
Hominy

Bruce Foods ⓘ
Bruce's Cut Okra
Bruce's Cut Okra and Tomatoes
Bruce's Cut Yam
Bruce's Okra, Tomatoes and Corn
Taylor Cut Yams
Taylor Whole Yams

Bush's Best
Bush's Best Products (All)

Carlita (Jewel-Osco)
Garbanzos Chick Peas

Casa Fiesta ⓘ
Green Chilies (Diced, Whole)

Cat Cora's Kitchen
Early Harvest Grape Leaves

Central Market Classics (Price Chopper)
Artichoke Hearts
Butternut Squash
Cocktail Onions
Green Asparagus
Italian Garlic Mushrooms
Marinated Mushrooms
Minced Garlic
Portabella Mushrooms
Sliced Water Chestnuts
Sweet Italian Mushrooms
White Asparagus
Whole Water Chestnuts

Christopher Ranch
Fresh Garlic Bulbs
Peeled Garlic Cloves

Clearly Organic (Best Choice)
Cut Green Beans
French Style Green Beans
Pieces & Stems Mushrooms
Sweet Peas
Whole Kernel Corn
Whole Kernel White Corn

Colavita
Vegetables in Oil (All)

Crest Top
Canned Products (All)

Cut 'N Clean
Cut 'N Clean (All)

Del Monte ⓘ
Canned Vegetables (All)

DeLallo
Artichoke Hearts ⓘ
Artichoke Hearts, Marinated ⓘ
Artichoke Portabella
Artichoke Prima Vera
Artichoke Quarters ⓘ
Artichoke, Marinated (Piccante, Royale)
Artichokes, Lemon Pesto
Artichokes, Roman Style
Baby Artichokes, Marinated
Balsamic Cipolline Onions
Cauliflower, Mild ⓘ
Cipolline Onions Agridolce
Fresh Garlic Fiesta
Garlic in Oil (Chopped, Roasted) ⓘ
Garlic, Imported Sliced in Water ⓘ
Garlic, Imported Whole Clove in Oil ⓘ
Garlic, Minced in Water ⓘ
Hearts of Palm (Salad Cut, Whole) ⓘ
Mediterranean Mushroom Medley
Mushroom & Red Pepper Cup
Mushrooms, Italian Garlic ⓘ
Portabella Mushroom Caps with
  Peppers
Portabella Mushrooms with Roasted
  Peppers ⓘ
Roman Medley
San Martino Italian Style Garlic
  Mushrooms
San Martino Portabella Mushrooms
  with Red Peppers
Yellow & Red Sun Dried Tomato
  Napolitano

Dietz & Watson ✓
Sweet Vidalia Onions in Sauce

East Texas Fair
Canned Products (All)

Eastern Star
Water Chestnuts, Whole

Eating Right ᕬ
Baby Arugula
Steamed and Peeled Beets Prepacked

Embasa
Sliced Carrots
Sliced Nopalitos
Whole Tomatillos

Farmer's Market ⓘ
Organic Butternut Squash
Organic Pumpkin
Organic Sweet Potato Puree

Fastco (Fareway)
Corn, Whole Kernel
Cream Corn
Peas

Flavorite (Cub Foods)
Split Green Peas
Yellow Split Peas

Food Club (Brookshire)
Asparagus Cuts and Tips
Asparagus Spears
Beets, Whole
Blackeye Peas with Snapped Peas
Blended Peas
Corn, Cream Style
Corn, Gold Cream Style
Corn, Mexican
Cream Peas Shelled
Dark Red Kidney Beans
Gold Corn, Whole Kernel
Gold Corn, Whole Kernel No Salt
    Added
Green Beans, French Style No Salt
    Added
Green Beans, Whole
Green Medium Lima Beans
Green Split Peas
Hominy, Golden Beans
Italian Cut Green Beans
Medium Green Lima Beans
Mixed Greens
Mixed Vegetables
Mixed Vegetables, No Salt Added
Mushroom Stems and Pieces
Mushrooms, Whole
Mushrooms, Whole Sliced
Mustard Greens
Peas & Sliced Carrots
Potato, Whole
Purple Hull Peas
Sliced Beets
Sliced Carrots
Sliced Carrots, No Salt Added
Spinach

Sweet & Crisp Corn
Sweet Cut Potato (Yam)
Sweet Peas
Sweet Peas, No Salt Added
Turnip Greens
White Sliced Potato
White Small Whole Potato

Food Club (Marsh)
Asparagus Spears
Beets, Sliced
Corn Gold Whole Kernel, No Salt
Corn Whole Kernel, Gold & White
Corn, Crisp & Sweet
Corn, Gold Cream Style
Corn, Gold Whole Kernel
Cut Green Beans, No Salt
Cut Green Beans, Veri Green
French Style Green Beans
French Style Green Beans, Veri Green
Green Beans French Style, No Salt
Green Beans, Cut
Green Beans, Whole
Mixed Vegetables
Mixed Vegetables, No Salt
Mushrooms Stems & Pieces, No Salt
Mushrooms, Stems & Pieces
Mushrooms, Whole
Mushrooms, Whole Sliced
Peas & Sliced Carrots
Pickled Beets, Whole
Sliced Carrots
Sliced Pickled Beets
Sliced White Potatoes
Small Peas
Spinach
Sweet Peas
Sweet Peas, No Salt
Sweet Potatoes, Cut (Yams)
White Corn, Whole Kernel
White Potatoes, Whole Small
Whole Beets, Small

Food You Feel Good About (Wegmans)
Brussels Sprouts
Cut Green Beans, No Salt
French Style Green Beans
French Style Green Beans, No Salt

Harvard Beets
Sliced Beets, No Salt
Sliced Carrots, No Salt Added
Sliced Pickled Beets
Small Sweet Peas
Sweet Peas
Sweet Peas, No Salt Added
Whole Kernel Corn, No Salt
Whole Kernel Sweet Corn
Whole Onions in Brine
Whole Pickled Beets

Freshlike
Canned Items (All)

Full Circle (Marsh)
Organic Garbanzo Beans

Full Circle (Price Chopper)
Organic Sweet Potatoes

Full Circle (Schnucks)
Black Beans & Corn
French Green Beans
Kernel Corn
Organic Green Beans
Organic Sweet Peas

Furmano's
Furmano's (All)

Gaea ()
Grape Leaves

Geisha
Artichoke Quarters
Bamboo Shoots
Bean Sprouts
Mixed Vegetables
Mushrooms
Water Chestnuts, Diced
Water Chestnuts, Sliced
Water Chestnuts, Whole

Genuardi's
Corn, Whole Golden

Giant
Artichoke Hearts, Whole
Carrots, Sliced
Cream Style Golden Corn
French Style Green Beans
Golden Corn, Whole Kernel
Green Beans, Cut
Mixed Vegetables
No Salt Added Cut Green Beans

No Salt Added French Style Green
   Beans
No Salt Added Sliced Carrots
No Salt Added Whole Kernel Golden
   Corn
Pickled Beets, Sliced
Spinach
Sweet Garden Mix (Cauliflower,
   Onions, Peppers & Pickles)

Ginger People, The ()
Organic Grated Ginger
Organic Minced Ginger
Organic Pickled Sushi Ginger

Glory Foods
Canned Vegetables (All)

Goya
Arracacha
Artichokes Hearts of Brine
Artichokes Marinated
Canned Yucca
Carrots, Sliced
Choclo Sliced
Crushed Tomatillo
Ensalada Encurtido
Field Peas with Snaps
Gandules
Gandules Verdes
Garlic, Chopped
Golden Hominy
Green Peas
Green Pigeon Peas
Hearts of Palm
Hominy
Huitlacoche
Jibarito Gandules
Lima Beans
Low Sodium Whole Kernel Corn
Minced Garlic
Mixed Vegetables
Nopalitos
Olluco
Papa Amarilla
Purple Corn
Recaito
Sliced Beets
Sweet Peas
Tender Sweet Peas

Tomato Cilantro Onion Garlic
White Asparagus
White Hominy
Whole Kernel Corn
Whole Tomatillo
Yautia Malanga
Yucca

Grand Selections (Hy-Vee)

Caribbean Blend Vegetables
Fancy Cut Green Beans
Fancy Whole Green Beans
Normandy Blend Vegetables
Petite Green Peas
Petite Whole Carrots
Riviera Blend Vegetables
Sugar Snap Peas
Super Sweet Cut Corn
White Shoepeg Corn
Whole Green Beans
Young, Early June Premium Peas

Great Value (Wal-Mart) 25

Asparagus Cut Spears
Asparagus Cuts & Tips
Beets, Sliced
Blackeye Peas
Collard Greens
Cream Style Corn
Cream Style Sweet Corn
Crinkle Cut Carrots
Diced Potatoes
French Style Green Beans
Golden Sweet Whole Kernel Corn
Green Beans
Green Split Peas
Italian Cut Green Beans
Minced Garlic
Mustard Greens
No Salt Added Cut Green Beans
No Salt Added French Style Green
    Beans
No Salt Added Golden Sweet Whole
    Kernel Corn
No Salt Added Sweet Peas
Nopalitos Sliced Tender Cactus,
    Bilingual
Peas & Carrots
Pieces & Stems Mushrooms

Sliced Carrots
Sliced Mushrooms
Sliced New Potatoes
Sliced Pickled Beets
Sweet Corn
Sweet Peas
Turnip Greens
White Hominy
Whole Green Beans
Whole Kernel Golden Corn
Whole Leaf Spinach
Whole New Potatoes
Whole Spear Asparagus
Yellow Hominy

GreenWise Market (Publix)

Organic Baby Carrots
Organic Carrot Chips
Organic Carrot Shreds
Organic Carrots
Organic Corn, Whole Kernel
Organic Green Beans
Organic Juicing Carrots
Organic Mushrooms
Organic Portabella Mushrooms
Organic Portabella Mushrooms, Sliced
Organic Snack Carrots
Organic Spinach
Organic Sweet Peas

Haggen

Beets (Sliced, Sliced Pickled, Whole)
Blackeye Peas
Carrots, Sliced
Corn (Cut, Super Sweet White)
Cream Corn
Green Beans, (Cut, French Style, No
    Salt)
Lentils
Peas (Blended No Salt, Plain)
Petite Peas & Carrots
Potatoes, Whole Small
Spinach
Split Peas (Green, Yellow)
Sweet Peas
Wax Beans, Cut

Hanover Foods

Blue Lake Cut Green Beans

Blue Lake Cut Green Beans and Whole
    Potatoes (in Ham Flavored Sauce)
Glazed Sweet Potatoes
Sliced White Potatoes
Small Whole White Potatoes
Superfine Triple Succotash
Vegetable Salad
Whole Boiled Onions

H-E-B
No Salt Sweet Peas

Hill Country Fare (H-E-B)
Cream Corn
Minced Garlic in Oil

Hy-Vee
Cream Style Corn
Fancy Diced Beets
Fancy Sliced Beets
French Style Green Beans
Green Beans, Cut
Green Split Peas
Mixed Vegetables
Sliced Carrots
Sliced Water Chestnuts
Sweet Peas
Whole Green Beans
Whole Kernel Corn
Whole Kernel Golden Corn
Whole Kernel White Sweet Corn

Italian Classics (Wegmans)
Artichoke Hearts In Brine
Balsamic Onions
Marinated Long-Stemmed Artichokes
Marinated Quartered Artichokes

Jewel-Osco
Green Peas
Quartered Artichoke Hearts

Juanitas
Mexican Style Hominy

Kroger
Candied Yams
Corn, Whole Kernel
Green Beans, Cut
Mixed Vegetables
White Potatoes (Sliced, Whole)

La Costena
Nopalitos

Las Palmas ⓘ
Crushed Tomatillos

Mancini
Onions (All)

Meijer
Asparagus (Cuts and Tips)
Beets Sliced, No Salt
Carrots Sliced
Carrots Sliced, No Salt
Chilies, Diced Mild Mexican Style
Corn, Cream Style
Hominy, White
Kale Greens, Chopped
Mixed Vegetable
Mushrooms (Sliced, Stems & Pieces,
    Stems & Pieces No Salt, Whole)
Mustard Greens, Chopped
Organic Corn, Sweet Golden
Organic Sweet Peas
Peas and Sliced Carrots
Pickled Beets (Sliced, Whole)
Pimentos (Pieces, Sliced)
Sauerkraut
Small Peas
Spinach
Spinach, Cut Leaf
Spinach, No Salt
Sweet and Sour Beets, Harvard
Sweet Peas
Sweet Peas, No Salt
Sweet Potatoes Cut, Light Syrup
Turnip Greens, Chopped
White Potatoes (Sliced, Whole)
Whole Kernel Corn, (Crisp and Sweet,
    Golden No Salt, Golden, White)
Whole Medium Beets

Mezzetta
Artichoke Hearts (All)
Cocktail Onions

Midwest Country Fare (Hy-Vee)
Broccoli Cuts
Brussel Sprouts
California Blend
Cauliflower Florets
Chopped Broccoli
Cream Style Golden Corn
Cut Golden Corn

Cut Green Beans
French Style Green Beans
Mixed Vegetables
Sweet Peas
Whole Kernel Golden Corn

Native Forest ✓
Artichoke Hearts (Marinated, Quartered, Whole)
Green Asparagus Cuts & Tips
Green Asparagus Spears
Organic Baby Corn
Organic Bamboo Shoots
Organic Hearts of Palm (Sliced, Whole)
Organic Mushroom Pieces & Stems

Nature's Promise (Giant)
Organic Sweet Peas
Organic Whole Kernel Corn

Nature's Promise (Stop & Shop)
Organic Cut Green Beans
Organic Sweet Peas
Organic Whole Kernel Corn

O Organics ⌒
Organic Cut Green Beans
Organic Sweet Peas
Organic Whole Kernel Corn

Our Family
Asparagus, Cut
Beets (Sliced, Whole)
Carrots (Diced, Sliced)
Corn, Cream Style
Corn, Whole Kernel
Corn, Whole Kernel No Salt Added
Garlic, Minced in Water
Mixed Vegetables
Mushroom Pieces & Stems
Mushrooms (Sliced, Whole)
No Salt Added Sweet Peas
Peas & Carrots
Peas (Medium, Very Small Early)
Potatoes, Diced
Spinach
Sweet Peas
Tex-Mex Corn with Peppers

Pastene
Artichoke Bottoms
Artichoke Hearts in Brine
Artichoke Quarters

Artichokes, Marinated
Baby Artichokes
Garlic, Minced
Mushrooms, Marinated
Straw Mushrooms, Broken

Peloponnese
Grape Leaves

Price Chopper
Cut Sweet Potato
Cut Yams
Imported Artichoke Hearts
Organic Roasted Red Pepper

Princella Sweet Potatoes
Canned Items (All)

Private Selection (Kroger)
Organic Green Beans
Organic Sweet Peas
Organic Whole Corn

Publix
Beets
Carrots
Corn - Cream Style Golden
Corn - Whole Kernel Golden Sweet
Green Beans - Veggi-Green
Green Beans
Mixed Vegetables
Potatoes - White
Spinach
Sweet Peas - Small
Sweet Peas

Rice River Farms ⓘ
Bistro Blend Mushrooms
Black Trumpet Mushrooms
Boletes Mushrooms, European Style
Chanterelle Mushrooms
Corn, Purple
Corn, Red
Corn, Sweet Freeze Dried
Corn, White
Cuitlacoche (Corn Smut)
European Mushroom Blend
Forest Mushroom Blend
Hen of the Woods Mushrooms
Lobster Mushrooms
Morel Mushrooms
Northwoods Mushroom Blend
Oyster Mushrooms

Porcini B (Cepes) Mushrooms
Porcini Extra A Mushrooms
Porcini Extra AA Mushrooms
Porcini Mushroom, Kibbled Standard
Portabella Mushrooms, Sliced
Posole, White Giant
Shiitake Mushrooms, First Quality
Shiitake Mushrooms, Sliced
Special Mushroom Blend
Steak Mushroom Blend
Stir Fry Mushroom Blend
Truffles, Black Summer Peelings
Truffles, Sliced Black
Truffles, Sliced Black Summer
Truffles, Sliced White Spring
Truffles, Sliced White Winter
Woodear Mushrooms, First Quality
Woodear Mushrooms, Shredded

Royal Prince Sweet Potatoes
Canned Items (All)

S&W Fine Foods ⓘ
Canned Vegetables (All)
Pickled Beets

Safeway ⌒
Asian Style Vegetables
Asparagus Spears
Beets, Sliced
Broccoli Spears
California Style Vegetables
Carrots Prepacked
Carrots, Sliced
Cauliflower
Cooked Squash
Corn on the Cob
Cream Style Corn
Crinkle Cut Carrots
Cut Corn
Cut Green Beans
Cut Leaf Spinach
Dark Red Low Sodium Kidney Beans
French Style Green Beans
Large Lima Beans
Medium Whole Beets
Mushrooms, Sliced Whole
No Salt Cut Green Beans
No Salt Green Peas
No Salt Whole Kernel Corn

Peas and Carrots
Pickled Beets, Sliced
Potatoes Red Prepacked
Sweet Peas
Tuscany Style Vegetables
White Potatoes Bag Prepacked
Whole Green Beans
Whole Kernel Corn
Whole Kernel Corn with Peppers
Whole Mushrooms
Winter Vegetables Mix

Safeway Select ⌒
Green Leaf Lettuce Prepacked
Petite Brussels Sprouts
Red Leaf Lettuce Prepacked
Romaine Leaf Lettuce Prepacked
Sweet White Corn
Whole Green Beans

Santiam
7 Mixed Vegetables
Curly Sliced Beets
Curly Sliced Carrots
Cut Green Beans
Cut Green Beans - No Salt Added
Golden Pumpkin
Pickled Curly Sliced Beets
Pickled Whole Beets
Sliced Green Beans
Sweet Peas
Sweet Peas - No Salt Added
Three Bean Salad
Whole Beets
Whole Kernel Corn
Whole Kernel Corn - No Salt Added

Schnucks
Artichokes, Grilled Italian
Asparagus, Cut
Asparagus, Whole
Beets, Pickled
Beets, Sliced
Beets, Small Sliced
Beets, Whole
Carrots, Sliced
Carrots, Sliced No Salt
Corn, Golden Whole Kernel
Corn, Whole Kernel
Corn, Whole Kernel (Vac Pack)

Corn, Whole Kernel Low Sodium
Cream Corn
Eggplant, Grilled Italian
Golden Hominy
Mixed Vegetables
Mixed Vegetables, Low Sodium
Mushrooms (Sliced, Stems & Pieces,
   Stems & Pieces No Salt, Whole)
Mushrooms, Grilled Italian
Peas, Low Sodium
Peas, Small
Peas, Tiny
Potato Sticks
Potatoes (Sliced, Whole)
Spinach
Spinach, No Salt
Sweet Peas
White Hominy
White Sweet Corn
Yams, Cut

Shaw's
Artichoke Quarters
China Water Chestnut
Marinated Artichoke Hearts
Whole Artichoke Heart

Shoppers Value (ACME)
Whole Kernel Corn

Shoppers Value (Albertsons)
Whole Kernel Corn

Shoppers Value (Jewel-Osco)
Cream Style Corn
Whole Kernel Corn

Stop & Shop
Asparagus, Cut
Cream Style Golden Corn
Dry Split Green Peas
No Salt Added Whole Kernel Corn
Sliced Beets, No Salt Added
Sliced Carrots
Sliced Carrots, No Salt Added
Sliced Pickled Beets
Sweet Crisp Whole Kernel Corn
Whole Kernel Corn
Whole Yams in Heavy Syrup

Sugary Sam
Sweet Potatoes (All)

Sun Luck
Baby Corn (Cut, Stir Fry, Whole)

Teasdale ⓘ ♻
Hominy (All)

Tosca
Garlic, Chopped
Garlic, Minced

Trader Joe's
Artichoke Hearts In Water
Crushed Garlic
Hearts Of Palm (All)
Marinated Mushrooms With Garlic
Minted Peas

Trappey ⓘ
Okra

Trappey's
Canned Items (All)

Valu Time (Brookshire)
Asparagus- Extra Long Spears
Beets, Diced
Gold Corn - Cream Style
Gold Corn - Whole Kernel
Mixed Vegetables
Mushroom Stems & Pieces
Mustard Greens, Chopped
Sliced Carrots
Sliced Potatoes
Spinach Leaf
Stuffed Pearl Onions
Sweet Peas
Turnip Green, Chopped
White Small Whole Potatoes

Valu Time (Marsh)
Chopped Green Turnips
Cut Green Beans
French Style Cut Green Beans
Gold Cream Style Corn
Gold Whole Kernel Corn
Mixed Vegetables
Short Cut Green Beans
Sliced Carrots
Small White Whole Potatoes
Sweet Peas

Valu Time (Schnucks)
Beets, Cut
Carrots, Sliced
Corn, Cream Style

Golden Corn, Whole Kernel
Green Beans, Cut
Green Beans, French Style
Mixed Vegetables
Small White Potatoes
Sweet Peas
Whole Leaf Spinach
Yellow Hominy

Veg-All
Canned Items (All)

Vons 〰
Asparagus, Cut
Golden Cream Style Corn
Golden Hominy
Lima Beans
Mushrooms Pieces and Stems
Southern Style Hash Brown Potatoes
Spinach
White Hominy
Whole Potatoes

Wegmans
Blackeye Peas
Bread & Butter Corn
Button Mushrooms
Creamed Corn
Crisp 'n Sweet Whole Kernel Corn
Cut Green Asparagus Spears & Tips
Cut Green Beans
Mixed Vegetables
Mushroom Pieces & Stems
Sliced Beets
Sliced Carrots
Sliced Mushrooms
Sliced Potatoes
Small Sweet Peas
Sweet Peas
Veggie-Green Cut Green Beans
Whole Beets
Whole Kernel Corn
Whole Potatoes
Whole Style Carrots

Winn-Dixie
Beets
Carrots (Length Cut, Sliced)
Corn, White Whole Kernel
Corn, Yellow Whole Kernel

Corn, Yellow Whole Kernel No Salt Added
Green Peas (Large, Medium, Small, Tiny)
Green Peas, No Salt Added
Mixed Vegetables
Mixed Vegetables, No Salt Added
Potatoes, White (Diced, Sliced, Whole)
Potatoes, Whole White No Salt Added
Spinach
Spinach, No Salt Added

Woeber ⓘ
Chopped Garlic (in Oil, in Water)

MISCELLANEOUS

Goya
Achiotina (Annatto in Lard)
Annatto in Lard
Banana Leaves
Flor de Calabaza
Flor de Izote
Garlic Paste
Habichuelas con Dulce

Porta Mangiare
Gluten-Free Meatball Mix

Rice River Farms ⓘ
Ancho Chile Paste
Chipotle Morita Paste
Guajillo Chile Paste
Kombu Seaweed
Nori (Seaweed) Sheets
Squash Blossoms

Tabasco ⓘ
Pepper Paste
Pepper Pulp

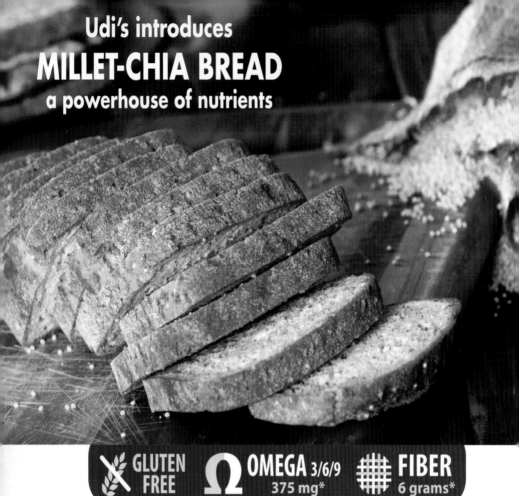

Udi's introduces

MILLET-CHIA BREAD
a powerhouse of nutrients

GLUTEN FREE   **Ω OMEGA 3/6/9** 375 mg*   **FIBER** 6 grams*

- Millet and Chia are naturally gluten free
- Chia is packed with protein, anti-oxidants, and omega-3
- Millet is a heart-healthy grain that delivers a deliciously crunchy texture
- 6 grams of fiber and 5 grams of protein per serving
- 12 grams of whole grain per serving

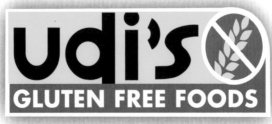

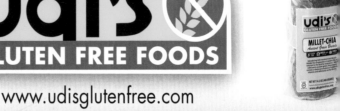

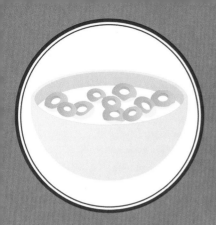

BREAD, CEREAL, PASTA, etc.

BREAD

Against the Grain 🥛 ✓
- Dairy-Free Cinnamon Raisin Bagel
- Dairy-Free Vermont Country Roll
- Original Baguette
- Original Rolls
- Pumpernickel Rolls
- Rosemary Baguette
- Rosemary Rolls
- Sesame Bagel
- Sun-Dried Tomato and Basil Bagel

Aimee's Livin' Magic
- Herbed Onion Bread
- Outrageous Onion Bread

Aleia's 🥛 ✓
- Cinnamon Raisin Bread
- Farmhouse White Sandwich Bread

Better Bread 🥛
- Sandwich Rolls

Bi Aglut
- Bi Aglut (All)

Bodhi's Bakehouse
- Gluten & Wheat Free Rolls
- Gluten & Yeast Free Loaf
- Gluten Free Chia Linseed Loaf
- Gluten Free Fruit Loaf
- Gluten Free Rice Loaf
- Maize & Soya Gluten Free Loaf
- Multi Grain Gluten Free Loaf
- Multi Grain Gluten Free Rolls

Canyon Bakehouse 🥛
- Cinnamon Raisin
- Colorado Caraway
- Hamburger Buns
- Mountain White
- Rosemary & Thyme Focaccia
- San Juan 7-Grain

Ener-G
- Brown English Muffins with Flax
- Brown Rice Hamburger Buns
- Brown Rice Loaf
- Corn Loaf
- Egg-Free Raisin Loaf
- English Muffins
- Four Flour Loaf
- High Fiber Loaf
- Light Brown Rice Loaf
- Light Tapioca Loaf
- Light White Rice Flax Loaf
- Light White Rice Loaf
- Papa's Loaf
- Rice Starch Loaf
- Seattle Brown Loaf
- Seattle Hamburger Buns
- Seattle Hot Dog Buns
- Tapioca Dinner Rolls
- Tapioca Hamburger Buns
- Tapioca Hot Dog Buns
- Tapioca Loaf, Regular Sliced
- Tapioca Loaf, Thin Sliced
- White Rice Flax Loaf
- White Rice Hamburger Buns
- White Rice Loaf
- Yeast-Free Brown Rice Loaf
- Yeast-Free Flax Meal Loaf
- Yeast-Free White Rice Loaf

Food for Life
- Gluten-Free English Muffins
- Wheat & Gluten-Free Bhutanese Red Rice Bread

Wheat & Gluten-Free Brown Rice Bread
Wheat & Gluten-Free China Black Rice Bread
Wheat & Gluten-Free Millet Bread
Wheat & Gluten-Free Raisin Pecan Bread
Wheat & Gluten-Free Rice Almond Bread
Wheat & Gluten-Free Rice Pecan Bread
Wheat & Gluten-Free White Rice Bread
Yeast-Free, Wheat & Gluten-Free Multi Seed Rice Bread

Foods by George
English Muffins, Cinnamon Currant
English Muffins, No-Rye Rye
English Muffins, Plain

French Meadow Bakery
Gluten-Free Cinnamon Raisin Bread
Gluten-Free Italian Rolls
Gluten-Free Multigrain Bread
Gluten-Free Sandwich Bread

Gillian's Foods
Gillian's Foods (All)

Glutano
Glutano (All)

Gluten Free Harvest, A
A Gluten Free Harvest (All)

Glutino
Genius By Glutino Multigrain Sandwich Bread
Genius By Glutino White Sandwich Bread
Multigrain Bagel
Premium Cinnamon & Raisin Bread
Premium Cinnamon 'N Raisin Bagels
Premium English Muffins
Premium Fiber Bread
Premium Flax Seed Bread
Premium Harvest Corn bread
Premium Plain Bagels
Premium Poppy Seed Bagels
Premium Sesame Bagels

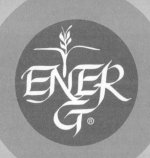
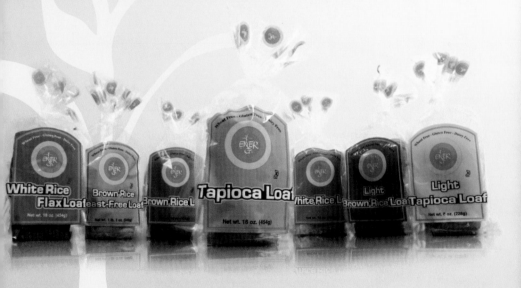

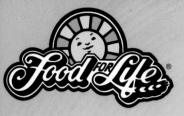

Start your day with

GLUTEN FREE
ENGLISH MUFFINS

Made with
Organic Brown Rice

- Fork Split
- No Added Oil

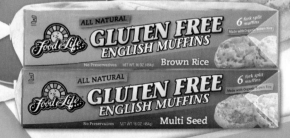

ALL NATURAL
GLUTEN FREE
ENGLISH MUFFINS
6 fork split muffins
Made with Organic Brown Rice
No Preservatives   NET WT. 16 OZ (454g)
Brown Rice

ALL NATURAL
GLUTEN FREE
ENGLISH MUFFINS
6 fork split muffins
Made with Organic Brown Rice
No Preservatives   NET WT. 16 OZ (454g)
Multi Seed

Available
natural & specialty foo
stores in the frozen sectio

(800) 797-509
www.foodforlife.cor

Food For Life Baking Co., Inc. • P.O. Box 1434 • Corona, CA 92878-1434

Gluten-Free, Goodness Loaded

Rudi's Gluten-Free Bakery bread is certified (GF) but very worthy of your ♡.
Each delicious slice has real fresh-bread taste to make the whole ✹✹ happy,
bring a ☺ to your day and add ☀ to your life.

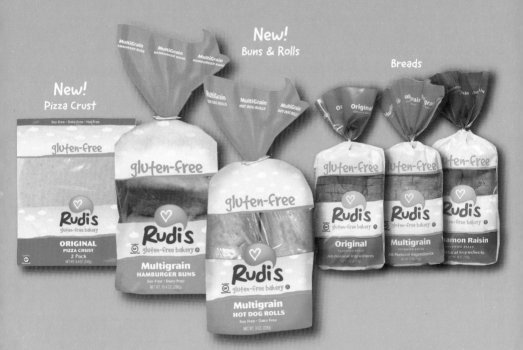

New!
Pizza Crust

New!
Buns & Rolls

Breads

All-natural ingredients. ♡ No artificial ingredients or preservatives.
Soy and dairy free. ♡ Soft delicious texture.

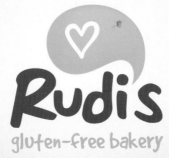

Rudis
gluten-free bakery

www.rudisglutenfreebakery.com /rudisglutenfree bakery

Gluuteny
Gluuteny (All)

Goya
Cassava Bread
Pandebono

Grainless Baker, The
The Grainless Baker (All)

Grindstone Bakery
Bedrock Cinnamon
Gluten Free 100% Quinoa Ciabatta
(Herbs, Plain)
Gluten Free High Flax Loaf
Gluten Free Quinoa & Millet Cinnamon
& Raisins Loaf
Gluten Free Quinoa & Millet Loaf with
Sprouted Seeds
Gluten Free Quinoa & Millet Plain Loaf
Pane Dolce Genoese

Joan's GF Great Bakes
Joan's GF Great Bakes (All)

Katz Gluten Free
Large Challah Rolls

Sandwich Rolls
Sliced Challah Bread
Small Challah Rolls
White Bread
Whole Grain Bread
Wholesome Bread

Kinnikinnick Foods
Kinnikinnick Foods (All)

Little Aussie Bakery, The
The Little Aussie Bakery (All)

Lydia's Organics
Lydia's Organics (All)

Mariposa Baking Company
12" Baguette
Bread Cubes for Stuffing
Cranberry Orange Nut Bread (Seasonal)
Focaccia
Hot Dog Buns
Multi-Grain Bread
Plain Bagels
Pull-Apart Rosemary Rolls (Seasonal)
Pumpkin Bread (Seasonal)

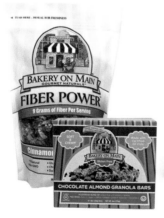
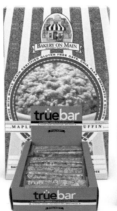
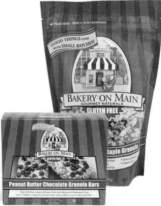

Rosemary Rolls
Sandwich Bread
Sandwich Rolls
Sesame Seed Bagels

Nu-World Amaranth
Amaranth Flatbread (All)

Orgran ⓘ 🍴
Crispibread Range (All)

Outside the Breadbox 🍴
Outside the Breadbox (All)

Rudi's Gluten-Free Bakery ⓘ 🍴 ✓
Gluten-Free Cinnamon Raisin Bread
Gluten-Free Multigrain Bread
Gluten-Free Original Bread
Multigrain Hamburger Buns
Multigrain Hot Dog Rolls

Schar 🍴
Baguettes, Par-Baked
Ciabatta Par-Baked Rolls
Classic White Bread (Shelf stable)
Classic White Rolls (Shelf stable)
Hearty Grain Bread (Frozen)
Hearty White Bread (Frozen)
Multigrain Bread (Shelf stable)
Sub Sandwich Par-Baked Rolls

Smart Treat 🍴
Smart Treat (All)

Trader Joe's
Gluten Free Bagels (Midwest)
Gluten Free French Rolls
Rye-less "Rye" Bread

Udi's Gluten Free Foods 🍴 ✓
Cinnamon Raisin Bagels
Cinnamon Raisin Bread
Classic Hamburger Buns
Classic Hot Dog Buns
Millet-Chia Bread
Omega Flax & Fiber Bread
Plain Bagels
White Sandwich Bread Loaf
Whole Grain Bagels
Whole Grain Bread Loaf
Whole Grain Hamburger Buns

Venice Bakery ✓
Gluten-Free Flatbread
Gluten-Free Focaccia

CEREAL & GRANOLA

ACME
Rice Biscuit Cereal

Aimee's Livin' Magic
Sprouted Granola
Superhero Cereal

Albertsons
Rice Biscuits Cereal

Arrowhead Mills
Maple Buckwheat Flakes Cereal
Rice & Shine Hot Cereal
Rice Flakes Sweetened Cereal
Yellow Corn Grits

Bakery on Main 🍴 ✓
Apple Raisin Walnut Granola
Cinnamon Raisin Fiber Power Granola
Cranberry Orange Cashew Granola
Extreme Fruit & Nut Granola
Nutty Cranberry Maple Granola
Rainforest Granola
Triple Berry Fiber Power Gluten-Free
Granola

Barbara's Bakery
Brown Rice Crisps ✓

Best Choice
Quick Grits
Toasted Rice

Black Lab Naturals ✓
Gluten-Free Granola (All)

Bob's Red Mill
Brown Rice Farina
GF Mighty Tasty Hot Cereal
GF Quick Cooking Oats
Organic Brown Rice Farina
Organic Buckwheat Berries
Organic Creamy Buckwheat
Sorghum Grain
Sorghum Grits
Soy Grits

Bora Bora ✓
Tribal Cinnamon Oatmeal

Brookfarm ⓘ
Gluten Free Muesli with Apricots
Gluten Free Muesli with Cranberries

Central Market (H-E-B)
Blue Blackwheat Gluten Free

Cerealvit ⓘ ✓
- Benevit Multigrain
- Choco Stars
- Coffee Flakes
- Corn Flakes

Chappaqua Crunch
- Gluten Free Granola with Fruit and Flax
- Gluten Free Granola with Vanilla and Flax

Chex
- Chocolate Chex
- Cinnamon Chex
- Corn Chex
- Honey Nut Chex
- Rice Chex

Cocoa Pebbles ⛃
- Cocoa Pebbles
- Cocoa Pebbles Treats

Crunchfuls ✓
- Crunchfuls (All)

Cub Foods
- Bite Size Rice Cereal

Eco-Planet ✓
- Gluten Free Instant Hot Cereal (Oatmeal Based)

Ener-G
- Rice Bran

Enjoy Life Foods ⛃ ✓
- Cinnamon Raisin Crunch Granola
- Crunchy Flax
- Crunchy Rice
- Double Chocolate Crunch Granola
- Very Berry Crunch Granola

EnviroKidz ⓘ ✓
- Amazon Frosted Flakes
- Gorilla Munch
- Koala Crisp
- Leapin Lemurs
- Peanut Butter Panda Puffs

Erewhon ⓘ ✓
- Cocoa Crispy Brown Rice Cereal
- Corn Flakes
- Crispy Brown Rice Gluten-Free Cereal
- Crispy Brown Rice with Mixed Berries
- Rice Twice Cereal

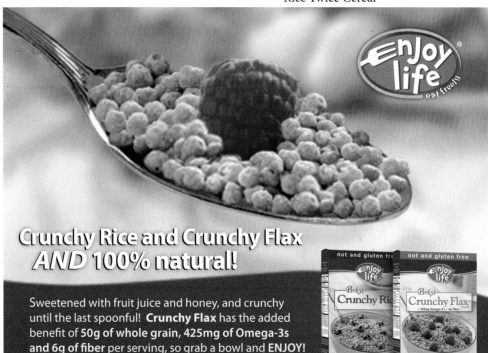

Strawberry Crisp Cereal

Farmo ✓
Farmo (All)

Fiona's Granola
Quinoa Crunch Cereal (All)

Free to Enjoy
Frosted Flakes
Honey Nut Flakes

Fruity Pebbles ⛭
Fruity Pebbles
Fruity Pebbles Treats

Giant
Quick Hominy Grits

Glutano
Glutano (All)

Gluten Free Sensations ⛭ ✓
Apple Crisp Granola
Cherry Vanilla Almond Granola
Chocolate Bliss Granola
Cranberry Pecan Granola
Cream of Brown Rice
French Vanilla Almond Granola

Glutenfreeda ⓘ ⛭
Granola (All)
Oatmeal (All)

Glutino
Apple Cinnamon Rings Cereal
Berry Sensible Beginnings
Frosted Sensible Beginnings
Honey Nut Cereal
Sensible Beginnings

Go Raw ✓
Go Raw (All)

GoGo Quinoa ✓
GoGo Quinoa (All)

Hail Merry
Grawnola (All)

Hodgson Mill
Gluten-Free Buckwheat Cereal with
Milled Flax Seed ⛭

Jessica's Natural Foods ✓
Almond Cherry Granola (Made with GF
Oats)
Chocolate Chip Granola (Made with GF
Oats)
Vanilla Maple Granola (Made with GF
Oats)

Jewel-Osco
Rice Biscuits Cereal

JK Gourmet
Granola (All)

Jules Gluten Free
Certified Gluten-Free Oats

Kallo
Organic Honey Puffed Rice Cereal
Organic Natural Puffed Rice Cereal

Katz Gluten Free
Oat Challah Rolls

Kay's Naturals ⛭ ✓
Cereals (All)

Kinnikinnick Foods ⛭
Kinnikinnick Foods (All)

Kookie Karma ✓
Cacao Crunch Krunchies
Goji Lime Coconut Krunchies
Walnut Raisin Krunchies

Living Intentions
SuperFood Cereal (All)

Love Grown Foods ✓
Oat Clusters & Love Granola (All)

Lundberg Family Farms ⛭
Purely Organic Hot Cereal

Lydia's Organics ⛭
Lydia's Organics (All)

Malt-O-Meal
Fruity Dyno-Bites

Marshmallow Pebbles ⛭
Marshmallow Pebbles

Maypo
Creamy Rice Hot Cereal

Meijer
Grits, Butter Flavored Instant
Grits, Quick

Nairn's
Gluten Free Oat Muesli
Gluten Free Oat Porridge (All)

Nature's Path ⓘ ✓
Crispy Rice
Crunchy Maple Sunrise
Crunchy Vanilla Sunrise
Fruit Juice Sweetened Cornflakes
Honey'd Cornflakes
Mesa Sunrise Flakes
Whole O's

New England Naturals ⓘ ✓
  Organic Gluten Free Crispy Fruity
  Cereal
Nu-World Amaranth
  Instant Puffed Hot Cereals (All)
Orgran ⓘ ⚜
  100% Amaranth Puffed Breakfast Cereal
  Itsy Bitsy Cocoa O's
  Multigrain Breakfast O's with Quinoa
  Rice O's Wild Berry Flavored
Oskri
  Cereal and Granola (All)
Pocono
  Cream of Buckwheat
Post ⓘ
  Cocoa Cupcake
  Fruity Cupcake
Puffins ✓
  Puffins Honey Rice Cereal
  Puffins Multigrain Cereal
Purely Elizabeth
  Purely Elizabeth (All)
Ralcorp
  Creamy Rice Hot Cereal
Ralston Foods ◌
  Rice Biscuits
Rice Krispies ⚜ ✓
  Gluten Free Rice Krispies
Rice River Farms ⓘ
  Hominy Grits, White
Ruth's Hemp Foods ✓
  Chia Goodness (All Flavors)
Seitenbacher
  Gluten-Free Muesli
  Gluten-Free Whole Grain Cornflakes
Shaw's
  Biscuit Cereal Rice
Simbree ✓
  Cocoa Almond Cherry Granola
  Gluten Free Plain Instant Oatmeal
  Gluten Free Premium Oats
  Gluten Free Raspberry Instant Oatmeal
Simpli ⓘ
  Gluten Free Apricot Instant Oatmeal
Smart Treat ⚜
  Smart Treat (All)

Trader Joe's
  Gluten Free Rolled Oats
Two Moms in the Raw ⓘ
  Cereals (All)
  Granola (Made with GF Oats) (All)
Udi's Gluten Free Foods ⚜ ✓
  Gluten Free Au Naturel Granola
  Gluten Free Cranberry Granola
  Gluten Free Original Granola
  Gluten Free Vanilla Granola
Whole Earth
  Organic Corn Flakes
  Organic Maple Frosted Flakes
Wolff's
  Cream of Buckwheat

PASTA & NOODLES

Ancient Harvest ⚜
  Gluten-Free Pasta
Andean Dream
  Quinoa Pasta, Fusilli
  Quinoa Pasta, Macaroni
  Quinoa Pasta, Shells
  Quinoa Pasta, Spaghetti
Barkat Rice Mills
  Alphabet Shapes Pasta
  Animal Shapes Pasta
  Macaroni Pasta
  Spaghetti Pasta
  Spirals Pasta
  Tagliatelle Pasta
Bi Aglut
  Bi Aglut (All)
Bionaturae
  Gluten Free Elbows ⚜
  Gluten Free Fusilli ⚜
  Gluten Free Linguine ⚜
  Gluten Free Penne ⚜
  Gluten Free Rigatoni ⚜
  Gluten Free Spaghetti ⚜
Casalare
  Gluten Free Pasta (All)
China Sun
  Brown Rice Vermicelli
  White Rice Vermicelli

DeBoles
Gluten Free Rice Spirals Plus Golden Flax
Gluten Free Whole Grain Penne
Gluten Free Whole Grain Spaghetti Style Pasta
Rice Angel Hair Pasta
Rice Fettuccine
Rice Lasagna
Rice Penne
Rice Spaghetti Style Pasta
Rice Spirals
Wheat Free Corn Elbow Style Pasta
Wheat Free Corn Spaghetti Style Pasta

Domata Living Flour ᵍ ✓
Gluten Free Pasta (All)

Eden Foods
Bifun (Rice) Pasta
Kuzu Pasta
Mung Bean Pasta (Harusame)

Ener-G
White Rice Lasagna
White Rice Macaroni
White Rice Small Shells
White Rice Spaghetti
White Rice Vermicelli

Fantastic
Gluten Free Glass Noodles, Beef
Gluten Free Glass Noodles, Chicken

Farmo ✓
Farmo (All)

Gillian's Foods ᵍ
Gillian's Foods (All)

Glutano
Glutano (All)

GoGo Quinoa ✓
GoGo Quinoa (All)

Goldbaum's
Pasta (All)

Heartland ⓘ
Gluten-Free Fusilli
Gluten-Free Penne
Gluten-Free Spaghetti

H-E-B
Gluten Free Fusilli Pasta
Gluten Free Penne Pasta
Gluten Free Spaghetti Pasta

Hodgson Mill
Gluten-Free Brown Rice Angel Hair with Milled Flaxseed ᵍ
Gluten-Free Brown Rice Elbows with Milled Flaxseed ᵍ
Gluten-Free Brown Rice Lasagna with Milled Flaxseed ᵍ
Gluten-Free Brown Rice Linguine with Milled Flaxseed ᵍ
Gluten-Free Brown Rice Penne with Milled Flaxseed ᵍ
Gluten-Free Brown Rice Spaghetti with Milled Flaxseed ᵍ

House Foods ⓘ
Tofu Shirataki

Il Macchiaiolo
100% Corn Fusilli Pasta
100% Corn Penne
100% Corn Riccioli
100% Rice Gigli Pasta
100% Rice Penne
100% Rice Riccioli

Jovial
Brown Rice Capellini
Brown Rice Caserecce
Brown Rice Fusilli
Brown Rice Penne Rigate
Brown Rice Spaghetti

Katz Gluten Free
Farfel

Konjac Foods
Konjac Pasta (All Varieties)

Leahey Gardens ⓘ
Gluten Free Macaroni & Cheese

Lundberg Family Farms ᵍ
Organic Elbow Brown Rice Pasta
Organic Penne Brown Rice Pasta
Organic Rotini Brown Rice Pasta
Organic Spaghetti Brown Rice Pasta

Manischewitz
Passover Noodles

Miracle Noodle
Miracle Noodle (All)

Mom's Place Gluten-Free ᵍ
Mom's Place Gluten-Free (All)

Mrs. Leeper's
Mrs. Leeper's (All)

Namaste Foods ⚇ ✓
  Pasta (All)
Notta Pasta
  Notta Pasta (All)
Orgran ⓘ ⚇
  Buontempo Pasta Range (All)
  Essential Fibre Pasta Range (All)
  Gourmet Pasta Range (All)
  Italian Style Pasta Range (All)
  Rice & Corn Pasta Range (All)
  Stoneground Pasta Range (All)
  Supergrains Pasta Range (All)
Pulmuone Wildwood ⚇
  Pasta Slim Alternatives
Rice River Farms ⓘ
  Cellophane Noodles/Bean Threads
  Pad Thai Noodles
Sam Mills ✓
  Gluten Free Corn Pasta For Kids (All)
  Gluten Free Pasta d'Oro (All)
Schar ⚇
  Anellini
  Multigrain Penne Rigate
  Penne
  Tagliatelle
Seitenbacher
  Gluten-Free Golden Ribbon Noodles
  Gluten-Free Rigatoni
Streit's ⓘ
  Chow Mein Noodles
Taste of Thai, A
  Taste of Thai, A (All)
Tinkyada
  Gluten-Free Rice Pasta (All)
Trader Joe's
  Organic Brown Rice Pasta (All)

PIZZA CRUST

Against the Grain ⚇ ✓
  Pizza Shell
Bay State Milling
  Gluten-Free Pizza Mix
Better Bread ⚇
  Pizza Crust
  Pizza Dough

Bodhi's Bakehouse
  Gluten Free Pizza Base
Ener-G
  Focaccia Crust
  Rice Pizza Shells
  Yeast-Free Rice Pizza Shells
French Meadow Bakery
  Gluten-Free Pizza Crust
Gillian's Foods ⚇
  Gillian's Foods (All)
Gluten-Free Naturals ⚇ ✓
  Gluten-Free Naturals (All)
Gluuteny ⚇
  Gluuteny (All)
Grainless Baker, The ⚇
  The Grainless Baker (All)
Joan's GF Great Bakes
  Joan's GF Great Bakes (All)
Katz Gluten Free
  Pizza Crust
Kinnikinnick Foods ⚇
  Kinnikinnick Foods (All)
Little Aussie Bakery, The
  The Little Aussie Bakery
Mariposa Baking Company
  Pizza Crust
Namaste Foods ⚇ ✓
  Pizza Crust Mix
Outside the Breadbox ⚇
  Outside the Breadbox (All)
Really Great Food ⚇
  Really Great Food (All)
Rudi's Gluten-Free Bakery ⓘ ⚇ ✓
  Gluten-Free Pizza Crust
Rustic Crust ✓
  Napoli Herb Gluten Free Pizza Crust
Schar ⚇
  Pizza Crusts
Toovaloo ⚇
  Pizza Crust
Udi's Gluten Free Foods ⚇ ✓
  9" Pizza Crusts
Venice Bakery ✓
  Gluten-Free Pizza Crusts

POLENTA

Bob's Red Mill
GF Corn Grits/Polenta
De La Estancia
Polenta (All)
DeLallo ⓘ
Instant Polenta ⓘ
Food Merchant Polenta ⚇
Basil & Garlic Polenta
Chili & Cilantro Polenta
Mushroom & Onion Polenta
Sundried Tomato Polenta
Traditional Polenta
Frontier Soups ⓘ
Roasted Corn Polenta a la Roma
Pastene
Instant Polenta
Polenta Valsugana
Instant Polenta Valsugana Express
Rice River Farms ⓘ
Corn Polenta
Corn Polenta, Coarse Italian Style
Corn Polenta, White Coarse
Corn Polenta, White Fine
Polenta, Fine Instant
Sam Mills ✓
Polenta
San Gennaro Foods ⚇
Pre-Cooked Polenta

POTATO, INSTANT & MIXES

ACME
Instant Dehydrated Potatoes
Instant Mashed Potatoes
Albertsons
Instant Mashed Potatoes
Always Save
Potato Flakes
Best Choice
4 Cheese Mash Potatoes
Au Gratin Potatoes
Butter & Herb Potatoes
Creamy Butter Mashed Potatoes
Mashed Potatoes
Roasted Garlic Potatoes

Sour Cream Mash Potatoes
Cub Foods
Dried Instant Potatoes
Edward & Sons ✓
Chreesy Mashed Potato Mix
Organic Home Style Mashed Potato Mix
Organic Roasted Garlic Mashed Potato Mix
Flavorite (Cub Foods)
Roasted Garlic Mashed Potatoes
Food Club (Brookshire)
Instant Mash Potatoes
Instant Mashed Potatoes, Roasted Garlic
Instant Potatoes, Butter & Herb Flavored
Instant Potatoes, Butter Flavored
Instant Potatoes, Four Cheese Flavored
Instant Potatoes, Roasted Garlic
Food Club (Marsh)
Dried Hash Browns
Instant Mashed Potatoes
Giant
Irish Potatoes, Whole
No Salt Added Whole White Potatoes
Sweet Potatoes, Cut
Goya
Chuno Negro
Papa Seca ◊
Great Value (Wal-Mart)
Instant Mashed Potatoes
Haggen
Instant Potatoes
Potatoes, Instant Mashed
Honest Earth
Baby Reds
Buttery Homestyle Mashed
Creamy Mashed
Yukon Golds
Hy-Vee
Four Cheese Mashed Potatoes
Hash Browns (Real Russet Potatoes)
Mashed Potatoes (Real Russet Potatoes)
Roasted Garlic Mashed Potatoes
Sour Cream & Chive Mashed Potatoes
Idaho Supreme
Buttery Homestyle
Four Cheese
Roasted Garlic

Idahoan
- Baby Reds
- Baby Reds Garlic & Parmesan
- Butter & Herb
- Buttery Golden Selects
- Buttery Homestyle
- Four Cheese
- Original Flakes
- Real Clubs
- Roasted Garlic
- Romano White Cheese
- Southwest

Jewel-Osco
- Dehydrated Mashed Potato Flakes
- Instant Mashed Potatoes

Kroger
- 3 Cheese Potatoes

Meijer
- Hash Browns
- Instant Mashed Potatoes

Mr. Dell's
- Potatoes

Our Family
- Butter & Herb Instant Potatoes
- Instant Potatoes
- Roasted Garlic Instant Potatoes
- Sliced Potatoes
- Sour Cream & Chive Instant Potatoes
- Whole Potatoes

Potato Buds
- Mashed Potatoes (All)

Price Chopper
- Hash Brown Potato
- Instant Potatoes

Schnucks
- Instant Potatoes

Shaw's
- Mashed Potato Flakes Box

Valu Time (Brookshire)
- Instant Mashed Potatoes

Vons 〰
- Instant Mashed Potatoes

Winn-Dixie
- Instant Potato Flakes

XXL Baking Potatoes ()
- XXL Baking Potatoes (All)

RICE & RICE MIXES

ACME
- Enriched Extra Fancy White Rice
- Extra Fancy Brown Rice
- Extra Fancy Medium White Rice
- Parboiled Long Grain Rice
- Parboiled Rice
- White Long Grain Rice

Albertsons
- Calrose Rice
- Long Grain Brown Rice
- Long Grain White Rice
- Parboiled Long Grain Rice

Alter Eco Fair Trade ⓘ
- Rice (All)

Always Save
- Long Grain Rice

Arrowhead Mills
- Brown Rice, Basmati
- Brown Rice, Long Grain

Best Choice
- Boil In Bag Rice
- Brown Rice
- Instant Brown Rice
- Instant Rice
- Long Grain Rice
- Medium Grain Rice

Bineshii Wild Rice
- Wild Rice

Blue Ribbon Golden
- Plain Rice ♗

Cajun Country Rice
- Cajun Country Rice (All)

Carlita (Jewel-Osco)
- Long Grain Rice

Casa Fiesta ⓘ
- Mexican Stye Rice Mix
- Mexican Style Rice

Central Market (H-E-B)
- Organic Long Grain White Rice
- Organic Short Grain Brown Rice

Clearly Organic (Best Choice)
- Brown Rice
- Long Grain White Rice

Cub Foods
- Long Grain Rice

Medium Grain Rice

DeLallo
Risotto Arborio Rice

Eden Foods
Brown Rice & Mugwort Mochi
Sprouted Brown Rice Mochi
Sweet Brown Rice Mochi
Wild Rice

Flavorite (ACME)
Brown Rice

Flavorite (Albertsons)
Brown Rice

Flavorite (Cub Foods)
Medium Grain Rice

Food Club (Brookshire)
Instant Boil in a Bag
Instant Brown Rice
Instant Rice
Long Grain Brown Rice
Long Grain Rice
Medium Grain Rice

Food Club (Marsh)
Rice Instant
Rice, Instant Brown

Food You Feel Good About (Wegmans)
Basmati Rice
Boil-In Bag Enriched Rice
Enriched Long Grain White Rice
Instant Brown Rice
Instant Rice
Jasmine Rice
Long Grain Brown Rice
Medium Grain Rice
Medium Grain White Rice

Full Circle (Price Chopper)
Basmati Rice
Long Grain Brown Rice
Long Grain White Rice

Full Circle (Schnucks)
Basmati Brown Rice
Basmati White Rice
Long Grain Brown Rice
Long Grain White Rice

Giant
Instant Long Grain Rice
Long Grain Brown Rice

Long Grain Rice

GoGo Rice ⅛
Organic Brown Rice
Organic Rice Medley
Organic White Rice
Sprouted Brown Rice

Goya
Basmati Rice ()
Brown Rice
Canilla Gaylord Rice
Canilla Rice
Chicken Flavored Rice ()
Curry Rice ()
Fiesta Rice ()
Golden Canilla Rice
Jasmine Rice ()
Low Sodium Yellow Rice ()
Medium Grain Rice
Mexican Rice ()
Organic Long Grain Brown Rice
Organic Long Grain White Rice
Primavera Rice ()
Spanish Rice ()
Valencia Rice ()
Yellow Rice ()

Great Value (Wal-Mart) 25
Brown Rice
Enriched Long Grain Rice, Extra Fancy
Parboiled Rice

Haggen
Brown Rice
Brown Rice, Long Grain
Rice, Instant
Rice, Instant Brown
Rice, Long Grain

Hinode
Dry Rice Items (All)
Microwavable Pouches (Brown, Jasmine, White)

Hy-Vee
Enriched Extra Long Grain Rice
Extra Long Grain Rice
Natural Long Grain Brown Rice
Natural Whole Grain Brown Rice
Rice (Boil in Bag)

Italian Classics (Wegmans)
Arborio Rice

Jewel-Osco
- Brown Long Grain Rice
- Domestic Long Grain Brown Rice
- Enriched Long Grain Rice
- Enriched White Rice
- Long Grain Rice
- Parboiled Rice

Konriko ⓘ ⛏
- Aix En Provence Brown Rice
- Artichoke Brown Rice Mix
- Hot 'n Spicy Brown Rice Pilaf
- Original Brown Rice
- Wild Pecan Rice

Lotus Foods
- Rice (All)

Louisiana Fish Fry ⓘ
- Dirty Rice Mix
- Jambalaya Mix

Lundberg Family Farms ⛏
- Butternut Squash Risottos
- Creamy Parmesan Risottos
- Garlic Primavera Risottos
- Heat & Eat Organic Countrywild Brown Rice Bowls
- Heat & Eat Organic Long Grain Brown Rice Bowls
- Heat & Eat Organic Short Grain Brown Rice Bowls
- Italian Herb Risottos
- Organic Alfredo Risottos
- Organic Florentine Risottos
- Organic Porcini Mushroom Risottos
- Organic Tuscan Risottos
- Rice (All Varieties)

Luzianne
- Jambalaya Dinner Kit

Meijer
- Rice, (Brown, Long Grain, Medium Grain)
- Rice, Instant (Boil in Bag, Brown)

Midwest Country Fare (Hy-Vee)
- Pre-Cooked Instant Rice

Nature's Promise (Giant)
- Organic Long Grain Brown Rice
- Organic Long Grain White Rice

Nature's Promise (Stop & Shop)
- Organic Long Grain Brown Rice
- Organic Long Grain White Rice

Nueva Cocina ⓘ
- Coconut Rice

O Organics 🌀
- Brown Basmati Rice
- Brown Rice
- Brown Rice Bowl
- Jasmine Rice
- Long Grain Brown Rice
- Thai Jasmine Rice
- White Rice Bowl

Ortega ⓘ
- Saffron Yellow Rice
- Spanish Rice

Our Family
- Brown Rice
- Garden Vegetable 90 Second Rice Mix
- Instant White Rice
- Long Grain & Wild 90 Second Rice Mix
- Long Grain White Rice
- Roasted Chicken 90 Second Rice Mix
- Whole Grain Brown 90 Second Rice Mix

Pastene
- Italian Arborio Rice

Publix
- Long Grain Brown Rice
- Long Grain Enriched Rice
- Medium Grain White Rice
- Precooked Instant Boil in Bag
- Precooked Instant Brown Rice
- Precooked Instant White Rice
- Yellow Rice Mix

Rice River Farms ⓘ
- Arborio Brown Rice
- Arborio Rice
- Asian Rice Blend
- Autumn Harvest Blend
- Bamboo Rice
- Banquet Blend
- Basmati Rice, Aged 2 Years
- Basmati Rice, Brown
- Basmati Rice, Indian White
- Basmati Rice, White
- Black Japonica Rice
- Botan Sushi Rice
- Brown Rice, Short Grain

Carnaroli Rice
Chef's Top Blend
Chinese Black Rice
Festival Blend
Festival Medley
French Gourmet Rice Blend
French Red (Camargue) Rice
Gaba Rice
Himalayan Red Rice (Bhutanese), Short
   Grain
Himalayan Red Rice, Medium Grain
Jasmine Rice
Jasmine Rice Blend
Kala Jeera Rice (Baby Basmati)
Kokuho Rice
Long Grain Brown Rice, Pecan Style
Mochi Rice
Par-Boiled Brown Rice
Par-Boiled White Rice
Premium Dry Roasted Wild Rice
Purple Sticky Rice (Black Thai)
Saffron Rice
Scarlet Rice Blend
Select Dry Roasted Wild Rice
Spanish Rice Blend
Speckled Sushi Rice Blend
Sunshine Blend
Wehani (Natural Red Rice)

Rice Select ⓘ ✓

Arborio (Risotto)
Jasmati
Kasmati
Royal Blend
Sushi Rice
Texmati Brown
Texmati Light Brown
Texmati Mushroom Medley
Texmati Vegetable Medley
Texmati White

Safeway ⌒

Instant Brown Rice
Instant Rice
Long Grain Brown Rice
Long Grain Rice
Long Grain White Rice
White Long Grain Rice

Schnucks

Instant Brown Rice
Instant Rice
Long Grain & Wild Rice
Long Grain Rice
Medium Grain Rice

Shaw's

Brown Long Grain Instant Rice
Extra Fancy White Rice
Long Brown Rice
Long Grain White Rice
Rice

Shoppers Value (Albertsons)

Long Grain Rice

Shoppers Value (Cub Foods)

Long Grain Rice

Stop & Shop

Boil N Bag Brown Rice
Enriched Long Grain Rice
Jasmine Rice

Success Rice

Jasmine Rice
White Rice
Whole Grain Brown Rice

Sun Luck

Jasmine Rice
Long Grain Rice
Niko Niko Brown Rice
Niko Niko Calrose Rice

Taste of China, A

Taste of China, A (All)

Taste of India, A

Taste of India, A (All)

Taste of Thai, A

Taste of Thai, A (All)

Tasty Bite ⓘ

Basmati Rice
Brown Rice
Garlic Brown Rice
Ginger Lentil Rice
Jasmine Rice
Tandoori Pilaf
Tehari Herb Rice

Trader Joe's

Biryani Curried Rice
Organic Brown Rice (Fully Cooked)
Organic Rice (All)

Rice (All)

TruRoots
Organic Germinated Brown Rice
Organic Haiga Mai Rice

Valu Time (Brookshire)
Long Grain Rice

Valu Time (Schnucks)
Long Grain Rice

Vietti ⓘ
Black Eye Peas and Rice
Pinto Beans and Rice
Red Beans and Rice
Sun Meadows Red Beans and Rice

Vons ᨆ
Brown Rice
Cal Rose Medium Grain Rice
Enriched Pre-Cooked Long Grain
   Instant Rice

Wegmans
Long Grain Rice

Wild Harvest (ACME)
Basmati Brown Rice
India Organic Basmati White Rice
Organic Jasmine Thai Rice
White Organic Long Grain Rice

Wild Harvest (Albertsons)
Domestic Long Grain Brown Rice
Organic Thai Jasmine Rice
Organic White Long Grain Rice

Wild Harvest (Cub Foods)
Basmati Brown Rice
Organic Jasmine Thai Rice
Organic White Long Grain Rice

Wild Harvest (Jewel-Osco)
Basmati Brown Rice
Domestic Long Grain Brown Rice
Organic India Basmati White Rice
Organic Jasmine Thai Rice
Organic White Long Grain Rice

Zatarain's
Black-Eyed Peas and Rice
Brown Rice Jambalaya Mix
Caribbean Rice Mix
Dirty Brown Rice Mix
Dirty Rice Mix
Dirty Rice with Cheese
Garden Vegetable Rice Mix

Garlic Butter Flavored Rice Mix
Jambalaya Mix
Jambalaya Mix with Cheese
Long Grain and Wild Rice
Mild Jambalaya Mix
Reduced Sodium Dirty Rice Mix
Reduced Sodium Jambalaya Mix
Rice Pudding Mix
Spanish Rice
Spicy Jambalaya Mix
Wild Brown Rice Mix
Yellow Rice

TACO SHELLS

Casa Fiesta ⓘ
Taco Shells
Taco Trays
Taco Tubs

Food Club (Brookshire)
Jumbo Taco Shells
Taco Shells

Food Club (Marsh)
Taco Shells

Guerrero
Taco Shells (Corn)
Tostadas (Corn)

Hy-Vee
Taco Shells

Meijer
Taco Shells

Ole Mexican Foods
Tostadas

Ortega ⓘ
Hard Shells - Yellow & White
Tostada Shells
Whole Grain Taco Shells

Taco Bell ᨆ
Taco Shells

Trader Joe's
Taco Shells

Valu Time (Brookshire)
Taco Shells

Vons ᨆ
Jumbo Taco Shells
Taco Shells, White Corn

TORTILLAS & WRAPS

Azteca ()
Corn Tortillas
Best Choice
Corn Tortillas, 6 inch
Chi-Chi's
Corn Tortillas
Food for Life
Wheat & Gluten-Free Brown Rice
Tortillas
French Meadow Bakery
Gluten-Free Tortilla
Giant Eagle
Corn Tortilla
Goya
Corn Tortillas
La Gordita Tortillas
Great Value (Wal-Mart) 25
Corn Tortillas
Guerrero
Corn Gorditas
Corn Tortillas
Sopes (Corn)
Konjac Foods
Konjac Tortillas
La Tortilla Factory ⓘ ✓
Smart & Delicious Gluten-Free Wraps
Mom's Place Gluten-Free ⓧ
Mom's Place Gluten-Free (All)
Ole Mexican Foods
Corn Tortilla
Price Chopper
Blue Tortilla (Corn/ Flax)
Tortilla (Yellow Corn/Flax/Soy)
Santa Fe ()
Corn Tortillas
Toovaloo ⓧ
Flatbread
Tortillas
Trader Joe's
Brown Rice Tortillas
Corn Tortillas (Hand Made & Original)
Tropical Cheese
Corn Tortilla
V & V Supremo
Sopes

Winn-Dixie
Corn Tortillas (Refrigerated)

MISCELLANEOUS

Bacchini
Gluten Free Corn Couscous
Gluten Free Corn-Rice Couscous
Goya
Hoja de Tamal
Montana Monster Munchies ⓘ ✓
Gluten Free Raw & Sproutable Oat
Groats
Gluten Free Whole Grain Quick Oats
Gluten Free Whole Grain Rolled Oats
Rice River Farms ⓘ
Corn Husks
Safeway Select ⌇
Brown and Wild Rice with Quinoa

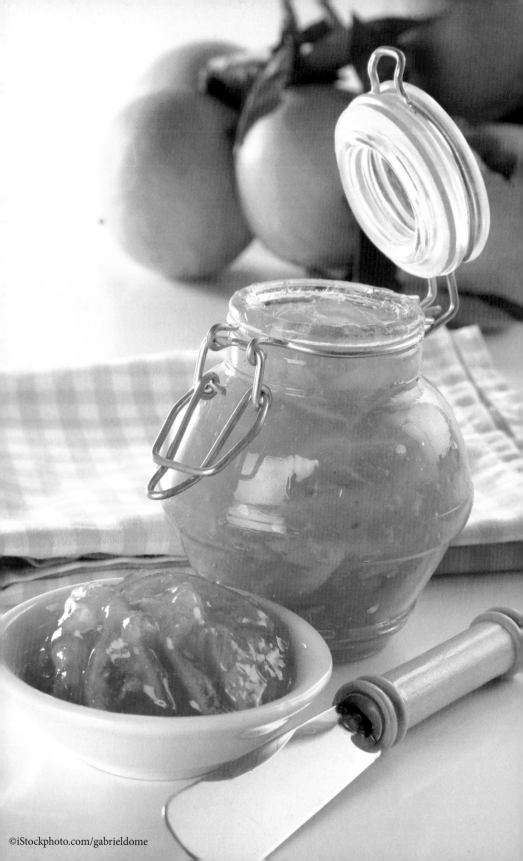

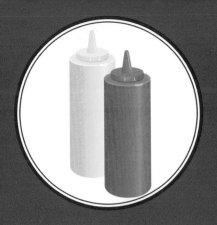

CONDIMENTS, SAUCES & DRESSINGS

Asian Sauces, Misc.

Ah So Sauces
Chinese Rib Sauce
Chinese Style BBQ Squeeze
Duck Sauce
Mandarin Duck Sauce
Sweet & Sour Sauce

Best Choice
Teriyaki Sauce

Bone Suckin' Sauce
Bone Suckin' Yaki ( )

China Pride
Duck Sauce

Chun's ( )
Chili Lemongrass Sauce
Chili Vinegar Sauce
Fish Sauce
Sweet and Sour Sauce

Dai-Day Oriental Sauces
Duck Sauce
Garlic Sparerib Sauce
Hunan Hot Duck Sauce

Earth Family ( )
Asian Sauce

Eden Foods
Mirin (Rice Cooking Wine)
Organic Dulse Flakes
Ume Plum Vinegar

Fischer & Wieser ⓘ
Asian Wasabi Plum Dipping Sauce

Ginger People, The ( )
Ginger Wasabi Sauce

Hy-Vee
Teriyaki Sauce

Jack Daniel's Sauces
EZ Marinader Teriyaki

Kikkoman
Dipping Sauce, Sweet and Sour ( )
Oyster Sauce (Red Label Only) ( )
Thai Red Curry Sauce ( )
Thai Yellow Curry Sauce ( )

Mee Tu Oriental Sauces
BBQ Hoisin Sauce
Chinese Marinade
Duck Sauce
Light Teri-Yaki Sauce
Sparerib Sauce
Teri-Yaki Sauce

Mitsukan
Mirin Sweet Cooking Seasoning

Organicville
Teriyaki Sauce (All) 𝍢 ✓

Polynesian Sauces
Hoisin Sauce
Oyster Sauce

Premier Japan ✓
Organic Gluten-Free Hoisin
Organic Gluten-Free Teriyaki

Really Great Food 𝍢
Really Great Food (All)

Robbie's Sauces
Sweet & Sour Sauce

San-J ⓘ ✓
Gluten Free Orange Sauce
Gluten Free Sweet and Tangy Sauce
Gluten Free Szechuan Sauce
Gluten Free Teriyaki Sauce
Gluten Free Thai Peanut Sauce

Saucy Susan
  Peking Duck
Schnucks Select
  Horseradish Wasabi
Snapdragon Pan-Asian Cuisine
  Japanese Black Sesame Dressing
  Java Ginger Sesame Dressing
  Kyoto Plum Dressing
  Passion Fruit Dressing
  Pineapple Chili Dressing
  Tangy Vietnamese Dressing
Sun Luck
  Black Bean Garlic Sauce
  Chili Garlic Sauce
  Chili Sauce (Hot, Sweet)
  Hot & Spicy Stir Fry Sauce
  Mirin Sweet Cooking Wine
  Plum Sauce
  Sweet & Sour Sauce
Taste of Thai, A
  Taste of Thai, A (All)
Trader Joe's
  Sweet Chili Sauce
  Thai Curry Sauce (Red or Yellow)
TryMe
  Oyster & Shrimp Sauce
Wegmans
  Sweet & Sour Stir Fry Sauce
  Sweet and Sour Sauce

ASIAN, SOY & TAMARI SAUCES

Best Choice
  Lite Soy Sauce
  Soy Sauce
Crystal
  Soy Sauce (Teriyaki is NOT gluten free)
Eden Foods
  Organic Tamari Soy Sauce, Brewed in U.S.
  Organic Tamari Soy Sauce, Imported
Hy-Vee
  Light Soy Sauce
  Soy Sauce
Kari-Out ✓
  Gluten Free Soy Sauce Packets

Kikkoman
  Gluten Free Soy Sauce ⓘ ✓
Meet Tu Oriental Sauces
  Light Soy Sauce
  Soy Sauce
San-J ⓘ ✓
  Organic Gluten Free Reduced Sodium Tamari Soy Sauce (Platinum Label)
  Organic Gluten Free Tamari Soy Sauce (Gold Label)
  Tamari Gluten Free Reduced Sodium Soy Sauce (White Label)
  Tamari Gluten Free Soy Sauce (Black Label)

BACON BITS

Best Choice
  Real Bacon Bits
  Real Bacon Pieces
Food Club (Brookshire)
  Imitation Bacon Flavored Chips
Gold Medal Spices ⟨⟩
  Bak'n Bits
Great Value (Wal-Mart) 🗓25
  Imitation Bacon Bits
Hormel
  Bacon Bits, Pieces & Crumbles
Sauer's ⟨⟩
  Bakin' Bits
Valu Time (Brookshire)
  Bacon Bits
Wellshire Farms
  Bacon Bits
  Salt Cured Bacon Bits

BARBEQUE SAUCE

Annie's Naturals
  Organic Annie's Original BBQ Sauce
  Organic Hot Chipotle BBQ Sauce
  Organic Smokey Maple BBQ Sauce
  Organic Sweet & Spicy BBQ Sauce
Austin's Own
  BBQ Sauce (All)
Bea's Gourmet Sauces
  Bea's Slammin' Honey Barbecue Sauce

Bone Suckin' Sauce
  Bone Suckin' Sauce (All)
Bull's Eye ⌒
  Barbecue Sauce, Original
  Barbecue Sauce, Regional Carolina Style
  Barbecue Sauce, Regional Kansas City
    Style
  Barbecue Sauce, Regional Memphis
    Style
  Barbecue Sauce, Regional Texas Style
Burnin' Love ⓘ ✓
  1919 Molasses Barbecue Sauce
  Sassy Mo'lassy
Burnt Sacrifice ()
  Burnt Sacrifice (All)
Butcher Block Sauces
  BBQ Sauce
Cattlemen's Barbecue
  Kansas City Classic Barbecue Sauce
  Memphis Sweet Barbecue Sauce
  Mississippi Honey Barbecue Sauce
Charlie Robinson's Barbecue Sauce
  Barbecue Sauce (Brown Sugar, Original,
    Hot)
Cub Foods
  Honey Barbecue Sauce
Dinosaur BBQ
  Creole Honey Mustard
  Devil's Duel
  Garlic Chipotle
  Jerk BBQ
  Mojito Marinade
  Roasted Garlic Honey
  Sensuous Slathering Sauce
  Wango Tango
EMERIL'S ⛊
  BBQ Sauces (All)
Encore Woodland
  Chicken Wing Sauce
  Chicken Wing Sauce, Extra Hot
Fischer & Wieser ⓘ
  Texas Pit BBQ Sauce
Flavorite (Cub Foods)
  Regular Barbecue Sauce
Food Club (Brookshire)
  BBQ Sauce, Hickory
  BBQ Sauce, Honey

  BBQ Sauce, Mesquite
  BBQ Sauce, Original
  BBQ Sauce, Regular
Food Club (Marsh)
  Hickory BBQ Sauce
  Honey BBQ Sauce
  Regular BBQ Sauce
Frank's
  Mississippi BBQ Sauce
Golding Farms ⓘ
  Lexington Style Barbeque Dip
GranoVita
  Barbeque Sauce
Hawkshead Relish
  BBQ Sauce
H-E-B
  Specialty Series BBQ Sauce, Carolina
  Specialty Series BBQ Sauce, Kansas City
  Specialty Series BBQ Sauce, Memphis
  Specialty Series BBQ Sauce, South Texas
Heinz
  Chicken & Rib BBQ Sauce
  Garlic BBQ Sauce
  Honey Garlic BBQ Sauce
  Original BBQ Sauce
Hy-Vee
  Hickory BBQ Sauce
  Honey Smoke BBQ Sauce
  Original BBQ Sauce
Jack Daniel's Sauces
  Hickory Brown Sugar BBQ Sauce
  Honey Smokehouse BBQ Sauce
  Original #7 BBQ Sauce
  Spicy BBQ Sauce
Jardine's ⓘ
  7J Carolina Midland Mustard BBQ
    Sauce
  7J City Slow Mo Molasses BBQ Sauce
  7J Louisiana Cajun Cayenne BBQ Sauce
  7J Texas Longhorn Peppercorn BBQ
    Sauce
  Chik'n Lik'n BBQ Sauce
  Killer BBQ Sauce
  Mesquite BBQ Sauce
  Texas Pecan BBQ Sauce
K.C. Masterpiece
  K.C. Masterpiece

Kraft Barbecue Sauce 〰
   Barbecue Sauce, Brown Sugar
   Barbecue Sauce, Char-Grill
   Barbecue Sauce, Hickory Smoke
   Barbecue Sauce, Honey
   Barbecue Sauce, Honey Hickory Smoke
   Barbecue Sauce, Honey Mustard
   Barbecue Sauce, Honey Roasted Garlic
   Barbecue Sauce, Hot
   Barbecue Sauce, Light Original
   Barbecue Sauce, Mesquite Smoke
   Barbecue Sauce, Original
   Barbecue Sauce, Spicy Honey

Midwest Country Fare (Hy-Vee)
   Hickory BBQ Sauce
   Honey BBQ Sauce
   Original BBQ Sauce

Mother's Mountain
   Aunt Ruby's Red BBQ Sauce
   Honey Hickory BBQ Sauce

Mrs. Bryant's
   Bone Doctor's Sweet & Spicy BBQ Sauce

Nando's Peri-Peri
   Garlic Sauce
   Wild Herb Sauce

Naturally Delicious
   Barbeque Sauce (Original, Honey)

NOH of Hawaii ()
   Hawaiian Barbecue Sauce
   Spicy Hawaiian Barbecue Sauce

Organicville
   BBQ Sauce (Original, Tangy) 𝄞 ✓

Pemberton Gourmet BBQ Sauce
   Pemberton Gourmet BBQ Sauce (All)

Polynesian Sauces
   Sparerib Sauce

Publix
   BBQ Sauce

Really Great Food 𝄞
   Really Great Food (All)

Robbie's Sauces
   BBQ Sauce (Hickory, Mild)

San-J ⓘ ✓
   Gluten Free Asian BBQ

Saz's
   Saz's (All)

Schnucks Select
   BBQ Sauce (Extreme Mesquite, Kansas
     City Style, Original)

Stokes Sauces
   Barbeque Sauce
   Brown Sauce
   Squeezy Brown Sauce

Stubb's
   Hickory Bourbon Bar-B-Q Sauce
   Honey Pecan Bar-B-Q Sauce
   Mild Bar-B-Q Sauce
   Moppin' Sauce
   Original Bar-B-Q Sauce
   Smokey Mesquite Bar-B-Q Sauce
   Spicy Bar-B-Q Sauce

Sweet Baby Ray's ⓘ
   Sweet Baby Ray's Barbeque Sauce (All)

Tiptree
   Tiptree (All)

Trader Joe's
   BBQ Sauce
   Kansas City BBQ Sauce

Trinity Hill Farms
   Zesty Barbeque Sauce

Valu Time (Brookshire)
   BBQ Sauce- Hickory
   BBQ Sauce- Regular
   Vienna Sausage- BBQ

Vita Foods ⓘ
   A&W BBQ Sauce
   Dr. Pepper BBQ Sauce
   Jim Beam Original Barbecue Sauce
   Jim Beam Spicy Barbecue Sauce

Walden Farms 𝄞
   Walden Farms (All)

Wegmans
   Brown Sugar BBQ Sauce
   Memphis Style BBQ Sauce

World Harbors
   Buccaneer Blends BBQ Sauces (All)

CHOCOLATE SYRUP

Bosco
   Chocolate Syrup (All)

Food Club (Brookshire)
   Chocolate Syrup

Hy-Vee
Chocolate Flavored Syrup
Chocolate Syrup
Meijer
Chocolate Syrup
Midwest Country Fare (Hy-Vee)
Chocolate Flavored Syrup
Nesquik
Syrup (All Flavors)
Price Chopper
Chocolate Syrup
Schnucks
Chocolate Syrup
Trader Joe's
Organic Chocolate Midnight Moo
Valu Time (Brookshire)
Chocolate Syrup
Wegmans
Chocolate Flavored Syrup
Winn-Dixie
Chocolate Syrup

CHUTNEYS

Bombay
Carrot Pickle
Chili Pickle
Chutneys (All)
Eggplant (Brinjal) Pickle
Garlic Pickle
Lime Pickle
Mango Pickle
Mixed Pickle
Burnin' Love ⓘ ✓
Sweet Onion Blues
Divine Brine ()
Divine Brine (All)
Hawkshead Relish
Chutneys (All)
McNulty's Chutney
Chutney (All)
Stokes Sauces
Chutney (All)
Tiptree
Tiptree (All)
Trader Joe's
Mango Ginger Chutney

Wild Thymes ⓘ
Apricot Cranberry Walnut Chutney
Caribbean Peach Lime Chutney
Mango Papaya Chutney
Plum Currant Ginger Chutney

COCKTAIL & SEAFOOD SAUCE

Best Choice
Cocktail Sauce
Cains
Cocktail Sauce
Ducktrap River of Maine
Mustard Dill Sauce
Food Club (Brookshire)
Seafood Cocktail Sauce
Food Club (Marsh)
Seafood Cocktail Sauce
Golding Farms ⓘ
Cocktail Sauce
Heinz
Cocktail Sauce (All Varieties)
Heluva Good
Cocktail Sauce
Hill Country Fare (H-E-B)
Cocktail Sauce
Hy-Vee
Cocktail Sauce For Seafood
Ken's Steak House Salad Dressing ⓘ
Cocktail Sauce (Refrigerated, Shelf
Stable)
Legal
Seafood Cocktail
Little River ⓘ
Bold & Spicy Cocktail Sauce
Cocktail Sauce
Louisiana Fish Fry ⓘ
Cocktail Sauce
Seafood Sauce
Price Chopper
Cocktail Sauce
Stokes Sauces
Cocktail Sauce
Stop & Shop
Cocktail Sauce for Seafood
Trader Joe's
Seafood Cocktail Sauce

Trinity Hill Farms
Seafood Cocktail Sauce
Vita Foods ⓘ
Vita Cocktail Sauce
Vons ᴧ
Cocktail Sauce for Seafood
Walden Farms ⚬
Walden Farms (All)
Wegmans
Remoulade Sauce
Wellshire Farms
Organic Cocktail Sauce
Woeber ⓘ
Cocktail Sauce
Seafood Sauce

CROUTONS

Aleia's ⚬ ✓
Classics Croutons
Parmesan Croutons
Ener-G
Plain Croutons
Gillian's Foods ⚬
Gillian's Foods (All)
Streit's ⓘ
Soup Croutons

DESSERT SYRUPS, SAUCES & GLAZES

Darbo
Berries Compotes
Black Currant
Black Elder
Elder Flower
Forest Raspberry
Herb and Ginger
Lemon Balm
Maraska Sour Cherry
Peach and Passion Fruit
Pomegranate
Rose Apricot Compotes
White Grape
Wild Blueberry
Wild Lingonberry
Goya
Cajeta de Guayaba

Cajeta de Leche
Cajeta de Mango
Cajeta de Membrillo
Hawkshead Relish
Fruit Compotes (All)
Sweet Sauces (All)
Hy-Vee
Strawberry Syrup
Lyle's Syrup
Black Treacle
Butterscotch Syrup
Chocolate Syrup
Golden Syrup
Mint Chocolate Syrup
Strawberry Syrup
Organic Nectars
Agave Syrups (All)
Raw Agave Dessert Syrups (All)
Trader Joe's
Fleur de Sel Caramel Sauce
Vita Foods ⓘ
A&W Topper
Dr. Pepper Topper
Jelly Belly Toasted Marshmallow Dessert
  Topper
Jelly Belly Very Cherry Dessert Topper
Orange Crush Topper
Stuckey's Chocolate Pecan Dessert
  Topper
Stuckey's Pecan Log Roll Dessert Topper
Walden Farms ⚬
Walden Farms (All)
Wegmans
Creamy Caramel Sauce
Milk Chocolate Sauce
Raspberry Chocolate Sauce
Triple Chocolate Sauce

DIP & DIP MIXES - SAVORY

Abby's Table
Dream Date
Nude Pudding
Nude Ranch
Turmeric Coconut
ACME
Cheese Dip

Alamo ⅄
   Gristmill Seasonings and Dips (All)
Aleia's ⅄ ✓
   Plain Stuffing Mix
   Savory Stuffing Mix
Barber's
   Party Dip
Best Choice
   French Onion Dip
   Green Onion Dip
   Ranch Style Dip
Broughton
   Chip Dip
Cabot
   Cabot Products (All)
Cantaré Foods
   Olive Tapenade Spreads
Casa Fiesta ⓘ
   Black Bean Dip
   Jalapeno Bean Dip
   Jalapeno Cheese Dip
Cheez Whiz ⌇
   Cheese Dip, Original
Chi-Chi's
   Con Queso
   Nacho Cheese Snackers
Country Fresh
   Dips
Creamland Dairies
   Dips (All)
Cugino's ()
   Cheesy Bacon Dip
   Fire Roasted Ranch Dip
   Garlic Schmarlic Dip
   Onion Wonion Dip
   Silly Dilly Dip
   Spinach Finach Dip
   Taco Schmaco Dip
   Veggie Weggie Dip
Davis & Davis
   Dipper Mixes (All BUT Ultimate Bacon)
Dean's
   Dips (All)
DeLallo
   Green Olive Tapenade
Dutch Farms
   French Onion Dip

EMERIL'S ⅄
   Dips (Guacamole, Classic Onion, Veggie Ranch)
Fischer & Wieser ⓘ
   Cilantro Pepito Pesto Appetizer Spread
   Guacamole Starter - Just Add Avocados
   Queso Starter - Just Add Cheese
Food Club (Brookshire)
   Original Bean Dip
Fritos
   Bean Dip ⓘ
   Chili Cheese Dip ⓘ
   Hot Bean Dip ⓘ
   Jalapeno & Cheddar Flavored Cheese Dip ⓘ
   Mild Cheddar Flavor Cheese Dip ⓘ
   Southwest Enchilada Black Bean Flavored Dip ⓘ
Fusion Flavors ⅄
   Dips (All)
Gaea ()
   Dips (All)
Garden Fresh Gourmet ⓘ
   Dips & Dip Mixes (All)
Giant
   French Onion Dip
Giant Eagle
   Buffalo Chicken Dip
   Mexicali Dip
   Queso Cheese Dip with Jalapeno
Goya
   Chimichurri
   Guacamole, Mild
   Guacamole, Spicy
Great Value (Wal-Mart) 🄬
   Homestyle Pimento Spread
Haggen
   Bean Dip, Medium
H-E-B
   Bean and Cheese Dip
   Bean Dip
   Chipotle Con Queso
   Hot Jalapeno Bean Dip
Heluva Good
   Dip (All)
Herr's ()
   French Onion Dip

Jalapeno Cheddar Dip
Mild Cheddar Dip

Hidden Valley
Dry Dip Mixes

Hiland Dairy
French Onion Dip
Light French Onion Dip
Southwest Ranch Dip
Vegetable Dip

Hill Country Fare (H-E-B)
Bean & Cheese Dip
Bean Dip
Hot Jalapeno Bean Dip
Jalapeno Bean Dip
Nacho Cheese Dip
Ranch Dry Dip Mix

Hy-Vee
Bacon & Cheddar Sour Cream Dip
French Onion Sour Cream Dip
Ranch & Dill Sour Cream Dip
Salsa Sour Cream Dip
Toasted Onion Sour Cream Dip
Vegetable Party Sour Cream Dip

Jewel-Osco
French Onion Dip

Jodie's Kitchen
Jodie's Kitchen (All)

Juanitas
Nacho Cheese Sauce

Lakeview Farms
Dill
Down Home Dill
Down Home Spinach
Fat Free Ranch Veggie
Fat Free Vegetable Dill
French Onion
Guacamole
Ranch
Sour Cream French Onion
Vegetable Ranch
Vegetable Spinach
Veggie
Zesty Guacamole

Lay's
Dip Creations Country Ranch Dry Dip
Mix ⓘ

Dip Creations Garden Onion Dry Dip
Mix ⓘ
French Onion Dip ⓘ
French Onion Flavored Dry Dip Mix ⓘ
Green Onion Flavored Dry Dip Mix ⓘ
Heavenly Baked Potato Flavored Dip ⓘ
Ranch Flavored Dry Dip Mix ⓘ
Smooth Ranch Dip ⓘ

Louis Trauth Dairy
French Onion Dip

Luisa's
Black Bean Dip
Fiesta Dip, Hot
Fiesta Dip, Medium
Fiesta Dip, Mild
Five Layer Fiesta Dip, Medium
Five Layer Fiesta Dip, Mild

Market District (Giant Eagle)
Roast Red Pepper and Feta Cheese Dip
Spinach and Artichoke Dip

Mayfield Dairy
French Onion Party Dip

Meadow Brook Dairy
Dip (All)

Oberweis Dairy
Roasted Pepper Dip

Ortega ⓘ
Guacamole Dip
Nacho Cheese Sauce (Pouch)

Our Family
French Onion Dip

Prairie Farms
Bacon Cheddar Dip
French Onion Dip
Jalapeno Fiesta Dip
Ranch Dip

Price's Creameries
Dip (All)

Publix
French Onion Dip
Guacamole Dip

Purity Dairies
French Onion Dip

Reiter Dairy
French Onion Dip

Ricos ✓
Cheese Sauce (All)

Santa Barbara Salsa
Santa Barbara Salsa (All)

Schnucks
Bean & Cheese Dip
Bean Dip
Dill Dip Pack
Onion Dip Pack

Shaw's
French Onion Cream Dip
Ranch Cream Dip/Spread
Real Cream Dip

Simply Organic
Chipotle Black Bean Dip ✓
Creamy Dill Dip ✓
French Onion Dip ✓
Guacamole Dip ✓
Ranch Dip ✓
Salsa Mix ✓
Spinach Dip ✓

Taco Bell 👓
Bean Con Queso
Chili Con Queso with Meat

Tostitos
Creamy Southwestern Ranch Dip ⓘ
Creamy Spinach Dip ⓘ
Dip Creations Freshly Made Guacamole
Dry Dip Mix ⓘ
Monterey Jack Queso ⓘ
Smooth & Cheesy Dip ⓘ
Spicy Nacho Dip ⓘ
Zesty Bean & Cheese Dip ⓘ

Trader Joe's
Blue Cheese With Roasted Pecan Dip
Cilantro And Chive Yogurt Dip
Eggplant Garlic Spread
Fat Free Spicy Black Bean Dip
Masala Lentil Dip
Queso Cheese Dip
Spinach & Sour Cream Dip
Sun-Dried Tomato Pesto Torta

Utz ☷
Cheddar & Jalapeno Dip
Mild Cheddar Cheese Dip

Walden Farms ☷
Walden Farms (All)

Wegmans
Salsa Con Queso (Cheddar Cheese Dip)

Wholly Guacamole ☷
Guacamole (All)

Wild Thymes ⓘ
Indian Vindaloo Curry Dipping Sauce
Moroccan Spicy Pepper Dipping Sauce
Thai Chili Roasted Garlic Dipping Sauce

Wise Snacks
Green Onion Dip Mix

DIP & DIP MIXES - SWEET

Baker's Chocolate 👓
Dipping Chocolate, Real Dark Semi-
Sweet
Dipping Chocolate, Real Milk

Jodie's Kitchen
Jodie's Kitchen (All)

Saco
Dolci Frutta Hard Chocolate Shell (All)

Simply Organic
Fruit Dip ✓

Walden Farms ☷
Walden Farms (All)

FRUIT BUTTERS & CURDS

Best Choice
Apple Butter

Eden Foods
Organic Apple Butter
Organic Apple Cherry Butter
Organic Cherry Butter, Montmorency
Tart

Elizabethan Pantry
Fruit Curds (All)

Fischer & Wieser ⓘ
Peach Pecan Butter
Pecan Apple Butter
Pumpkin Pie Butter

Food You Feel Good About
(Wegmans)
Jammin' Strawberry Fruit Spread

Giant
Apple Butter

Great Value (Wal-Mart) 🔲
Spiced Apple Butter

Hawkshead Relish
  Flavored Butters (All)
  Fruit Curds (All)
H-E-B
  More Fruit Blackberry Spread
  More Fruit Cherry/ Blueberry Spread
  More Fruit Four Berry Spread
  More Fruit Peach Mango Spread
  More Fruit Strawberry Spread
Honey Acres
  Honey Spread Crème (All)
Manischewitz
  Apple Butter
Simon Fischer ()
  Apricot Butter
  Prune Lekvar
Trader Joe's
  Lemon Curd
  Mango Butter
  Pumpkin Butter (Seasonal)
White House
  White House (All)

GRAVY & GRAVY MIXES

Full Flavor Foods ✓
  Gravy Mixes (All)
Leahey Gardens ⓘ
  Gluten Free Homestyle Creamy Gravy
  Gluten Free Mushroom Gravy
  Gluten Free No Beef Brown Gravy
  Gluten Free No Beef Mexican Style
    Gravy
  Gluten Free No Chicken Golden Gravy
Maxwell's Kitchen
  Brown Gravy Mix
  Chicken Gravy Mix
  Pork Gravy Mix
  Turkey Gravy Mix
Organic Gourmet
  Vegan Brown Gravy Mix
Orgran ⓘ ⚇
  Gravy Mix
Riega Foods ⓘ ✓
  Alfredo Cheese Sauce Mix
  Pepper Jack Cheese Sauce Mix
  White Cheddar Cheese Sauce Mix

  Yellow Cheddar Cheese Sauce Mix
Road's End Organics ✓
  Organic Golden Gravy Mix
  Organic Savory Herb Gravy Mix
  Organic Shiitake Gravy Mix
Seitenbacher
  Gluten-Free Gravies (All)
Simply Organic
  Brown Gravy Mix ✓
  Hollandaise Sauce Mix ✓
  Mushroom Sauce Mix ✓
  Roasted Chicken Gravy Seasoning Mix ✓
  Roasted Turkey Gravy Seasoning Mix ✓
  Vegetarian Brown Gravy ✓
Trader Joe's
  All Natural Turkey Gravy (Seasonal)
  Turkey Gravy (Seasonal)

HORSERADISH

Atomic Horseradish
  Atomic Horseradish
Beano's ⓘ
  Heavenly Horse Radish Sauce
Boar's Head
  Condiments (All)
Bubbies ⚇
  Beet Horseradish (All)
  Prepared Horseradish (All)
**Central Market Classics
(Price Chopper)**
  Horseradish Spread
  Smokey Horseradish
Di Lusso
  Horseradish Sauce
Dietz & Watson ✓
  Cranberry Horseradish Sauce
  Hot and Chunky Horseradish Sauce
  Red Horseradish Sauce
  Smoky Horseradish Sauce
Ducktrap River of Maine
  Horseradish Sauce
Heinz
  Horseradish Sauce
Heluva Good
  Horseradish

Hy-Vee
All Natural Prepared Horseradish
Manischewitz
Horseradish (All)
Morehouse
Horseradish (All)
Price Chopper
Beet Horseradish
White Horseradish
Saag's ⓘ
Saag's (All)
Schnucks Select
Creamy Horseradish
Dijon Horseradish
Stokes Sauces
Creamed Horseradish Sauce
Vita Foods ⓘ
Vita Beet Horseradish
Vita Cream Style Horseradish
Vita Prepared Horseradish
Wegmans
Horseradish Cream Sauce
Prepared Horseradish
Wellshire Farms
Organic Horseradish
Woeber ⓘ
Pure Horseradish
Reserve Smoky Horseradish Sauce
Sandwich Pal Cranberry Horseradish
Sauce
Sandwich Pal Horseradish Sauce
Sandwich Pal Smoky Horseradish Sauce
Southwest Horseradish Sauce

Hot Sauce

Always Save
Hot Sauce
Best Choice
Chicken Wing Sauce
Louisiana Hot Sauce
Bone Suckin' Sauce
Bone Suckin' Habanero Sauce
Burnin' Love ⓘ ✓
Heatbreak Sauce
Torch-ered Heartbreak Sauce

Casa Fiesta ⓘ
Hot Pepper Sauce
Cholula Hot Sauce
Cholula Hot Sauce (All)
Crystal
Hot Sauce (All)
Wing Sauce (All)
Dave's Gourmet
Dave's Gourmet (All)
Jump Up and Kiss Me Hot Sauce
Dr. Gonzo's Uncommon Condiments
Dr. Gonzo's Uncommon Condiments
(All)
El Pinto ♨
El Pinto (All)
Encore Woodland
Hot Sauce
Fischer & Wieser ⓘ
Four Star Black Raspberry Chipotle
Sauce
Mango Ginger Habanero Sauce
Original Roasted Raspberry Chipotle
Sauce, The
Papaya Lime Serrano Sauce
Pomegranate & Mango Chipotle Sauce
Roasted Blackberry Chipotle Sauce
Roasted Blueberry Chipotle Sauce
Food Club (Brookshire)
Louisiana Hot Sauce
Food Club (Marsh)
Chili Sauce
Louisiana Hot Sauce
Frank's RedHot
Buffalo Wings Sauce
Chile 'n Lime Hot Sauce
HOT Buffalo Wings Sauce
Original Cayenne Pepper Sauce
Sweet Chili Sauce
Sweet Heat BBQ Wings Sauce
Thick Cayenne
Xtra Hot Sauce
Giant
Chili Sauce
Gifts of Nature ✓
Sriracha Hot Sauce with a Touch of
Wasabi

Ginger People, The ()
- Hot Ginger Jalapeno Sauce
- Sweet Ginger Chili Sauce
- Thai Green Curry Sauce

Goya
- Ancho Salsita
- Arbol Salsita
- Habanero Salsita
- Hot Sauce

Great Value (Wal-Mart) 📅
- Chili Sauce
- Louisiana Hot Sauce

Heinz
- Chili Sauce (All Varieties)

Huy Fong
- Chili Garlic Sauce
- Sambal Oelek
- Sriracha Chili Sauce

Hy-Vee
- Chili Sauce

Jardine's ⓘ
- Blazin' Saddle XXX Hot Sauce
- Texas Champagne Cayenne Pepper Sauce
- Texas Kicker XX Hot Sauce

Juanitas
- Pico Pica Hot Sauce
- Pico Pica Mild Sauce

Ken's Steak House Salad Dressing ⓘ
- Buffalo Wing Sauce Marinade

La Victoria
- Jalapeno Hot Sauce
- Salsa Brava Hot Sauce

Louisiana Fish Fry ⓘ
- Hot Sauce

Louisiana Gold 🍴
- Hot Sauce

Louisiana Hot Sauce ⓘ
- Louisiana Chipotle Flavor Hot Sauce
- Louisiana Habanero Flavor Hot Sauce
- Louisiana Jalapeno Flavor Hot Sauce
- Louisiana Red Chili Flavor Hot Sauce
- Louisiana Red Hot Sauce
- Louisiana Roasted Garlic Flavor Hot Sauce
- Louisiana Wing Sauce

Meijer
- Chili Sauce

Moore's
- Buffalo Wing Sauce
- Honey BBQ Wing Sauce

Nando's Peri-Peri
- Extra Hot Sauce
- Hot Sauce

Organicville
- Organic Chili Sauce 🍴 ✓

Price Chopper
- Hot Sauce

Red Rooster Hot Sauce ⓘ
- Hot Sauce

Safeway 〰
- Chili Sauce

Schnucks
- Hot Sauce

Shiloh's ✓
- Caribbean Hot Sauce
- Harissa Spicy Sauce

Slap Ya Mama
- Etouffee Sauce
- Pepper Sauce

Sontava! ⓘ
- XX Habanero Hot Sauce
- XXX Habanero Hot Sauce

Stokes Sauces
- Sweet Chilli Sauce

Stop & Shop
- Hot Sauce

Stubb's
- Original Wing Sauce

Tabasco ⓘ
- Chipotle Pepper Sauce
- Garlic Pepper Sauce
- Green Pepper Sauce
- Habanero Pepper Sauce
- Pepper Sauce

Tapatio
- Tapatio Hot Sauce

Trader Joe's
- Jalapeño Hot Sauce

Trappey ⓘ
- Hot Sauces

TryMe
- Yucatan Sunshine Habanero Sauce

Valu Time (Brookshire)
Hot Sauce
Vita Foods ⓘ
Jim Beam Hot Sauce
Jim Beam Original Hot Sauce
Sauza Hot Sauce
Scorned Woman Hot Sauce
Wizard's, The ✓
Organic Hot Stuff
Woeber ⓘ
Sandwich Pal Wasabi Sauce

Hummus

DeLallo
Prince Omar Hummus (Original, with Roasted Garlic, with Roasted Peppers)
Garden Fresh Gourmet ⓘ
Hummus (All)
Goya
Chipotle Hummus
Classic Hummus
Garlic Hummus
Mediterranean Hummus
H-E-B
Four Pepper Hummus
Mediterranean Olive Hummus
Roasted Garlic Hummus
Roasted Red Pepper Hummus
Traditional Hummus
Private Selection (Kroger)
Garlic & Chive Hummus
Hummus
Roasted Red Pepper Hummus
Pulmuone Wildwood ⓘ
Hummus (All)
Simply Enjoy (Giant)
Artichoke and Spinach Hummus
Original Hummus
Red Pepper Hummus
Roasted Garlic Hummus
Simply Enjoy (Stop & Shop)
Artichoke and Spinach Hummus
Original Hummus
Red Pepper Hummus
Roasted Garlic Hummus

Trader Joe's
Hummus (All BUT White Bean Hummus and White Bean & Basil Hummus)
Wild Garden
Hummus Products (All)

Jams, Jellies & Preserves

Bineshii Wild Rice
Jams (All)
Bionaturae
Fruit Spreads (All) ⓘ
Central Market (H-E-B)
Organic Apricot Preserve
Organic Blueberry Preserve
Organic Morello Cherry Preserve
Organic Raspberry Preserve
Organic Strawberry Preserve
Crofter's
Crofter's (All)
Cub Foods
Red Raspberry Preserves
Darbo
Apricot Fruchtikus
Apricot Preserve (Diabetic)
Balm and Ginger Jelly
Black Cherry Preserve
Black Cherry Preserve (Diabetic)
Black Currant Jelly
Black Currant, Finely Strained Preserve
Blackberry and Black Currant Finely Strained Preserve
Blueberry Preserve (Diabetic)
Elder Flower Jelly
Elder Plum Preserve
Forest Berries Preserve
Fruit in Rum Preserve
Garden Strawberry Preserve
Garden Strawberry, Finely Strained Preserve
Gravensteiner Apple Jelly
Lingonberry Preserve (Diabetic)
Maraska Sour Cherry Preserve
Orange Preserve (Diabetic)
Plum, Finely Strained Preserve
Raspberry and Rhubarb Preserve

Raspberry Preserve
Raspberry Preserve (Diabetic)
Raspberry, Finely Strained Preserve
Red Currant, Finely Strained Preserve
Red Fruits Fruchtikus
Rose Apricot Preserve
Rose Apricot, Finely Strained Preserve
Rosehip, Finely Strained Preserve
Seville Bitter Orange Preserve
Strawberry and Vanilla Fruchtikus
Strawberry and Vanilla Preserve
Strawberry Preserve (Diabetic)
Tropical Fruchtikus
Wild Blueberry Preserve
Wild Lingonberry Preserve

E.D. Smith
E.D. Smith (All)

Elizabethan Pantry
Fruit Preserves (All)
Golden Mint Jelly
Marmalades (All)

Fischer & Wieser ⓘ
Almond Cherry Jubilee Jam
Amaretto Peach Pecan Preserves
Apricot Orange Marmalade
Jalapeno Peach Preserves
Mild Green Jalapeno Jelly
Old Fashioned Peach Preserves
Red Hot Jalapeno Jelly
Southern Style Preserves
Strawberry Rhubarb Preserves
Whole Lemon & Fig Marmalade

Food Club (Brookshire)
Apple Jelly
Apricot Preserves
Concord Grape Preserves
Grape Jelly
Orange Marmalade Preserves
Peach Preserves
Red Plum Preserves
Seedless Tumbler Blackberry Preserves
Strawberry Preserves

Food Club (Marsh)
Apricot Preserves
Grape Jam
Grape Jelly
Grape Jelly, Squeezable

Orange Marmalade Preserves
Strawberry Preserves
Strawberry Spread, Squeezable

Food You Feel Good About (Wegmans)
Organic Jammin' Red Raspberry Fruit Spread

Full Circle (Price Chopper)
Cherry Conserve
Grape Jelly

Full Circle (Schnucks)
Apricot Fruit Spread
Blueberry Fruit Spread
Cherry Fruit Spread
Grape Jelly
Raspberry Fruit Spread
Strawberry Fruit Spread

Giant
Apricot Preserves
Grape Jelly
Orange Marmalade
Strawberry Preserves

Goya
Guava Marmalade

Griffin Foods
Griffin Foods (All)

Hawkshead Relish
Savory Jams (All)
Savory Jellies (All)
Savory Marmalades (All)
Sweet Jams (All)
Sweet Jellies (All)
Sweet Marmalades (All)

H-E-B
More Fruit Apricot Spread
More Fruit Grape Spread
More Fruit Peach Spread
More Fruit Pineapple Spread
More Fruit Red Raspberry

Hill Country Fare (H-E-B)
Apple Jelly
Apricot Preserves
Grape Jam
Grape Jelly
Peach Preserves
Pineapple Preserves
Red Raspberry Preserves
Strawberry Jam

Strawberry Preserves

Honey Acres
Honey Apricot (All)

Hy-Vee
Apple Jelly
Apricot Preserves
Blackberry Jelly
Cherry Jelly
Cherry Preserves
Concord Grape Jelly
Concord Grape Preserves
Grape Jelly
Orange Marmalade
Peach Preserves
Red Plum Jelly
Red Raspberry Jelly
Red Raspberry Preserves
Strawberry Jelly
Strawberry Preserves

Kissel's Spiced Jam
Apricot Rosemary
Blueberry Lavender
Cherry Fennel
Peach Coriander
Plum Tarragon
Strawberry Basil

Marsh
Concord Grape Jam

Meijer
Apple Jelly
Apricot Fruit Spread
Apricot Preserves
Blackberry Seedless Fruit Spread
Blackberry Seedless Preserves
Grape Jam
Grape Jelly
Orange Marmalade Preserves
Peach Preserves
Red Raspberry Fruit Spread
Red Raspberry Preserves
Red Raspberry with Seeds Preserves
Strawberry Fruit Spread
Strawberry Preserves

Nature's Promise (Giant)
Organic Grape Jelly
Organic Raspberry Fruit Spread
Organic Strawberry Fruit Spread

Nature's Promise (Stop & Shop)
Organic Grape Jelly
Organic Strawberry Fruit Spread

O Organics ✑
Blackberry Preserve
Blueberry Preserve
Raspberry Preserve

Oskri
Jam and Preserves (All)

Polaner ⓘ
All Fruit (All)
Jams (All)
Jellies (All)
Preserves (All)
Sugar Free (All)

Price Chopper
Apple Jelly
Apricot Preserve
Blueberry Preserves
Cherry Preserves
Concord Grape Jelly
Currant Jelly
Grape Jelly
Mint Jelly
Orange Marmalade
Peach Preserves
Pineapple Preserve
Raspberry Jelly
Red Raspberry Preserves
Seedless Red Raspberry Preserves
Seedless Strawberry Jam
Strawberry French Toast Spread
Strawberry Jelly
Strawberry Preserves
Sugar Free Raspberry Preserves
Sugar Free Strawberry Preserves

Publix
Jams (All Flavors)
Jellies (All Flavors)
Preserves (All Flavors)

Purity
Jam, Partridge and Apple

Safeway Select ✑
Apricot Jam
Blackberry Jam
Blueberry Jam
Boysenberry Jam

- Mint Jelly
- Raspberry Jam
- Seville Orange Marmalade

Sorrell Ridge
- 100% Specialty Flavors - Black Cherry
- 100% Specialty Flavors - Black Raspberry
- 100% Specialty Flavors - Blackberry
- 100% Specialty Flavors - Cherry
- 100% Specialty Flavors - Plum Good
- 100% Specialty Flavors - Strawberry Rhubarb
- 100% Specialty Flavors - Wild Blueberry
- 100% Spreadable Fruit - Apricot
- 100% Spreadable Fruit - Boysenberry
- 100% Spreadable Fruit - Concord Grape
- 100% Spreadable Fruit - Orange Marmelade
- 100% Spreadable Fruit - Peach
- 100% Spreadable Fruit - Raspberry
- 100% Spreadable Fruit - Seedless Raspberry
- 100% Spreadable Fruit - Seedless Strawberry
- 100% Spreadable Fruit - Strawberry
- Organic Apricot Fruit Spread
- Organic Blueberry Fruit Spread
- Organic Orange Marmalade Fruit Spread
- Organic Raspberry Fruit Spread
- Organic Strawberry Fruit Spread

St. Dalfour
- Black Cherry Spread
- Black Currant Spread
- Black Raspberry Spread
- Cranberry Blueberry Spread
- Four Fruit Spread
- Fruit Conserves (All)
- Ginger Orange Spread
- Gold Peach Spread
- Mirabelle Plum Spread
- Orange Marmalade Spread
- Pear William Preserve Spread
- Pineapple Mango Spread
- Red Raspberry and Pomegranate Spread
- Red Raspberry Spread
- Royal Fig Spread
- Strawberry Spread
- Wild Blueberry Spread

Stokes Sauces
- Apple and Ginger Sauce
- Blackcurrant Extra Jam
- Blueberry Extra Jam
- Bramley Apple Sauce
- Cranberry and Orange Sauce
- Cranberry Sauce
- Cumberland Sauce
- Mint Sauce
- Raspberry Extra Jam
- Redcurrant Jelly
- Seville Orange Marmalade
- Seville Orange Marmalade No 7
- Strawberry Extra Jam

Stop & Shop
- Apple Jelly
- Apricot Preserves
- Mint Jelly
- Seedless Red Raspberry Preserves
- Seedless Strawberry Preserves
- Strawberry Preserves

Suzanne's Specialties
- Jellies and Preserves

Tiptree
- Tiptree (All)

Valu Time (Brookshire)
- Apple Jelly
- Grape Jelly
- Strawberry Preserves

Valu Time (Marsh)
- Grape Jelly
- Strawberry Preserves

Vons
- Apricot Pineapple Preserves
- Boysenberry Preserves
- Grape Jam
- Grape Jelly
- Red Raspberry Preserves
- Seedless Blackberry Preserves
- Strawberry Jelly
- Strawberry Preserves

Walden Farms
- Walden Farms (All)

Wall's Berry Farm
- Wall's Berry Farm (All)

Wegmans
Apple Jelly
Apricot Preserves
Apricot, Peach & Passion Fruit Spread - Sugar Free
Apricot, Peach & Passion Fruit Spread
Blackberry (Seedless) Preserves
Blueberry, Cherry & Raspberry Fruit Spread
Cherry Jelly
Cherry Preserves
Grape Jelly
Grape Preserves
Orange Marmalade
Peach Preserves
Pineapple Preserves
Raspberry, Strawberry & Blackberry Fruit Spread
Raspberry, Wild Blueberry & Blackberry Fruit Spread - Sugar Free
Raspberry, Wild Blueberry & Blackberry Fruit Spread
Red Currant Jelly
Red Raspberry Jelly
Red Raspberry Preserves
Strawberry Jelly
Strawberry Preserves
Strawberry, Plum & Raspberry Fruit Spread - Sugar Free
Strawberry, Plum & Raspberry Fruit Spread

Welch's
Welch's (All)

KETCHUP

ACME
Blended Squeeze Bottle Tomato Catsup
Inverted Bottle Ketchup
Squeeze Bottle Tomato Catsup

Albertsons
Ketchup Inverted Bottle
Ketchup Squeeze Bottle

Always Save
Squeeze Ketchup

Best Choice
EZ Squeeze Ketchup

Ketchup
Squeeze Ketchup
Squeeze Ketchup Bonus

Central Market (H-E-B)
Organic Ketchup

Clearly Organic (Best Choice)
Ketchup

Cub Foods
Ketchup

Del Monte ⓘ
Tomatoes & Tomato Products (All BUT Spaghetti Sauce Flavored with Meat)

E.D. Smith
E.D. Smith (All)

Flavorite (Cub Foods)
Ketchup

Food Club (Brookshire)
Ketchup

Food Club (Marsh)
Ketchup

Food You Feel Good About (Wegmans)
Organic Tomato Ketchup

Frank's
Frank's Ketchup

French's
Fancy Tomato Ketchup

Full Circle (Price Chopper)
Ketchup

Full Circle (Schnucks)
Organic Ketchup
Squeeze Ketchup

Giant
Tomato Ketchup

Giant Eagle
Ketchup

Goya
Ketchup

GranoVita
Chilli Ketchup

Great Value (Wal-Mart) 🔲25
Ketchup

GreenWise Market (Publix)
Organic Ketchup

Haggen
Ketchup

Hanover Foods
Catsup (Ketchup)
Hawkshead Relish
Ketchup (All)
H-E-B
Tomato Ketchup
Heinz
Hot Ketchup
Ketchup
No Sodium Added Ketchup
Organic Ketchup
Reduced Sugar Ketchup
Simply Heinz Ketchup
Hill Country Fare (H-E-B)
Ketchup
Hunt's
Ketchup (All Varieties)
Hy-Vee
Thick & Rich Tomato Ketchup
Jewel-Osco
Ketchup
Tomato Catsup
Karma Sauce
Tomato Katsup
Kroger
Tomato Ketchup
Meijer
Ketchup
Ketchup (Squeeze)
Organic Tomato Ketchup
Midwest Country Fare (Hy-Vee)
Tomato Ketchup
Mother's Mountain
Tomato Catchup
Nature's Basket (Giant Eagle)
Organic Tomato Ketchup USDA
Nature's Promise (Giant)
Organic Ketchup
Nature's Promise (Stop & Shop)
Organic Ketchup
O Organics ⌀
Tomato Ketchup
Organicville
Organic Ketchup ♀ ✓
Our Family
Ketchup

Publix
Ketchup
Red Gold
Tomato Products (All)
Robbie's Sauces
Ketchup
Schnucks
Ketchup
Shaw's
Bottled Catsup
Inverted Ketchup
Ketchup Squeeze Bottle
Tomato Ketchup
Shoppers Value (ACME)
Squeeze Tomato Ketchup
Shoppers Value (Albertsons)
Squeeze Ketchup
Shoppers Value (Cub Foods)
Squeeze Tomato Ketchup
Shoppers Value (Jewel-Osco)
Squeeze Tomato Ketchup
Stokes Sauces
Bloody Mary Tomato Ketchup
Chilli Ketchup
Tomato Ketchup
Stop & Shop
Tomato Ketchup
Tiptree
Tiptree (All)
Trader Joe's
Organic Ketchup
Trinity Hill Farms
Gourmet Ketchup
Valu Time (Brookshire)
Ketchup
Valu Time (Marsh)
Ketchup
Valu Time (Schnucks)
Ketchup
Vita Foods ⓘ
Jim Beam Original Ketchup
Vons ⌀
Squeeze Ketchup
Walden Farms ♀
Walden Farms (All)
Wegmans
Tomato Ketchup

Whole Earth
Organic Tomato Ketchup
Winn-Dixie
Ketchup

Maraschino Cherries

ACME
Maraschino Cherries
Maraschino Cherries With Stems
Albertsons
Maraschino Cherries
Maraschino Cherries Pitted
Maraschino Cherries Stem
Always Save (Price Chopper)
Maraschino Cherries
Cub Foods
Maraschino Red Cherries
Flavorite (Cub Foods)
Maraschino Cherries
Food Club (Brookshire)
Maraschino Green Cherries
Maraschino Red Cherries
Red Maraschino Cherries with Stems
Giant
Maraschino Cherries
Great Value (Wal-Mart) 25
Maraschino Cherries
Haggen
Maraschino Cherry (Plain, with Stem)
Hy-Vee
Red Maraschino Cherries
Red Maraschino Cherries with Stems
Jewel-Osco
Maraschino Cherries
Meijer
Maraschino Cherry, Red
Maraschino Cherry, Red with Stem
Midwest Country Fare (Hy-Vee)
Maraschino Cherries
Our Family
Maraschino Cherries
Maraschino Cherries with Stems
Maraschino Cherries, Green
Salad Cherries
Price Chopper
Cherries with Stems

Maraschino Cherries
Publix
Maraschino Cherries
Schnucks Select
Maraschino Cherries (Red, with Stem)
Shaw's
Maraschino Cherries
Stop & Shop
Maraschino Cherries with Stems
Thrifty Maid (Winn-Dixie)
Maraschino Cherries
Valu Time (Schnucks)
Maraschino Cherries
Vons 🖑
Maraschino Cherries
Maraschino Cherries with Stems
Wegmans
Jumbo Maraschino Cherries - Without Stems
Maraschino Cherries - With Stems
Maraschino Cherries - Without Stems
Winn-Dixie
Maraschino Cherries

Marinades & Cooking Sauces

Best Choice
59 A-P Sauce
Boar's Head
Condiments (All)
Bragg
Bragg (All)
Cains
Franklin Italian Marinade
Cajun Injector ⓘ
Barbeque Mesquite
Creole Butter
Creole Garlic and Herb
Hickory BBQ
Honey Bacon BBQ
Hot N' Spicy Butter
Jalapeno Butter
Lemon Butter Garlic
Roasted Garlic
Turkey Supreme
Cat Cora's Kitchen
Corfu Sauce

Cretan Sauce
Cyprus Sauce
Santorini Sauce
Central Market (H-E-B)
All Natural Island Habanero Marinade
All Natural Remoulade Marinade
**Central Market Classics
(Price Chopper)**
Burgundy Cooking Wine
Sherry Cooking Wine
Chun's ()
Sweet Chili Marinade
Coconut Secret ⓘ
Coconut Aminos Soy-Free Seasoning
  Sauce
Concord Foods
Lemon Juice
Lime Juice
Contadina ⓘ
Sweet & Sour Sauce
Cugino's ()
Authentic Italian Marinade
Lemon Mediterranean Marinade
Culinary Circle (Cub Foods)
Marinara Sauce
Fischer & Wieser ⓘ
¡Especial! Pasilla de Oaxaca
All Purpose Vegetable & Meat Marinade
Charred Pineapple Bourbon Sauce
Plum Chipotle Grilling Sauce
Sweet & Savory Onion Glaze
Traditional Steak & Grilling Sauce
Food Club (Brookshire)
Garlic & Herb Marinade
Lemon Juice
Lemon Pepper Marinade
Lime Juice
Mesquite Marinade
Food Club (Marsh)
Lemon Juice
Lemon Juice Squeeze Bottle
Lime Juice Squeeze Bottle
Gaea ()
Cooking Sauces (All)
Gia
Anchovy Paste
Black Olive Paste

Garlic Paste
Green Pesto Paste
Sun Dried Tomato Pesto Paste
Gifts of Nature ✓
Cranberry Chipotle Sauce
Ginger People, The ()
Ginger Lemon Grass Sauce
Golding Farms ⓘ
Chipotle Ranch Sauce
Goodness Gardens
World Sauces (All)
Goya
Chipotle Mojo
Cooking Wine, Red
Cooking Wine, White
Edmundo Cooking Wine
La Vina Cooking Wine
Lemon Juice
Mojo Criollo
Naranja Agria
Hawkshead Relish
Savory Sauces (All)
H-E-B
Beef Stew Mix
Sloppy Joe Mix
Hill Country Fare (H-E-B)
Herb & Garlic Marinade
Lemon Pepper Marinade
Mesquite Lime Marinade
Holland House
Cooking Wines
Howard's
Howard's (All)
Hy-Vee
Citrus Grill Marinade
Herb & Garlic Marinade
Lemon Pepper Marinade
Mesquite Marinade
J&D's
Bacon Ranch
Jack Daniel's Sauces
EZ Marinader Garlic & Herb
EZ Marinader Steakhouse
Jardine's ⓘ
Buckin' Berry Raspberry Chipotle Sauce
Pineapple Chipotle Sauce

Johnny's Fine Foods ⓘ
Jamaica Me Sweet Hot & Crazy
Dressing/Marinade
Jamaica Mistake Dressing/Marinade
Jamaica Mistake Lite Dressing/Marinade
Salmon Finishing Sauce

K.C. Masterpiece
K.C. Masterpiece (All BUT Honey
Teriyaki with Sesame, Spiced
Caribbean Jerk)

Ken's Steak House Salad Dressing ⓘ
Herb & Garlic Marinade

Kikkoman
Gluten Free Teriyaki Marinade and
Sauce
Tikka Masala Curry Sauce ⟨⟩

Kitchen Bouquet
Kitchen Bouquet

Lea & Perrins
White Wine Marinade

Marukan
Ponzu Natural Citrus Marinade (NOT
Ponzu Soy Dressing)

Maya Kaimal ⓘ
Butter Masala Sauce
Classic Korma Refrigerated Sauce
Coconut Curry Refrigerated Sauce
Kashmiri Curry Sauce
Madras Curry Sauce
Spicy Ketchup
Tamarind Curry Refrigerated Sauce
Tikka Masala Sauce
Tikki Masala Refrigerated Sauce
Vindaloo Refrigerated Sauce

Meijer
Garlic & Herb Marinade
Lemon Pepper Marinade
Mesquite Marinade

Moore's
Original Marinade
Teriyaki Marinade

Mother's Mountain
Atantic Maine Marinade
Cajun Maine Marinade
Dijon Dill Maine Marinade
Original Maine Marinade

Nando's Peri-Peri
Curry Coconut Cooking Sauce
Fresh Lemon Cooking Sauce
Lime and Cilantro Marinade
Roasted Reds Cooking Sauce
Sundried Tomato and Basil Marinade
Sweet Apricot Cooking Sauce
Zesty Barbeque Marinade

Napa Valley Naturals ⟨⟩
Cooking Wines (All)

Ojai Cook, The
Bite Back Marinade
Carne Asada Marinade
Chipotle Marinade
Sesame Ginger Teriyaki with Sugar

Olde Cape Cod
Caribbean Marinade
Chipotle Grilling Sauce
Honey Orange Grilling Sauce
Lemon & Pepper Marinade
Lemon Ginger Grilling Sauce
Steakhouse Marinade
Sweet & Bold Grilling Sauce

Our Family
Lemon Juice

Polynesian Sauces
Chicken Nugget Sauce
Ham Glaze

Pompeian
Cooking Wines (All)

Price Chopper
BBQ Marinade
Beef Marinade
Chicken BBQ Marinade
Italian Supreme Marinade
Lemon Garlic Marinade
Lemon Juice
Pork Marinade
Southwest Grill Marinade
Southwest Smokin Hot Marinade
Spiedie Marinade
Wine Vinegar

Really Great Food ⛏
Really Great Food (All)

Regina ⓘ
Cooking Wines (All)

Sauce Goddess ✓
- Big & Tangy Sauce
- Sticky Sweet Grill Glaze
- Sweet & Spicy Grill Glaze
- Sweet Red Devil Sauce

Saucy Susan
- Ham Glaze
- Peach Apricot, Original
- Peach Apricot, Spicy

Sauer's ()
- Chipotle Pepper Marinade
- Mesquite Marinade
- Peppercorn & Garlic Marinade
- Zesty Herb Marinade

Schnucks
- Lemon Juice

Schnucks Select
- Lemon Dill Marinade
- Original Marinade
- Rosemary Thyme Marinade

Seeds of Change ⓘ
- Jalfrezi Simmer Sauce
- Korma Simmer Sauce
- Madras Simmer Sauce
- Tikka Masala Simmer Sauce

Soy Vay
- Toasted Sesame Dressing and Marinade

Squeez-Eez
- Lemon Juice
- Lime Juice

Stubb's
- Beef Marinade
- Burger Rub
- Chicken Marinade
- Pork Marinade
- Texas Steakhouse Marinade

Sun Luck
- Teriyaki Marinade

Tasty Bite ⓘ
- Good Korma Simmer Sauce
- Pad Thai Simmer Sauce
- Rogan Josh Simmer Sauce
- Satay Partay Simmer Sauce
- Tikka Masala Simmer Sauce

Tiptree
- Cumberland Sauce
- Hot Mango Sauce
- Tiptree Brown Sauce

Trader Joe's
- Organic Tomato Basil Marinara

Trinity Hill Farms
- Sweet Chili Sauce and Marinade
- Teriyaki Sauce and Marinade

TryMe
- Cajun Sunshine
- Tennessee Sunshine
- Tiger Sauce

Vita Foods ⓘ
- 7-Up Marinade
- Biltmore Apple Rosemary Marinade
- Dr. Pepper Marinade
- Jim Beam Original Wing Sauce
- Jim Beam Wing Sauce
- Sauza Cilantro Lime Marinade

Weber
- Black Peppercorn Marinade
- Chipotle Marinade
- Italian Herb Marinade
- Tequila Lime Marinade
- White Wine and Herb Marinade

Wegmans
- Chicken BBQ Marinade
- Citrus Dill Marinade
- Fajita Marinade
- Greek Marinade
- Honey Mustard Marinade
- Lemon & Garlic Marinade
- Mojo Marinade
- Rosemary Balsamic Marinade
- Santa Fe Marinade
- Spiedie Marinade
- Steakhouse Peppercorn Marinade
- Tangy Marinade
- Zesty Savory Marinade
- Zesty Thai Marinade

Wild Thymes ⓘ
- Chili Ginger Honey Marinade
- New Orleans Creole Marinade
- Tropical Mango Lime Marinade

Woeber ⓘ
- Reconstituted Lemon Juice

World Harbors
- Fajita Marinade
- Honey Dijon Marinade

Island Mango Marinade
Italian Grill Marinade
Lemon Pepper Marinade
Mojo Marinade
Steakhouse Marinade
Thai Marinade

Mayonnaise

Always Save
Salad Dressing
Sandwich Spread
Best Choice
Light Mayo, Jar
Light Mayo, Squeeze
Best Foods
Mayonnaise Products (All)
Best Maid/Del-Dixi
Best Maid (All)
Blue Plate
Low Fat Mayonnaise
Mayonnaise
Sandwich Spread
Sugar Free Mayonnaise
Cains
All-Natural Mayonnaise
Fat Free Mayonnaise
Kitchen Recipe Mayonnaise
Light Mayonnaise
Cub Foods
Mayonnaise
Dietz & Watson ✓
Mixed Pepper Mayo
Smoky Chipotle Mayo
Sweet Red Pepper Mayo
Duke's ()
Cholesterol Free Mayonnaise
Light Mayonnaise
Mayonnaise
Earth Balance
Earth Balance (All)
Flavorite (Albertsons)
Mayonnaise
Follow Your Heart
Grapeseed Vegenaise
Organic Vegenaise
Original Vegenaise

Reduced Fat Vegenaise
Soy-Free Vegenaise
Food Club (Brookshire)
Mayonnaise
Food Club (Marsh)
Mayonnaise
Mayonnaise, Light
Giant
Light Mayonnaise
Real Mayonnaise
Goya
Mayonnaise
Mayonnaise with Lime
GranoVita
Mayola! Egg Free Mayonnaise - Garlic
Mayola! Egg Free Mayonnaise - Lemon
Mayola! Egg Free Mayonnaise - Original
Haggen
Lite Mayonnaise
Mayonnaise
Hellmann's
Mayonnaise Products (All)
Hill Country Fare (H-E-B)
Mayonnaise
J&D's
Baconnaise ()
Lite Baconnaise ()
JFG Mayonnaise
Mayonnaise
Reduced Fat Mayonnaise
Sandwich Spread
Squeeze Mayonnaise
Kraft Mayonnaise ∾
Mayonnaise, Fat Free
Mayonnaise, Light
Mayonnaise, Light Mayo
Mayonnaise, Real Mayo
Mayonnaise, Sandwich Shop Chipotle
Mayonnaise, Sandwich Shop Garlic & Herb
Mayonnaise, Sandwich Shop Horseradish-Dijon
Mayonnaise, Sandwich Shop Hot & Spicy
Mayonnaise, with Olive Oil
La Costena
Mayonnaise with Lime Juice

Meijer
  Mayonnaise
  Mayonnaise Light
Miracle Whip ⟲
  Dressing, Fat Free
  Dressing, Light
  Dressing, Original
Miso Mayo ✓
  Miso Mayo- Garlic 'N' Dill
  Miso Mayo- Original
  Miso Mayo- Spicy Red Peppers
Mrs. Filbert's
  Mrs. Filbert's Real Mayonnaise
Naturally Delicious
  Mayonnaise
Ojai Cook, The
  Chipotle Lemonaise
  Fire & Spice Lemonaise
  Garlic Herb Lemonaise
  Green Dragon Lemonaise
  Latin Lemonaise
  Light Lemonaise
  Original Lemonaise
Olde Cape Cod
  Mayonnaise
Organicville
  Non Dairy Organic Mayo � ✓
Price Chopper
  Mayonnaise
Pulmuone Wildwood ☘
  Aioli
Safeway ⟲
  Squeeze Mayonnaise
Smart Balance
  Smart Balance (All)
Stokes Sauces
  Mayonnaise (All)
  Squeezy Mayonnaise
Stop & Shop
  Real Mayonnaise
Trader Joe's
  Mayonnaise (Real, Reduced Fat,
    Organic)
Valu Time (Brookshire)
  Mayonnaise
Valu Time (Marsh)
  Mayonnaise

Vegenaise
  Grapeseed
  Organic
  Original
  Reduced Fat
  Soy-Free
Walden Farms ☘
  Walden Farms (All)
Wegmans
  Classic Mayonnaise
  Light Mayonnaise
  Mayonnaise

MEXICAN, MISC.

Calavo
  Guacamole (All)
Casa Fiesta ⓘ
  Enchilada Sauce
  Enchilada Sauce (Hot, Mild)
  Habanero Sauce
Food Club (Brookshire)
  Green Enchilada Sauce
  Red Enchilada Sauce
Hill Country Fare (H-E-B)
  Carne Guisada Sauce
  Enchilada Sauce, Hot
  Enchilada Sauce, Medium
  Enchilada Sauce, Mild
Hy-Vee
  Diced Green Chilies
  Mild Diced Tomatoes & Green Chilies
  Mild Enchilada Sauce
  Original Diced Tomatoes & Green
    Chilies
  Sliced Hot Jalapenos
  Spanish Rice Mexican Style
  Taco Mix
  Whole Green Chilies
La Victoria
  Green Enchilada Sauce - Mild
  Red Chili Sauce
  Red Enchilada Sauce - Hot
  Red Enchilada Sauce - Mild
Las Palmas ⓘ
  Red Chile Sauce
  Red Enchilada Sauce

Meijer
Taco Seasoning
Our Family
Red Enchilada Sauce, Mild
Stop & Shop
Chili Sauce
Trader Joe's
Guacamole (All)
Guacamole with Spicy Pico de Gallo
Tropical Cheese
Uno Dos Tres Individual
Vita Foods ⓘ
Scorned Woman Chipotle & Garlic
Pepper Sauce
Vons ⌁
Fajita Seasoning Mix

MUSTARD

Always Save
Squeeze Mustard
Annie's Naturals
Organic Dijon Mustard
Organic Honey Mustard
Organic Yellow Mustard
Beano's ⓘ
Bold & Tangy Deli Mustard
Honey Mustard
Bertman's Mustard
Bertman's Mustard (All)
Best Choice
Brown Mustard
Mustard
Salad Mustard
Squeeze Honey Mustard
Squeeze Horseradish Mustard
Squeeze Mustard
Best Foods
Mustard Products (All)
Best Maid/Del-Dixi
Best Maid (All)
Boar's Head
Condiments (All)
Bone Suckin' Sauce
Bone Suckin' Mustard (All)

Central Market Classics (Price Chopper)
Country Dijon Mustard
Cranberry Honey Mustard
Dijon Mustard
Honey Mustard
Horseradish Mustard
Southwestern Mustard
Wasabi Mustard
Whole Grain Dijon
Di Lusso
Chipotle Mustard
Cranberry Honey Mustard
Deli Style Mustard
Dijon Mustard
Honey Mustard
Jalapeno Mustard
Dietz & Watson ✓
Champagne Dill Mustard
Chipotle Mustard
Cranberry Honey Mustard
Jalapeno Mustard
Spicy Brown Mustard
Sweet and Hot Mustard
Wasabi Mustard
Whole Grain Dijon Mustard
Yellow Mustard
Dr. Gonzo's Uncommon Condiments
Moose River Adirondack Blackfly
Mustard
XX Mustard Plaster XX
Eden Foods
Organic Brown Mustard
Organic Yellow Mustard
EMERIL'S ⚱
Mustard (Smooth Honey, Dijon, Kicked
Up Horseradish, NY Deli Style,
Yellow)
Fischer & Wieser ⓘ
Smokey Mesquite Mustard
Sweet Heat Mustard
Sweet, Sour & Smokey Mustard Sauce
Food Club (Brookshire)
Dijon Mustard
Honey Mustard
Salad Mustard
Spicy Brown Mustard

Food Club (Marsh)
Dijon Mustard
Honey Mustard
Mustard Salad
Spicy Brown Mustard

Food You Feel Good About (Wegmans)
Spicy Brown Mustard

French's
Honey Mustard Sauce
Prepared Mustards (All)

Full Circle (Price Chopper)
Yellow Mustard

Full Circle (Schnucks)
Spicy Brown Mustard
Yellow Mustard

Giant
Dijon Mustard
Original Yellow Mustard
Spicy Brown Mustard

Golding Farms ⓘ
Dijon Gourmet Mustard
Honey Dijon Mustard
Honey Mustard
Horseradish Gourmet Mustard
Three Pepper Mustard

Great Value (Wal-Mart) 25
Course Ground Mustard
Honey Mustard
Prepared Dijon Mustard
Prepared Mustard
Southwest Spicy Sweet, Hot Mustard
Spicy Brown Mustard
Squeeze Prepared Mustard

GreenWise Market (Publix)
Organic Creamy Yellow Mustard
Organic Spicy Brown Mustard
Organic Tangy Dijon

Grey Poupon 〰
Mustard, Country Dijon
Mustard, Deli
Mustard, Dijon
Mustard, Harvest Coarse Ground
Mustard, Hearty Spicy Brown
Mustard, Honey
Mustard, Savory Honey
Mustard, Spicy Brown

Griffin Foods
Griffin Foods (All)

Haggen
Mustard
Mustard, Dijon
Mustard, Spicy Brown

Hawkshead Relish
Mustards (All)

H-E-B
Dijon Mustard

Heinz
Mustard (All Varieties)

Hellmann's
Mustard Products (All)

Hill Country Fare (H-E-B)
Honey Mustard
Spicy Brown Mustard
Yellow Mustard

Honey Acres
Honey Mustards (All)

Hy-Vee
Dijon Mustard
Honey Mustard
Mustard
Spicy Brown Mustard

Jardine's ⓘ
Bronco Mustard

Koops'
Mustards (All)

Meijer
Dijon Mustard (Squeeze Bottle)
Honey Mustard (Squeeze Bottle)
Horseradish Mustard (Squeeze Bottle)
Hot N' Spicy Brown Mustard (Squeeze Bottle)
Salad Mustard
Salad Mustard (Squeeze Bottle)
Spicy Brown Mustard

Meijer Gold
Bavarian Mustard
Blueberry Honey Mustard
Champagne Dill Mustard
Cherry Honey Mustard
Zesty Whole Grain Mustard

Meijer Organics
Dijon Mustard
Mustard

Spicy Brown Mustard (Meijer Organic)

Midwest Country Fare (Hy-Vee)
Yellow Mustard

Morehouse
Mustard Products (All)

Mother's Mountain
Classic Honey Mustard
Peppercorn Dijon Mustard
Portland Beer Mustard
Spiced Apple Mustard
Zesty Honey Mustard

O Organics 〰
Dijon Mustard
Yellow Mustard

Olde Cape Cod
Mustards

Organicville
Mustard (Dijon, Stone Ground, Yellow)
🏅 ✔

Our Family
Dijon Mustard
Honey Mustard
Horseradish Mustard
Spicy Brown Mustard
Squeeze Mustard

Price Chopper
Brown Mustard
Dijon Mustard
Honey Mustard
Mustard
Organic Spicy Mustard
Organic Yellow Mustard

Publix
Classic Yellow Mustard
Deli Style Mustard
Dijon Mustard
Honey Mustard
Spicy Brown Mustard

Raye's Mustard
Raye's Mustard (All BUT Beer
Mustards)

Really Great Food 🏅
Really Great Food (All)

Saag's ⓘ
Saag's (All)

Safeway 〰
Coarse Ground Dijon Mustard

Honey Mustard

Safeway Select 〰
Stoneground Mustard with Horseradish

Schnucks
Honey Mustard
Horseradish Mustard
Mustard
Spicy Brown Mustard
Yellow Mustard

Schnucks Select
Chipotle Mustard
Dijon Mustard
Sweet 'N Hot Mustard
Whole Grain Garlic Mustard

Spence & Co. Ltd.
Mustard Dill Sauce

Stokes Sauces
Mustard and Dill Sauce
Mustards (All)

Trader Joe's
Mustard (Dijon, Whole Grain or
Organic Yellow)

True Natural Taste
True Natural Taste (All)

Valu Time (Brookshire)
Salad Mustard

Valu Time (Marsh)
Salad Mustard

Vita Foods ⓘ
Jim Beam Original Mustard

Vons 〰
Mustard
Spicy Deli Mustard
Squeeze Mustard

Wegmans
Classic Yellow Mustard
Dijon Traditional Mustard
Dijon Whole Grain Mustard
Honey Mustard
Horseradish Mustard
Mustard Sauce
Yellow Mustard

Wellshire Farms
Organic Dill Mustard
Organic Horseradish Mustard

Wild Harvest (Albertsons)
Organic Creamy Peanut Butter

Winn-Dixie
- Dijon Mustard
- Honey Mustard
- Horseradish Mustard
- Spicy Brown Mustard
- Yellow Mustard

Woeber ⓘ
- Dijon Mustard
- Dusseldorf Mustard
- Organic Deli Mustard
- Organic Spicy Brown Mustard
- Organic Yellow Mustard
- Reserve Champagne Dill Mustard
- Reserve Cranberry Honey Mustard
- Reserve Honey Mustard
- Reserve Southwest Mustard
- Reserve Whole Grain Dijon Mustard
- Sandwich Pal Horseradish Mustard
- Sandwich Pal Hot & Spicy Mustard
- Sandwich Pal Jalapeno Mustard
- Sandwich Pal Sweet & Spicy Mustard
- Spicy Brown Mustard
- Supreme Honey Mustard
- Wasabi Mustard
- Yellow Salad Style Mustard

NUT BUTTERS

Algood
- Peanut Butter (All)

Always Save
- Peanut Butter, Creamy
- Peanut Butter, Crunchy

Arrowhead Mills
- Creamy Almond Butter
- Creamy Cashew Butter
- Creamy Valencia Peanut Butter
- Crunchy Valencia Peanut Butter
- Organic Creamy Valencia Peanut Butter
- Organic Crunchy Valencia Peanut Butter
- Organic Sesame Tahini

Artisana 🍴
- Artisana Organic Nut Butters (All)
- Sattva Organic Nut/Seed Butters (All)

Barney Butter
- Almond Butter (All)

Best Choice
- Creamy Peanut Butter
- Crunchy Peanut Butter

Blue Diamond Growers 🍴
- Homestyle Almond Butter (Creamy, Crunchy, Honey)
- Ready Spread Almond Butter (Creamy, Crunchy, Honey)

Central Market (H-E-B)
- All Natural Cashew Butter
- All Natural Peanut Butter Crunchy
- All Natural Peanut Butter Smooth
- Peanut Butter With Honey

Clearly Organic (Best Choice)
- Creamy Peanut Butter
- Crunchy Peanut Butter

Cub Foods
- Chunky Peanut Butter
- Creamy Peanut Butter

Earth Balance
- Earth Balance (All)

East Wind Nut Butters
- Almond Butter
- Cashew Butter
- Peanut Butter

Eden Nuts
- Eden Nuts (All)

Fastco (Fareway)
- Peanut Butter (Creamy, Crunchy)

Fisher Nuts ()
- Peanut Butter, Chunky
- Peanut Butter, Creamy

Food Club (Brookshire)
- Apple Butter
- Peanut Butter, Creamy
- Peanut Butter, Crunchy

Food Club (Marsh)
- Peanut Butter, Creamy
- Peanut Butter, Crunchy

Food You Feel Good About (Wegmans)
- Natural Peanut Butter, Creamy
- Natural Peanut Butter, Crunchy
- Organic Creamy Peanut Butter, No Stir
- Organic Crunchy Peanut Butter, No Stir

Full Circle (Price Chopper)
- Almond Butter

Cashew Butter
Creamy Peanut Butter
Sunflower Butter Crunch

Full Circle (Schnucks)
Almond Butter Spread
Creamy Peanut Butter
No Sugar Creamy Peanut Butter
Sunflower Butter

Giant
Creamy All Natural Peanut Butter
Creamy Peanut Butter
Crunchy Peanut Butter

Great Value (Wal-Mart) 25
Creamy Peanut Butter
Crunchy Peanut Butter
Peanut Free Smooth Soy Butter

Hill Country Fare (H-E-B)
Creamy Peanut Butter
Crunchy Peanut Butter
Smooth Peanut Butter

Hy-Vee
Creamy Peanut Butter
Crunchy Peanut Butter
Reduced Fat Creamy Peanut Butter

I.M. Healthy
SoyNut Butter (All)

Justin's
Justin's (All)

Koeze
Peanut Butter (All Varieties)

Kroger
Hazelnut Spread
Honey Roasted Peanut Butter, Creamy
Honey Roasted Peanut Butter, Crunchy
Peanut Butter
Peanut Butter, Crunchy
Peanut Butter, Reduced Fat Creamy
Super Crunchy Peanut Butter

Maisie Jane's
Almond Butter

Maple Grove Farms
Peanut Butter (All Varieties)

Meijer
Peanut Butter (Creamy, Crunchy)
Peanut Butter and Jelly
Peanut Butter, Reduced Fat Creamy
Peanut Butter, Reduced Salt Creamy

Meijer Naturals
Peanut Butter (Creamy, Crunchy)

Meijer Organics
Peanut Butter, Organic (Creamy, Crunchy)

Midwest Country Fare (Hy-Vee)
Creamy Peanut Butter
Crunchy Peanut Butter

Naturally Nutty
Naturally Nutty (All)

Nature's Basket (Giant Eagle)
Organic Creamy Peanut Butter (Nutco)
Organic Creamy Peanut Butter, No Salt
Organic Crunchy Peanut Butter (Nutco)

Nature's Promise (Giant)
Organic Almond Butter
Organic Crunchy Peanut Butter
Organic Sodium Free Peanut Butter

Nature's Promise (Stop & Shop)
Organic Almond Butter
Organic Sodium Free Peanut Butter

Nutella
Nutella Hazelnut Spread

O Organics
Old Fashioned Creamy Peanut Butter
Old Fashioned Crunchy Peanut Butter
Organic Crunchy Peanut Butter

Peanut Butter & Co
Peanut Butters (All)

Peter Pan
Peanut Butter (All Varieties)

Price Chopper
Chunky Peanut Butter
Creamy Peanut Butter
Organic Creamy Peanut Butter
Sunflower Butter Crunch

Publix
Fresh Ground Peanut Butter

Richfood (Cub Foods)
Creamy Peanut Butter

Safeway
Reduced Fat Chunky Peanut Butter
Reduced Fat Creamy Peanut Butter

Schnucks
Peanut Butter (Chunky, Creamy)

Simple Food
Organic Soynut Butter (All Flavors)

Smart Balance
Smart Balance (All)

Stop & Shop
Chunky Peanut Butter
Creamy Peanut Butter

SunButter
Sunflower Seed Spreads (All)

Teddie
Teddie (All)

Trader Joe's
Nut Butters (All)
Sunflower Seed Butter

Valu Time (Brookshire)
Peanut Butter- Creamy
Peanut Butter- Crunchy

Valu Time (Marsh)
Peanut Butter, Creamy
Peanut Butter, Crunchy

Valu Time (Schnucks)
Chunky Peanut Butter
Smooth Peanut Butter

Vons ✍
Chunky Peanut Butter
Creamy Peanut Butter
Reduced Fat Chunky Peanut Butter
Reduced Fat Creamy Peanut Butter

Walden Farms ⛲
Walden Farms (All)

Wegmans
Creamy Peanut Butter
Creamy Peanut Spread (Reduced Fat)
Crunchy Peanut Butter
Organic Natural Creamy Peanut Butter,
with Peanut Skins
Organic Natural Crunchy Peanut Butter,
with Peanut Skins

Whole Earth
Organic Crunchy Peanut Butter
Organic Smooth Peanut Butter
Original Crunchy Peanut Butter
Original Smooth Peanut Butter

Wild Harvest (ACME)
Creamy Organic Peanut Butter
Crunchy Organic Peanut Butter
Natural Creamy Peanut Butter

Wild Harvest (Albertsons)
Organic Crunchy Peanut Butter

Wild Harvest (Cub Foods)
Natural Creamy Peanut Butter
Organic Creamy Peanut Butter

Wild Harvest (Jewel-Osco)
Natural Creamy Peanut Butter
Organic Creamy Peanut Butter
Organic Crunchy Peanut Butter

Wilderness Poets
Wilderness Poets (All)

OLIVES

Albertsons
Manzanilla Stuffed Spanish Olives
Stuffed Queen Spanish Olives

Always Save
Broken Pitted Olives
Salad Olives
Stuffed Manzanilla Olives

B&G Foods ⓘ
Black Olives
Green Olives

Bell View
Bell View (All)

Bell-Carter
Olives (All)

Best Choice
Placed Stuffed Manzanilla Olives
Ripe Jumbo Olives
Ripe Large Olives
Ripe Medium Olives
Ripe Olive Slices
Ripe Olives, Chopped
Ripe Small Olives
Sliced Salad Olives
Stuffed Manzanilla Olives
Stuffed Queen Olives
Tossed Manzanilla Olives
Tossed Queen Olives

Cat Cora's Kitchen
Garlic Stuffed Olives
Kalamata Olives
Natural Pimento Stuffed Olives
Olympian Pitted Olives
Organic Kalamata Olives
Organic Mixed Olives
Organic Olympian Olives

Organic Pitted Kalamata Olives
Pitted Green Olives with Oregano & Lemon Snack Pack
Pitted Kalamata Olives
Pitted Kalamata Olives Snack Pack
Sundried Olives Snack Pack
Whole Kalamata Olives Snack Pack

Central Market Classics (Price Chopper)

Pitted Queen Olives
Stuffed Blue Cheese Olives
Stuffed Garlic Olives
Stuffed Jalapeno Olives

DeLallo

Alexandros Olives
Almond Stuffed Olives
Arbequina Olives
Black Bella Di Cerignola Olives
Black Greek Olives in Brine
Black Greek Olives, Mammoth in Brine
Black Greek Olives, Seasoned
Black Greek Olives, Seasoned in Oil
Black Greek Pitted Olives
Black Olives, Sliced
Calabrese Olives in Brine
Calabrese Olives, Super Colossal
Calamata Olives, Colossal in Brine
Calamata Olives, Colossal in Oil
Calamata Olives, Garlic Stuffed
Calamata Olives, Jumbo Pitted in Brine
Calamata Olives, Piccante Pitted
Calamata Olives, Pitted X-Large
Calamata Olives, X-Jumbo
California Mix
Castelvetrano Olives
European Style Party Mix
French Moroccan Nicoise Olives
French Moroccan Picholine Olives
French Style Party Medley
Fresh Garlic Stuffed Olives
Gaeta Black Olives
Garlic & Jalapeno Stuffed Olives
Garlic Stuffed Olives
Greek Green Olives, Pitted (with Garlic, with Hot Peppers)
Greek Olives, Super Colossal Black

Green & Black Bella Di Cerignola Salad with Garlic
Green Greek Cut Freestone
Green Naflion Olives
Green Olives Stuffed with Blue Cheese in Oil
Green Olives Stuffed with Feta
Green Olives, Aglio Pitted in Oil
Green Olives, Bella Di Cerignola in Oil
Green Olives, Colossal Pitted in Brine
Green Olives, Piccante in Oil
Green Olives, Piccante Pitted
Green Olives, Super Supreme Whole
Green Olives, Super Supreme Whole in Brine
Halkidiki Olives, Super Mammoth
Hot Pitted Olive Salad
Italian Aglio Green Pitted Olives
Italian Sun Dried Olives
Italian Vinegar Olives
Jalapeno Stuffed Olives
Maddelena Olives
Manzanilla Olives, Stuffed
Manzanilla Olives, Stuffed in Brine
Mediterranean Mix
Mixed Greek Olives, Marinated
Mixed Medley Salad
Nicoise Olives in Brine
Oil Cured Pitted Olives
Olive Medley in Brine
Olive Medley, Seasoned
Olives, Anchovy Stuffed
Olives, Garlic Stuffed in Brine
Olives, Gigante Pitted in Oil
Olives, Jalapeno Stuffed in Brine
Olives, Pitted (Colossal, Extra Large, Jumbo, Large, Medium)
Olives, Pitted Gigante
Olives, Roasted Garlic Stuffed
Olives, Seasoned Oil Cured
Organic Argentine Manzanilla Nero
Organic Argentine Manzanilla Olives
Organic Arrabbiata Olives, Hot
Organic Bella Di Cerignola in Brine
Organic Calamata Olives, Extra Large Pitted
Organic Calamata Olives, Jumbo

Organic Cordoba Mix
Organic Extra Large Pitted Calamata
   Olives in Oil
Organic Hot Arrabbiata in Oil
Organic Jumbo Calamata Cup (Brine)
Organic Olives Jubilee
Organic Olives, Garlic Seasoned
Organic Olives, Pitted Grande
Organic Peruvian Verde Olives
Organic Verde Grande Olives
Pepperazzi
Piccante Green Pitted Olives
Queen Olives, Stuffed
Queen Olives, Stuffed in Brine
San Remo Olives in Oil
Seasoned Jumbo Pitted Calamata Olives
Seasoned Olive Medley
Sicilian Green Cracked Olives in Brine
Sicilian Marinated Mix with Garlic
Sicilian Marinated Olive Mix without
   Garlic
Sicilian Olives, Cracked Jumbo in Brine
Sicilian Style Olives, Cracked Jumbo
Small Pitted Olives
Super Colossal Pitted Olives
Taggiasca Olives in Oil

Di Lusso
Green Ionian Olives
Mediterranean Mixed Olives

Early California ⚇
Olives (All)

Food Club (Brookshire)
Large Ripe Pitted Olives
Manzanilla Stuffed Olives, Thrown
Medium Ripe Pitted Olives
Queen Stuffed Olives, Thrown
Ripe Olives, Chopped
Ripped Buffet Sliced Olives
Salad Olives
Salad Olives with Minced Pimento
Sliced Ripe Olives
Small Ripe Pitted Olives

Food Club (Marsh)
Olives Manzanilla Stuffed Thrown
Olives Ripe Pitted Large
Olives Ripe Pitted Medium
Olives Ripe Sliced Buffet

Stuffed Thrown Queen Olives
Fragata
Olives (All)
Gaea ()
Olives (All)
Genuardi's ↝
Small Ripe Pitted Olives
Giant
Extra Large Ripe Pitted Olives
Large Pitted Olives
Olives Medley
Ripe Olives, Sliced
Salad Olives
Small Ripe Pitted Olives
Stuffed Placed Queen Olives
Stuffed Queen Olives
Stuffed Spanish Manzanilla Olives
Stuffed Thrown Manzanilla Olives
Goya
Aceituna Botija
Aceitunas Verde Rodajas
Alcaparrado
Alcaparrado with Pimientos
Black Olives (Pitted)
Black Olives (Small Ripe)
Jumbo Olives
Jumbo Salad Olives
Manzanilla Lisas Olives
Manzanilla Plain Olives
Manzanilla Rellenas Olives
Manzanilla Stuffed Olives
Olives Cocktail Pitted
Olives Stuffed with Anchovy
Olives Stuffed with Garlic
Olives Stuffed with Hot Pimientos
Olives Stuffed with Jalapeño
Olives Stuffed with Lemon
Olives Stuffed with Salmon
Olives Stuffed with Tuna
Perdigon Olives
Pitted Alcaparrado
Queen Stuffed Olives
Salad Olives
Tejocote/Manzanilla
Great Value (Wal-Mart) 25
Chopped Ripe Olives
Jumbo Pitted Ripe Olives

Large Pitted Ripe Olives
Medium Pitted Ripe Olives
Minced Pimento Stuffed Manzanilla
  Olives
Minced Pimento Stuffed Queen Olives
Sliced Ripe Olives
Sliced Salad Olives

Haggen
Olives, Chopped Ripe
Olives, Green (Sliced, Stuffed)
Olives, Green Salad
Olives, Jumbo
Olives, Ripe (Large, Medium, Sliced)
Olives, Spanish Queen
Olives, Stuffed Spanish
Sliced Ripe Olives

Hy-Vee
Manzanilla Olives
Queen Olives
Ripe Olives (Chopped, Large Pitted,
  Medium Pitted, Sliced)
Sliced Salad Olives

Jardine's ⓘ
Texas Caviar Olives
Texas Martini Olives

Lindsay Olives
Olives (All)

Mario
Mario (All)

Meijer
Jumbo Ripe Pitted Olives
Large Ripe Olives
Medium Ripe Olives
Olives Manzanilla Stuffed, Tree
Olives Ripe
Olives Ripe, Pitted
Olives Ripe, Sliced
Olives Salad
Olives Salad, Sliced
Olives, Manzanilla Stuffed (Placed,
  Thrown)
Olives, Queen Stuffed Placed
Olives, Queen Whole Thrown

Mezzetta
Olives (All)

Midwest Country Fare (Hy-Vee)
Large Ripe Black Olives

Sliced Ripe Black Olives

Our Family
Chopped Black Olives
Garlic Stuffed Olives in Chardonnay &
  Herb Marinade
Jalapeno Stuffed Olives in Chardonnay
  & Herb Marinade
Manzanilla Spanish Olives Stuffed with
  Minced Pimentos
Pimento Stuffed Olives in Chardonnay
  & Herb Marinade
Pitted Kalamata Olives in Herb
  Marinade
Pitted Ripe Olives (Large, Jumbo,
  Medium, Small)
Salad Olives
Sliced Ripe Olives
Sliced Ripe Olives, Buffet Size
Stuffed Manzanilla Olives
Stuffed Manzanilla Olives, Thrown
Stuffed Queen Olives, Thrown

Pastene
Black Greek Olives
Gaeta Olives
Kalamata Olives
Kalamata Olives, Pitted
Manzanilla Olives, Stuffed
Olives, Extra Large Pitted
Olives, Oil Cured
Plain Olives, Stuffed
Queen Olives, Stuffed
Ripe Olives, Sliced
Salad Olives

Pearls ♘
Olives (All)

Peloponnese
Antipasto Party Olives
Country Gourmet Mixed
Country Olives
Cracked Green Olives
Cracked Olives
Greek Green (Stuffed)
Ionian Olives
Kalamata Olive Spread
Kalamata Olives

Pinnaroo Hill
Table Olives (All)

Price Chopper
Olive Stuffed Manzanilla Thrown
Olive Stuffed Queen Thrown
Salad Olives
Sliced Spanish Olives
Stuffed Manzanilla Olives
Stuffed Spanish Olives

Publix
Colossal Olives
Green Olives (All Sizes & Styles)
Large Olives
Ripe Olives
Small Olives

Safeway ⌇
Manzanilla Stuffed Olives
Queen Green Olives

Safeway Select ⌇
Queen Olives Stuffed with Garlic
Queen Olives Stuffed with Pimento

Santa Barbara Olive Co.
Santa Barbara Olive Co. (All)

Shotgun Willie's ⓘ
Jalapeno Stuffed Olives

Stop & Shop
Large Ripe Pitted Olives
Medium Ripe Pitted Olives
Sliced Ripe Olives
Small Ripe Pitted Olives
Spanish Manzanilla Olives
Spanish Queen Olives
Stuffed Spanish Manzanilla Olives

Tassos
Olives (All)

Trader Joe's
Colossal Olives Stuffed With Garlic
  Cloves
Colossal Olives Stuffed With Jalapeno
  Peppers
Green Olive Tapenade
Nonpareil Capers
Pitted Kalamata Olives
Stuffed Queen Sevillano Olives

Valu Time (Brookshire)
Jalapeno Stuffed Olives
Medium Broken Ripe Olives- Pitted
Stuffed Manzanilla Olives- Thrown

Valu Time (Marsh)
Salad Olives
Stuffed Olives

Vons ⌇
Colossal Ripe Olives
Extra Large Pitted Olives
Large Pitted Olives
Manzanilla Stuffed Olives
Medium Pitted Olives
Olives, Chopped
Olives, Sliced
Ripe Olives, Sliced

Wegmans
Colossal Ripe Olives - Pitted
Greek Mix Olives
Kalamata Olives - Pitted
Kalamata Olives - Whole
Manzanilla Olives - with Pimento
Medium Ripe Olives - Pitted
Olives - Stuffed with Almonds
Olives - Stuffed with Garlic
Olives - Stuffed with Red Peppers
Queen Stuffed Olives
Ripe Olives - Sliced
Salad Olives
Spanish Salad Olives - Sliced
X Large Ripe Olives

Winn-Dixie
Green Olives (All Varieties)
Ripe Olives (All Varieties)

PASTA & PIZZA SAUCE

Alpino
Spicy Pizza Topping

Amy's Kitchen ✓
Family Marinara Pasta Sauce
Light in Sodium Family Marinara Pasta
  Sauce
Light in Sodium Tomato Basil Pasta
  Sauce
Tomato Basil Pasta Sauce

Bea's Gourmet Sauces
Marinara Sauce
Roasted Garlic Sauce
Tomato Basil Sauce
Vodka Sauce

Best Choice
- Garlic and Herb Sauce
- Meat Spaghetti Sauce
- Mushroom Spaghetti Sauce
- Pizza Sauce
- Traditional Spaghetti Sauce
- Vegetable Spaghetti Sauce

Boboli
- Pizza Sauce

Bove's of Vermont ᵧ
- Sauces (All)

Casa Visco
- Casa Visco (All)

Central Market (H-E-B)
- Organic Garlic Lover's Pasta Sauce
- Organic Mushroom Pasta Sauce
- Organic Primavera Pasta Sauce
- Organic Tomato & Basil Pasta Sauce

Classico
- Alfredo Sauces (All)
- Bruschetta Toppings (All)
- Pesto Sauces (All)
- Red Sauces (All)

Colavita
- Sauce (All)

Contadina ⓘ
- Pizza Sauces (All)
- Pizza Squeeze

Cub Foods
- Traditional Spaghetti Sauce

Cugino's ⌀
- Classic Marinara

Culinary Circle (ACME)
- Italian Sausage Pasta Sauce
- Puttanesca Vegetable Pasta Sauce
- Tomato Florentine Pasta Sauce

Culinary Circle (Albertsons)
- Arrabbiata Pasta Sauce
- Italian Sausage Pasta Sauce
- Puttanesca Vegetable Pasta Sauce

Culinary Circle (Cub Foods)
- Italian Sausage Pasta Sauce
- Three Mushroom Pasta Sauce

Culinary Circle (Jewel-Osco)
- Arrabbiata Pasta Sauce
- Italian Sausage Pasta Sauce
- Marinara Sauce

- Puttanesca Vegetable Pasta Sauce
- Three Mushroom Pasta Sauce
- Tomato Florentine Pasta Sauce

Dave's Gourmet
- Dave's Gourmet (All)

Dei Fratelli ⓘ
- Dei Fratelli (All)

Del Monte ⓘ
- Tomatoes & Tomato Products (All BUT Spaghetti Sauce Flavored with Meat)

DeLallo
- Arrabbiata Sauce, Imported ⓘ
- Bruschetta Sauce, Imported ⓘ
- Fancy Pizza Sauce ⓘ
- Garlic, Oil, & Hot Pepper Sauce, Imported ⓘ
- Italian Pizza Sauce, Imported ⓘ
- Marinara Sauce, Fat Free ⓘ
- Marinara Sauce, Imported ⓘ
- Pesto Sauce in Olive Oil ⓘ
- Pink Vodka Sauce ⓘ
- Porcini Mushroom Sauce, Imported ⓘ
- Primavera Sauce, Imported ⓘ
- Puttanesca Sauce, Imported ⓘ
- Red Clam Sauce ⓘ
- Roasted Garlic Marinara Sauce ⓘ
- Roasted Garlic Sauce, Imported ⓘ
- Spaghetti Sauce with Meat ⓘ
- Spaghetti Sauce with Mushrooms ⓘ
- Sun Dried Tomato Pesto ⓘ
- Three Cheese Sauce, Imported ⓘ
- Tomato Basil Sauce ⓘ
- Tomato Basil Sauce, Imported ⓘ
- Traditional Spaghetti Sauce ⓘ
- White Clam Sauce ⓘ

Dell'Amore ᵧ
- Dell'Amore (All)

Dement's ᵧ
- Dement's (All)

Eden Foods
- Organic No Salt Added Spaghetti Sauce
- Organic Pizza Pasta Sauce
- Organic Spaghetti Sauce

EMERIL'S ᵧ
- Cacciatore Dinner Sauce
- Chunky Marinara Pasta Sauce
- Eggplant & Gaaahlic

Home Style Marinara Pasta Sauce
Italian Style Tomato & Basil
Kicked Up Tomato Pasta Sauce
Roasted Gaaahlic Pasta Sauce
Roasted Red Pepper Pasta Sauce
Sicilian Gravy Pasta Sauce
Three Cheeses
Vodka Pasta Sauce

Fastco (Fareway)
Marinara Spaghetti Sauce
Meat Spaghetti Sauce
Mushroom Spaghetti Sauce
Traditional Spaghetti Sauce

Food Club (Brookshire)
Extra Chunky Pepper Spaghetti Sauce
Garlic and Onions Spaghetti Sauce
Meat Flavor Pasta Sauce
Meat Spaghetti Sauce
Mushroom Pasta Sauce
Mushroom Spaghetti Sauce
Pizza Sauce
Plain Pasta Sauce
Spaghetti Sauce, Extra Chunky Garden
    Combo
Spaghetti Sauce, Four Cheese
Spaghetti Sauce, Garlic & Herb
Traditional Pasta Sauce
Traditional Spaghetti Sauce

Food Club (Marsh)
Pizza Sauce

Food You Feel Good About (Wegmans)
Chunky Pizza Sauce
Mushroom Spaghetti Sauce
Parmesan Romano Spaghetti Sauce
Smooth Marinara Spaghetti Sauce
Spaghetti Sauce Flavored with Meat
Tomato Basil Pasta Sauce

Francesco Rinaldi ⓘ
Garden Style Sauces (All)
Hearty Sauces (All)
Traditional Sauces (All)

Full Circle (Price Chopper)
Garlic Pasta Sauce
Parmesan Pasta Sauce
Pasta Sauce, Basil

Full Circle (Schnucks)
Parmesan Pasta Sauce
Portobello Mushroom Sauce
Roasted Garlic Sauce
Tomato Basil Sauce

Full Flavor Foods ✓
Sauce Mixes (All)

Furmano's ♨
Furmano's (All)

Gaea ◌
Pasta Sauce (All)

Giant
Thick and Rich Spaghetti Sauce with
    Meat
Thick and Rich Traditional Spaghetti
    Sauce

Giant Eagle
Chunky Garden Pasta Sauce
Meat Flavored Pasta Sauce
Mushroom Pasta Sauce
Onion and Garlic Pasta Sauce
Parmesan and Romano Pasta Sauce
Roasted Garlic Pasta Sauce
Savory Cheese Combo Sauce
Traditional Pasta Sauce
Traditional Pizza Sauce

Great Value (Wal-Mart) 25
Italian Garden Combination Chunky
    Pasta Sauce
Mushrooms & Green Peppers Spaghetti
    Sauce
Onions & Garlic Chunky Pasta Sauce
Pizza Sauce
Traditional Spaghetti Sauce

Hanover Foods
Spaghetti Sauce

Harvest Traditions ♨
All Natural Pasta Sauce (All)

H-E-B
Four Cheese Pasta Sauce
Garlic & Herb Pasta Sauce
Mushroom/ Onion Pasta Sauce
Puttanesca Pasta Sauce
Spicy Red Pepper Pasta Sauce
Spinach and Cheese Marinara
Tomato Basil Pasta Sauce
Vegetable Primavera Pasta Sauce

Hill Country Fare (H-E-B)
Four Cheese Pasta Sauce
Garden Medley Pasta Sauce
Meat Pasta Sauce
Mushroom Pasta Sauce
Parmesan & Romano Pasta Sauce
Sauteed Onion & Garlic Pasta Sauce
Tomato/Garlic/Onion Pasta Sauce
Traditional Pasta Sauce
Traditional Pasta Sauce with Meat
Traditional Pasta Sauce with Mushroom

Hy-Vee
3 Cheese Spaghetti Sauce
Garden Spaghetti Sauce
Mushroom Spaghetti Sauce
Pizza Sauce
Spaghetti Sauce with Meat
Traditional Spaghetti Sauce

Isola
Pasta Sauces (All)

Italian Classics (Schnucks)
Four Cheese Pasta Sauce
Puttanesca Sauce
Red Pepper Sauce
Tomato Basil Pasta Sauce

Italian Classics (Wegmans)
Alfredo Sauce
Arrabbiata Sauce
Bolognese Sauce
Bruschetta Topping, Artichoke Asiago
Bruschetta Topping, Roasted Red Pepper
Bruschetta Topping, Traditional Tomato
Diavolo Sauce
Grandma's Pomodoro Sauce
Italian Sausage & Roasted Pepper Sauce
Marinara Sauce
Mushroom Marsala Sauce
Portabello Mushroom Sauce
Puttanesca Sauce
Sunripened Dried Tomato Sauce
Vodka Sauce
White Clam Sauce

Kroger
Garlic and Herb Sauce
Marinara Sauce
Mushroom Sauce

Six Cheese Pasta Sauce
Traditional Pasta Sauce

Lucini Italia
Pasta and Pizza Sauces (All)

Luigi Giovanni
Luigi Giovanni (All)

Market District (Giant Eagle)
Arrabiatta
Marinara
Tomato Basil
Tomato Vodka

Meijer
3 Cheese Spaghetti Sauce, Extra Chunky
Four Cheese Pasta Sauce
Garden Combo Spaghetti Sauce, Extra Chunky
Garlic and Cheese Spaghetti Sauce, Extra Chunky
Marinara Select Pasta Sauce
Mushroom and Green Pepper Spaghetti Sauce, Extra Chunky
Mushroom and Olive Select Pasta Sauce
Onion and Garlic Select Pasta Sauce
Pizza Sauce
Plain Spaghetti Sauce
Spaghetti Sauce with Meat
Spaghetti Sauce with Mushrooms

Mezzetta
Napa Valley Bistro Pasta Sauces (All)
Pesto

Midwest Country Fare (Hy-Vee)
All Natural Garlic and Onion Spaghetti Sauce
Four Cheese Spaghetti Sauce
Garden Vegetable Spaghetti Sauce
Garlic and Herb Spaghetti Sauce
Meat Flavor Spaghetti Sauce
Mushroom Spaghetti Sauce
Traditional Spaghetti Sauce

Mom's
Artichoke Heart & Asiago Cheese Pasta Sauce
Garlic & Basil Spaghetti Sauce
Martini Pasta Sauce
Puttanesca Spaghetti Sauce
Special Marinara Spaghetti Sauce
Spicy Arrabbiata

Monte Bene ⓘ
  Monte Bene (All)
Nature's Basket (Giant Eagle)
  Organic Marinara Sauce
  Organic Mushroom Pasta Sauce
  Organic Pizza Sauce
  Organic Roasted Garlic Pasta Sauce
  Organic Three Cheese Pasta Sauce
  Organic Tomato Basil Pasta Sauce
  Organic Vodka Cream Pasta Sauce
Nature's Promise (Giant)
  Organic Pasta Sauce, Garden Vegetable
  Organic Pasta Sauce, Parmesan
O Organics ⌁
  Organic Marinara Pasta Sauce
  Organic Roasted Garlic Pasta Sauce
  Organic Tomato Basil Pasta Sauce
Organicville
  Pasta Sauce (All) 🍸 ✔
  Pizza Sauce (All) 🍸 ✔
Paolo's 🍸
  Paolo's (All)
Pastene
  Artichoke Pasta Sauce
  Chateau Marinara Sauce
  Italian (Basil) Pesto
  Kitchen Ready Spaghetti Sauce
  Pizza Sauce
  Tomato Basil Sauce
  White Clam Sauce
Prego
  Chunky Garden Combo
  Chunky Garden Mushroom & Green
    Pepper
  Chunky Garden Mushroom Supreme
    with Baby Portobello
  Chunky Garden Tomato, Onion &
    Garlic
  Flavored with Meat
  Fresh Mushroom
  Heart Smart Mushroom
  Heart Smart Ricotta Parmesan
  Heart Smart Roasted Red Pepper &
    Garlic
  Heart Smart Traditional
  Italian Sausage & Garlic
  Marinara

  Mushroom & Garlic
  Roasted Garlic & Herb
  Roasted Garlic Parmesan
  Three Cheese
  Tomato Basil Garlic
  Traditional
Price Chopper
  Organic Marinara Pasta Sauce
  Organic Tomato Basil Sauce
Publix
  Chunky Mushroom
  Garden Style
  Parmesan and Romano
  Pizza Pasta Sauce
  Premium Basil and Tomato
  Premium Creamy Vodka
  Premium Six Chesse
  Tomato, Garlic, and Onion
  Traditional
  Tradtional, Meat
Red Gold
  Tomato Products (All)
Sacla
  Pesto
  Premium Tomato Sauces with Whole
    Cherry Tomatoes
Santa Barbara Salsa
  Santa Barbara Salsa (All)
Sauces 'n Love
  Pasta and Pizza Sauces (All BUT
    Alfredo)
Sauer's ()
  Pesto Sauce
  Spaghetti Sauce
Schnucks
  3 Cheese Pasta Sauce
  4 Cheese Spaghetti Sauce
  Garden Combination Pasta Sauce
  Garden Vegetable Pasta Sauce
  Garlic & Onion Pasta Sauce
  Garlic Herb Pasta Sauce
  Pasta Sauce with Meat
  Pasta Sauce with Mushroom
  Pizza Sauce
  Plain Pasta Sauce
  Tomato Onion Garlic Pasta Sauce
  Traditional Pasta Sauce

Seeds of Change ⓘ
  Arrabiatta di Roma
  Marinara di Venezia
  Romagna Three Cheese
  Tomato Basil Genovese
  Tuscan Roasted Tomato & Garlic
  Vodka Americano
Simply Enjoy (Giant)
  Fra Diavolo Pasta Sauce
  Marinara Pasta Sauce
  Tomato Basil Pasta Sauce
Simply Enjoy (Stop & Shop)
  Pasta Sauce, Fra Diavolo
  Pasta Sauce, Marinara
  Pasta Sauce, Tomato Basil
  Pasta Sauce, Vodka
Simply Organic
  Alfredo Sauce ✓
  Garden Vegetable Spaghetti Sauce ✓
  Italian Herb Spaghetti Sauce ✓
  Roasted Garlic Spaghetti Sauce ✓
  Sweet Basil Pesto ✓
  Tomato Basil Spaghetti Sauce ✓
Taste of Thai, A
  Taste of Thai, A (All)
Trader Joe's
  Arrabiata Sauce
  Marinara Sauce
  Organic Marinara Sauce
  Organic Marinara Sauce, No Salt Added
  Organic Spaghetti Sauce
  Organic Vodka Sauce
  Pesto Alla Genovese Basil Pesto
  Pizza Sauce, Fat Free
  Roasted Garlic Marinara
  Rustico Pasta Sauce
  Three Cheese Pasta Sauce
  Tomato Basil Marinara
  Tuscan Marinara Sauce, Low Fat
Tuscan Traditions ♘
  Tuscan Traditions (All)
Tuttorosso
  Tomato Products
Valu Time (Brookshire)
  Meat Pasta Sauce
  Mushroom Pasta Sauce
  Original Pasta Sauce

  Plain Pasta Sauce
Valu Time (Marsh)
  Meat Pasta Sauce
  Mushroom Pasta Sauce
  Original Pasta Sauce
Value (Kroger)
  Garlic Herb Pasta Sauce
  Mushroom Pasta Sauce
  Traditional Pasta Sauce
Vietti ⓘ
  Second Harvest Spaghetti Sauce with
    Beef
Walden Farms ♘
  Walden Farms (All)
Wegmans
  Bolognese Sauce
  Organic Marinara Pasta Sauce
  Organic Roasted Garlic Pasta Sauce
  Organic Tomato Basil Pasta Sauce
Winn-Dixie
  Classic Fra Diavolo Pasta Sauce
  Classic Home Style Pasta Sauce
  Classic Marinara
  Classic Peppers & Onions Pasta Sauce
  Classic Style Double Garlic Pasta Sauce
  Classic Style Fat Free Pasta Sauce
  Classic Tomato Basil Pasta Sauce
  Garden Vegetable Combination Pasta
    Sauce
  Garlic & Onion Pasta Sauce
  Meat Pasta Sauce
  Mushroom Pasta Sauce
  Parmesan & Romano Pasta Sauce
  Pizza Sauce
  Traditional Pasta Sauce

PEPPERS

Alpino
  Sport Peppers
B&G Foods ⓘ
  Peppers
Bell View
  Bell View (All)
Best Choice
  Diced Chilis, Lime
  Diced Chilis, Mild

Diced Chilis, Original
Diced Pimento
Sliced Pimento

Casa Fiesta ⓘ

Chipotle Peppers in Adobo Sauce
Diced Jalapeno Peppers
Nacho Sliced Jalapeno Peppers
Serrano Peppers
Whole Chipotle Peppers

Chi-Chi's

Green Chilis
Red Jalapenos

DeLallo

Banana Peppers, Whole (Hot, Mild) ⓘ
Curly Peppers, Imported ⓘ
Fried Peppers with Onions ⓘ
Green Cherry Peppers with Prosciutto
Hot Pepper, Sliced
Pepperoncini, Hot ⓘ
Pepperoncini, Sliced Mild
Pepperoncini, Whole Mild ⓘ
Pimentos (Diced, Sliced) ⓘ
Piquillo Peppers, Grilled ⓘ
Piquillo Peppers, Roasted ⓘ
Red Cherry Peppers with Prosciutto
Red Peppers (Roasted, Roasted with
    Garlic) ⓘ
Red Peppers, Roasted in Brine ⓘ
Red Peppers, Roasted with Garlic in Oil
    ⓘ
Red Peppers, Whole Roasted in Water
    ⓘ
Sweet Piquante Peppadew Peppers ⓘ
Whole Mild Pepperoncini
Wild Hot Pepper, Diced in Olive Oil ⓘ
Yellow & Red Peppers (Roasted, Roasted
    with Garlic) ⓘ
Yellow Peppers, Roasted ⓘ

Di Lusso

Roasted Red Peppers

Dietz & Watson ✓

Jalapeno Spread
Jalapeno, Sliced
Pepperoncini
Sweet Roasted Red Peppers

Embasa

Chiles Gueritos

Chipotle Peppers
Nacho Sliced Jalapenos
Sliced Jalapenos
Whole Jalapenos

Food Club (Brookshire)

Diced Mild Chiles
Green Chiles, Whole
Mild Banana Pepper Rings
Pepperoncini
Sliced Jalapenos

Food Club (Marsh)

Banana Pepper Rings, Hot
Banana Pepper Rings, Mild
Diced Chilies, Mild
Jalapeno Peppers, Sliced
Pepperoncini

Gaea ⟨⟩

Peppers (All)

Goya

Aji Amarillo
Aji Amarillo En Salmuera
Aji Colombiano Dulce
Aji Rocoto
Cascabel/Guajillo
Chile Ancho
Chile Arbol
Chile Limon
Chile Pasilla
Chile Pulla
Chiles Chipotles
Chiltepe/Piquin
Fancy Red Pimientos
Green Peppers
Jalapeño Pickled Nachos
Jalapeño Whole
Jalapeño, Sliced
Pasta de Aji Mirasol
Pasta de Aji Panca
Pasta de Huacatay
Pasta de Rocoto
Red Peppers
Serrano Peppers

Great Value (Wal-Mart) 25

Fire Roasted Green Chiles, Bilingual
Nacho Sliced Jalapenos, Bilingual
Sliced Jalapenos
Whole Jalapenos, Bilingual

Hatch
Chile (All)

Heinz
Peppers (All Varieties)

Hy-Vee
Green Salad Pepperoncini
Hot Banana Peppers
Mild Banana Peppers
Whole Green Chilies

Jardine's ⓘ
Texas Tornados Sweet & Spicy Jalapeno Slices

La Costena
Peppers (All BUT Chipotles in Adobo Sauce)

La Victoria
Green Chiles - Diced & Whole
Jalapeno Peppers - Diced
Jalapeno Peppers - Sliced

Las Palmas ⓘ
Jalapenos

Mancini
Peppers (All)

Meijer
Banana Pepper Rings (Hot, Mild)
Pepperoncini

Mezzetta
Peppers (All)

Mount Olive Pickle Company
Mount Olive Pickle Company (All)

Mrs. Renfro's
Mrs. Renfro's

Ortega ⓘ
Chiles & Jalapenos

Osage
Pimentos, Pieces
Pimentos, Sliced

Our Family
Banana Pepper Rings, Mild
Green Chilies, Chopped
Jalapeno Peppers, Sliced

Pastene
Chipotle Peppers in Adobo Sauce
Gourmet Peppers
Green Vinegar Peppers
Hot Cherry Peppers
Hot Crushed Peppers

Hot Finger Peppers
Hot Pepper Rings
Jalapeno Peppers
Pepper Poppers
Pepper Salad
Pepperoncini (Sliced, Whole)
Piquillo Peppers
Red Peppers, Sliced
Roasted Peppers
Sweet Banana Peppers
Sweet Cherry Peppers
Sweet Garlic Peppers

Peloponnese
Roasted Florina Sweet Peppers
Roasted Sweet Pepper Spread

Rice River Farms ⓘ
Aji Amarillo Chiles, Destemmed
Aji Panca Chiles
Aleppo Pepper
Ancho Chiles, First Quality
Ancho Chiles, First Quality Destemmed
Cascabel Chiles
Chile Threads
Chipotles in Adobo
Chipotles, Brown
Chipotles, Morita
Chipotles, Morita Destemmed First Quality
De Arbol Chiles, First Quality
Ghost Chiles
Green Bell Pepper, Diced 1/4
Guajillo Chiles
Guajillo Chiles, Destemmed
Habanero, Crushed
Habaneros
Mulato Chiles
New Mexico Chiles
New Mexico Chiles, Destemmed
Pasilla Negro Chiles
Pasilla Negro Chiles, Destemmed
Pequin Chiles
Pimentos, Sun Dried
Red Bell Pepper, Diced 1/4
Serrano Chiles, Smoked
Thai Chiles

Safeway Select ∿
Fire Roasted Red Peppers

Schnucks
Pepperoncini
Spicy Roasted Peppers

Shotgun Willie's ⓘ
Jalapeno Slices

Tassos
Peppers (All)

Trader Joe's
Fire Roasted Red Peppers (Regular or Sweet & Yellow)
Marinated Red Peppers

Trappey ⓘ
Peppers

Vons ⌇
Diced Green Chili Peppers

Wegmans
Roasted Red Peppers - Whole

Winn-Dixie
Jalapenos
Pepperoncini
Sliced Banana Peppers (Hot, Mild)

Zocalo Gourmet
Costa Peruana Chili Pastes (All)

Picante Sauce

Chi-Chi's
Picante

Food Club (Brookshire)
Picante Sauce, Medium
Picante Sauce, Mild

Haggen
Picante Sauce (Medium, Mild)

Hill Country Fare (H-E-B)
Hot Picante Sauce
Medium Picante Sauce
Mild Picante Sauce
Picante Sauce

Hy-Vee
Medium Picante Sauce
Mild Picante Sauce

Ortega ⓘ
Picante - Hot
Picante - Medium
Picante - Mild

Pace
Picante Sauce (Extra Mild, Hot, Medium, Mild)

Schnucks
Picante Sauce (Medium, Mild)

Pickles

Always Save
Hamburger Dill Slices
Kosher Dill Spears
Kosher Dills
Sweet Pickle Chips
Whole Sweet Pickles

B&G Foods ⓘ
Capers
Pickles

Bay Valley Foods
Pickles (All)

Bell View
Bell View (All)

Best Choice
Bread & Butter Pickles
Bread & Butter Slices
Extra Hot Dills
Hamburger Dill Slices
Kosher Baby Dill
Kosher Dill Pickles
Kosher Dill Slices
Kosher Spears
Midget Dills
Polish Spears
Sweet Gherkins
Whole Kosher Dills
Whole Sweet Midgets
Whole Sweet Pickles
Zesty Dill Spears

Best Maid/Del-Dixi
Best Maid (All)

Boar's Head
Pickles (All)

Bubbies ⚱
Bread & Butter Chips (All)
Pure Kosher Dills (All)

Central Market Classics (Price Chopper)
Champagne Dill

Gourmet Capers
DeLallo
  Capers, Capote ⓘ
  Capers, Non Pareil ⓘ
Dietz & Watson ✓
  Kosher Spear Pickles
  New Half Sours Pickles
  Sour Garlic Pickles
Divine Brine ()
  Divine Brine (All)
Food Club (Brookshire)
  Bread & Butter Pickle Chips
  Bread & Butter Sandwich Sliced Pickles
  Bread and Butter Slickles
  Dill Hamburger Pickle Slices
  Dill Kosher Pickle Spears
  Dill Kosher Sandwich Pickles
  Kosher Dill Sandwich Slickles
  Kosher Whole Dill Pickle
  Polish Spears Dill Pickles
  Sweet Gherkin Whole Pickles
  Sweet Midgets Pickles
  Sweet Whole Pickles
Food Club (Marsh)
  Bread & Butter Pickle Chips
  Bread & Butter Pickle Slickles
  Bread & Butter Pickle Sticks Fresh Pack
  Dill Hamburger Pickles, Sliced
  Dill Kosher Pickle Spears
  Dill Kosher Pickles, Whole
  Dill Kosher Sandwich Pickle Slickles
  Dill Pickle Spears
  Dill Polish Pickle Spears
  Polish Dill Pickles
  Sweet Gherkin Whole Pickles
  Sweet Whole Pickles
Full Circle (Schnucks)
  Bread & Butter Pickles
  Kosher Baby Dills
  Whole Dill Pickles
Gedney
  Pickles (All)
Genuardi's ᐸᐳ
  Bread and Butter Chips
Giant
  Capers
  Hamburger Chip Dill Pickles

Whole Kosher Dill Pickles
GoyaAlcaparron
  Curtido Salvadoreno
  Loroco
  Pacaya
  Spanish Capers
Great Value (Wal-Mart) 🔲
  Baby Dill Pickles
  Bread & Butter Pickles
  Dill Spears Pickles
  Garlic Dill Slicers Pickles
  Hamburger Dill Chips Pickles
  Kosher Baby Dill Pickles
  Kosher Dill Spears Pickles
  Kosher Whole Dill Pickles
  Sweet Gherkin Pickles
  Sweet Whole Pickles
  Whole Dill Pickles
Haggen
  Baby Kosher Dills
  Baby Kosher Fresh
  Bread & Butter Sandwich Slices
  Cucumber Chips
  Hamburger Dill Sliced
  Kosher Dill Spears
  Kosher Sandwich Sliced
  Sweet Whole
  Whole Kosher Dills
  Zesty Kosher Dills Spears
Hawkshead Relish
  Indian-Style Pickles (All)
Heinz
  Pickles (All Varieties)
Hermann's Pickles
  Pickles (All)
Hill Country Fare (H-E-B)
  Hamburger Chips
  Sweet Dill Spears
Hy-Vee
  Bread & Butter Sandwich Slices
  Bread & Butter Sweet Chunk Pickles
  Bread & Butter Sweet Slices
  Dill Kosher Sandwich Slices
  Fresh Pack Kosher Baby Dills
  Hamburger Dill Slices
  Kosher Baby Dills
  Kosher Cocktail Dills

Kosher Dill Pickles
Kosher Dill Spears
Low Sodium Kosher Spears
No Salt Bread and Butter Chips
Polish Dill Pickles
Polish Dill Spears
Refrigerated Kosher Dill Sandwich
 Slices
Special Recipe Baby Dills
Special Recipe Bread & Butter Slices
Special Recipe Hot & Spicy Zingers
Special Recipe Hot & Sweet Zinger
 Chunks
Special Recipe Jalapeno Baby Dills
Special Recipe Sweet Garden Crunch
Sugar Free Bread and Butter Chips
Sugar Free Sweet Pickle Spears
Sugar Free Sweet Relish
Sweet Gherkins
Whole Sweet Pickles
Zesty Kosher Dill Spears
Zesty Sweet Chunks

Italian Classics (Wegmans)
Capers, Capote
Capers, Nonpareil
Lemon & Caper Sauce

Meijer
Bread and Butter Chips
Bread and Butter Chips, Sugar Free
Bread and Butter Sandwich Slices
Dill Hamburger Pickle Slices
Dill Kosher Pickles (Baby, Whole)
Dill Kosher Pickles Spears
Dill Polish Pickle Spears
Dill Polish Pickles
Dill Whole Pickles
Kosher Baby Dills
Kosher Dill Halves, Refrigerated
Kosher Dill Sandwich Slice
Kosher Dill Sandwich Slice Slickles
Kosher Dill Zesty Sandwich Slice
Kosher Dills
Kosher Whole Dills, Refrigerated
No Garlic Dill Pickle Spears
Pepper Rings (Hot, Mild)
Polish Dill Sandiwch Slice Slickles

Sweet Pickles (Gherkin Whole, Midget
 Whole, Whole)
Sweet Pickles, Sugar Free
Sweet Relish, Sugar Free
Whole Refrigerated Pickles
Zesty Dill Spears

Mezzetta
Capers

Midwest Country Fare (Hy-Vee)
American Sandwich Slices
Fresh Pack Kosher Dill Whole Pickles
Fresh Pack Whole Dill Pickles
Hamburger Dill Slices
Sweet Relish
Whole Sweet Pickles

Mount Olive Pickle Company
Mount Olive Pickle Company (All)

Mrs. Renfro's
Mrs. Renfro's

Our Family
Baby Dill Pickles (Fresh Pack)
Bread & Butter Sandwich Stackers
Cocktail Dill Pickles
Cocktail Dills (Fresh Pack)
Dill Hamburger Slices
Dill Relish
Dill Salad Cubes
Kosher Baby Dills (Fresh Pack)
Kosher Dill Gerkins (Fresh Pack)
Kosher Dill Pickles (Fresh Pack)
Kosher Dill Spears (Fresh Pack)
Kosher Sandwich Stackers
No Garlic Dill Pickles (Fresh Pack)
Polish Dill Pickles (Fresh Pack)
Sweet Bread & Butter Chips
Sweet Bread & Butter Chunks (Fresh
 Pack)
Sweet Bread & Butter Slices (Fresh Pack)
Sweet Gerkins
Sweet Midget Pickles
Sweet Relish
Sweet Salad Cubes
Sweet Whole Pickles

Pastene
Caperberries
Capers, Imported

Publix
Pickles (All Varieties)
Puckered Pickle
Puckered Pickle (All)
Safeway ᗰ
Sweet Midgets
Sweet Pickles
Sweet Whole Gherkins
Safeway Select ᗰ
Nonpareil Capers
Schnucks
Bread & Butter Chips
Bread & Butter Slices
Bread & Butter Spears
Dill Halves
Dill Hamburger Slices
Dill Kosher Spears
Fresh Kosher Pickles
Kosher Sandwich Slices
Kosher Spears
Polish Dill Spears
Sweet Gerkins
Sweet Midget Pickles
Sweet Pickles
Whole Sweet Pickles
Zesty Dill Sandwich Slices
Sechler's
Pickle Products (All)
Stop & Shop
Hamburger Chips Dill Pickles
Strub's
Strub's (All)
Talk O' Texas
Crisp Okra Pickles (Hot, Mild)
Trader Joe's
Organic Kosher Sandwich Pickles
Organic Sweet Butter Pickles
Pickles (All)
Valu Time (Brookshire)
Hamburger Sliced Dill Pickles
Whole Kosher Dill Pickles
Valu Time (Marsh)
Dill Hamburger Pickle Slices
Dill Kosher Pickle Whole
Valu Time (Schnucks)
Hamburger Chips

Vons ᗰ
Dill Pickle Slicers
Dill Pickle Slices
Dills Pickle Relish
Hamburger Dill Pickle Chips
Kosher Pickle Spears
Sweet Bread and Butter Chips
Zesty Dill Pickle Slicers
Wegmans
Hamburger Dill Slices
Kosher Dill Spears - Fresh Pack
Kosher Dills Whole - Fresh Pack
Polish Dill Spears - Fresh Pack
Polish Dills Whole - Fresh Pack
Refrigerated Kosher Dill Mini Pickles
Refrigerated Kosher Dill Pickle Halves
Refrigerated Kosher Dill Pickle
  Sandwich Slices
Refrigerated Kosher Dill Pickle Spears
Refrigerated Kosher Dill Whole Pickles
Sweet Bread & Butter Chips - Fresh Pack
Sweet Gherkins
Sweet Midgets
Sweet Sandwich Slices - Fresh Pack
Winn-Dixie
Dill Pickles (All Varieties)
Sweet Pickles (All Varieties)

RELISH

Always Save
Sweet Relish
B&G Foods ⓘ
Relishes
Best Choice
Dill Pickle Relish
Hot Dog Relish
Sweet Pickle Relish
Sweet Relish
Best Maid/Del-Dixi
Best Maid (All)
Bubbies ♀
Pure Kosher Dill Relish (All)
Central Market Classics
(Price Chopper)
Cranberry Apple Relish

DeLallo
Giardiniera, Mild ⓘ
Dr. Gonzo's Uncommon Condiments
Hot Pepper Mashes (All)
Food Club (Brookshire)
Dill Relish
Sweet Relish
Food Club (Marsh)
Dill Relish
Hot Dog Relish
Sweet Relish
Full Circle (Schnucks)
Sweet Relish
Genuardi's ᏉᎵ
Sweet Relish
Giant
Sweet & Tangy Relish
Sweet Relish
Grandmother's
Corn Relish
Hot Pepper Relish
Onion Relish
Sweet Pepper Relish
Great Value (Wal-Mart) 🔲25
Sweet Pickle Relish
Haggen
Dill Relish
Sweet Relish
Hawkshead Relish
Relishes (All)
Heinz
Relish (All Varieties)
Hill Country Fare (H-E-B)
Dill Relish
Sweet Relish
Howard's
Howard's (All)
Hy-Vee
Dill Relish
Squeeze Sweet Relish
Sweet Relish
Meijer
Dill Relish
Sweet Relish
Mount Olive Pickle Company
Mount Olive Pickle Company (All)

Mrs. Campbell's ⓘ
Hot Chow Chow
Sweet Chow Chow
Mrs. Renfro's
Mrs. Renfro's
Organicville
Organic Sweet Relish
Pastene
Giardinera
Puckered Pickle
Puckered Pickle (All)
Schnucks
Sweet Relish
Sweet Relish, Sugar Free
Stokes Sauces
Relishes (All)
Stop & Shop
Sweet Relish
Tiptree
Tiptree (All)
Trader Joe's
Organic Sweet Relish
Valu Time (Brookshire)
Sweet Relish
Valu Time (Marsh)
Sweet Relish
Valu Time (Schnucks)
Sweet Relish
Wegmans
Dill Relish
Hamburger Relish
Hot Dog Pickle Relish
Sweet Relish
Winn-Dixie
Dill Relish
Sweet Relish
Woeber ⓘ
Sandwich Pal Mustard Relish

SALAD DRESSING & MIXES

Annie's Naturals
Artichoke Parmesan Dressing
Balsamic Vinaigrette
Cowgirl Ranch Dressing
Fat Free Mango Vinaigrette
Fat Free Raspberry Balsamic Vinaigrette

Lemon & Chive Dressing
Lite Goddess Dressing
Lite Herb Balsamic
Lite Honey Mustard Vinaigrette
Lite Poppy Seed Dressing
Lite Raspberry Vinaigrette
Organic Balsamic Vinaigrette
Organic Buttermilk Dressing
Organic Caesar Dressing
Organic Cowgirl Ranch Dressing
Organic Creamy Asiago Cheese
  Dressing
Organic French Dressing
Organic Green Garlic Dressing
Organic Green Goddess Dressing
Organic Oil & Vinegar
Organic Papaya Poppyseed Dressing
Organic Pomegranate Vinaigrette
Organic Red Wine & Olive Oil
  Vinaigrette
Organic Roasted Garlic Vinaigrette
Organic Sesame Ginger Vinaigrette
Organic Thousand Island Dressing
Roasted Red Pepper Vinaigrette
Tuscany Italian Dressing

Aunt Mid's
Salad Dressings (All)

Best Choice
Salad Dressing
Squeeze Salad Dressing

Best Maid/Del-Dixi
Best Maid (All)

Bineshii Wild Rice
Wild Rice Apple Walnut Salad Mix

Bolthouse Farms ⓘ ✔
Bolthouse Farms Dressing (All)

Bragg
Bragg (All)

Briannas Fine Salad Dressings
Briannas Fine Salad Dressings (All BUT
  Asiago Caesar, Chipotle Cheddar,
  Ginger Mandarin, Lemon Tarragon)

Burnin' Love ⓘ ✔
My Honey L.O.V.es. Me Vinaigrette

Cains
Balsamic Vinaigrette Dressing
Bellisimo Italian Dressing

Blue Cheese Dressing
Blush Wine Vinaigrette Fat Free
Caesar Country Fat Free
Chipotle Ranch Dressing
Creamy Caesar
Creamy Italian Dressing
Deluxe Buttermilk Ranch
Fat Free Italian Dressing
Fat Free Raspberry Vinaigrette Dressing
French Dressing
Honey Dijon Fat Free
Italian Cheese Trio
Italian Country Dressing
Italian Dressing
Light Blush Wine Vinaigrette
Light Caesar Dressing
Light French Dressing
Light Italian
Light Ranch
Light Raspberry Vinaigrette Dressing
Peppercorn Parmesan Dressing
Peppercorn Ranch Fat Free
Ranch Dressing
Ranch with Bacon
Raspberry Vinaigrette Country
Robust Italian Dressing
White Balsamic with Honey Dressing
Zesty Tomato & Onion French

Central Market (H-E-B)
Organic Balsamic Vinegar

**Central Market Classics
(Price Chopper)**
Balsamic & Oil
Balsamic Vinaigrette

Cub Foods
Bacon Ranch Salad Dressing
Creamy Ranch Salad Dressing
Italian Salad Dressing
Salad Dressing
Sweet Spicy French Salad Dressing
Western Salad Dressing

DeLallo
Balsamic Vinaigrette Dressing
Classic Italian Dressing
Italian House Dressing
Sweet Italian House Dressing

Drew's All Natural
Buttermilk Ranch Natural Dressing
Garlic Italian Natural Dressing
Greek Olive Natural Dressing
Honey Dijon Natural Dressing
Organic Aged Balsamic Dressing
Organic Peppercorn Ranch Dressing
Poppy Seed Natural Dressing
Raspberry Natural Dressing
Roasted Garlic & Peppercorn Natural
    Dressing
Romano Caesar Natural Dressing
Rosemary Balsamic Natural Dressing
Smoked Tomato Natural Dressing

Duke's ()
Salad Dressing

Durkee
Buttermilk Ranch Dressing

Eating Right
Balsamic Red Wine Fat Free Salad
    Dressing
Blue Cheese Yogurt Dressing
Caesar Yogurt Dressing
Herb Balsamic Fat Free Salad Dressing
Light Ranch Salad Dressing
Ranch Yogurt Dressing

EMERIL'S
Balsamic Vinaigrette Dressing
Bam It Salad Seasoning
Caesar Dressing
House Herb Vinaigrette Dressing
Italian Vinaigrette Dressing
Raspberry Balsamic Vinaigrette

Fanny's Italian Dressing
Salad Dressings (All)

Fischer & Wieser (i)
Citrus, Herb, & Truffle Oil Vinaigrette
Original Roasted Raspberry Chipotle
    Vinaigrette
Southwestern Herb & Tomato
    Vinaigrette
Spicy Coriander & Lime Dressing
Sweet Corn & Shallots Dressing

Flavorite (Cub Foods)
Fat-Free Raspberry Vinaigrette Salad
    Dressing
Ranch Salad Dressing

Follow Your Heart
Caesar with Parmesan Dressing
Creamy Garlic Dressing
High Omega Vegan Ranch Dressing
Lemon Herb Dressing
Low Fat Ranch Dressing
Organic Balsamic Vinaigrette Dressing
Organic Chipotle Lime Ranch Dressing
Organic Chunky Bleu Cheese Dressing
Organic Creamy Caesar Dressing
Organic Creamy Miso Ginger Dressing
Organic Creamy Ranch Dressing
Organic Italian Vinaigrette Dressing
Organic Oil-Free Tamari Miso
    Vinaigrette
Organic Thick and Chunky Bleu Cheese
Organic Thick and Creamy Caesar
Organic Thick and Creamy Ranch
Organic Vegan Caesar Dressing
Sesame Dijon Dressing
Sesame Miso Dressing
Spicy Southwest Ranch Dressing
Thousand Island Dressing
Vegan Caesar Dressing
Vegan Honey Mustard Dressing

Food Club (Brookshire)
Bleu Cheese Dressing
California French Dressing
Fat Free Italian Dressing
Fat Free Ranch Dressing
French Dressing
Honey Dijon Dressing
Italian Dressing
Jalapeno Ranch Dressing
Lite Ranch Dressing
Peppercorn Ranch Dressing
Ranch Dressing
Robust Italian Dressing
Salad Dressing
Thousand Island Dressing
Western Style Dressing
Zesty Italian Dressing

Food Club (Marsh)
Bleu Cheese
California French
California French Fat Free
Classic Caesar

French Western
Italian
Italian Fat Free
Jalapeno Ranch
Ranch
Ranch Fat Free
Ranch Lite
Salad Dressing
Salad Dressing Lite Whipped
Thousand Island
Western Style
Zesty Italian

Food You Feel Good About (Wegmans)
Fat Free Roasted Red Pepper Dressing

Foods Alive 🍴
Organic Meg's Sweet & Sassy Flax Oil Super Dressing
Organic Meg's Sweet & Sassy Hemp Oil Super Dressing
Organic Mike's Special Flax Oil Super Dressing
Organic Sweet Mustard Flax Oil Super Dressing

Four Brothers
Greek House Dressing

Fresh Express
Caesar
Caesar Lite
Caesar Supreme
Coleslaw
Pear Gorgonzola
Strawberry Fields

Full Circle (Price Chopper)
Fat Free Balsamic Vinegar
Feta Dressing
Italian Dressing
Pomegranate Dressing
Ranch Dressing
Raspberry Vinaigrette

Full Circle (Schnucks)
Organic Balsamic Vinaigrette
Organic Buttermilk Ranch
Organic Pomegranate Vinaigrette
Organic Raspberry Vinaigrette
Organic Tuscan Italian

Galassi Foods
Salad Dressing (All)

Golding Farms ⓘ
Balsamic Vinaigrette Dressing
Creamy Cucumber Dressing
Honey Dijon Dressing
Pomegranate Raspberry Vinaigrette Dressing
Poppy Seed Vinaigrette Dressing
Raspberry Walnut Vinaigrette Dressing
Tuscan Tomato Vinaigrette Dressing
Vidalia Onion Vinaigrette Dressing

Good Seasons 〰
Cruet Kit, Italian 2 Pack
Dressing, Classic Balsamic Vinaigrette With Extra Virgin Olive
Dressing, Italian Vinaigrette With Extra Virgin Olive Oil
Dressing, Light Honey Dijon with Grey Poupon Mustard
Dressing, Red Raspberry Vinaigrette With Poppyseed
Dressing, Sun Dried Tomato Vinaigrette With Roasted Red Pepper
Salad Dressing & Recipe Mix, Italian
Salad Dressing Mix, Cheese Garlic
Salad Dressing Mix, Garlic & Herb
Salad Dressing Mix, Mild Italian
Salad Dressing Mix, Zesty Italian

GranoVita
Salad Cream

H-E-B
Carmelized Onion and Bacon Salad Dressing
Light Balsamic Dressing
Light Ranch Dressing

Henri's
Salad Dressings (All)

Hidden Valley
Bottled Salad Dressings (All BUT Crushed Garlic Caesar, Farmhouse Roasted Onion Parmesan, Farmhouse Creamy Parmesan)
Dry Dressing Mixes
Spinach Salad Kit

Hill Country Fare (H-E-B)
Bacon Bites

Bacon Ranch Dressing
Coleslaw Dressing
Dry Italian Salad Dressing
Fat Free Ranch Dressing
Honey Mustard Salad Dressing
Italian Salad Dressing
Ranch Salad Dressing Mix
Thousand Island Dressing
XL Pourable Italian
XL Pourable Ranch
Zesty Italian Salad Dressing

Homemade Dressings
Homemade Dressings (All)

Hy-Vee
Bacon Ranch Dressing
Buttermilk Ranch Dressing
French Dressing
Italian Dressing
Light French Salad Dressing
Light Italian Dressing
Light Ranch Dressing
Light Thousand Island Dressing
Peppercorn Ranch Dressing
Ranch Dressing
Raspberry Vinaigrette Dressing
Thousand Island Dressing
Zesty Italian Dressing

JFG Mayonnaise
Salad Dressing

Jimmy's
Jimmy's (All BUT Thousand Island and
Thousand Island Lite)

Johnny Fleeman's
Honey French Salad Dressing
Honey Mustard Salad Dressing

Johnny's Fine Foods ⓘ
Great! Caesar Dressing
Ranch Dressing & Dip

Ken's Steak House Salad Dressing ⓘ
3 Cheese Italian
Balsamic & Basil
Buttermilk Ranch
Caesar
Chef's Reserve Blue Cheese with
Gorgonzola
Chef's Reserve Creamy Greek

Chef's Reserve Farm House Ranch with
Buttermilk
Chef's Reserve French with Applewood
Smoked Bacon
Chef's Reserve Golden Vidalia Onion
Chef's Reserve Honey Balsamic
Chef's Reserve Honey Dijon
Chef's Reserve Italian with Garlic and
Asiago Cheese
Chef's Reserve Ranch
Chef's Reserve Russian
Chunky Blue Cheese
Country French with Orange Blossom
Honey
Creamy Balsamic
Creamy Caesar
Creamy French
Creamy Italian
Fat Free Raspberry Pecan
Fat Free Sun Dried Tomato
Greek
Honey Mustard
Italian and Marinade
Italian with Aged Romano
Italian with Extra Virgin Olive Oil
Light Options Balsamic Vinaigrette
Light Options Caesar
Light Options Honey Dijon
Light Options Honey French
Light Options Italian with Romano and
Red Pepper
Light Options Olive Oil and Vinegar
Light Options Parmesan and
Peppercorn
Light Options Ranch
Light Options Raspberry Walnut
Light Options Sweet Vidalia Onion
Vinaigrette
Lite Balsamic & Basil
Lite Balsamic Vinaigrette
Lite Caesar
Lite Chunky Blue Cheese
Lite Country French with Orange
Blossom Honey
Lite Creamy Caesar
Lite Creamy Parmesan with Cracked
Peppercorn

Lite Honey Mustard
Lite Italian
Lite Northern Italian
Lite Olive Oil Vinaigrette
Lite Poppyseed
Lite Ranch
Lite Raspberry Pomegranate
Lite Raspberry Walnut
Lite Red Wine Vinaigrette
Lite Sun Dried Tomato Vinaigrette
Lite Sweet Vidalia Onion
Lite Thousand Island
Peppercorn Ranch
Ranch
Red Wine Vinegar & Olive Oil
Russian
Sweet Vidalia Onion
Thousand Island
Zesty Italian

Kraft Salad Dressing 🖐

Salad Dressing, Balsamic Vinaigrette
Salad Dressing, Buttermilk Ranch
Salad Dressing, Caesar Vinaigrette With
Parmesan
Salad Dressing, Caesar With Bacon
Salad Dressing, Catalina
Salad Dressing, Classic Caesar
Salad Dressing, Classic Italian
Vinaigrette
Salad Dressing, Creamy French
Salad Dressing, Creamy Italian
Salad Dressing, Creamy Poppyseed
Salad Dressing, Free Caesar Italian
Salad Dressing, Free Catalina
Salad Dressing, Free Classic Caesar
Salad Dressing, Free French Style
Salad Dressing, Free Honey Dijon Fat
Free
Salad Dressing, Free Italian
Salad Dressing, Free Ranch Fat Free
Salad Dressing, Free Zesty Italian
Salad Dressing, Garlic Ranch
Salad Dressing, Greek Vinaigrette
Salad Dressing, Honey Dijon
Salad Dressing, Honey Dijon
Vinaigrette

Salad Dressing, Light Balsamic
Vinaigrette
Salad Dressing, Light Balsamic
Vinaigrette Parmesan Asiago
Salad Dressing, Light Balsamic
Vinaigrette Sicilian Roasted Garlic
Salad Dressing, Light Creamy French
Style
Salad Dressing, Light Done Right Red
Wine Vinaigrette
Salad Dressing, Light Ranch Reduced Fat
Salad Dressing, Light Raspberry
Vinaigrette with Extra Virgin Olive
Oil
Salad Dressing, Light Thousand Island
Salad Dressing, Light Three Cheese
Ranch
Salad Dressing, Peppercorn Ranch
Salad Dressing, Ranch
Salad Dressing, Ranch With Bacon
Salad Dressing, Roasted Red Pepper
Italian with Parmesan
Salad Dressing, Roka Blue Cheese
Salad Dressing, Roka Brand Blue Cheese
Salad Dressing, Special Collection
Parmesan Romano
Salad Dressing, Sun Dried Tomato
Vinaigrette
Salad Dressing, Sweet Honey Catalina
Salad Dressing, Tangy Tomato Bacon
Salad Dressing, Thousand Island
Salad Dressing, Thousand Island With
Bacon
Salad Dressing, Three Cheese Ranch
Salad Dressing, Tuscan House Italian
Salad Dressing, Vidalia Onion
Vinaigrette With Roasted Red Pepper
Salad Dressing, Zesty Italian

Kroger

Coleslaw Dressing

La Martinique

Balsamic Vinaigrette
Blue Cheese Vinaigrette
Original Poppy Seed
True French Vinaigrette

Lily's Gourmet Dressings ⓘ

Balsamic Vinaigrette

Gourmet Caesar
Northern Italian
Poppyseed with Vidalia Onion
Raspberry Walnut Vinaigrette

Living Intentions
Salad Booster (All)

Lucini Italia
Salad Dressing (All)

Maple Grove Farms ⚕ ✔
Asiago & Garlic
Caesar Lite
Champagne Vinaigrette
Fat Free Balsamic Vinaigrette
Fat Free Caesar
Fat Free Cranberry Balsamic
Fat Free Greek
Fat Free Honey Dijon
Fat Free Lime Basil Vinaigrette
Fat Free Poppyseed
Fat Free Raspberry Vinaigrette
Fat Free Vidalia Onion
Fat Free Wasabi Dijon
Ginger Pear Vinaigrette
Honey Mustard
Honey Mustard Lite
Maple Balsamic
Strawberry Balsamic
Sugar Free Balsamic Vinaigrette
Sugar Free Italian with White Balsamic
Sugar Free Raspberry Vinaigrette
Sweet & Sour

Midwest Country Fare (Hy-Vee)
French Dressing
Italian Dressing
Ranch Dressing
Thousand Island Dressing

Mount Olive Pickle Company
Mount Olive Pickle Company (All)

Mrs. May's Naturals
Fruit & Nut Toppers (All)

Naturally Delicious
Balsamic
Blue Cheese
Chipotle Ranch
French
Honey Mustard
Italian

Light Blush Wine
Light Italian
Light Raspberry
Peppercorn Parmesan

Nature's Basket (Giant Eagle)
Organic Balsamic Dressing
Organic Italian Dressing
Organic Ranch Dressing
Organic Raspberry Vinaigrette
Organic Roasted Red Pepper Dressing
Organic Sesame Ginger Dressing

Nature's Promise (Giant)
Organic Ranch Dressing

Nature's Promise (Stop & Shop)
Organic Balsamic Vinaigrette Salad
Dressing

O Organics ✍
Balsamic Vinaigrette Dressing
Caesar Dressing
Champagne Vinaigrette
Ranch Dressing

O'Charley's
Signature Salad Dressings (All)

Olde Cape Cod
Balsamic
Balsamic with Olive Oil
Chipotle Ranch
Honey Dijon
Honey French Lite
Lemon and Mint with Green Tea
Vinaigrette
Lemon Poppyseed
Lite Blush Wine Vinaigrette
Lite Caesar
Lite Raspberry Vinaigrette
Lite Sweet & Sour Poppyseed
Orange Poppyseed
Parmesan & Peppercorn
Sundried Tomato Lite
Zesty Mango Vinaigrette

Organicville
Salad Dressing (All) ⚕ ✔
Vinaigrette (All) ⚕ ✔

Oxford
Italian
Ranch

Price Chopper
Balsamic Vinaigrette Garlic
Balsamic Vinaigrette Salad Dressing
Blue Cheese Dressing
Cheese Ranch Dressing
Creamy Italian Dressing
French Dressing
Light Blue Cheese Dressing
Lite Caesar Dressing
Red Wine Vinaigrette
Tropical French Salad
Zesty Italian Dressing

Publix
Balsamic Vinaigrette
California French
Chunky Blue Cheese
Creamy Parmesan
Fat Free Italian
Fat Free Thousand Island
Italian
Lite Caesar
Lite Honey Dijon
Lite Ranch
Lite Raspberry Walnut
Ranch
Thousand Island
Zesty Italian

Richfood (Cub Foods)
Ranch Light Salad Dressing
Sweet Spicy French Light Salad Dressing

Rooties
Blue Cheese

Safeway ⌇
Balsamic Vinaigrette Salad Dressing
  Spray
Italian Vinaigrette Salad Dressing Spray
Raspberry Vinaigrette Salad Dressing
  Spray

Safeway Select ⌇
Italian Parmesan Herb Salad Dressing

San-J ⓘ ✔
Gluten Free Tamari Ginger Dressing
Gluten Free Tamari Peanut Dressing
Gluten Free Tamari Sesame Dressing

Sauer's ◖◗
Salad Toppings

Sbarro
Balsamic
Creamy French
Italian (Golden, Classico)
Lite Olive Oil Balsamic
Ranch

Schnucks Select
Balsamic Basil Vinaigrette
Blue Cheese Bacon Dressing
Caesar Dressing
Honey Dijon Dressing
Parmesan Ranch
Poppy Seed Dressing
Raspberry Vinaigrette

Seven Seas ⌇
Salad Dressing, Green Goddess
Salad Dressing, Red Wine Vinaigrette

Simply Organic
Classic Caesar Dressing ✔
Garlic Vinaigrette Dressing ✔
Italian Dressing ✔
Orange Ginger Vinaigrette ✔
Pineapple Cilantro Vinaigrette ✔
Ranch Dressing ✔

Stokes Sauces
Balsamic Sauce
Dressings (All)

Trader Joe's
Balsamic Vinaigrette (Regular, Fat Free
  or Organic)
Low Fat Parmesan Ranch Dressing
Organic Red Wine And Olive Oil
  Vinaigrette
Pear Champagne Vinaigrette
Romano Caesar Dressing
Tuscano Italian Dressing With Balsamic
  Vinegar

Valu Time (Brookshire)
French Dressing
Italian Dressing
Light Italian Dressing
Light Ranch Dressing
Ranch Dressing
Salad Dressing
Thousand Island Dressing

Valu Time (Marsh)
French Dressing

Italian Dressing
Ranch Dressing

Virginia's Live a Little ()
Salad Dressings (All BUT Ginger Sesame)

Vita Foods (i)
Biltmore Asiago Salad Dressing
Biltmore Buttermilk Dill Ranch Salad Dressing
Biltmore Caesar Salad Dressing
Biltmore Honey Mustard Salad Dressing
Biltmore Italian Herb Vinaigrette Salad Dressing
Biltmore Orange Poppy Seed Salad Dressing
Oak Hill Farms Raspberry Vinaigrette
Virginia Brand Vidalia Onion French Royale
Virginia Brand Vidalia Onion Frontier Ranch
Virginia Brand Vidalia Onion Honey Mustard

Vons
California French Salad Dressing
Lite Italian Salad Dressing
Lite Ranch Salad Dressing

Walden Farms
Walden Farms (All)

Wegmans
Basil Vinaigrette Salad Dressing
Caramelized Onion & Bacon Dressing
Cracked Pepper Ranch Dressing
Creamy Curry & Roasted Red Pepper Dressing
Creamy Italian Dressing
Creamy Ranch Dressing
Fat Free Parmesan Italian Dressing
Light Garlic Italian Dressing
Light Golden Caesar Dressing
Light Parmesan Peppercorn Ranch Dressing
Light Ranch Dressing
Organic Balsamic Vinaigrette
Organic Creamy Caesar Dressing
Organic Honey Mustard Dressing
Organic Italian Dressing
Organic Raspberry Vinaigrette

Organic Sun-Dried Tomato Vinaigrette
Parmesan Italian Dressing
Roasted Red Bell Pepper & Garlic Dressing
Salad Dressing - Whip
Thousand Island Dressing
Three Spice Garden French Dressing
Traditional Italian Dressing

Wild Thymes (i)
Black Currant Salad Refresher
Fig Walnut Balsamic Vinaigrette
Mandarin Orange Basil Vinaigrette
Mango Salad Refresher
Mediterranean Balsamic Vinaigrette
Meyer Lemon Salad Refresher
Morello Cherry Salad Refresher
Parmesan Walnut Caesar Vinaigrette
Passion Fruit Salad Refresher
Pomegranate Salad Refresher
Raspberry Pear Balsamic Vinaigrette
Raspberry Salad Refresher
Roasted Apple Shallot Vinaigrette
Tahitian Lime Ginger Vinaigrette
Tangerine Salad Refresher
Tuscan Tomato Basil Vinaigrette

Winn-Dixie
Balsamic Vinaigrette
California French
Chunky Blue Cheese
Creamy French
Creamy Ranch
Fat Free Italian
Fat Free Ranch
Fat Free Thousand Island
Garden Ranch
Honey Dijon
Italian
Lite Italian
Lite Ranch
Robust Italian
Thousand Island
Zesty Italian

Woeber (i)
Sandwich Pal Sandwich Dressing

SALSA

Amy's Kitchen ✓
Black Bean & Corn Salsa
Medium Salsa
Mild Salsa

Bone Suckin' Sauce
Bone Suckin' Salsa (All)

Casa Fiesta ⓘ
Chili Salsa
Jalapeno Cheese Salsa
Salsa Dip
Salsa Picante
Thick and Chunky Salsa

Central Market (H-E-B)
All Natural Hatch Salsa - Roja

Chi-Chi's
Fiesta Salsa
Garden Salsa
Natural Salsa
Original Salsa

Clint's Salsa
Clint's Salsa (All)

Cugino's ⟨⟩
Tomato Lime Salsa

Dei Fratelli ⓘ
Dei Fratelli (All)

Drew's All Natural
Organic Salsa (All)

El Pinto ⚇
El Pinto (All)

Embasa
Salsa Casera - Hot
Salsa Mexicana - Medium

EMERIL'S ⚇
Gaaahlic Lovers Medium Salsa
Kicked Up Chunky Hot Salsa
Original Recipe Medium Salsa
Southwest Style Medium Salsa

Fischer & Wieser ⓘ
Artichoke & Olive Salsa
Black Bean & Corn Salsa
Chipotle & Corn Salsa
Cilantro & Olive Salsa
Das Peach Haus Peach Salsa
Hatch Chile & Pineapple Salsa
Havana Mojito Salsa

Hot Habanero Salsa
Salsa A La Charra
Salsa Muy Rica
Salsa Verde Ranchera
Silican Tomato Pesto Salsa

Food Club (Brookshire)
Thick and Chunky Salsa, Medium
Thick and Chunky Salsa, Mild

Food Club (Marsh)
Chunky Medium Salsa
Chunky Mild Salsa

Food You Feel Good About (Wegmans)
Hot Salsa
Medium Salsa
Mild Salsa
Roasted Chipotle Salsa
Roasted Salsa Verde
Roasted Sweet Pepper Salsa
Roasted Tomato Salsa
Santa Fe Style Salsa

Frontera ⟨⟩
Salsa (All)

Full Circle (Price Chopper)
Roasted Medium Salsa

Full Circle (Schnucks)
Organic Salsa, Hot
Organic Salsa, Medium
Organic Salsa, Mild

Garden Fresh Gourmet ⓘ
Salsa (All)

Giant
Festingos Medium Salsa
Fresh Mango Salsa
Fresh Salsa
Fresh Verde Salsa
Mild Salsa

Giant Eagle
Black Bean and Corn Salsa
Fiesta Salsa
Fire Roasted Tomato Salsa
Guacamole
Hot Mexican Style Salsa
Mexican Style Medium Salsa
Mexican Style Salsa
Peach Mango Salsa
Salsa

Spicy Guacamole
Sweet Onion Salsa
Thick and Chunky Salsa

Goldwater
Goldwater (All)

Goya
Chipotle Salsita
Jalapeño Salsa
Salsa Botanita
Salsa Hot
Salsa Mild
Salsa Pico de Gallo Hot
Salsa Roja Mexicano Casera
Salsas - Pico De Gallo
Salsas - Taquera
Salsas - Verde

Grand Selections (Hy-Vee)
Medium Black Bean & Corn Salsa
Mild Black Bean & Corn Salsa

Grande ⓘ
Salsas (All)

Great Value (Wal-Mart) 25
Salsa Con Queso
White Salsa Con Queso

GreenWise Market (Publix)
Organic Medium Salsa
Organic Mild Salsa

Haggen
Salsa (Medium, Mild)

Hatch
Sauces & Salsa (All)

Hawkshead Relish
Salsas (All)

H-E-B
Chipotle Salsa
Chunky Hot Salsa Picante
Chunky Salsa, Medium
Chunky Salsa, Mild
Habanera Salsa
Medium Salsa Dip
Mild Salsa Dip
Roasted Restaurant Style Salsa
Salsa Con Queso

Herr's ()
Chunky Salsa (Hot, Medium, Mild)
Salsa Con Queso Dip
Southwestern Black Bean & Corn Salsa

Hill Country Fare (H-E-B)
Salsa Con Queso

Hy-Vee
Chunky Medium Salsa
Chunky Mild Salsa
Hot Picante Salsa
Thick and Chunky Hot Salsa
Thick and Chunky Medium Salsa
Think and Chunky Mild Salsa

Jardine's ⓘ
7J Campfire Roasted Salsa
7J Chipotle Salsa
7J Chipotle Tomatillo Salsa
7J Garden Original Salsa
7J Hint of Habanero Salsa
7J Lightly Roasted Salsa
7J Mi Queso Su Queso
7J Pineapple Chipotle Salsa
7J Prairie Peach Salsa
7J Queso Amarillo
7J Salsa Serrano
7J Salsa Verde
7J Southwest Cilantro Salsa
7J Texasalsa (Hot, Medium, Mild)
7J Tomatillo Salsa
Cilantro & Green Olive Salsa
Cilantro Lime Salsa
Cowpoke Artichoke Salsa
Fresh From Home Authentic Salsa
Fresh From Home Naturally Fresh Salsa
Fresh From Home Pinch of Habanero
  Salsa
Fresh From Home Ranch Roasted Salsa
Fresh From Home Smoky Tomatillo
  Salsa
Fresh From Home Tumbleweed Verde
  Salsa
Frijole Chipotle Salsa
Habanero Salsa
Mango Mariachi Salsa
Ole Chipotle Salsa
Peach Salsa
Pineapple Chipotle Salsa
Pineapple Habanero Salsa
Pineapple Salsa
Pomegranate Salsa
Queso Caliente

Queso Loco
Raspberry Chardonnay Salsa
Raspberry Chipotle Salsa
Raspberry Salsa
Roasted Garlic Salsa
Roasted Tomatillo Salsa
Salsa Bobos
Texacante Salsa

Joe T. Garcia's
Salsa Picante (All)
Salsa Verde (All)

Jose Pedro ⚱
Jose Pedro (All)

La Victoria
Cilantro - Medium
Cilantro - Mild
Green Salsa Jalapena - Extra Hot
Red Salsa Jalapena - Extra Hot
Salsa Ranchera - Hot
Salsa Suprema - Medium
Salsa Suprema - Mild
Salsa Victoria - Hot
Thick 'N Chunky - Hot
Thick 'N Chunky - Mild
Thick 'N Chunky Verde - Medium
Thick 'N Chunky Verde - Mild

Meijer
Restaurant Style Salsa (Hot, Medium, Mild)
Salsa (Hot, Medium, Mild)
Santa Fe Style Salsa (Hot, Medium, Mild)
Thick and Chunky Salsa (Hot, Medium, Mild)

Mother's Mountain
New England Chili Salsa

Mrs. Renfro's
Mrs. Renfro's (All BUT Nacho Cheese Sauce)

Nature's Basket (Giant Eagle)
Organic Corn & Black Bean Salsa
Organic Hot Salsa
Organic Medium Salsa
Organic Mild Salsa
Organic Pineapple Salsa

Nature's Promise (Giant)
Organic Chipotle Salsa
Organic Medium Salsa
Organic Mild Salsa

Nature's Promise (Stop & Shop)
Organic Mild Salsa

O Organics ⟿
Chunky Bell Pepper Salsa
Organic Chipotle Salsa
Organic Fire Roasted Salsa
Organic Mild Salsa

Old Dutch Foods
Restaurant Style Cocina Del Norte Salsa
Restaurant Style Monterey Jack Queso Supreme
Restaurant Style Salsa Con Queso Dip
Restaurante Style Fruit Salsa
Restaurante Style Salsa (Medium, Mild)

Organicville
Organic Salsa (All) ⚱ ✓

Ortega ⓘ
Black Bean & Corn (Mexican)
Garden - Medium
Garden - Mild
Original - Medium
Original - Mild
Roasted Garlic
Salsa con Queso
Salsa Verde
Thick & Chunky - Medium
Thick & Chunky - Mild

Pace
Chunky Salsa (Medium, Mild)
Pico de Gallo
Pineapple Mango Chipotle Salsa
Salsa Dip (Medium, Mild)
Salsa Verde
Thick & Chunky Salsa (Extra Mild, Hot, Medium, Mild)

Publix
All Natural Hot Salsa
All Natural Medium Salsa
All Natural Mild Salsa
Southwestern Black Bean and Corn Salsa
Thick & Chunky - Hot Salsa
Thick & Chunky - Medium Salsa
Thick & Chunky - Mild Salsa

Red Gold
Tomato Products (All)
Safeway 〰
Salsa Con Queso Medium
Three Bean and Pepper Salsa
Safeway Select 〰
Chunky Classic Medium Salsa
Peach Pineapple Salsa
Pico De Gallo with Fresh Cilantro
Southwest Hot Salsa
Southwest Medium Salsa
Southwest Mild Salsa
Salba Smart
Organic Salsa ⓘ
Sally's 🏅
Sally's (All)
Santa Barbara Salsa
Santa Barbara Salsa (All)
Schnucks
Salsa (Hot, Medium, Mild)
Sorrell Ridge
Pineapple Salsa - Medium
Stop & Shop
All Natural Authentic Homestyle Mild
  Salsa
Fresh Mild Salsa
Southwest Hot Salsa
Southwest Medium Salsa
Southwest Mild Salsa
Taco Bell 〰
Salsa Con Queso, Medium
Salsa Con Queso, Mild
Salsa, Thick 'N Chunky Medium
Salsa, Thick 'N Chunky Mild
TGI Friday's (Heinz)
Salsa (All Varieties)
Timpone's
Salsa Muy Rica
Tostitos
All Natural Hot Chunky Salsa ⓘ
All Natural Medium Chunky Salsa ⓘ
All Natural Mild Chunky Salsa ⓘ
Restaurant Style Salsa ⓘ
Salsa Con Queso ⓘ
Trader Joe's
Black Bean & Roasted Corn Salsa
Chunky Salsa

Corn And Chili Tomato-less Salsa
Double Roasted Salsa
Fire Roasted Tomato Salsa
Fresh Salsa (All BUT Avocado Salsa)
Garlic Chipotle Salsa
Hot And Smoky Chipotle Salsa
Pineapple Salsa
Salsa (Autentica or Verde)
Spicy, Smoky, Peach Salsa
Utz 🏅
Mt. Misery Mike's Salsa Dip
Sweet Salsa Dip
Valu Time (Brookshire)
Medium Salsa
Mild Salsa
Valu Time (Marsh)
Salsa Medium
Salsa Mild
Valu Time (Schnucks)
Medium Salsa
Mild Salsa
Vita Foods ⓘ
Sauza Salsa Traditional
Wegmans
Organic Hot Salsa
Organic Mango Salsa
Organic Medium Salsa
Organic Mild Salsa
Wholly Salsa 🏅
Salsa (All BUT Queso)

SAUERKRAUT

Always Save
Sauerkraut
B&G Foods ⓘ
Sauerkraut
Best Choice
Fancy Sauerkraut
Bubbies 🏅
Sauerkraut (All)
Dei Fratelli ⓘ
Dei Fratelli (All)
Dietz & Watson ✓
Sauerkraut
Food Club (Brookshire)
Sauerkraut

Food Club (Marsh)
Sauerkraut
Food You Feel Good About (Wegmans)
Sauerkraut
Frank's
Frank's Sauerkraut
Giant
Sauerkraut
Great Value (Wal-Mart) 🔲25
Sauerkraut
Haggen
Sauerkraut
Hatfield ()
Sauerkraut
Hy-Vee
Shredded Kraut
Our Family
Sauerkraut
Price Chopper
Sauerkraut
Schnucks
Kraut
Sauerkraut
Valu Time (Brookshire)
Shredded Sauerkraut
Valu Time (Schnucks)
Sauerkraut

SLOPPY JOE SAUCE

ACME
Sloppy Joe Sauce
Best Choice
Sloppy Joe Mix
Sloppy Joe Sauce
Dei Fratelli ⓘ
Sloppy Joe Sauce
Food Club (Brookshire)
Sloppy Joe Sauce
Food Club (Marsh)
Sloppy Joe Sauce
Giant Eagle
Sloppy Joe Sauce
Heinz
Sloppy Joe Sauce

Hormel
Not-So-Sloppy-Joe Sauce
Hy-Vee
Sloppy Joe Sauce
Jewel-Osco
Original Sloppy Joe Sauce
Kroger
Sloppy Joe Sauce
Meijer
Sloppy Joe Sauce
Our Family
Sloppy Joe Sauce
Schnucks
Sloppy Joe Sauce
Shaw's
Sloppy Joe Sauce
Valu Time (Brookshire)
Sloppy Joe Sauce

STEAK SAUCE

A.1. Steak Sauces and Marinades ⌒
Steak Sauce
Steak Sauce, Bold & Spicy With Tobasco
Steak Sauce, Carb Well
Steak Sauce, Chicago Steakhouse
Steak Sauce, Classics
Steak Sauce, Jamaican Jerk
Steak Sauce, New Orleans Cajun
Steak Sauce, New York Steakhouse
Steak Sauce, Smoky Mesquite
Steak Sauce, Steak House Cracked
Peppercorn
Steak Sauce, Supreme Garlic
Steak Sauce, Sweet Hickory With Bull's
Eye BBQ Sauce
Steak Sauce, Teriyaki
Steak Sauce, Thick &Hearty
Best Choice
Steak Sauce
Steak Seasoning Sauce
Crystal
Steak Sauce (All)
Dave's Gourmet
Steak Sauce
Food Club (Brookshire)
Steak Seasoning Sauce

Thick and Zesty Steak Sauce
Food Club (Marsh)
Steak Sauce
Golding Farms ⓘ
Golden Steak Sauce
Premium Steak Sauce
Vidalia Onion Steak Sauce
Great Value (Wal-Mart) 🔲25
Steak Sauce
Hawkshead Relish
Steak Sauce
Heinz
Traditional Steak Sauce
Hy-Vee
Classic Steak Sauce
Jack Daniel's Sauces
Steak Sauce (Both Varieties)
Lea & Perrins
Traditional Steak Sauce
Meijer
Steak Sauce (Plastic Bottle)
Really Great Food ⛹
Really Great Food (All)
Rio Grande
Steak Sauce
Safeway 👓
Bold Steak Sauce
Schnucks
Zesty Steak Sauce
Schnucks Select
New York Steak Sauce
Shiloh's ✔
Chimichurri Steak Sauce
Original Steak Sauce
Parisian BBQ Steak Sauce
Trinity Hill Farms
Gourmet Steak Sauce and Marinade
TryMe
Bullfighter Steak & Burger Sauce
Valu Time (Brookshire)
Steak Sauce
Vita Foods ⓘ
Jim Beam Original Steak Sauce
Zip Sauce
Zip Sauce (All)

SYRUP, PANCAKE & MAPLE

Aunt Jemima ()
Syrups (All)
Bineshii Wild Rice
Syrups (All)
Cary's
Pure Maple Syrup
Sugar Free Syrup
Central Market (H-E-B)
Organic Dark Maple Syrup
Organic Medium Maple Syrup
Central Market Classics (Price Chopper)
Blueberry Syrup
Dark Amber Maple Syrup
Strawberry Syrup
Crosby's ⛹
Table Syrup
Darbo
3-Herb Tea Syrup
Apple and Ginger Tea Syrup
Black Currant Tea Syrup
Blood Orange Tea Syrup
Lemon Balm and Ginger Tea Syrup
Lingonberry Tea Syrup
Peppermint Tea Syrup
Red Fruits Tea Syrup
Rosehip Tea Syrup
E.D. Smith
E.D. Smith (All)
Food Club (Brookshire)
100% Amber Leaf Maple Syrup
2% Maple Syrup
Butter Flavored Syrup
Lite Syrup
Food Club (Marsh)
Butter Flavored Syrup
Chocolate Syrup
Lite Butter Syrup
Strawberry Syrup
Food You Feel Good About (Wegmans)
Dark Amber Pure Maple Syrup
Pure Maple Syrup
Full Circle (Price Chopper)
Maple Syrup

Full Circle (Schnucks)
100% Maple Syrup
Giant
Pancake Syrup
Pure Maple Syrup
Ginger People, The ()
Organic Ginger Syrup
Grand Selections (Hy-Vee)
100% Pure Maple Syrup
Griffin Foods
Griffin Foods (All)
Haggen
Lite Pancake & Waffle Syrup
Highland Sugarworks
Maple Syrup
Hill Country Fare (H-E-B)
Butter Pancake/Waffle Syrup
Lite Butter Syrup
Lite Pancake/Waffle Syrup
Lite Syrup
Original Syrup
Pancake/Waffle Syrup
Rich Butter Syrup
Sugar Free Syrup
Howard's
Howard's (All)
Hy-Vee
Artificial Butter Flavored Syrup
Lite Pancake Syrup
Low Calorie Sugar Free Syrup
Pancake & Waffle Syrup
Karo
Karo Syrups (All)
Maple Grove Farms ⚇ ✔
Honey Maple Spread
Maple Blend Spread
Pure Maple Cream
Syrups (All Varieties)
Market District (Giant Eagle)
Pure Maple Syrup
Meijer
Butter Flavored Syrup
Lite Butter Syrup
Lite Syrup
Regular Syrup

Midwest Country Fare (Hy-Vee)
Pancake and Waffle Syrup
Mrs. Renfro's
Mrs. Renfro's
Nature's Promise (Giant)
Organic Maple Syrup
Nature's Promise (Stop & Shop)
Organic Maple Syrup
O Organics ⌇
Grade A Dark Amber 100% Pure Maple
Syrup
Organics Are For Everyone
Date Syrup
Oskri
Date Syrup
Price Chopper
Maple Syrup
Publix
Pancake Syrup
Pancake Syrup, Sugar Free
Purity
Raspberry Syrup
Strawberry Syrup
Safeway ⌇
Lite Butter Syrup
Lite Syrup
Old Fashioned Syrup
Original Flavored Syrup
Original Syrup
Sugar Free Syrup
Safeway Select ⌇
Pure Maple Syrup
Sohgave
Agave Nectar (Amber, Light, Raw)
Flavored Agave Nectars
Flavored Agave Syrups
Spring Tree
Pure Maple Syrup
Sugar Free Syrup
Stop & Shop
Pancake & Waffle Syrup
Reduced Calorie Lite Table Syrup
Trader Joe's
Maple Syrup (All)
Valu Time (Brookshire)
Regular Syrup

Valu Time (Marsh)
   Butter Flavor Syrup
   Regular Flavor Syrup
Vermont Maid ⓘ
   Vermont Maid Syrup (All Varieties)
Vita Foods ⓘ
   Jelly Belly French Vanilla Pancake Syrup
   Jelly Belly Tuitti-Fruitti Pancake Syrup
   Jelly Belly Very Cherry Pancake Syrup
   Jim Beam Pancake Syrup
   Stuckey's Maple Pecan Pancake Syrup
Vons ⌒
   Butter Flavored Syrup
Walden Farms ⚇
   Walden Farms (All)
Wegmans
   2% Real Maple Pancake Syrup
   Lite Pancake Syrup
   Maraschino Cherry Syrup
   Organic Maple Syrup
Winn & Lovette (Winn-Dixie)
   Maple Syrup (All Varieties)
Winn-Dixie
   Butter Flavor Syrup
   Lite Syrup
   Regular Syrup
Xagave
   Agave Nectar (All)

Taco Sauce

Casa Fiesta ⓘ
   Green Taco Sauce
   Taco Sauce
Chi-Chi's
   Taco Sauce
Food Club (Marsh)
   Taco Sauce, Mild
Great Value (Wal-Mart) 🏷️25
   Red Taco Sauce
Hy-Vee
   Medium Taco Sauce
   Mild Taco Sauce
La Victoria
   Green Taco Sauce - Medium
   Green Taco Sauce - Mild
   Red Taco Sauce - Medium
   Red Taco Sauce - Mild
Ortega ⓘ
   Green Taco Sauce
   Taco Sauce - Hot
   Taco Sauce - Medium
   Taco Sauce - Mild
Pace
   Taco Sauce (Medium, Mild)
Taco Bell ⌒
   Taco Sauce, Medium
   Taco Sauce, Mild

Tartar Sauce

Best Maid/Del-Dixi
   Best Maid (All)
Cains
   Tartar Sauce
Food Club (Marsh)
   Tartar Sauce
Golding Farms ⓘ
   Tartar Sauce
Heinz
   Tartar Sauce
Ken's Steak House Salad Dressing ⓘ
   Tartar Sauce (Refrigerated, Shelf Stable)
Legal
   Tartar Sauce
Little River ⓘ
   Tangy Tartar Sauce
Louisiana Fish Fry ⓘ
   Remoulade Dressing
   Tartar Sauce
Ojai Cook, The
   Tartar Sauce
Organic Gourmet
   Organic Tartar Sauce & Dip
Stokes Sauces
   Tartare Sauce
Stop & Shop
   Tartar Sauce
Vita Foods ⓘ
   Vita Tartar Sauce
Wegmans
   Tartar Sauce

VINEGAR

Always Save
Cider Vinegar
White Vinegar

B.R. Cohn
Wine Vinegars (All)

Barengo
Balsamic Vinegar
Red Wine Vinegar

Best Choice
Balsamic Vinegar
Cider Vinegar
Red Wine Vinegar
White Distilled Vinegar
White Vinegar

Bionaturae
Balsamic Vinegar ᛦ

Bragg
Bragg (All)

Cat Cora's Kitchen
Oxymelo Barrel Aged Vinegar with
Thyme Honey

Coconut Secret ⓘ
Coconut Vinegar

Colavita
Vinegar (All)

DeLallo
Balsamic Vinegar ⓘ
Balsamic Vinegar Spray ⓘ
Garlic Wine Vinegar ⓘ
Golden Balsamic Vinegar ⓘ
Private Stock Balsamic Vinegar ⓘ
Raspberry Balsamic Vinegar ⓘ
Red Wine Vinegar ⓘ
Red Wine Vinegar, Imported ⓘ
White Wine Vinegar, Imported ⓘ

Eden Foods
Organic Apple Cider Vinegar
Organic Brown Rice Vinegar
Red Wine Vinegar

Food Club (Brookshire)
5% Cider Vinegar
Cider Vinegar
Red Wine Vinegar
White Vinegar

Food Club (Marsh)
Cider Vinegar
White Vinegar

Food You Feel Good About (Wegmans)
Fat Free Red Wine Vinegar

Full Circle (Price Chopper)
Balsamic Vinegar

Gaea ⟨⟩
Vinegar (All)

Goya
Cider Vinegar
White Vinegar
Wine Vinegar

Grand Selections (Hy-Vee)
Red Wine Vinegar
White Wine Vinegar

Great Value (Wal-Mart)
Apple Cider Vinegar
Balsamic Vinegar
Distilled White Vinegar
Premium Garlic Flavored Red Wine
Vinegar
Premium Red Wine Vinegar

GreenWise Market (Publix)
Organic Balsamic Vinegar
Organic Red Wine Vinegar

Haggen
Vinegar (Apple Cider, Cider, Distilled)

Hawkshead Relish
Vinegars (All)

Heinz
Apple Cider Flavored Vinegar
Apple Cider Vinegar
Distilled White Vinegar
Garlic Wine Vinegar
Red Wine Vinegar

Hy-Vee
All Natural White Distilled Vinegar
Apple Cider Flavored Distilled Vinegar
White Distilled Vinegar

Isola
Cream of Balsamic (All Varieties)

Italian Classics (Schnucks)
Red Wine Vinegar
White Wine Vinegar

Italian Classics (Wegmans)
Balsamic Vinegar, Four Leaf
Balsamic Vinegar, Three Leaf
Balsamic Vinegar, Two Leaf
Chianti Red Wine Vinegar
Tuscan White Wine Vinegar

Kikkoman
Rice Vinegar ()
Seasoned Rice Vinegar ()

Lorenzi ()
Balsamic Vinegar

Lucini Italia
Vinegar (All)

Marukan
Genuine Brewed Rice Vinegar
Lite Seasoned Gourmet Rice Vinegar
Organic Rice Vinegar
Organic Seasoned Rice Vinegar
Seasoned Gourmet Rice Vinegar

Meijer
Balsamic 12 Year Aged Vinegar
Balsamic 4 Years Aged Vinegar
Balsamic Vinegar
Cider Vinegar
Red Wine Vinegar
Vinegar
White Distilled Vinegar
White Vinegar
White Wine Vinegar

Mitsukan
Rice Vinegar
Seasoned Rice Vinegar

Morehouse
Vinegar

Nakano
Rice Vinegars (All)
Seasoned Rice Vinegars (All)

Napa Valley Naturals ()
Balsamic Vinegar

Newman's Own Organics ⓘ
Balsamic Vinegar

O Olive Oil
Vinegars (All)

O Organics
Organic Balsamic Vinegar

Ortalli
Ortalli (All)

Our Family
Apple Cider Vinegar 5%
White Vinegar 5%

Pastene
Balsamic Cream
Balsamic Vinegar
Organic Red Wine Vinegar

Pompeian
Vinegar (All)

Price Chopper
Cider Vinegar

Publix
Apple Cider Vinegar
Balsamic Vinegar
Red Wine Vinegar
White Distilled Vinegar

Regina ⓘ
Vinegars (All)

Safeway Select
Red Wine Vinegar
Seasoned Rice Vinegar
Verdi Balsamic Vinegar
White Wine Vinegar

Schnucks
Balsamic Vinegar, Italian

Schnucks Select
Balsamic Vinegar

Sun Luck
Rice Vinegar (Natural, Seasoned)

Tosca
Balsamic White Vinegar

Trader Joe's
Orange Muscat Champagne Vinegar

Valu Time (Brookshire)
Cider Flavored Vinegar
White Distilled Vinegar

Vons
Apple Cider Vinegar
Cider Vinegar
Distilled White Vinegar
White Vinegar

Wegmans
Apple Cider Vinegar
Balsamic Vinegar Spray, Two Leaf
Cider Vinegar
Red Wine Vinegar
White Distilled Vinegar

White House
White House (All)
Woeber ⓘ
Cider Flavored Vinegar
Distilled White Vinegar
Pure Apple Cider Vinegar
Real Red Wine Vinegar
Tarragon Vinegar

WORCESTERSHIRE SAUCE

Best Choice
Worcestershire Sauce
Crystal
Worcestershire Sauce (All)
Food Club (Brookshire)
Worcestershire Sauce
Food Club (Marsh)
Worcestershire Sauce
French's
Worcestershire Sauce (Extra
Tenderizing, Reduced Sodium)
Golding Farms ⓘ
Worcestershire Sauce
Great Value (Wal-Mart) 🗓25
Worcestershire Sauce
Heinz
Worcestershire Sauce
Hill Country Fare (H-E-B)
Worcestershire Sauce
Hy-Vee
Worcestershire Sauce
Lea & Perrins
Worcestershire Sauce (All Varieties)
Meijer
Worcestershire Sauce
Robbie's Sauces
Worcestershire Sauce
Schnucks
Worcestershire Sauce
TryMe
Wine & Pepper Worcestershire
Valu Time (Brookshire)
Worcestershire Sauce
Vons 〰
Worcestershire Sauce

Wizard's, The ✓
Organic Gluten-Free Vegan
Worcestershire

MISCELLANEOUS

Alpino
Hot Pepper Mix Giardiniera
Mild Pepper Mix Giardiniera
Muffalata
Beano's ⓘ
"When Buffaloes Fly" Chicken Wing
Sauce
All American Sandwich Spread
Buffalo Sandwich Sauce
Italian Submarine Dressing
Original Submarine Dressing
Smokey Bacon Sandwich Sauce
Southwest Sandwich Sauce
Wasabi Sandwich Sauce
Best Foods
Sandwich Spread
Best Maid/Del-Dixi
Sandwich Spread
Bombay
Garlic Paste
Ginger Garlic Paste
Ginger Paste
Tandoori Paste
Bragg
Liquid Aminos (All)
Cat Cora's Kitchen
Feta Cheese Tapenade
Green Olive Tapenade
Kalamata Olive Tapenade
Smoked Eggplant Spread
Cub Foods
Sandwich Spread
Cugino's ()
Garlic Spread
Darbo
Lingonberry Sauce
Stewed Plums
DeLallo
Prince Omar Baba Ghannouj
Di Lusso
Sandwich Spread

Sweet Onion Sauce

Dietz & Watson ✓
Hoagie Dressing
Muffaletta Mix
Sandwich Spread

Divine Brine ()
Beet Caviar

East Wind Nut Butters
Tahini

Essie's South American Style Sauce
Essie's South American Style Sauce

Food Club (Brookshire)
Chili Sauce
Sandwich Spread

Gaea ()
Tapenades (All)

Galassi Foods
Sauces (All)

Garlic Valley Farms
Garlic Juice (All)

Ginger People, The ()
Ginger Spread

Goya
Sofrito

GranoVita
Mushroom Savoury Pâté
Mushroom Savoury Pâté (Chubb Pack)
Olive Savoury Pâté
Organic Brown Sauce
Organic Ready Spready (Herb, Original)
Organic Tofu Pâté (Yeast Free Tomato, Yeast Free Spicy Mexican)
Ready Spready (Herb Provence, Mushroom, Original)
Shiitake Mushroom Savoury Pâté
Vegetable Savoury Pâté

Hellmann's
Sandwich Spread

Jewel-Osco
Sandwich Spread

Joyva
Sesame Tahini

Karma Sauce
Bad Karma Sauce
Curry Karma Sauce
Good Karma Sauce
Smokey Karma Sauce

Kevala
Tahini

Kroger
Sandwich Spread

Leahey Gardens ⓘ
Gluten Free Cheese Sauce

Louisiana Fish Fry ⓘ
Wings Sauce

Market District (Giant Eagle)
Cheddar Horseradish

Organic Gourmet
Bearnaise Sauce Mix
Hollandaise Sauce Mix
Savoury Spread Nutritional Yeast Extract

Oskri
Tahini

Peloponnese
Baba Ghanoush
Eggplant Spread

Robbie's Sauces
Garlic Sauce

Sbarro
Garlic Sauce

Schnucks
Garlic Wing Sauce
Wing Sauce (Hot, Medium, Mild)

Schnucks Select
Sweet Onion Sauce

Shiloh's ✓
Bearnaise Sauce
Chimichurri Aioli

Stokes Sauces
Coronation Sauce

Stop & Shop
Fat Free Grated Topping

Tassos
Spreads (All)

Trader Joe's
Artichoke Red Pepper Tapenade
Bruschetta Sauce
Chili Pepper Sauce
Curry Simmer Sauce
Masala Simmer Sauce
Red Pepper Spread With Garlic And Eggplant
Tahini Sauce

Valu Time (Brookshire)
Sandwich Spread
Vietti ⓘ
Hot Dog Sauce
Rays Coney Island Sauce
Rudy's Hot Dog Sauce
Texas Pete Meatless Hot Dog Sauce
Tony Packo Hot Dog Sauce
Wagners
Hollandaise
Wild Thymes ⓘ
Cranberry Apple Walnut Sauce
Cranberry Fig Sauce
Cranberry Raspberry Sauce
Wilderness Poets
Hempspreads (All)
Tahini (All)

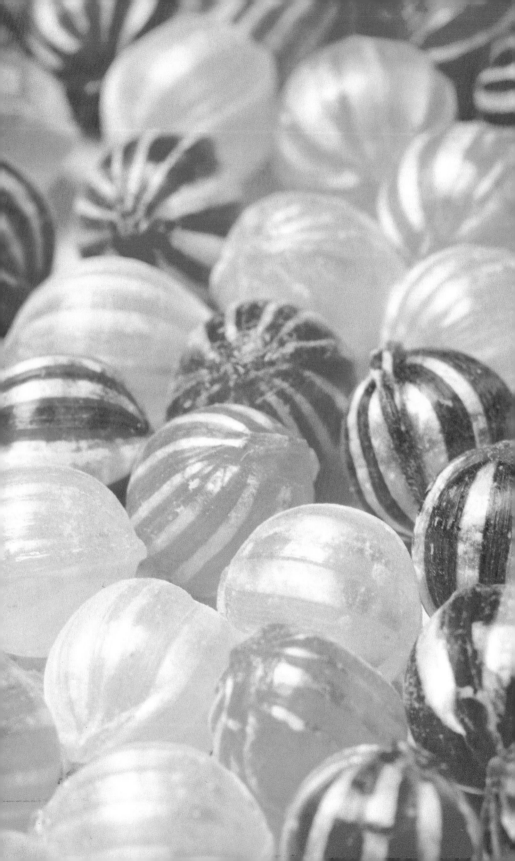

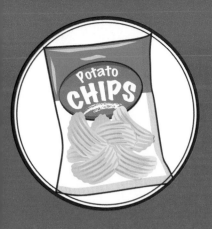

SNACKS & CONVENIENCE FOODS

APPLESAUCE

ACME
Applesauce
Cinnamon Applesauce
Natural Applesauce
Sweetened Applesauce

Albertsons
Applesauce
Cinnamon Applesauce
Strawberry Applesauce

Always Save
Applesauce

Best Choice
Applesauce
Cinnamon Applesauce
Natural Applesauce
Sweetened Applesauce

Cub Foods
Cinnamon Applesauce
Original Applesauce
Regular Applesauce
Strawberry Applesauce
Unsweetened Applesauce

Darbo
Applesauce

Eden Foods
Organic Applesauce
Organic Cherry Applesauce
Organic Cinnamon Applesauce
Organic Strawberry Applesauce

Flavorite (Cub Foods)
Applesauce
Cinnamon Applesauce
Regular Applesauce

Unsweetened Applesauce

Food Club (Brookshire)
Applesauce
Cinnamon Applesauce
Mixed Berry Applesauce
Natural Applesauce
Strawberry Applesauce

Food Club (Marsh)
Applesauce
Chunky Applesauce
Cinnamon Applesauce
Mixed Berry Applesauce
Natural Applesauce
Regular Applesauce
Strawberry Applesauce

Food You Feel Good About (Wegmans)
Applesauce with Vitamin C and Calcium
Chunky Natural Applesauce
Natural Applesauce

Full Circle (Price Chopper)
Applesauce
Natural Applesauce
Organic Natural Applesauce

Full Circle (Schnucks)
Cinnamon Applesauce
Organic Applesauce
Sweetened Applesauce

Giant
Applesauce
Chunky Applesauce
Cinnamon Applesauce
Natural Applesauce

Giant Eagle
Applesauce
Applesauce with Vitamins and Calcium
Chunky Applesauce
Cinnamon Applesauce
Mixed Berry Applesauce
Strawberry Applesauce
Unsweetened Applesauce
Unsweetened Applesauce with Vitamins

GoGo SqueeZ
GoGo Squeez (All)

Great Value (Wal-Mart) 25
Applesauce
Cinnamon Applesauce
Natural Applesauce
No Sugar Added Applesauce Sweetened
with Splenda
Strawberry Flavored Applesauce
Unsweetened Applesauce

GreenWise Market (Publix)
Organic Apple Sauce - Original
Organic Apple Sauce - Unsweetened

Haggen
Cinnamon Applesauce
Natural Applesauce
Regular Applesauce

Hy-Vee
Applesauce
Cinnamon Applesauce
Natural Applesauce
Unsweetened Applesauce

Jewel-Osco
Applesauce
Chunky Applesauce
Cinnamon Applesauce
Natural Applesauce
Sweetened Applesauce

Leroux Creek
Apple Sauce (All)

Meijer
Chunky Applesauce
Cinnamon Applesauce
Mixed Berry Applesauce
Natural Applesauce
Organic Cinnamon Applesauce
Organic Sweetened Applesauce
Organic Unsweetened Applesauce

Original Applesauce
Strawberry Applesauce

Midwest Country Fare (Hy-Vee)
Applesauce with Peaches
Applesauce with Raspberries
Applesauce with Strawberries
Home Style Applesauce
Unsweetened Applesauce

Mrs. Bryant's
Orchard Fresh Gourmet™ Blueberry
Applesauce (No Sugar Added)
Orchard Fresh Gourmet™ Cherry
Applesauce (No Sugar Added)
Orchard Fresh Gourmet™ Cranberry
Applesauce
Orchard Fresh Gourmet™ Original
Cinnamon Applesauce
Orchard Fresh Gourmet™ Strawberry
Applesauce (No Sugar Added)

Nature's Promise (Giant)
Organic Applesauce
Organic Applesauce Cups

Nature's Promise (Stop & Shop)
Organic Applesauce
Organic Applesauce Cups
Organic Cinnamon Applesauce Cups

Our Family
Cinnamon Applesauce (Cups)
Natural Unsweetened Applesauce
Original Applesauce
Strawberry Applesauce (Cups)

Price Chopper
Tropical Fruit Applesauce

Publix
Chunky Applesauce
Cinnamon Applesauce
Old Fashioned Applesauce
Unsweetened Applesauce

Safeway
Applesauce
Chunky Sweetened Apple Sauce in
Glass Jar
Cinnamon Applesauce
Natural Applesauce
Squeezable Applesauce Pouches
Squeezable Banana Applesauce Pouches

Squeezable Cinnamon Applesauce Pouches
Squeezable Strawberry Applesauce Pouches
Sweetened Applesauce in a Glass Jar
Unsweetened Applesauce in a Glass Jar

Schnucks
Applesauce
Chunky Applesauce
Cinnamon Applesauce
Mixed Berry Applesauce
Natural Applesauce
Strawberry Applesauce

Shaw's
Applesauce
Cinnamon Applesauce
Natural Applesauce

Stop & Shop
Applesauce
Applesauce Cups
Cinnamon Applesauce Cups
Natural Applesauce
Natural Style Applesauce

Sunflower Markets ☒
Applesauce

Valu Time (Schnucks)
Applesauce

Vons ∽
Applesauce
Cinnamon Applesauce
Gravenstein Applesauce

Wacky Apple ☒
Applesauce

Wegmans
Cinnamon Applesauce
Cinnamon Applesauce with Calcium and Vitamin C
MacIntosh Applesauce - Sweetened
Mixed Berry Applesauce
Peach Mango Applesauce
Sweetened Applesauce
Sweetened Chunky Applesauce
Sweetened with Calcium and Vitamin C Applesauce

White House
White House (All)

Winn-Dixie
Cinnamon Applesauce
Sweetened Applesauce
Unsweetened Applesauce

BAKED GOODS

Aimee's Livin' Magic
Livin' the Good Life Brownie
Wild Vanilla Blondie

Amy's Kitchen ✓
Gluten Free Chocolate Cake

Bi Aglut
Bi Aglut (All)

Biscuiterie de Provence ⓘ
Délice de l'Amandier
Délice du Chataigner

Bodhi's Bakehouse
Lupin Loaf

Caffe Portofino ☒
Gluten Free Cheesecakes

Canyon Bakehouse ☒
Cranberry Crunch Muffins

Cookies... for Me? ☒
Baked Goods (All)

Crave Bakery ✓
Crave Bakery (All)

Earth Café ☒ ✓
Earth Café (All)

Ener-G
Brownies
Cinnamon Rolls
Plain Doughnut Holes
Plain Doughnuts
Poundcake

Farmo ✓
Farmo (All)

Foods by George ☒
Blueberry Muffins
Brownies
Corn Muffins
Crumb Cake
Pound Cake

Frankly Natural Bakers
Gluten-Free Carob Almondine Brownie
Gluten-Free Cherry Berry Brownie
Gluten-Free Java Jive Brownie

Gluten-Free Misty Mint Brownie
Gluten-Free Wacky Walnut Brownie
Free to Enjoy
Mini Jaffa Cakes
French Meadow Bakery
Gluten-Free Fudge Brownie
Gilbert's Goodies ⓘ ✓
Gilbert's Goodies (All)
Gillian's Foods ⛧
Gillian's Foods (All)
Glenny's ✓
Brown Rice Marshmallow Treats,
    Chocolate
Brown Rice Marshmallow Treats, Peanut
    Caramel
Brown Rice Marshmallow Treats,
    Raspberry Jubilee
Brown Rice Marshmallow Treats,
    Vanilla
Gluten Free Cookie Jar Baking Co, The
The Gluten Free Cookie Jar (All)
Gluten Free Harvest, A
A Gluten Free Harvest (All)
Glutenfreeda ⓘ ⛧
Cheesecakes (All)
Glutino
Glazed Chocolate Donuts
Glazed Original Donuts
Gluuteny ⛧
Gluuteny (All)
Grainless Baker, The ⛧
The Grainless Baker (All)
Hail Merry
Miracle Tarts (All)
Inspired Cookie, The ✓
Chocolate Chunk Brownies
Jennies
Pound Cake Minis (All)
JK Gourmet
Muffin Loaves (All)
Joan's GF Great Bakes
Joan's GF Great Bakes (All)
Katz Gluten Free
Apricot Tart
Chocolate Chip Cookies
Chocolate Cupcakes
Chocolate Dipped Cookies

Chocolate Rugelech
Chocolate Strip
Cinnamon Rugelech
Cinnamon Strip
Colored Sprinkle Cookies
Honey Loaf
Honey Muffins
Kishka Kugel
Marble Cake
Raspberry Tart
Sugar Free Vanilla Cookies
Vanilla Cookies
Vanilla Cupcakes
Kookie Karma ✓
Holisitic Choco Lot
Holistic Chocolate Chip
Raw Banana Bread
Raw Carob Truffle
Raw Cherry Cashew
Raw Lemon Fig
Lakeview Farms
Cherry Cheesecake
Strawberry Cheesecake
Little Aussie Bakery, The
The Little Aussie Bakery (All)
Margarita's
Strawberry Cheesecake
Mariposa Baking Company
Cinnamon Rolls
Coconut Lemon Squares
Corn Bread (Seasonal)
Mini Pecan Pie (Seasonal)
Mocha Truffle Brownies
Penguino Cupcakes
Polar Bear Cupcakes
Sour Cream Coffeecake
Truffle Brownies
Walnut Truffle Brownies
Mrs. Bryant's
Blueberry Apple Bread
Cherry Apple Bread
Cranberry Apple Bread
Raisin Apple Bread
Strawberry-Cherry-Cranberry Apple
    Bread
Nature's Promise (Giant)
Organic Cinnamon Applesauce Cups

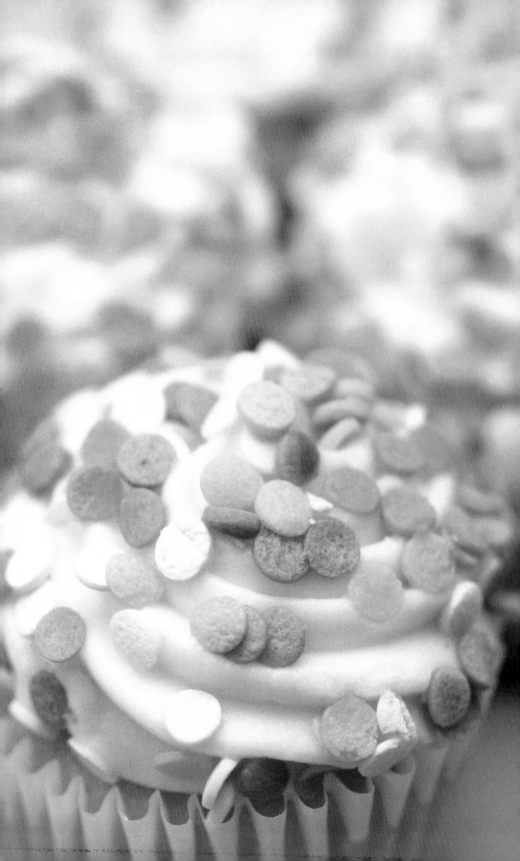

GLUTEN-FREE JOY.

REAL FRUIT. WHOLE SOY. ALL JOY.

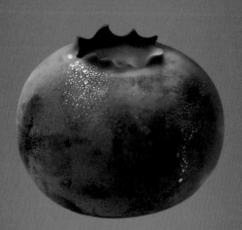

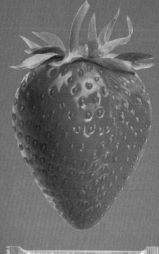

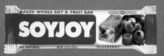

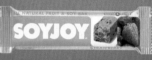

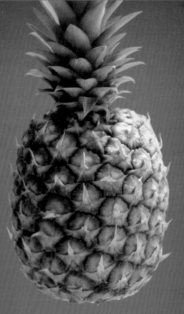

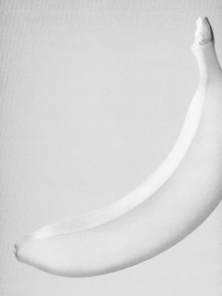

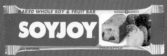

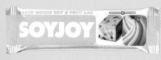

LEARN MORE OR BUY ONLINE AT SOYJOY.COM

Nina's Nutritious Cookies ⓘ
- Chocolate Cookie
- Orange Cake

Outside the Breadbox ⚥
- Outside the Breadbox (All)

Pamela's Products ⓘ
- Agave Sweetened New York Cheesecake
- Chocolate Fudge Cake
- Coffee Cake
- Hazelnut Cheesecake with Chocolate Crust
- White Chocolate Raspberry Cheesecake
- Zesty Lemon Cheesecake

Shabtai Gourmet Gluten-Free Bakery ⚥
- Gluten Free & Egg Free Bon Bons
- Gluten Free 7 inch Occasion Layer Cake
- Gluten Free Apricot Roll
- Gluten Free Brownie Bites
- Gluten Free Devils Food Seven Layer Cake
- Gluten Free Devils Stix (Baby Swiss Rolls)
- Gluten Free Fudge Brownie
- Gluten Free Honey Loaf Cake
- Gluten Free Marble Loaf Cake
- Gluten Free Raspberry Roll
- Gluten Free Ring Ting Cupcakes
- Gluten Free Seven Layer White Cake
- Gluten Free Sponge Cake Loaf
- Gluten Free Swiss Chocolate Roll

Smart Treat ⚥
- Smart Treat (All)

Sweet Cake Bake Shop ⚥
- Gluten Free Brownies and Bars (All)

Tate's Bake Shop ⓘ ✓
- Gluten Free Brownies

Trader Joe's
- Flourless Chocolate Cake

Tropical Cheese
- Arepa Amarilla
- Arepa Blanca
- Arepa de Choclo
- Arepa de Queso

Udi's Gluten Free Foods ⚥ ✓
- Blueberry Muffins
- Chocolate Chia Fortified Muffin Tops
- Cinnamon Rolls

- Dark Chocolate Brownie Bites
- Double Chocolate Muffins
- Lemon Streusel Muffins
- Oat & Blueberry Fortified Muffin Tops

BARS

22 Days
- Energy Bars (All)
- Protein Bars (All)

ALPSNACK ✓
- Bars (All)

Amazing Grass ⓘ ✓
- Energy Bars (All)

ANDI ⚥
- Protein Bars (All)

Attune ⓘ ✓
- Dark Chocolate Probiotic Bar
- Milk Chocolate Crisp Probiotic Bar
- Mint Chocolate Probiotic Bar

Bakery on Main ⚥ ✓
- Apple Cinnamon Soft & Chewy Granola Bars
- Apple Pie Flavor Instant Oatmeal
- Apricot Almond Chai Truebar
- Chocolate Almond Soft & Chewy Bars
- Coconut Cashew Truebar
- Cranberry Maple Nut Granola Bars
- Extreme Trail Mix Granola Bars
- Fruit & Nut Truebar
- Hazelnut Chocolate Cherry Truebar
- Maple Multigrain Muffin Flavor Instant Oatmeal
- Peanut Butter & Jelly Soft & Chewy Granola Bars
- Peanut Butter Chocolate Chips Granola Bars
- Raspberry Chocolate Almond Truebar
- Strawberry Shortcake Flavor Instant Oatmeal
- Walnut Cappuccino Truebar

Balance Bar ()
- Peanut Butter Bar

Bellybar
- Lemoney Lovey Bellybar

Bi Aglut
- Bi Aglut (All)

Black Lab Naturals ✓
Gluten-Free Date Bars (All)
BoomiBar ⚇
Boomi Bar (All)
Bora Bora ✓
Exotic Coconut Almond Superfood Bar
Hula Cacao Hazelnut Antioxidant Bar
Island Brazil Nut Almond Energy Bar
Native Walnut Acai Superfood Bar
Pacific Mango Macadamia
Antioxidant Bar
Paradise Walnut Pistachio
Antioxidant Bar
Tiki Blueberry Flax Antioxidant Bar
Tropical Sesame Cranberry Superfood
Bar
Volcanic Chocolate Banana Energy Bar
Wild Pomegranate Pecan Superfood Bar
Brookfarm ⓘ
Gluten Free Muesli Bar
BumbleBar ⚇
BumbleBar (All)

Byron Bay Cookies ⓘ
White Chocolate Macadamia Nut
Cookie Bar
Can Do Kid ✓
Can Do Kid Bars (All)
Coconut Secret ⓘ
Coconut Snack Bars (All)
Crispy Cat Candy Bars ✓
Chocolate Sundae
Mint Coconut
Toasted Almond
Ener-G
Chocolate Chip Snack Bars
Enjoy Life Foods ⚇ ✓
Caramel Apple Chewy Bars
Cocoa Loco Chewy Bars
Sunbutter Crunch Chewy Bars
Very Berry Chewy Bars
EnviroKidz ⓘ ✓
Cheetah Berry Crispy Rice Bars
Koala Chocolate Crispy Rice Bars
Lemur Peanut Choco Drizzle Crispy
Rice Bars

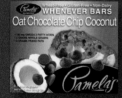
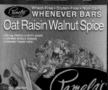
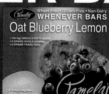
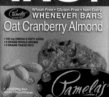

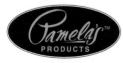

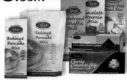

Panda Peanut Butter Crispy Rice Bars
Penguin Fruity Burst Crispy Rice Bars

Figamajigs ⓘ
Figamajigs (All)

Fiona's Granola
Quinoa Bars (All)

Frankly Natural Bakers
Gluten-Free Apricot Energy Bar
Gluten-Free Date Nut Energy Bar
Gluten-Free Raisin Energy Bar
Gluten-Free Tropical Energy Bar

Glenny's ✓
Cashew & Almond Bar
Cherry & Almond Bar
Cranberry & Almond Bar
Fruit & Nut Classic Bar

Gluten Free Café
Chocolate Sesame Bar
Cinnamon Sesame Bar
Lemon Sesame Bar

Glutino
Apple Breakfast Bars
Blueberry Breakfast Bars
Cherry Breakfast Bars
Chocolate Banana Organic Bar
Chocolate Peanut Butter Organic Bar
Strawberry Breakfast Bars
Wildberry Organic Bar

Go Raw ✓
Go Raw (All)

GoMacro ✓
Almond Butter with Carob Macrobar
Banana Almond Macrobar
Cashew Butter Macrobar
Cashew Caramel Macrobar
Cherries N' Berries Macrobar
Chocolate Crunch Macrobar
Granola with Coconut Macrobar
Peanut Butter Chocolate Chip Macrobar
Peanut Protein Macrobar
Tahini Date Macrobar

Greens +
Chia Bar Natural
Energy Bar Natural
Protein Bar Natural
Whey Krisp
Wildberry Energy Bar

Wildberry Protein Bar

Honey Stinger ⓘ
Energy Bars

JK Gourmet
Granola Bars (All)

JustFruit
JustFruit (All)

Kaia Foods ✓
Gluten-Free Sprouted Buckwheat
Granola Bars (All Flavors)

KIND ⚇ ✓
KIND Snacks (All)

Kookie Karma ✓
Raw Granola Bar

Larabar
Larabar (All)

Luna
Luna Protein, Chocolate
Luna Protein, Chocolate Cherry
Almond
Luna Protein, Chocolate Peanut Butter
Luna Protein, Cookie Dough
Luna Protein, Mint Chocolate Chip

Lydia's Organics ⚇
Lydia's Organics (All)

Manischewitz
Raspberry Jell Bars

Meijer
Extreme Snack Bars

Mrs. May's Naturals
Sesame Strips Bars (All)
TRIO Bars (All)

Nature's Promise (Giant)
Organic Honey Roasted Cranberry
Snack Bar

Nature's Promise (Stop & Shop)
Organic Honey Roasted Cranberry
Snack Bar

Nugo Nutrition ⓘ ✓
Nugo 10 - Apple Cinnamon
Nugo 10 - Cranberry
Nugo 10 - Lemon
Nugo Dark - Chocolate Pretzel
Nugo Dark - Mint Chocolate Chip
Nugo Dark - Peanut Butter Cup
Nugo Free - Carrot Cake
Nugo Free - Dark Chocolate Crunch

Nugo Free - Dark Chocolate Trail Mix

Omega Smart Bar
Omega Smart Bar (All)

Organic Nectars
Raw Cacao Chocolate Bars (All)

Oskri
Bars (All)

Pamela's Products ⓘ
Oat Blueberry Lemon Whenever Bars
Oat Chocolate Chip Coconut Whenever Bars
Oat Cranberry Almond Whenever Bars
Oat Raisin Walnut Spice Whenever Bars

POM Wonderful
POM Wonderful (All)

PranaBar ♀
PranaBar (All)

Promax ⓘ
Bars (All BUT Cookies n' Cream, Always Verify Gluten-Free Printed on Label)

Pure Bar ⓘ
Pure Bars (All)

PureFit ✓
PureFit (All)

Raw Revolution ✓
Raw Revolution (All)

RiseBar ♀
RiseBar (All)

Ruth's Hemp Foods ✓
Flax Bars (All)
Hemp Bars (All)
MacaPower Bars (All)

Safeway Select ∾
72 % Dark Chocolate Blueberry Almond Bar
72% Dark Chocolate Cranberry Orange Bar
Lemonade Fruit Bars
Lime Fruit Bars
Orange Fruit Bars
Strawberry Fruit Bars

Schar ♀
Chocolate Hazelnut Bars

SoyJoy
SoyJoy Bars (All)

Tanka
Tanka Bar

Taste of Nature
Argentina Peanut Plains Bar
Brazilian Nut Fiesta Bar
California Almond Valley Bar
Niagara Apple Country Bar
Quebec Cranberry Carnival

thinkThin ✓
thinkThin Bites (All)
thinkThin Crunch (All)
thinkThin Dessert Bars (All)
thinkThin Protein Bars (All)

Tiger's Milk ◌
Peanut Butter & Honey
Peanut Butter
Protein Rich

Trader Joe's
Gluten Free Granola
Golden Roasted Flaxseed With Blueberries
Golden Roasted Whole Flaxseed

Two Moms in the Raw ⓘ
Chia Bars (All)
Granola Bars (Made with GF Oats) (All)
Nut Bars (All)

Zing ⓘ ✓
Zing Bars (All)

ZonePerfect
Blueberry
Chocolate Almond Raisin
Chocolate Caramel Cluster
Chocolate Chip Cookie Dough
Chocolate Coconut Crunch
Chocolate Peanut Butter
Dark Chocolate Caramel Pecan
Double Dark Chocolate
Fudge Graham

BEEF JERKY & OTHER MEAT SNACKS

Cheyenne Brand ◌
Beef & Cheese
Hot Snack Stick
Mild Snack Stick
Original
Peppered

Red Hot Sausage
Spicy Snack Stick
Teriyaki
Food Club (Brookshire)
Honey BBQ Beef Jerky
Original Beef Jerky
Original Beef Steak Nuggets
Peppered Beef Jerky
Full Circle (Schnucks)
Organic Beef Jerky, Original
Organic Beef Jerky, Teriyaki
Golden Valley Natural
BBQ Turkey Jerky
Organic Beef Jerky (All)
J&D's
Cheddar BaconPOP
Regular BaconPOP
Old Dutch Foods
Original Beef Jerky
Old Wisconsin ⓘ 🔲25
Beef Summer Sausage
Original Summer Sausage
Snack Bites — Beef
Snack Bites — Pepperoni
Snack Bites — Turkey
Snack Sticks — Beef
Snack Sticks — Pepperoni
Snack Sticks — Spicy Beef
Snack Sticks — Turkey
Our Family
Beef Sticks
Price Chopper
Beef Jerky- Original
Beef Jerky- Peppered
Beef Jerky- Teriyaki
Seltzer's
Beef Jerky ()
Beef Sticks ()
Dried Beef ()
Shelton's ⓘ
Beef Jerky
Pepperoni Turkey Sticks
Regular Turkey Sticks
Turkey Jerky, Hot
Turkey Jerky, Regular
Tanka
Tanka Bites

Tanka Wild Sticks
Tasty Eats
Original Vegetarian Jerky
Tandoori Vegetarian Jerky

CANDY & CHOCOLATE

Aimee's Livin' Magic
Brazilian Beauty
Faerie Hearts
Hot Hearts & Roses Aphrodisiac Elixir
Life by Chocolate
Maca Mamma's Hazelnut Cups
Magic Hearts
Magic Walnut Clusters
Masala Dark Chocolate Leaves
Nipples of Venus
Peppermint Bliss Creme-Filled Bon-Bons
Pistachio Dreams
Purple Velvet Rosebuds
Reishi Peanut Butter Cups
Smart Chocolate
Superhero Peppermint Swirls
Superhero Spheres
Superhero Sunbursts Cosmic Chocolates
Alter Eco Fair Trade ⓘ
Chocolate (All)
Andes
Andes (All)
Annabelle's
Big Hunk Bar (2 oz.) ☒
Big Hunk Bar (Miniatures) ()
Atomic FireBall
Atomic Fireball (All)
Baby Bottle Pop
Baby Bottle Pop (All)
Baby Ruth
Baby Ruth
Bernod Group ☒
Organic Cotton Candy
Best Choice
Blow Pops
Chocolate Peanuts
Chocolate Stars
Circus Peanuts
Gummi Bears

Gummy Sour Worms
Gummy Worms
Jawbreakers
Laffy Taffy
Lemon Drops
Orange Slices
Runts
Smarties
Spearmint
Starlight Mints

Bit-O-Honey
Bit-O-Honey

Black Forest Gummies
Black Forest Gummies (All)
Fruit Snacks (All)

Bogdon Candy
Bogdon Candy (All)

Bosco
Chocolate Bars (All)

Boston Baked Beans
Boston Baked Beans

Butterfinger
Butterfinger (NOT BF Crisp, BF Giant Bar, BF Snackerz, BF Medallions, BF Jingles, BF Hearts, BF Pumpkins)

Candy Tree, The ✓
Cherry Bites
Cherry Laces
Cherry Twists
Gluten Free Bites
Gluten Free Black Twists
Gluten Free Lariats
Lollipops (All Flavors)
Raspberry Bites
Raspberry Laces
Raspberry Twists
Strawberry Bites
Strawberry Laces
Strawberry Twists

Caramel Apple Pops
Caramel Apple Pops (All)

Caring Candies
Sucrose Free Chocolate
Sugar Free BonBons
Sugar Free Candy Canes
Sugar Free Doc's Pops Lollipops
Sugar Free Hard Boiled Candy
Sugar Free Mini Round Lollipops
Sugar Free Sour Spiralz Lollipops

Cella Cherries
Dark Chocolate Covered Cherries
Milk Chocolate Covered Cherries

Charbonnel et Walker
Bittermints
Bucks Fizz Truffles
Cappuccino Truffles
Caramel Truffles
Cocoa Dusted Milk Truffles
Dark Apricot Creams
Dark Brazil Nut
Dark Butter Foure
Dark Café Charbonnel
Dark Caramel Chocolate
Dark Caramel Vanilla
Dark Cecily
Dark Chocolate Solid Hearts
Dark Coffee Walnut
Dark Crown
Dark English Rose
Dark English Violet
Dark Enrobed Ginger
Dark Falstaff
Dark Fraise
Dark Framboise
Dark Fudge Chocolate
Dark Fudge Vanilla
Dark Gianduja
Dark Ginger Marzipan
Dark Ginger Sticks
Dark Ginger Thins
Dark Lemon
Dark Mandarin
Dark Marc de Champagne Hearts
Dark Marc de Champagne Truffles
Dark Marzipan Armande
Dark Menthe
Dark Mint Thins
Dark Montelimar
Dark Noisette Cream
Dark Orange Cointreau
Dark Orange Cream
Dark Orange Sticks
Dark Orange Thins
Dark Pomponette

Dark Praline Noisette
Dark Romano
Dark Rum Foure
Dark Thins
Dark Truffle Café
Lemon Truffles
Milk Apricot Creams
Milk Banoffee Truffles
Milk Brazil Nut
Milk Butter Foure
Milk Café Charbonnel
Milk Caramel Chocolate
Milk Caramel Vanilla
Milk Cecily
Milk Chocolate Solid Hearts
Milk Chocolate Truffles
Milk Crown
Milk Falstaff
Milk Fudge Chocolate
Milk Fudge Vanilla
Milk Ginger Marzipan
Milk Marc de Champagne Truffles
Milk Marzipan Armande
Milk Montelimar
Milk Noisette Cream
Milk Orange Cointreau
Milk Orange Cream
Milk Praline Noisette
Milk Romano
Milk Rum Foure
Milk Rum 'n' Raisin Barrel
Milk Thins
Milk Truffle Café
Mint Truffles
Pink Marc de Champagne Hearts
Pink Marc de Champagne Truffles
Plain Chocolate Truffles
Plain Gold Leaf Truffles
Port & Cranberry Truffles
Strawberry Truffles
Strawberry White Truffles
Vanilla Truffles
Vodka Truffles
White Chocolate Solid Hearts

Charleston Chew
Charleston Chew (All)

Charms
Charms Candy Carnival (All)
Charms Sour Balls (All)
Charms Squares (All)

Charms Blow Pops
Charms Blow Pops (All)
Charms Pops (All)
Super Blow Pops (All)

Child's Play
Child's Play (All)

Chocolate Dream
Dark Chocolate Dream, Almond
Dark Chocolate Dream, Pure Dark
Dark Chocolate Dream, Raspberry
Dark Chocolate Dream, Rice Crunch
Sweet Chocolate Dream, Creamy Sweet

CocoMira ✓
Toffee Crunch (All Flavors)

Concord Foods
Caramel Apple Kit
Caramel Apple Wrap

Crows
Crows (All)

Dots
Dots (All)
Tropical Dots (All)

Dryden & Palmer
Rock Candy (All)

Earth's Sweet Pleasures
Earth's Sweet Pleasures (All)

Empress Chocolate
Empress Chocolate (All)

Endangered Species Chocolate ✓
Bite-Sized Chocolates (All)
Chocolate Bars (All)

Enjoy Life Foods 🍴 ✓
Boom Choco Boom Crispy Rice Bar
Boom Choco Boom Dark Chocolate Bar
Boom Choco Boom Rice Milk Bar

Equal Exchange ⓘ
Chocolate Bars (All)

Ferrara Pan Candy Company
Assorted Fruit Discs
Butter Toffee
Butterscotch Discs
Cherry Sours
Cinnamon Discs

www.TheHersheyCompany.com

French Burnt Peanuts
Fruit Cocktails
Gummies (All)
Jellies (All)
Jelly Beans (All)
Jujus (All)
Lemon Drops
Root Beer Barrels
Sour Heads
Sour Jacks
Sour Watermelon
Starlight Mints (Chocolate, Peppermint, Spearmint)
Swirly Peppermint

Figamajigs ⓘ
Figamajigs (All)

Flavorite (ACME)
Spice Drops

Flavorite (Albertsons)
Spice Drops

Flavorite (Cub Foods)
Spice Drops

Fluffy Stuff Cotton Candy
Fluffy Stuff (All)

Food Club (Brookshire)
Chocolate Caramel Mini Cups
Chocolate Peanut Butter Cups

Frooties
Frooties (All)

Fruit Smoothie Pops
Fruit Smoothie Pops (All)

Gifts of Nature ✓
Dark Chocolate Coated Cranberries
Milk Chocolate Coated Cranberries
Tri Mix Coated Cranberries
White Silk Coated Cranberries

Gimbal's Fine Candies
Gimbal's (All)

Ginger People, The ()
Baker's Cut Crystallized Ginger Chips
Crystallized Ginger
Crystallized Ginger Medallions
Gin Gin's Boost Ultra Strength Ginger Candy
Gin Gin's Hard Candy
Ginger Chews (All)
Organic Crystallized Ginger

Premium Cut Crystallized Ginger

Go Raw ✓
Go Raw (All)

Goobers
Goobers

Goody Good Stuff ✓
Goody Good Stuff Gummies (All)

Goya
Chocolate "El Sol"
Chocolate Amargo
Chocolate Dulce
Chocolate Menier Bar
Chocolate Panela

Great Value (Wal-Mart) 25
Butterscotch Discs
Candy Corn
Cinnamon Disc
Cinnamon Discs
Fruit Smiles (Sour Apple, Watermelon, Blue Raspberry, Tropical Punch)
Fruit Smiles (Strawberry, Grape, Orange, Lemon)
Gummy Bears
Gummy Worms
Jelly Beans
Orange Slices
Peppermint Starlight Mints
Spearmint Starlight Mints
Spice Drops
Starlight Mints

Haribo
Haribo (All BUT Black Licorice Wheels, Red Licorice Wheels, Sour S'ghetti, Fruity Pasta, Brixx, Konfekt and Pontefract Cakes)

Hint Mint
Hint Mint (All)
Petit Hint Mint (All)

Hoffman's ()
Solid Chocolate Pieces

Holy Chocolate ()
Holy Chocolate (All)

Honees Candies
Honees (All)

Honey Acres
Honey Mints (All)

Hy-Vee
Chocolate Caramel Clusters
Chocolate Stars
Classic Starlight Mints
Double Dipped Chocolate Covered
Peanuts
Lemon Drops

JawBusters
JawBusters

Joyva
Halvah
Jell Rings
Marshmallow Twists
Sesame Crunch

Juicy Drop Pop
Juicy Drop Pop (All)

Junior Mints
Junior Caramel (All)
Junior Mints (All)

Justin's
Justin's (All)

Koeze
Caramel Crunch (All Varieties)
Cashew Brittle (All Varieties)
Clusters (All Varieties)
Puddles (All Varieties)

Laffy Taffy
Laffy Taffy
Laffy Taffy Fruitarts Chews
Laffy Taffy Rope

Landgarten
Berries Love a Mix of Chocolate
Cranberries Love Orange Chocolate
Ginger Loves Dark Chocolate
Gojiberries Love Dark Chocolate
Hazelnuts Love Milk Chocolate
Pineapples Love Milk Chocolate
Raspberries Love Dark Chocolate
Strawberries Love Milk Chocolate

Lang's Chocolates ()
Brittle
Chocolate Covered Nuts
Chocolates
Dessert Cups
Turtles

Lemonhead & Friends
Lemonhead & Friends (All)

Let's Do…Organic ✓
Organic Classic Gummi Bears
Organic Jelly Gummi Bears
Organic Super Sour Gummi Bears

Lik-M-Aid Fun Dip
Lik-M-Aid Fun Dip

Manischewitz
Caramel Cashew Patties
Chocolate Frolic Bears
Hazelnut Truffles
Max's Magic Lollycones
Peppermint Patties
Swiss Chocolate Mints
Viennese Crunch

Maple Grove Farms 🍾 ✓
Candy (All Varieties)

Marzipan House, The
The Marzipan House (All)

Mentos
Mentos (All)

Mike and Ike
Mike and Ike

Milka Chocolate ✍
Milk Chocolate Confection, Alpine Milk

Nestlé
Milk Chocolate

Newman's Own Organics ⓘ
Chocolate Bars (All)
Chocolate Cups (All)
Mint Rolls
Mints in Tins

Nips
Regular
Sugar Free

Oh Henry!
Oh Henry!

Old Dominion Peanut Company
Basket Candies (Butter Peanut Crunch,
Peanut Crunch)
Butter Toasted Pecans
Chocolate Coated (Dipped Peanuts,
Coated Brittle)
Old-Fashioned Brittle (Peanut, Cashew)
Peanut Candies (Bars, Butter Peanut
Crunch, Butter Toffee Peanuts,
Peanuts Squares)

Orgran ⓘ ⚊
   Molasses Licorice
Oskri
   Candy and Chocolate (All)
Our Family
   After Dinner Mints
   Apple Rings
   Assorted Rolls
   Bubble Gum
   Butterscotch Buttons
   Candy Corn
   Cherry Slices
   Cherry Sours
   Chocolate Almond Bark
   Chocolate Caramel Clusters
   Chocolate Peanuts
   Chocolate Stars
   Cinnamon Bears
   Circus Peanuts
   Fruit Slices
   Giant Jells
   Gummi Bears
   Gummi Burgers & Hot Dogs
   Gummi Worms
   Jaw Breakers
   Jelly Beans
   Orange Slices
   Peach Rings
   Peppermint Lozenges
   Rainbow Pops
   Salt Water Taffy
   Sour Neon Worms
   Spice Drops
   Starlight Mints
   Tootsie Midgees
   Vanilla Almond Bark
   Wintergreen Lozenges
Pearson Candy Company
   Pearson Candy Company (All)
PEZ
   PEZ Candy (All)
Piedmont Candy Co.
   Piedmont Candy (All)
Pixy Stix
   Pixy Stix
Poco Dolce
   Poco Dolce (All)

Pop Rocks
   Pop Rocks
Pops Galore
   Pops Galore (All)
Premium Chocolatiers
   Chocolates (All)
Price Chopper
   Canada Mints
   Cinnamon Buttons
   Circus Peanuts
   Gummi Worms
   Jelly Beans
   Laffy Taffy
   Mary Janes
   Milk Chocolate Raisins
   Pixy Stix
   Starlight Spearmint
   Tootsie Role
   Vanilla Caramel
Private Selection (Kroger)
   Gourmet Jelly Beans
Publix
   Butterscotch Discs
   Chocolate Brittle
   Chocolate Covered Peanut Brittle
   Double Dipped Chocolate Covered
    Peanuts
   Gummi Worms
   Lollipops
   Peanut Brittle
   Smarties Candy
   Sour Worms
   Starlight Mints Candy
Purity
   Bull's Eyes
   Candy Barrels
Push Pop
   Push Pop (All)
Raisinets
   Raisinets (All)
Red Bird
   Red Bird (All)
Red Hots
   Red Hots
Red Rocker Candy
   Brittles (All)
   Toffees (All)

Reed's
 Ginger Candy
Rendez Vous
 All Natural Hard Candies
Richardson Brands Company
 Gourmet Chocolate Mints
 Soft Sugar Mints
 Specialty Mints
Ring Pop
 Ring Pop (All)
River Street Sweets
 Bear Claws
 Brittle (All Flavors)
 Chocolate Barks
 Divinity
 Pralines
Safeway ᜂ
 Candy Corn
 Indian Corn
 Peanut Butter Cups
 Peanut Butter Cups Dark Chocolate
 Pumpkins
Schnucks
 Bit-O-Honey
 Bubble Gum
 Butterscotch Discs
 Candy Corn
 Cherry Sours Candy
 Cinnamon Bears
 Circus Peanuts
 Dum Dum Drops
 Giant Jells Candy
 Gum Balls
 Gummi Bears
 Gummi Burgers
 Gummi Worms
 Laffy Taffy
 Lemon Drops
 Orange Slices
 Salt Water Taffy
 Sour Neon Worms
 Spearmint Leaves
 Spearmint Starlight
 Spice Drops
 Starlight Mints
 Tootsie Rolls

Smarties
 Smarties (All)
Sno-Caps
 Sno-Caps
Sour Patch Kids ᜂ
 Candy, Soft & Chewy Sour Then Sweet
  Blue Raspberry
 Candy, Soft & Chewy Sour Then Sweet
  Cherry
 Candy, Soft & Chewy Sour Then Sweet
  Chillerz
 Candy, Soft & Chewy Sour Then Sweet
  Extreme
 Candy, Soft & Chewy Sour Then Sweet
  Fruits
 Candy, Soft & Chewy Sour Then Sweet
  Kids
 Candy, Soft & Chewy Sour Then Sweet
  Peach
 Candy, Soft & Chewy Sour Then Sweet
  Watermelon
Spangler Candy Company
 Candy Canes (All)
 Dum Dums (All)
 Marshmallow Products (All)
 Saf-T-Pops (All)
Spice Rack Chocolates
 Spice Rack Chocolates (All BUT
  Enfuego Collection)
Sugar Babies
 Sugar Babies
Sugar Daddy
 Sugar Daddy Pops
Sugar Mama
 Sugar Mama Caramels
Surf Sweets
 Surf Sweets (All)
SweetRiot
 Chocolate Products (All)
Taza Chocolate
 Chocolate Bars (All)
Tea Forte
 Minteas
Terrys ᜂ
 Chocolate, Orange Dark
 Chocolate, Orange Milk
 Chocolate, Pure Milk

Theo Chocolate ( )
45% Milk Chocolate
70% Dark Chocolate
85% Dark Chocolate
Apple Cider Caramel
Chai Tea Milk Chocolate
Cherry & Almond
Cherryfest Caramel
Coconut Curry Milk Chocolate
Coffee
Coffee Salted Caramel
Dominican Republic 84%
Fig, Fennel & Almond
Ghost Chile Salted Caramel
Grey Salted Vanilla Caramel
Hazelnut Crunch Milk Chocolate
Lavender Caramel
Madagascar 74%
Mint
Orange
Pink Salted Vanilla Caramel
Roasted Cacao Nibs
Salted Almond Dark Chocolate
Salted Almond Milk Chocolate
Spicy Chile
Taste of Washington Caramel Collection
Theo & Audubon 91% Costa Rica Dark Chocolate
Theo & EMP 70% Dark Chocolate
Theo & Jane Goodall 45% Milk Chocolate
Theo & Jane Goodall 70% Dark Chocolate
Theo Th'mores
Toasted Coconut

Tic Tac
Tic Tac Mints (All)

Toblerone
Candy, Minis Swiss Chocolate With Honey & Almond Nougat
Candy, Minis Swiss Milk Chocolate With Honey & Almond Nougat
Candy, Minis White Confection With Honey & Almond Nougat
Candy, Swiss Bittersweet With Honey & Almond Nougat

Candy, Swiss Milk Chocolate With Honey & Almond Nougat
Candy, Swiss White Confection With Honey & Almond Nougat
Candy, Truffle Peaks

Too Tarts
Too Tarts (All)

Tootsie Pops
Tootsie Peppermint Pop
Tootsie Pops (All)

Tootsie Rolls
Tootsie Rolls (All)

Trader Joe's
70% Dark Chocolate Bar, Caramel with Black Sea Salt
70% Dark Chocolate Bar, Toffee with Walnuts & Pecans
Black Licorice Scottie Dogs
CarbSafe Sugar Free Chocolate Bars (Milk, Dark)
Chocolate Covered Blueberries
Chocolate Sunflower Seed Drops
Dark Chocolate Almonds Sea Salt and Sugar
Dark Chocolate Covered Caramels
Dark Chocolate Covered Cherries
Dark Chocolate Covered Espresso Beans
Dark Chocolate Covered Ginger
Dark Chocolate Covered Pomegranate Seeds
Dark Chocolate Covered Power Berries
Dark Chocolate Covered Raisins
Dark Chocolate Covered Toffee
Dark Chocolate Mint Creams
Dark Chocolate Peanut Butter Cups
English Toffee
Fair Trade Swiss Chocolate Bars (Milk, Dark)
Green Tea Mints
Milk And Dark Chocolate Covered Almonds
Milk Chocolate Covered Raisins
Milk Chocolate Peanut Butter Cups
Mini Milk Chocolate Peanut Butter Cups
Organic Chocolate Bars
Organic Pops

Ounce Plus 3pk Chocolate Bars
Peach Pops
Pound Plus Chocolate Bars
Yogurt Raisins
Tropical Source
Mint Crunch Dark Chocolate Bar
Raspberry Dark Chocolate Bar
Rice Crisp Dark Chocolate Bar
Rich Dark Chocolate Bar
Toasted Almond Dark Chocolate Bar
Tropical Stormz Pops
Tropical Stormz Pops (All)
Twinkle Candy
Twinkle Pops (All)
Two Moms in the Raw ⓘ
Truffles (All)
Valu Time (Brookshire)
Butterscotch Disks
Candy Corn
Circus Peanuts
Fruit Slices Candy
Gummi Bears
Gummi Worms
Hot Shots Candy
Jelly Beans
Orange Slices Candy
Root Beer Barrels
Smarties
Sour Worms
Spice Drops
Starlight Mints
VerMints ⚇
VerMints (All)
Warheads
Hard Candies (All)
Wegmans
Chocolate Covered Virginia Peanuts
Xan Confections ()
Xan Confections (All BUT Milk & Dark
Chocolate S'mores)
YC Chocolate
Almond Buttercrunch ()
Caramel Nut Clusters ()
Chocolate Bars
Truffles ()
Zip-A-Dee Mini Pop
Zip-A-Dee-Mini Pop (All)

Zotz
Zotz (All)

CHEESE PUFFS & CURLS

Always Save
Cheese Puffs
Barbara's Bakery
Cheese Puff Bakes (Original, White
Cheddar) ()
Cheese Puffs ()
Cheetos ⓘ
Crunchy Cheddar Jalapeno Cheese
Flavored Snacks
Crunchy Cheese Flavored Snacks
Crunchy Cheesy Cheddar BBQ Cheese
Flavored Snacks
Crunchy Fiery Fusion Cheese Flavored
Snacks
Crunchy Flamin' Hot Cheese Flavored
Snacks
Crunchy Flamin' Hot Limon Cheese
Flavored Snacks
Natural White Cheddar Puffs Cheese
Flavored Snacks
Puffs Cheese Flavored Snacks
Puffs Cheesy Poofs Cheese Flavored
Snacks
Puffs Flamin' Hot Cheese Flavored
Snacks
Puffs Honey BBQ Cheese Flavored
Snacks
Puffs Natural White Cheddar Cheese
Flavored Snacks
Twisted Cheese Flavored Snacks
Clearly Organic (Best Choice)
Cheese Puffs
EatSmart Naturals ⓘ
Whole Grain Cheese Curls
Fastco (Fareway)
Cheese Crunchy
Cheese Puffs
Food Club (Brookshire)
Snack Cheese Puffs
Great Value (Wal-Mart) 🔲25
Cheddar Cheese Crunch
Cheddar Cheese Puffs

Cheddar Flavor Cheese Sensations

Herr's ()
Buffalo Blue Cheese Curls
Crunchy Cheese Sticks
Honey Cheese Curls
Hot Cheese Curls
Hot Honey Cheese Curls
Jalapeno Poppers Cheese Curls
Regular Cheese Curls

Hill Country Fare (H-E-B)
Cheese Crunchy
Cheese Puffs

Kroger
Baked Cheese Balls
Baked Cheese Curls
Crunchy Cheese Curls
Value Cheese Curls

Meijer
Cheese Pops
Cheese Puffs
Cheezy Treats
White Cheddar Puffs

Neal Brothers
Organic Cheese Pops
Organic Cheese Puffs
Organic Cheese Twists

Old Dutch Foods
Bac'N Puffs (Hot & Spicy, Regular)
Baked Cheese Stix
Baked Crunchy Curls

Our Family
Baked Cheese Puffs

Pik-Nik ☃
Cheese Balls
Cheese Curls

Pirate's Booty ⓘ
Pirate's Booty (All)

Price Chopper
Cheese Balls

Publix
Crunchy Cheese Curls
Crunchy Cheese Puffs

Rancho Berenda ✓
Cheese Puffs
Smokin' Hot Cheese Puffs

Real McCoy's ✓
Jalapeno Cheddar Rice Puffs

Vermont White Cheddar Rice Puffs

Schnucks
Baked Cheese Puffs
Crunchy Cheese Snacks

Snikiddy ✓
Baked Cheese Puffs (All)

Snyder's of Hanover ⓘ
Cheese Twists

Trader Joe's
Buccaneer Joes White Cheddar Corn
Puffs
Crunchy Curls
Jalapeño Cheese Crunchies
Reduced Fat Cheese Crunchies

Utz ☃
Baked Cheese Balls
Baked Cheese Curls
Crunchy Cheese Curls
White Cheddar Cheese Curls

Valu Time (Brookshire)
Baked Cheese Puffs

Valu Time (Marsh)
Baked Cheese Puffs

Valu Time (Schnucks)
Cheese Flavor Crunchy

Value (Kroger)
Cheese Curls

Wellaby's
Cheese Ups, Classic Cheese
Cheese Ups, Parmesan
Cheese Ups, Smoked Cheese

Wise Snacks
Crunchy Cheese Doodles
Doodle O's
Puff Cheese Doodles

CHIPS & CRISPS, OTHER

Aimee's Livin' Magic
Apple Cinnamon Snappers
Crisps of Avalon
Hot Mama's Zucchini Chips
Over the Top! Onion Crisps
Over the Top! Onion Crisps Nama
Shoyu Free!
Walnut-Hemp Sun-Dried Tomato
Crispers

Always Save
- BBQ Corn Chips
- Big Dip Chips
- Corn Chips

Arico Natural Foods Company
- Cassava Chips (All)

Beanitos ⓘ ✔
- Bean Chips (All)

Brothers All Natural ⚱
- Fruit Crisps (All)

Byron Bay Cookies ⓘ
- Original Crisp Bread
- Rosemary & Sea Salt Crisp Bread

Calbee ⓘ
- Original Flavor Snapea Crisps
- Snapea Crisps Caesar

Cheetos ⓘ
- Fantastix Chili Cheese Flavored Baked Corn/Potato Snacks
- Fantastix Flamin' Hot Flavored Baked Corn/Potato Snacks

Chester's ⓘ
- Chili Cheese Flavored Fries
- Flamin' Hot Flavored Puffcorn Snacks
- Flamin' Hot Flavored Fries

Chifles
- Plantain Chips (All)

Classic Foods ⓘ
- Baked Classics
- California Classics

Corn Nuts ⌒
- Crunchy Corn Snacks, Barbecue
- Crunchy Corn Snacks, Chile Picante
- Crunchy Corn Snacks, Chile Picante Con Limon
- Crunchy Corn Snacks, Chorizo Chipotle
- Crunchy Corn Snacks, Limon
- Crunchy Corn Snacks, Nacho Cheese
- Crunchy Corn Snacks, Original
- Crunchy Corn Snacks, Ranch
- Crunchy Corn Snacks, Salsa Jalisco
- Crunchy Corn Snacks, Variety Pack 24 Ct

Crunchfuls ✔
- Crunchfuls (All)

Danielle Chips
- Danielle Chips (All)

EatSmart Naturals ⓘ
- Garden Veggie Crisps
- Gluten Free Pretzel Sticks

El's Kitchen ✔
- Gluten Free Bagel Snaps (All)

Fastco (Fareway)
- Blue Corn Chips
- Corn Chips
- Corn Pop

Fritos
- Flavor Twists Honey BBQ Flavored Corn Chips ⓘ
- Lightly Salted Corn Chips ✔
- Original Corn Chips ✔
- Scoops! Corn Chips ✔
- Tapatio Flavored Corn Chips ⓘ

Funyuns ⓘ
- Flamin' Hot Onion Flavored Rings
- Onion Flavored Rings

Glenny's ✔
- Organic Soy Crisps, Barbeque
- Organic Soy Crisps, Creamy Ranch
- Organic Soy Crisps, Sea Salt
- Organic Soy Crisps, White Cheddar
- Peanuts & Peanut Butter Bar
- Soy Crisps, Apple Cinnamon
- Soy Crisps, Barbeque
- Soy Crisps, Caramel
- Soy Crisps, Cheddar
- Soy Crisps, Creamy Ranch
- Soy Crisps, Lightly Salted
- Soy Crisps, Olive Oil
- Soy Crisps, Onion & Garlic
- Soy Crisps, Salt & Pepper
- Soy Crisps, White Cheddar
- Unsalted Soy Crisps

Go Raw ✔
- Super Chips (All)

Good Health Natural Products
- Apple Chips ()
- Humbles Olive, Lemon, & Feta Chips ()
- Humbles Sea Salt Chips ()

GoPicnic
- Banks Cassava Pepper Vegetable Chips

Goya
- Cassava Chips
- Garlic Plantain Chips

No Salt Plantain Chips
Plantain Chips
Plantain Strips
Sweet Plantain Chips
Grace Island Specialty Foods
Cheese Crisps (All)
Great Lakes International Trading ⓘ
Banana Crisps
Great Value (Wal-Mart)
Bigger Corn Chips
Corn Chips
Green Tree
Apple Chips (All)
H-E-B
Rice and Adzuki Bean Chips - Chipotle
Cheese Flavored
Rice and Adzuki Bean Chips - Salted
Herr's ⟨⟩
BBQ Corn Chips
BBQ Popped Chips
Cheddar Snack Friez
Cheesy Bacon Ranch Snack Friez
Hot Snack Friez
Ketchup Snack Friez
Sea Salt Popped Chips
Veggie Crisps
Hill Country Fare (H-E-B)
Corn Chips
Hot Kid
BBQ Rice Crisps
Cheese Rice Crisps
Masala Rice Crisps (International
Flavors)
Natural Rice Crisps
Pizza Rice Crisps
Seaweed Rice Crisps
Sesame Rice Crisps
Sundried Tomato Rice Crisps
(International Flavors)
Sweet Chili Rice Crisps
Thai Spice Rice Crisps (International
Flavors)
Unsalted Rice Crisps
Wasabi Rice Crisps
Kaia Foods ✓
Kale Chips

Kay's Naturals ✓
Protein Chips (All)
Kookie Karma ✓
Cheezy Kale Krackers
Herb Vegetables Krackers
Lundberg Family Farms
Fiesta Lime Rice Chips
Honey Dijon Rice Chips
Pico de Gallo Rice Chips
Santa Fe Barbecue Rice Chips
Sea Salt Rice Chips
Sesame & Seaweed Rice Chips
Wasabi Rice Chips
Mediterranean Snacks ⓘ
Baked Lentil Chips (All Flavors)
Mike-Sell's
Puffcorn (Cheddar, Movie Theater,
Original)
Nature's Promise (Giant)
Vegetable Chips
Nature's Promise (Stop & Shop)
Vegetable Chips
Newman's Own Organics ⓘ
Soy Crisps (Barbeque, Cinnamon Sugar,
Lightly Salted, White Cheddar)
Nonni's
Rissoto Chips
Old Dutch Foods
Arriba Tortilla Chips, Nacho Cheese
Restaurante Tortilla Chips, Bite Size
Restaurante Tortilla Chips, Bite Size
Nacho
Restaurante Tortilla Chips, Dip Strips
Restaurante Tortilla Chips, Restaurante
Style
Restaurante Tortilla Chips, Tostados
Restaurante Tortilla Chips, White Corn
Orgran ⓘ
Crispibites
Our Family
Corn Chips
Pirate's Booty ⓘ
Pirate's Booty (All)
Plocky's
Hummus Chips (All)
Popcorners ✓
Popcorners (All)

Publix
Corn Chips - King Size
Real McCoy's ✔
Sea Salt Rice Chips
Sweet and Spicy Rice Chips
Worcester and Chives Rice Chips
Sabritas ⓘ
Pizzerolas Flavored Corn Chips
Rancheritos Flavored Corn Chips
Safeway Select 〰
Banana Chips
Original Kettle Chip
Schnucks
BBQ Corn Chips
Caramel Corn Mini Rice Crisps
Cheddar Cheese Mini Rice Crisps
Corn Chip Ribbons
King Corn Chips
Ranch Mini Rice Crisps
Seneca Farms
Apple Chips
Crisp Onions
Snapdragon Pan-Asian Cuisine
Bangkok Sweet Chili Rice Crisps
Japanese Wasabi Rice Crisps
Sea Salt & Vinegar Rice Crisps
Sour Cream & Wasabi Rice Crisps
Teriyaki Spice Rice Crisps
Whole Grain Brown Rice Crisps
The Good Bean 🍴 ✔
Good Bean Snacks
Trader Joe's
Calbee Snapea Crisps
Cassava Chips
Organic Corn Chip Dippers
Roasted Plantain Chips
Sea Salt & Pepper Rice Crisps
Vacuum Fried Banana Chips
Vegetable Root Chips
Veggie Chips
Utz 🍴
Corn Chips (Barbeque, Plain)
Valu Time (Brookshire)
Crunchy Cheese Snacks
Regular Corn Chips
Valu Time (Schnucks)
BBQ Corn Chips

Corn Chips
Want-Want
Black Sesame Super Slim Brown Rice
Crisps
Garden Vegetable Super Slim Brown
Rice Crisps
Lime Super Slim Crinkles Rice Chips
Multigrain Super Slim Brown Rice
Crisps
Original Super Slim Brown Rice Crisps
Sea Salt Super Slim Crinkles Rice Chips
Sea Salt Super Slim Rice Crisps
Sesame Super Slim Rice Crisps
Sun Ripened Tomato Super Slim
Crinkles Rice Chips
Wegmans
Corn Chips
Wise Snacks
Dipsy Doodles
Onion Rings

CHIPS & CRISPS, POTATO

Always Save
BBQ Potato Chips
Black Pepper Chips
Cheddar & Sour Cream Chips
Regular Potato Chips
Sour Cream & Onion Chips
Wavy Chips
Best Choice
BBQ Oven Chips
Cheddar Oven Chips
Original Oven Chips
Shoestring Potato Sticks
Brothers All Natural 🍴
Potato Crisps (All)
Cape Cod ⓘ
Potato Chips (All)
Corazonas
Potato Chips
Cub Foods
Twin Ripple Potato Chips
Fastco (Fareway)
BBQ Chips
Kettle Chips
Kettle Jalapeno Chips

Kettle Salt & Vinegar Chips
Potato Chips
Rippled Chips
Sour Cream & Onion Chips

Food Club (Brookshire)
BBQ Kettle Potato Chips
BBQ Potato Chips
Cheddar & Sour Cream Potato Chips
Jalapeno Kettle Potato Chips
Kettle Potato Chips
Potato Sticks
Regular Potato Chips
Ripple Potato Chips
Salt and Pepper Kettle Potato Chips
Salt and Pepper Potato Chips
Sour Cream and Onion Potato Chips
Wavy Potato Chips

Food Club (Marsh)
BBQ Kettle Potato Chips
Original Kettle Potato Chips
Potato Sticks
Regular Potato Chips

Full Circle (Schnucks)
BBQ Chips
Regular Chips
Regular Kettle Chips
Ripple Chips
Salt & Vinegar Kettle Chips

Giant
Potato Sticks

Good Health Natural Products
Avocado Oil Potato Chips, Barcelona Barbeque ☻
Avocado Oil Potato Chips, Chilean Lime ☻
Avocado Oil Potato Chips, Sea Salt ☻
Glories Sweet Potato Chips ☻
Olive Oil Potato Chips, Cracked Pepper & Sea Salt ☻
Olive Oil Potato Chips, Garlic ☻
Olive Oil Potato Chips, Rosemary ☻
Olive Oil Potato Chips, Sea Salt ☻

Goya
Sweet Potato Chips

Herr's ()
1853 BBQ Kettle Chips
1853 Buttermilk & Herb Kettle Chips

1853 Kettle Chips
Baby Back Ribs Potato Chips
BBQ Low Salt Baked Crisps
Cheddar & Sour Cream Baked Crisps
Cheddar & Sour Cream Potato Chips
Cheddar Horseradish Kettle Chips
Cheddar Horseradish Potato Chips
Creamy Dill Potato Chips
Firemen's Chicken BBQ Potato Chips
Fire-Roasted Sweet Corn Potato Chips
Honey BBQ Potato Chips
Hot BBQ (Chillicothe) Potato Chips
Hot Chips Potato Chips
Jalapeno Kettle Chips
Jane's Krazy Mixed-Up Natural Kettle Chips
KC Prime Potato Chips
Ketchup Potato Chips
Lightly Salted Potato Chips
Loaded Baked Potato Chips
Natural Kettle Chips
New Yorker Potato Chips
No Salt Added Potato Chips
Old Bay Potato Chips
Old Fashioned Potato Chips
Original Baked Crisps
Pizza Potato Chips
Potato Stix Regular
Ragin' Ranch Potato Chips
Reduced Fat Kettle Chips
Regular BBQ (Low Salt)
Regular Kettle Chips
Regular Potato Chips
Ripple Kettle Chips
Ripple Potato Chips
Russet Kettle Chips
Salt & Pepper Potato Chips
Salt & Vinegar Potato Chips
Sea Salt & Cracked Pepper Kettle Chips
Sweet Potato Chips
Swiss Chocolate Covered Potato Chips
Tangy BBQ Baked Crisps
Texas Pete Hot Sauce Potato Chips
Texas Pete Hot Sauce Ripple Kettle Chips

Jay's ⓘ
BBQ Potato Chips

Curly Waves
Kettle Cooked Old Fashioned Potato
Chips
Open Pit BBQ Chips
Potato Chips
Ridges Sour Cream & Cheddar Potato
Chips

Kettle Brand
Potato Chips (All)

Kruncher! ⓘ
Hot Buffalo Wing Kettle Chips
Jalapeno Kettle Chips
Kosher Dill Kettle Chips
Original Kettle Chips
Sea Salt & Cracked Pepper Kettle Chips
Sweet Hawaiian Onion Kettle Chips

Lay's
Baked! Original Potato Crisps ✓
Baked! Parmesan & Tuscan Herb
Flavored Potato Crisps ⓘ
Baked! Sour Cream & Onion Artificially
Flavored Potato Crisps ⓘ
Baked! Southwestern Ranch Flavored
Potato Crisps ⓘ
Balsamic Sweet Onion Flavored Potato
Chips ⓘ
Cajun Herb & Spice Flavored Potato
Chips ⓘ
Cheddar & Sour Cream Artificially
Flavored Potato Chips ⓘ
Chile Limon Potato Chips ⓘ
Chipotle Ranch Flavored Potato Chips ⓘ
Classic Potato Chips ✓
Creamy Garden Ranch Flavored Potato
Chips ⓘ
Deli Style Potato Chips ✓
Dill Pickle Flavored Potato Chips ⓘ
Garden Tomato & Basil Flavored Potato
Chips ⓘ
Honey BBQ Flavored Potato Chips ⓘ
Honey Mustard Flavored Potato Chips ⓘ
Hot & Spicy Barbecue Flavored Potato
Chips ⓘ
Kettle Cooked Creamy Mediterranean
Herb Flavored Potato Chips ⓘ
Kettle Cooked Crinkle Cut Spice
Rubbed BBQ Potato Chips ⓘ

Kettle Cooked Harvest Ranch Flavored
Potato Chips ⓘ
Kettle Cooked Jalapeno Flavored Potato
Chips ⓘ
Kettle Cooked Maui Onion Flavored
Potato Chips ⓘ
Kettle Cooked Original Potato Chips ⓘ
Kettle Cooked Reduced Fat Original
Potato Chips ⓘ
Kettle Cooked Sea Salt & Cracked
Pepper Flavored Potato Chips ⓘ
Kettle Cooked Sea Salt & Vinegar
Flavored Potato Chips ⓘ
Kettle Cooked Sharp Cheddar Flavored
Potato Chips ⓘ
Kettle Cooked Spicy Cayenne & Cheese
Flavored Potato Chips ⓘ
Light Original Potato Chips ⓘ
Lightly Salted Potato Chips ✓
Limon Flavored Potato Chips ⓘ
Natural Sea Salt Flavored Thick Cut
Potato Crisps ✓
Salt & Vinegar Flavored Potato Chips ⓘ
Sour Cream & Onion Flavored Potato
Chips ⓘ
Southwest Cheese & Chiles Flavored
Potato Chips ⓘ
Stax Cheddar Flavored Potato Crisps ✓
Stax Mesquite Barbecue Flavored Potato
Crisps ✓
Stax Original Potato Crisps ✓
Stax Ranch Flavored Potato Chips ⓘ
Stax Salt & Vinegar Flavored Potato
Crisps ✓
Stax Sour Cream & Onion Flavored
Potato Crisps ✓
Sweet Southern Heat BBQ Flavored
Potato Chips ⓘ
Tangy Carolina BBQ Flavored Potato
Chips ⓘ
Wavy Au Gratin Flavored Potato Chips ⓘ
Wavy Hickory BBQ Flavored Potato
Chips ⓘ
Wavy Original Potato Chips ✓
Wavy Ranch Flavored Potato Chips ⓘ

Manischewitz
Potato Chips (All Varieties)

Martin's Potato Chips
Potato Chip Products (All)

Maui Style ⓘ
Regular Potato Chips
Salt & Vinegar Flavored Potato Chips

Meijer
Potato Sticks

Mike-Sell's
Bold Bahama Kettle Chips
Creamy Sweet Onion Kettle Chips
Good N' Hot Potato Chips
Green Onion Potato Chips
Mesquite Smoked Bacon Potato Chips
Salt & Pepper Potato Chips
Zesty Barbeque Potato Chips

Miss Vickie's ⓘ
Hand Picked Jalapeno Kettle Cooked
  Flavored Potato Chips
Sea Salt & Cracked Pepper Flavored
  Potato Chips
Sea Salt & Vinegar Kettle Cooked
  Flavored Potato Chips
Simply Sea Salt Kettle Cooked Potato
  Chips

Mrs. Bryant's
Route 11 BBQ Potato Chips
Route 11 Dill Pickle Potato Chips
Route 11 Lightly Salted Potato Chips
Route 11 Sweet Potato Chips

Munchos ⓘ
Regular Potato Crisps

Old Dutch Foods
Baked Potato Crisps, Cheddar & Sour
  Cream
Baked Potato Crisps, Original
Dutch Crunch Chips, Hot Buffalo
  Wings
Dutch Crunch Chips, Jalapeno &
  Cheddar
Dutch Crunch Chips, Low Sodium
Dutch Crunch Chips, Mesquite Bar-B-Q
Dutch Crunch Chips, Original
Dutch Crunch Chips, Parmesan &
  Garlic
Dutch Crunch Chips, Salt & Vinegar
Dutch Gourmet Chips, Honey Dijon
Dutch Gourmet Chips, Sea Salt

Dutch Gourmet Chips, Slow Cooked
  Ribs
Dutch Gourmet Chips, Szechwan
Potato Chips, Bar-B-Q
Potato Chips, Cheddar & Sour Cream
  Rip-L
Potato Chips, Dill Pickle
Potato Chips, Low Sodium Rip-L
Potato Chips, Onion & Garlic
Potato Chips, Original
Potato Chips, Rip-L
Potato Chips, Sour Cream & Onion
Ripples Chips, Cheddar & Sour Cream
Ripples Chips, Creamy Dill
Ripples Chips, French Onion
Ripples Chips, Loaded Spud
Ripples Chips, Mesquite Bar-B-Q
Ripples Chips, Original

Our Family
Barbecue Potato Chips
Classic Potato Chips
Sour Cream & Onion Flavored Potato
  Chips
Wavy Potato Chips

Pik-Nik ⛾
50% Reduced Salt Shoestring Potatoes
Fabulous Fries
Original (Salted, Unseasoned)
  Shoestring Potatoes

Pirate's Booty ⓘ
Pirate's Booty (All)

Popchips
Popchips (All)

Pringles
Fat Free Original
Fat Free Sour Cream & Onion

Publix
Dip Style Potato Chips
Original Thins Potato Chips
Salt & Vinegar Potato Chips

Rachel's
Barbecue Baked Chips
Buffalo Wing Kettle Chips
Cheddar & Sour Cream Baked Chips
Gourmet Kettle Chips
Grilled Kettle Chips
Jalapeno Kettle Chips

Maui Kettle Chips
Parmesan & Garlic Kettle Chips
Plain Baked Thins
Plain Kettle Chips
Reduced Fat Plain Kettle Chips
Salt & Cracked Pepper Kettle Chips
Salt & Vinegar Kettle Chips
Sea Salt Kettle Chips
Sour Cream & Onion Baked Chips
Steak & Onion Kettle Chips
Traditional Kettle Chips

Ruffles
Authentic Barbecue Flavored Potato
   Chips ⓘ
Baked! Original Potato Crisps ✔
Cheddar & Sour Cream Flavored Potato
   Chips ⓘ
Double Fisted Bacon Cheeseburger
   Flavored Potato Chips ⓘ
Light Original Potato Chips ⓘ
Loaded Chili & Cheese Flavored Potato
   Chips ⓘ
Molten Hot Wings Flavored Potato
   Chips ⓘ
Natural Reduced Fat Sea Salted Potato
   Chips ✔
Original Potato Chips ✔
Queso Flavored Potato Chips ⓘ
Queso Jalapeno Flavored Potato Chips ⓘ
Reduced Fat Original Potato Chips ✔
Sour Cream & Onion Flavored Potato
   Chips ⓘ
Tapatio Limon Flavored Potato Chips ⓘ

Sabritas ⓘ
Adobadas Flavored Potato Chips

Safeway Select ⌒
Jalapeno Kettle Chips
Salt and Pepper Kettle Chips

Salba Smart
Potato Crisps ⓘ

Schnucks
BBQ Chips
BBQ Kettle Chips
Cheddar & Sour Cream Chips
Classic Chips
Jalapeno Kettle Chips
Original Kettle Chips

Ridged Chips
Sour Cream Chips

Seneca Farms
Sweet Potato Chips

Snikiddy ✔
Baked Fries (All)

Snyder's of Hanover ⓘ
BBQ Potato Chips
Habanero Potato Chips
Hot Buffalo Wing Potato Chips
Jalapeno Potato Chips
Kosher Dill Potato Chips
Regular Potato Chips
Ripple Potato Chips
Salt & Vinegar Potato Chips
Sour Cream & Onion Potato Chips

Trader Joe's
Baked Potato Chips (Salted & Salt and
   Vinegar)
BBQ Chips
Kettle Cooked Olive Oil Potato Chips
Kettle Cooked Potato Chips with Sea Salt
Popped Potato Chips (Barbecue, Salted)
Potato Trio
Red Bliss Potato Chips
Sweet Potato Chips

Utz ⚎
All Natural Kettle Cooked, Dark Russet
All Natural Kettle Cooked, Gourmet
   Medley
All Natural Kettle Cooked, Lightly
   Salted
All Natural Kettle Cooked, Sea Salt &
   Vinegar
Barbeque Potato Chips
Carolina BBQ Potato Chips
Cheddar & Sour Cream Potato Chips
Crab Potato Chips
Grandma Utz Kettle Cooked, Barbeque
Grandma Utz Kettle Cooked, Plain
Homestyle Kettle Cooked, Plain
Honey BBQ Potato Chips
Kettle Classics, Dark Russet
Kettle Classics, Jalapeno
Kettle Classics, Plain
Kettle Classics, Smokin' Sweet BBQ
Kettle Classics, Sour Cream & Chive

Kettle Classics, Sweet Potato
Mystic Kettle Cooked Potato Chips
  (Dark Russet, Plain, Sea Salt &
  Vinegar)
No Salt BBQ Potato Chips
No Salt Potato Chips
Red Hot Potato Chips
Reduced Fat Potato Chips
Regular Potato Chips (Flat, Ripple,
  Wavy Cut)
Salt & Pepper Potato Chips
Salt & Vinegar Potato Chips
Sour Cream & Onion Potato Chips

Valu Time (Brookshire)
BBQ Potato Chips
Cheddar & Sour Cream Potato Chips
Regular Potato Chips
Ripple Potato Chips
Salt & Vinegar Potato Chips
Sour Cream & Onion Potato Chips

Valu Time (Marsh)
BBQ Potato Chips
Sour Cream & Onion Potato Chips

Wegmans
Wavy Potato Chips

Wise Snacks
All Natural Flats
Cheddar & Sour Cream Ridgies
Lightly Salted Chips
New York Deli Jalapeno Kettle Chips
New York Deli Kettle Chips
Onion & Garlic Chips
Ridgies
Salt & Vinegar Chips
Sour Cream & Onion Ridgies
Unsalted Chips
Wavy Chips

CHIPS, TORTILLA

Always Save
Bite Size Tortilla Chips
Round White Tortilla Chips
Round Yellow Tortilla Chips
White Restaurant-Style Tortilla Chips

Azteca ⟨⟩
Corn Tortilla Chips

Casa Fiesta ⓘ
Nach-Ole Tortilla Chips

Central Market (H-E-B)
Organic Thin Tortilla Chips, Salted
Organic Ultra Thin Tortilla Chips,
  Unsalted
Organic White Corn Tortilla Chips

Chi-Chi's
Chips (All Varieties)

Classic Foods ⓘ
Kettle Classics
Stoned Classics

Corazonas
Whole Grain Tortilla Chips

Doritos ⓘ
1st Degree Burn Blazin' Jalapeno
  Flavored Tortilla Chips
2nd Degree Burn Fiery Buffalo Flavored
  Tortilla Chips
3rd Degree Burn Scorchin' Habanero
  Flavored Tortilla Chips
Blazin' Buffalo & Ranch Flavored
  Tortilla Chips
Cool Ranch Flavored Tortilla Chips
Fiery Fusion Flavored Tortilla Chips
Flamas Flavored Tortilla Chips
Four Cheese Flavored Tortilla Chips
Late Night All Nighter Cheeseburger
  Flavored Tortilla Chips
Pizza Supreme Flavored Tortilla Chips
Reduced Fat Cool Ranch Flavored
  Tortilla Chips
Reduced Fat Nacho Cheese Flavored
  Tortilla Chips
Reduced Fat Spicy Nacho Flavored
  Tortilla Chips
Salsa Verde Flavored Tortilla Chips
Spicy Nacho Flavored Tortilla Chips
Stadium Nacho Flavored Tortilla Chips
Taco Flavored Tortilla Chips
Tailgate BBQ Flavored Tortilla Chips
Tangy Buffalo Wing Flavored Tortilla
  Chips
Tapatio Flavored Tortilla Chips
Toasted Corn Tortilla Chips ✓

EatSmart Naturals ⓘ
Whole Grain Tortilla Chips

Tortilla Chips

Fastco (Fareway)
White Round Bite Size Tortilla Chips
White Round Tortilla Chips
Yellow Round Tortilla Chips

Food Club (Brookshire)
Nacho Style Tortilla Chips
White Corn Restaurant Style Tortilla
Chips
White Mini Rounds, Snack Bite Size
White Round Tortilla Chips
Yellow Round Tortilla Chips

Food Club (Marsh)
Bite Sized White Mini Rounds
Yellow Round Tortilla Chips

Food Should Taste Good ⓘ ✔
Tortilla Chips (All)

**Food You Feel Good About
(Wegmans)**
Organic Blue Tortilla Chips, Made with
Organic Corn
Organic White Tortilla Chips, Made
with Organic Corn
Organic Yellow Tortilla Chips, Made
with Organic Corn

Fresh Gourmet ()
Tortilla Strips (Lightly Salted, Santa Fe
Style, Tri-Color)

Full Circle (Schnucks)
Blue Restaurant Style Tortilla Chips
White Restaurant Style Tortilla Chips
Yellow Restaurant Style Tortilla Chips

Garden Fresh Gourmet ⓘ
Tortilla Chips (All BUT Pita Chips)

Goya
Tortilla Chips

Grande ⓘ
Restaurant Style Tortilla Chips
Salsa Limon Tortilla Chips
Tortilla Chips

GreenWise Market (Publix)
Blue Tortilla Chips
Yellow Tortilla Chips

Guerrero
Corn Tortilla Chips

Guiltless Gourmet ()
Baked Tortilla Chips (All)

Herr's ()
Bite Size Dippers Tortilla Chips
Nachitas
Restaurant Style Tortilla Chips
Sesame Rice Tortilla Chips

Hippie Chips ()
Hippie Chips (All)

Kroger
Bite Size Tortilla Chips
Nacho Tortilla Chips
Radical Ranch Tortilla Chips
Santa Fe Tortilla Strips
Spicy Salsa Tortilla Chips
Thin Restaurant Style Tortilla Chips
Traditional Tortilla Chips
Yellow Traditional Tortilla Chips

Nature's Promise (Giant)
Blue Corn Tortilla Chips
Yellow Tortilla Chips

Nature's Promise (Stop & Shop)
Blue Corn Tortilla Chips
Yellow Tortilla Chips

O Organics ᔕ
Blue Corn Tortilla Chips with Flax
Blue Corn Tortilla Chips with Sesame
Seeds
White Corn Tortilla Chips
Yellow Corn Tortilla Chips

Ortega ⓘ
Round Tortilla Chips

Our Family
Restaurant Style Tortilla Chips
Tostada Chips

Pan de Oro ✔
Tortilla Chips (All)

Price Chopper
Organic Blue Tortilla Chips
Organic Vegetable Tortilla
Organic Yellow Tortilla

Publix
White Corn Tortilla Chips - Restaurant
Style
Yellow Corn Tortilla Chips - Round
Style

Rancho Berenda ✔
White Triangle Tortilla Chips

Ricos ✓
  Chips (All)
Ruth's Hemp Foods ✓
  Hemp Tortilla Chips
Salba Smart
  Organic Tortilla Chips ♀
Santitas ✓
  White Corn Triangles Tortilla Chips
  Yellow Corn Tortilla Chips (Rounds,
    Strips, Triangles)
Schnucks
  Classic Tortilla Chips
  Round Tortilla Chips
  White Round Tortilla Bites
  Yellow Round Tortilla Chips
Snyder's of Hanover ⓘ
  Restaurant Style Tortilla Chips
  White Corn Tortilla Chips
  Yellow Corn Tortilla Chips
Tostitos
  Baked! Scoops Tortilla Chips ✓
  Bite Size Rounds Tortilla Chips ✓
  Crispy Rounds Tortilla Chips ✓
  Dipping Strips Tortilla Chips ✓
  Multigrain Scoops! Tortilla Chips ⓘ
  Natural Blue Corn Restaurant Style
    Tortilla Chips ✓
  Natural Yellow Corn Restaurant Style
    Tortilla Chips ✓
  Restaurant Style Tortilla Chips ✓
  Restaurant Style with A Hint of Jalapeno
    Flavored Tortilla Chips ⓘ
  Restaurant Style with A Hint of Lime
    Flavor Tortilla Chips ⓘ
  Restaurant Style with A Hint of Pepper
    Jack Flavored Tortilla Chips ⓘ
  Salsa Verde Flavored Tortilla Chips ⓘ
  Scoops! Tortilla Chips ✓
  Thick & Hearty Rounds Tortilla Chips ✓
Trader Joe's
  Blue Corn Tortilla Chips
  Organic Baked Blue Corn Tortilla Chips
  Organic Baked Nacho Tortilla Chips
  Organic Blue Corn Tortilla Chips
  Organic Tortilla Longboard Chips
  Organic White Corn Tortilla Chips

  Organic Yellow Corn Tortilla Chips,
    Round
  Reduced Guilt Tortilla Strips
  Restaurant Style Organic White Corn
    Tortilla Chips
  Salsa Tortilla Chips
  Soy & Flaxseed Tortilla Chips (Spicy &
    Regular)
  Super Seeded Tortilla Chips
  Veggie & Flaxseed Tortilla Chips
  White Corn Tortilla Strips
  Yellow Corn Tortilla Chips
Utz ♀
  Baked Tortilla Chips
  Cheesier Nacho Tortilla Chips
  Restaurant Style Tortilla Chips
  White Corn Tortilla Chips
Valu Time (Brookshire)
  Nacho Chips
  Round Yellow Tortilla Chips
Valu Time (Marsh)
  Round Yellow Tortilla Chips
Valu Time (Schnucks)
  Yellow Tortilla Chips
Wegmans
  Authentic Tortilla Chips (100% White
    Corn)
  Lime Flavored Tortilla Chips
  Round Tortilla Bite-Size Chips (100%
    White Corn)
  Round Tortilla Chips
  Round Tortilla Chips (100% White
    Corn)

COOKIES

Aleia's ♀ ✓
  Almond Horn Cookies
  Chocolate Chip Cookies
  Chocolate Coconut Macaroons
  Coconut Macaroons
  Ginger Snap Cookies
  Oatmeal & Golden Raisin Cookies
  Peanut Butter Cookies
  Snickerdoodle Cookies
Amaretti del Chiostro
  Amaretti del Chiostro

Amy's Kitchen ✓
Gluten Free Almond Shortbread Cookies
Gluten Free Chocolate Chip Shortbread Cookies
Gluten Free Classic Shortbread Cookies

Andean Dream
Chocolate Chip Quinoa Cookies
Cocoa-Orange Quinoa Cookies
Coconut Quinoa Cookies
Orange Essence Quinoa Cookies
Raisins & Spice Quinoa Cookies

Annie's Homegrown
Gluten Free Cocoa & Vanilla Bunny Cookies
Gluten Free Ginger Snap Bunny Cookies
Gluten Free SnickerDoodle Bunny Cookies

Aunt Gussie's 🍴 ✓
Gluten Free Cookies (Regular & Sugar Free)

Bi Aglut
Bi Aglut (All)

Biscottea ✓
Gluten-Free Blueberry with White Tea Shortbread
Gluten-Free Chai Spices Shortbread
Gluten-Free Earl Grey Tea Shortbread

Biscuiterie de Provence ⓘ
Macarons de Baronnies

Bodhi's Bakehouse
Gluten Free Chocolate Latte Cookies
Gluten Free Chocolate Macadamia Cookies
Gluten Free Chocolate Orange Jaffa Cookies
Gluten Free Lemon Shortbread Cookies
Gluten Free Lupin Cookies
Sweetheart Cookie Tray
Vegan Anzac Cookie Tray

Byron Bay Cookies ⓘ
Chocolate Orange Cookie
Sticky Date & Ginger Cookie
Triple Chocolate Fudge Cookie
White Chocolate Macadamia Nut Cookie

Caffe Portofino 🍴
Carcagnole Cookie
Pignoli Cookies

Caveman Cookies ✓
Caveman Cookies (All)

Clarine's Florentines ()
Florentines

Coffaro's Baking Co.
Gluten Free Chocolate Chip Biscotti
Gluten Free Cranberry Almond Biscotti
Gluten Free Lemon Vanilla Biscotti

Cookies... for Me? 🍴
Cookies (All)

Crave Bakery ✓
Crave Bakery (All)

Domata Living Flour 🍴 ✓
Gluten Free Cookies (All)

Dr. Lucy's Cookies 🍴
Dr. Lucy's Cookies (All)

Ener-G
Chocolate Biscotti
Chocolate Chip Biscotti
Chocolate Chip Potato Cookies
Chocolate Cookies
Cinnamon Cookies
Cranberry Biscotti
Ginger Cookies
Raisin Biscotti
Sunflower Cookies
Vanilla Cookies
White Chocolate Chip Cookies

Enjoy Life Foods 🍴 ✓
Chocolate Chip Crunchy Cookies
Chocolate Chip Soft Baked Cookies
Double Chocolate Brownie Soft Baked Cookies
Double Chocolate Crunchy Cookies
Gingerbread Spice Soft Baked Cookies
Happy Apple Soft Baked Cookies
Lively Lemon Soft Baked Cookies
No-Oats "Oatmeal" Soft Baked Cookies
Snickerdoodle Soft Baked Cookies
Sugar Crisp Crunchy Cookies
Vanilla Honey Graham Crunchy Cookies

EnviroKidz ⓘ ✓
Vanilla Animal Cookies

Farmo ✓
Farmo (All)

Gilbert's Goodies ⓘ ✓
Gilbert's Goodies (All)

Gillian's Foods ⚇
Gillian's Foods (All)

Glenny's ✓
Gluten Free Oatmeal Cookies, Chocolate Chip
Gluten Free Oatmeal Cookies, Oatmeal Raisin

Glutano
Glutano (All)

Gluten Free Cookie Jar Baking Co, The
The Gluten Free Cookie Jar (All)

Gluten Free Harvest, A
A Gluten Free Harvest (All)

Glutino
Chocolate Chip Cookies
Chocolate Vanilla Cream Cookies
Chocolate Wafers
Lemon Wafers
Vanilla Cream Cookies
Vanilla Wafers

Gluuteny ⚇
Gluuteny (All)

Go Raw ✓
Super Cookies (All)

GoGo Quinoa ✓
GoGo Quinoa (All)

GoMacro ✓
Almonds with Vanilla MacroTreat
Cashews with Vanilla MacroTreat
Granola and Chocolate MacroTreat
Peanut Butter and Banana MacroTreat
Walnuts and Cranberries MacroTreat
Wild Blueberry with Lemon MacroTreat

Goya
Gluten Free Maria Cookies

Grainless Baker, The ⚇
The Grainless Baker (All)

Grindstone Bakery ⚇
Gluten Free Coconut Crunch Cookie
Gluten Free Dark Chocolate Cookie
Gluten Free Toasted Sesame Cookie

Hail Merry
Macaroons (All)

Inspired Cookie, The ✓
Espresso Lemon Chocolate Chunk Cookies
Lemon Lavender Cookies
Peppermint Chocolate Chunk Cookies

Jennies
Macaroons (All)

JK Gourmet
Biscotti (All)

Joan's GF Great Bakes
Joan's GF Great Bakes (All)

Jo-Sef ⚇
Chocolate Animal Cookies
Sandwich Chocolate O's
Sandwich Cinnamon O's
Sandwich Vanilla O's
Square Chocolate Cookies
Square Cinnamon Cookies
Square Vanilla Cookies
Vanilla Animal Cookies

Jovial
Chocolate Chocolate Cream Cookies
Chocolate Vanilla Cream Cookies
Fig Fruit Filled Cookies

Kay's Naturals ⚇ ✓
Cookie Bites (All)

Kinnikinnick Foods ⚇
Kinnikinnick Foods (All)

Lily Bloom's Kitchen
Gluten Free Macaroons

Little Aussie Bakery, The
The Little Aussie Bakery (All)

Liz Lovely
Gluten Free Chocolate Chip
Gluten Free Chocolate Fudge
Gluten Free German Chocolate Cake Cookies
Gluten Free Ginger Molasses
Gluten Free Lemon Coconut
Gluten Free Oatmeal Raisin
Gluten Free Snickerdoodle
Gluten Free Triple Chocolate Mint

Manischewitz
Tender Coconut Patties

Mariposa Baking Company
Almond Biscotti
Cinnamon Toast Biscotti

Ginger Spice Biscotti

Mary's Gone Crackers

Mary's Gone Crackers (All)

Mi-Del ✓

Gluten-Free Arrowroot Cookies

Gluten-Free Chocolate Caramel Cookies

Gluten-Free Chocolate Chip Cookies

Gluten-Free Chocolate Sandwich
Cookies

Gluten-Free Cinnamon Snaps

Gluten-Free Ginger Snaps

Gluten-Free Pecan Cookies

Gluten-Free Royal Vanilla Sandwich
Cookies

Gluten-Free S'mores

Miss Meringue ⓘ

Meringue Cookies (All)

Montana Monster Munchies ⓘ ✓

Legacy Valley Gluten-Free Original
Cookies

Legacy Valley Gluten-Free Silver Dollar
Cookies

Mrs. Bryant's

Chocolate Chip Oatmeal Almond
Crunch Cookies

Chocolate Chip Peanut Butter Oatmeal
Cookies

Orgran ⓘ ⚕

Amaretti Biscotti Biscuits

Biscotti Range (All)

Classic Chocolate Biscotti

Dinosaur Wholefruit Cookies

Itsy Bitsy Bears

Outback Animals Cookies Range (All)

Premium Shortbread Hearts

Wild Raspberry Fruit Filled Biscuits

Outside the Breadbox ⚕

Outside the Breadbox (All)

Pamela's Products ⓘ

Almond Anise Biscotti

Butter Shortbread

Chocolate Chip Walnut Cookies

Chocolate Chunk Pecan Shortbread

Chocolate Walnut Biscotti

Chunky Chocolate Chip Cookies

Dark Chocolate-Chocolate Chunk
Cookies

Espresso Chocolate Chunk Cookies

Ginger Cookies with Sliced Almonds

Lemon Almond Biscotti

Lemon Shortbread

Old Fashion Raisin Walnut Cookies

Peanut Butter Chocolate Chip Cookies

Pecan Shortbread

Shortbread Swirl

Simplebites Chocolate Chip Mini
Cookies

Simplebites Extreme Chocolate Mini
Cookies

Simplebites Ginger Mini Snapz

Spicy Ginger Cookies

Schar ⚕

Chocolate O's

Chocolate Sandwich Cremes

Cocoa Wafers

Hazelnut Wafers

Ladyfingers

Vanilla Sandwich Cremes

Vanilla Wafers

Shabtai Gourmet Gluten-Free Bakery ⚕

Gluten Free Chocolate Chip Biscotti

Gluten Free Chocolate Chip Cookies

Gluten Free Florentine Lace Cookies

Gluten Free Lady Fingers

Gluten Free Meltaway Crumb Sandies

Gluten Free Mini Black & White
Cookies

Gluten Free Rainbow Cookie Squares

Smart Treat ⚕

Smart Treat (All)

Streit's ⓘ

Macaroons (All Flavors)

Sweet Cake Bake Shop ⚕

Gluten Free Cookies (All)

Taste of Thai, A

Taste of Thai, A (All)

Tate's Bake Shop ⓘ ✓

Gluten Free Chocolate Chip Cookies

Trader Joe's

Gluten Free Ginger Snaps

Meringue Cookies (All)

Snickerdoodle Soft Baked Cookies

Udi's Gluten Free Foods ⚕ ✓

Chocolate Chip Cookies

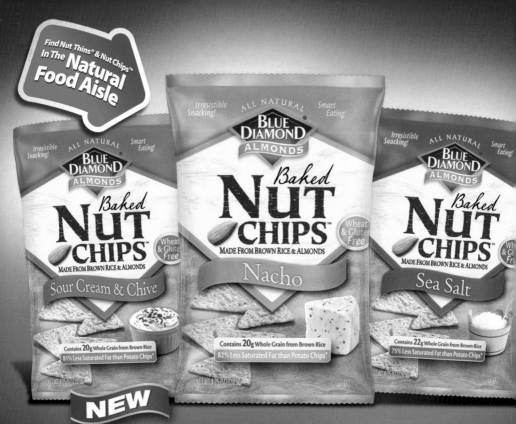

Find Nut Thins® & Nut Chips™ In The **Natural Food Aisle**

Irresistible Snacking! ALL NATURAL Smart Eating!

BLUE DIAMOND ALMONDS

Baked **Nut CHIPS™**
MADE FROM BROWN RICE & ALMONDS

Sour Cream & Chive

Wheat & Gluten Free

Contains **20g** Whole Grain from Brown Rice
81% Less Saturated Fat than Potato Chips*

BLUE DIAMOND ALMONDS

Baked **Nut CHIPS™**
MADE FROM BROWN RICE & ALMONDS

Nacho

Wheat & Gluten Free

Contains **20g** Whole Grain from Brown Rice
82% Less Saturated Fat than Potato Chips*

BLUE DIAMOND ALMONDS

Baked **Nut CHIPS™**
MADE FROM BROWN RICE & ALMONDS

Sea Salt

Contains **22g** Whole Grain from Brown Rice
75% Less Saturated Fat than Potato Chips*

NEW

Nut Chips™ • Less fat and fewer calories than potato chips,‡ baked not fried

The Newest Crunch
In Our Tasty Wheat & Gluten Free* Bunch

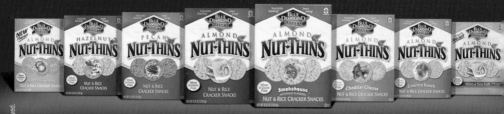

More Than Great Taste From the Almond People™

www.BlueDiamond.com

PROUD SPONSOR of Celiac Disease Foundation

Proud Sponsor of the Celiac Disease Foundation

*Each production run is sampled and tested to confirm gluten levels do not exceed 20 PPM.

‡ According to the USDA Nutritional Database, 2010, SR23 Baked Nut Chips contain at least 75% less fat than potato chips, and less fat and fewer calories than tortilla chips.

Oatmeal Raisin Cookies
Snickerdoodle Cookies
WOW Baking ♀
Cookies (All)
Wright's Farm ()
Almond Crescent Cookie

CORN CAKES

Kallo
Organic Thin Salted Corn Cakes

CRACKERS

Aimee's Livin' Magic
Curry, 'Kraut Chia Crackers
Dill Kimchi Crackers
Rosemary Kimchi Crackers
BHUJA
Cracker Mix
Original Mix
Biscuiterie de Provence ⓘ
Les Aristocades Apéritives
Les Aristocades Gourmandes
Blue Diamond Growers ♀
Almond Nut Thins
Barbeque Nut Thins
Cheddar Cheese Nut Thins
Country Ranch Nut Thins
Hazelnut Nut Thins
Hint of Sea Salt Nut Thins (Low
Sodium)
Pecan Nut Thins
Smokehouse Nut Thins
Corn Thins ♀
Corn Thins (All)
Crunchmaster ♀
Crunchmaster (All)
Doctor in the Kitchen ♀
Flackers Flax Seed Crackers (All)
Eden Foods
Brown Rice Crackers
Nori Maki Rice Crackers
Edward & Sons ✓
Brown Rice Snaps, Black Sesame (with
organic brown rice)

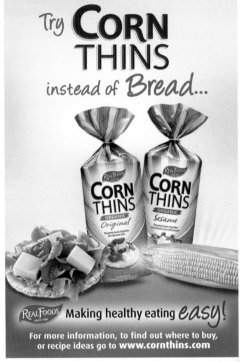

Brown Rice Snaps, Cheddar (with
organic brown rice)
Brown Rice Snaps, Onion Garlic
Brown Rice Snaps, Tamari Seaweed
Brown Rice Snaps, Tamari Sesame
Brown Rice Snaps, Toasted Onion (with
organic brown rice)
Brown Rice Snaps, Unsalted Plain (with
organic brown rice)
Brown Rice Snaps, Unsalted Sesame
Brown Rice Snaps, Vegetable (with
organic brown rice)
Exotic Rice Toast, Jasmine Rice &
Spring Onion
Exotic Rice Toast, Purple Rice & Black
Sesame
Exotic Rice Toast, Thai Red Rice &
Flaxseeds
Rice Snax, Bar-B-Que
Rice Snax, Lightly Salted
Rice Snax, Onion Garlic
Rice Snax, Salt & Vinegar
Ener-G
Broken Melba Toast

Cinnamon Crackers
Communion Wafers
Flax Crackers
Gourmet Crackers
Seattle Crackers

Fantastic
Delites Rice Snacks
Original Rice Crackers

Farmo ✓
Farmo (All)

Foods Alive ☃
Organic BBQ Flax Crackers
Organic Hemp Flax Crackers
Organic Italian Zest Flax Crackers
Organic Maple & Cinnamon Flax
Crackers
Organic Mexican Harvest Flax Crackers
Organic Mustard Flax Crackers
Organic Onion Garlic Flax Crackers
Organic Original Flax Crackers

Free to Enjoy
Mini Cheesey Crackers

Glutano
Glutano (All)

Glutino
Cheddar Crackers
Multigrain Crackers
Original Crackers
Table Crackers
Vegetable Crackers

Go Raw ✓
Flax Snax (All)

Grainless Baker, The ☃
The Grainless Baker (All)

Hol-Grain ⓘ ☃
Brown Rice Crackers - Lightly Salted
Brown Rice Crackers - No Salt
Brown Rice Crackers - Onion & Garlic
Flavor
Brown Rice Crackers - Sesame Lightly
Salted

KA-ME
Brown Rice Crisps (All)
Rice Crackers (All)

Kathy's Krackers
Flax Crackers (All)

Kinnikinnick Foods ☃
Kinnikinnick Foods (All)

Late July
Multigrain Snacks

Lydia's Organics ☃
Lydia's Organics (All)

Mariposa Baking Company
Crostini

Mary's Gone Crackers
Mary's Gone Crackers (All)

Mediterranean Snacks ⓘ
Lentil Crackers

Nairn's
Gluten Free Oat Cakes (All)

Natural Nectar
Cracklebred (All)

Orgran ⓘ ☃
Deli Crackers - Multigrain with
Poppyseed
Essential Fibre Crispibread
Essential Fibre Rotondo Biscuits

Outside the Breadbox ☃
Outside the Breadbox (All)

Rice Thins ☃
Rice Thins (All)

Safeway Select ⌇
Original Rice Crackers

San-J ⓘ ✓
Gluten Free Brown Sesame Rice
Crackers
Gluten Free Tamari Black Sesame Rice
Crackers
Gluten Free Tamari Rice Crackers
Gluten Free Teriyaki Sesame Rice
Crackers

Schar ☃
Cheese Bites
Crispbread
Snack Crackers
Table Crackers

SESMARK ⓘ
Rice Thins (All)

Sezme Sesame
Honey Snaps
Vanilla Snaps

Skinny Crisps ☃
Skinny Crisps (All)

Trader Joe's
Wasabi Roasted Seaweed Snack
Two Moms in the Raw ⓘ
Sea Crackers (All)
Wellaby's
Crackers, Feta Oregano & Olive Oil
Crackers, Original
Crackers, Parmesan & Sun Dried
Tomato
Crackers, Rosemary & Onion
Mini Crackers, Grated Parmesan
Mini Crackers, Original Cheese

DRIED FRUIT

Aimee's Livin' Magic
Really Raw Hunza Raisins
Albertsons
Mini Snack Raisins
Raisins
Always Save
Raisins
Bare Fruit Snacks
Dried Fruit (All)
Best Choice
Dried Apricot
Dried Blueberries
Dried Cherries
Dried Cranberries
Raisin Canister
Seedless Raisins
Crispy Green ⓘ
Crispy Green (All)
Crunchies ⓘ
Crunchies (All)
Eden Foods
Dried Montmorency Tart Cherries
Montmorency Dried Tart Cherries
Organic Dried Cranberries
Organic Dried Wild Blueberries
Organic Wild Berry Mix
Flavorite (Cub Foods)
Dried Plums
Natural Raisins
Raisin Canister
Food Club (Brookshire)
Raisins

Seedless Raisins
Food Club (Marsh)
Raisins
Seedless Raisins
Seedless Thompson Raisins
**Food You Feel Good About
(Wegmans)**
Raisins
Sweetened Dried Cherries
Sweetened Dried Cranberries
Foods Alive ⚭
Organic Raw Goji Berries
Fresh Gourmet ⟨⟩
Cranberries - Dried & Sweet
Golden Raisins - Plump & Sweet
Fruit d'Or
Dried Cranberries, Sweetened
(Flavored, Original)
Dried Cranberries, Sweetened with
Apple Juice
Dried Mixed Berries, Sweetened with
Apple Juice
FruitziO ⓘ
FruitziO (All)
Full Circle (Schnucks)
Raisins
Funky Monkey Snacks
Funky Monkey Snacks (All)
Giant
Seedless Raisins
Goya
Mocochinchi
Ponche Dried Fruit Mix
Great Lakes International Trading ⓘ
Dried Fruit (All)
Great Value (Wal-Mart) 📓
California Pitted Prunes
California Sun-Dried Raisins
Haggen
Apricot Mango
Raisins
Hy-Vee
California Sun Dried Raisins
Kroger
Raisins
L'Esprit de Campagne
Dried Fruit (All)

Maisie Jane's
Dried Fruit (Chocolate, Natural)
Mariani ⓘ
Dried Fruits (All BUT Cinnamon Raisin
Bread Raisins)
Meijer
Prunes, Pitted
Raisins, Seedless
Mrs. May's Naturals
Freeze Dried Fruit Chips (All)
Nature's Promise (Giant)
Organic California Raisins
Organic Dried Cranberries
Yogurt Covered Raisins
Nature's Promise (Stop & Shop)
Organic California Raisins
Organic Dried Cranberries
Organic Thompson Raisins
Yogurt Covered Raisins
Newman's Own Organics ⓘ
Berry Blend
Dried Apples
Dried Apricots
Dried Cranberries
Dried Pitted Prunes
Raisins
Nutra Fig ⓘ
Dried Figs (All)
O Organics 〰
Raisins
Ocean Spray
Craisins (Original ONLY)
Oskri
Dried Fruits (All)
Peeled Snacks ✓
Peeled Snacks (All)
Publix
Raisins
Rice River Farms ⓘ
Apple Rings
Apples, 3/8 Diced Natural
Apples, Cinnamon Diced
Apples, Diced
Apricots, Diced
Apricots, Turkish Whole
Banana Chips, Organic
Banana Chips, Sweetened

Blackberries
Blueberries
Blueberries, Wild
Cantaloupe
Cherries, Bing
Cherries, Rainier
Cherries, Tart
Coconut Chips, Toasted Unsweetened
Coconut, Macaroon
Cranberries
Cranberries, Whole
Currants, Zante
Dates, Deglet (Pitted)
Dates, Diced
Dates, Medjool (with Pits)
Figs, Black Mission
Figs, Black Mission Diced
Figs, Calimyrna White
Figs, Calimyrna White Diced
Fruit Fusion
Ginger, Crystallized
Ginger, Crystallized Diced
Goji Berries
Health Club Fruit Blend
Island Fruit Mix
Jackfruit
Mango, Diced
Mango, Sliced
Mango, Sliced Low Sugar
Nectarine, White
Papaya Spears, Sliced Natural
Papaya Spears, Sweetened
Papaya, Diced Sweetened
Peaches
Pears
Persimmon, Sliced
Pineapple Mango Coins
Pineapple Rings
Pineapple Rings, Unsweetened
Pineapple, Diced
Plums, Red
Pluots
Prunes, No Pits
Raisins, Golden
Raisins, Thompson Seedless Select
Raspberries
Salad Topper, Autumn Harvest

Special Fruit Blend
Starfruit
Strawberries
Tropical Fruit Mix
Richfood (Cub Foods)
Seedless Raisins
Safeway Select 〰
Philippine Mango
Sensible Foods
Sensible Foods (All)
St. Dalfour ⓘ
Dried Fruits (All)
Stop & Shop
Pitted Prunes
Sun Dried California Raisins
Sun-Maid ()
Sun-Maid Natural Sun-Dried Raisins
Zante Currants
Sunsweet
Sunsweet (All BUT Chocolate Covered
PlumSweets)
Trader Joe's
Dried Fruit (All BUT Black Currants)
Tropi Treats
Dried Pineapple Bites
Value (Kroger)
Raisins
Wegmans
Pitted Prunes
Sweetened Dried Philippine Mango
Sweetened Dried Tropical Pineapple
Sweetened Dried Wild Blueberries
Unsweetened Dried Apricots
Welch's
Welch's (All)
Winn-Dixie
Raisins

FRUIT CUPS

Best Choice
Mixed Berry
Pineapple Tidbits
Strawberry
Tropical Fruit
Cub Foods
Dinosaurs Fruit Snacks

Mixed Fruit Cups
Pineapple Fruit Cups
Del Monte ⓘ
Fruit Snack Cups (Metal or Plastic)
Flavorite (Cub Foods)
Mixed Fruit Cup
Pineapple Fruit Cup
Fruit Roll-Ups
Flavor Wave
Hy-Vee
Diced Peaches in Light Syrup Fruit Cups
Diced Pears in Light Syrup Fruit Cups
Mandarin Oranges in Light Syrup Fruit
Cups
Mandarin Oranges in Orange Gel Fruit
Cups
Mixed Fruit in Light Syrup Fruit Cups
Peaches in Strawberry Gel Fruit Cups
Pineapple Tidbit Fruit Cups
Tropical Fruit Cups
Kroger
Peaches in Strawberry Gelatin
Our Family
Diced Mixed Fruit Cup
Diced Peaches Fruit Cup
Mandarin Oranges Fruit Cup
Safeway 〰
Mandarin Oranges in Light Syrup
Mandarin Oranges in Light Syrup Fruit
Cups
Pineapple in Pineapple Juice Fruit Cups

FRUIT SNACKS

ACME
Dried Fruit Snack
Maya N Miguel Fruit Snacks
Sharks Fruit Snacks
Veggie Tales Fruit Snack
Albertsons
Curious George Dried Fruit Snack
Peanuts Fruit Snacks
Tropical Fruit Snacks
Veggie Tales Fruit Snacks
Annie's Homegrown
Organic Bunny Fruit Snacks, Berry
Patch

Organic Bunny Fruit Snacks, Grapes Galore
Organic Bunny Fruit Snacks, Pink Lemonade
Organic Bunny Fruit Snacks, Summer Strawberry
Organic Bunny Fruit Snacks, Sunny Citrus
Organic Bunny Fruit Snacks, Tropical Treat
Organic Orchard Fruit Bites, Apple
Organic Orchard Fruit Bites, Cherry
Organic Orchard Fruit Bites, Grape
Organic Orchard Fruit Bites, Strawberry

Clif
Clif Kid Twisted Fruit (All)

Cub Foods
Veggie Tales Fruit Snacks

Ferrara Pan Candy Company
Fruit Snacks (All)

Flavorite (Cub Foods)
Curious George Fruit Snacks
Dinosaur Fruit Snacks
Veggie Tales Fruit Snacks

Food Club (Marsh)
Fruit Snacks, Build-A-Bear Workshop
Fruit Snacks, Curious George
Fruit Snacks, Dinosaurs
Fruit Snacks, Sharks
Fruit Snacks, Veggie Tales

Food You Feel Good About (Wegmans)
Cherry Fruit Flats
Grape Fruit Flats
Raspberry Fruit Flats
Strawberry Fruit Flats

Fruit by the Foot
Berry Blast
Berry Tie-Dye
Color By the Foot
iCarly
Strawberry
Tropical Twist
Variety Pack

Fruit Gushers
Blue Raspberry
Flavor Shock

Mood Morphers
Mouth Mixers Punch Berry
Strawberry
Triple Berry Shock
Tropical
Tropical Flavors
Value Pack (Strawberry, Tropical)
Variety Pack (Strawberry, Watermelon, Tropical)
Watermelon Blast

Fruit Roll-Ups
Blastin' Berry Hot Colors
Minis, Strawberry Craze
Minis, Wildberry Punch
Scoops Fruity Ice Cream Flavors
Stickerz Mixed Berry
Stickerz Tropical Berry Flavor
Stickerz Variety Pack
Strawberry
Strawberry Sensation
Tropical Tie-Dye
Value Pack (Strawberry/Berry Cool Punch)
Variety Pack (Strawberry/Tie-Dye/Wildfire)

Fruit Shapes
Care Bears
Comics
Create-A-Bug
Dora the Explorer
Dreamworks
My Little Pony
Nickelodeon
Scooby-Doo
Shark Bites
Spiderman
Sponge Bob
Sunkist Mixed Fruit
Transformers
Value Pack Sunkist
Variety Pack Scooby-Doo

Giant
Dinosaur Fruit Snacks
Shark Fruit Snacks

Goodness Gardens
Squeezy Fruit (All)

GoPicnic
Tasty Brand Organic Fruit Snacks

Honey Stinger ⓘ
Energy Chews

Hy-Vee
Dinosaurs Fruit Snacks
Sharks Fruit Snacks
Snoopy Fruit Snacks
Veggie Tales Fruit Snacks

Jewel-Osco
Curious George Mixed Fruit Snack
Fruit Snack
Maya & Miguel Fruit Snack
Tropical Fruit Snacks

Kaia Foods ✔
Fruit Leathers (All Flavors)

Meijer
African Safari Fruit Snacks
Curious George Fruit Snacks
Dinosaurs Fruit Snacks
Fruit Roll (Justice League Berry, Rescue
   Heroes, Strawberry, Strawberry
   Garfield, Wildberry Rush)
Jungle Adventure Fruit Snacks
Justice League Fruit Snacks
Mixed Fruit Snacks
Peanuts Fruit Snacks
Sharks Fruit Snacks
Underwater World Fruit Snacks
Veggie Tales Fruit Snacks

Our Family
Star Wars Fruit Snacks

Richfood (ACME)
Dinosaurs Fruit Snack

Safeway ᗡ
Curious George Assorted Fruit Snacks
Fruit Shapes Fruit Snacks
Fruity Sprockets Fruit Snacks

Sharkies ⚱
Sharkies (All)

Shaw's
Build-a-Bear Fruit Snacks
Dinosaur Fruit Snacks
Dried Fruit Snack
Dried Tropical Fruit Snack
Fruit Snacks
Mixed Fruit Character Fruit Snacks

Mixed Fruit Dried Fruit Snack
Mixed Fruit Shark Box Fruit Snacks

Stop & Shop
Shark Fruit Snacks

Trader Joe's
Fruit Leathers (All)

Vons ᗡ
Fruit Snacks Multi Pack

Wacky Apple ⚱
Flat Fruit

Welch's
Welch's (All)

GELATIN SNACKS & MIXES

ACME
Lime Gelatin
Orange Gelatin
Raspberry Sugar-Free Gelatin
Strawberry Gelatin
Sugar-Free Cherry Gelatin Mix
Sugar-Free Orange Gelatin
Sugar-Free Strawberry Gelatin
Sugar-Free Strawberry Gelatin Mix

Albertsons
Cherry Gelatin Mix
Lime Gelatin Mix
Orange Gelatin Mix
Raspberry Gelatin Mix
Strawberry Gelatin Mix
Sugar Free Cherry Gelatin Mix
Sugar Free Orange Gelatin Mix
Sugar Free Raspberry Gelatin Mix
Sugar Free Strawberry Gelatin Mix

Always Save
Cherry Gelatin
Orange Gelatin
Raspberry Gelatin
Strawberry Gelatin

Angelica's Gelatina
Single Serve Gelatin (All)

Best Choice
Cherry Gelatin
Lemon Gelatin
Lime Gelatin
Orange Gelatin
Raspberry Gelatin

Strawberry Banana Gelatin
Strawberry Gelatin
Sugar Free Cherry Gelatin
Sugar Free Lime Gelatin
Sugar Free Orange Gelatin
Sugar Free Strawberry Gelatin

D'Gari
D'Gari (All)

Eating Right ✺
Orange and Lemon Lime Sugar Free
  Gelatin
Strawberry and Cherry Sugar Free
  Gelatin

Fastco (Fareway)
Apricot Gelatin
Black Cherry Gelatin
Cherry Gelatin
Lemon Gelatin
Lime Gelatin
Orange Gelatin
Peach Gelatin
Raspberry Gelatin
Strawberry Gelatin
Sugar Free Cherry Gelatin
Sugar Free Orange Gelatin
Sugar Free Raspberry Gelatin
Sugar Free Strawberry Gelatin
Wild Strawberry Gelatin

Flavorite (Cub Foods)
Orange Gelatin
Raspberry Gelatin
Sugar-Free Black Cherry Gelatin
Sugar-Free Cherry Gelatin
Sugar-Free Lime Gelatin
Sugar-Free Raspberry Gelatin
Sugar-Free Strawberry Gelatin

Food Club (Brookshire)
Cherry Gelatin Dessert
Lime Gelatin Dessert
Orange Gelatin Dessert
Raspberry Gelatin Dessert
Strawberry Banana Gelatin Dessert
Strawberry Gelatin Dessert
Sugar Free Cherry Gelatin Dessert
Sugar Free Lime Gelatin Dessert
Sugar Free Orange Gelatin Dessert
Sugar Free Raspberry Gelatin Dessert

Sugar Free Strawberry Gelatin Dessert
Unflavored Gelatin Dessert

Food Club (Marsh)
Cherry Gelatin Dessert
Lemon Gelatin Dessert
Lime Gelatin Dessert
Orange Gelatin Dessert
Raspberry Gelatin Dessert
Strawberry Gelatin Dessert
Sugar Free Orange Gelatin Dessert
Sugar Free Raspberry Gelatin Dessert
Sugar Free Strawberry Gelatin Dessert
Unflavored Gelatin Dessert

Goya
Guava Jelly Center

Great Value (Wal-Mart) 📅25
Cherry Gelatin Dessert
Lemon Gelatin Dessert
Lime Gelatin Dessert
Orange Gelatin Dessert
Peach Gelatin Dessert
Strawberry Banana Gelatin Dessert
Strawberry Gelatin Dessert
Sugar Free Cherry Gelatin Dessert
Sugar Free Lime Gelatin Dessert
Sugar Free Orange Gelatin Dessert
Sugar Free Peach Gelatin Dessert
Sugar Free Raspberry Gelatin Dessert
Sugar Free Strawberry Banana Gelatin
  Dessert
Sugar Free Strawberry Gelatin Dessert

Hy-Vee
Cherry Gelatin
Cranberry Gelatin
Lemon Gelatin
Lime Gelatin
Orange Gelatin
Raspberry Gelatin
Strawberry Gelatin
Sugar Free Cherry Gelatin
Sugar Free Cranberry Gelatin
Sugar Free Lime Gelatin
Sugar Free Orange Gelatin
Sugar Free Raspberry Gelatin
Sugar Free Strawberry Gelatin

Jell-O ✺
Cheesecake Snacks, Original Strawberry

Gel Cups, Sugar Free Variety 6 Strawberry/4 Raspberry/2 Orange Low Calorie

Gel Cups, X-Treme Cherry & Blue Raspberry

Gel Cups, X-Treme Watermelon & Green Apple

Gelatin Dessert, Apricot Artificial Flavor

Gelatin Dessert, Berry Blue

Gelatin Dessert, Black Cherry

Gelatin Dessert, Blackberry Fusion

Gelatin Dessert, Cherry

Gelatin Dessert, Cranberry

Gelatin Dessert, Grape

Gelatin Dessert, Island Pineapple

Gelatin Dessert, Lemon

Gelatin Dessert, Lime

Gelatin Dessert, Margarita Limited Edition

Gelatin Dessert, Melon Fusion

Gelatin Dessert, Orange

Gelatin Dessert, Peach

Gelatin Dessert, Peach Artificial Flavor

Gelatin Dessert, Pina Colada Limited Edition

Gelatin Dessert, Raspberry

Gelatin Dessert, Strawberry

Gelatin Dessert, Strawberry Banana

Gelatin Dessert, Strawberry Kiwi

Gelatin Dessert, Sugar Free Black Cherry Low Calorie

Gelatin Dessert, Sugar Free Cherry Low Calorie

Gelatin Dessert, Sugar Free Cranberry Low Calorie

Gelatin Dessert, Sugar Free Lemon Low Calorie

Gelatin Dessert, Sugar Free Lime Low Calorie

Gelatin Dessert, Sugar Free Orange Low Calorie

Gelatin Dessert, Sugar Free Peach Low Calorie

Gelatin Dessert, Sugar Free Raspberry Low Calorie

Gelatin Dessert, Sugar Free Strawberry Banana Low Calorie

Gelatin Dessert, Sugar Free Strawberry Low Calorie

Gelatin Dessert, Tropical Fusion

Gelatin Dessert, Watermelon

Gelatin Snacks, Peach & Watermelon Sugar Free

Gelatin Snacks, Pear Chunks In Cherry Pomegranate Gelatin

Gelatin Snacks, Real Chunks Of Pineapple In Tropical Fusion Sugar Free Gelatin

Gelatin Snacks, Strawberry

Gelatin Snacks, Strawberry & Orange

Gelatin Snacks, Strawberry & Raspberry

Gelatin Snacks, Sugar Free Cherry & Black Cherry Low Calorie

Gelatin Snacks, Sugar Free Raspberry & Orange Low Calorie

Gelatin Snacks, Sugar Free Strawberry Low Calorie

Gelatin Snacks, Sugar Free Variety 12 Strawberry/4 Raspberry/2 Orange Low Calorie

Gelatin Snacks, Sugar Free Variety Lemon-Lime/Orange Low Calorie

Gelatin Snacks, Sugar Free Variety Strawberry-Kiwi/Tropical Berry Low Calorie

Mousse Temptations, Caramel Creme Sugar Free

Mousse Temptations, Chocolate Indulgence Sugar Free

Mousse Temptations, Dark Chocolate Decadence Sugar Free

Smoothie Snacks, Mixed Berry

Smoothie Snacks, Strawberry Banana

Jewel-Osco

Cherry Gelatin

Lime Gelatin

Orange Gelatin

Raspberry Gelatin

Strawberry Gelatin

Sugar-Free Banana Strawberry Gelatin

Sugar-Free Cherry Gelatin

Sugar-Free Lime Gelatin

Sugar-Free Orange Gelatin
Sugar-Free Raspberry Gelatin
Sugar-Free Strawberry Gelatin

Kool-Aid Gels ∽
Gel Snacks, Cherry Tropical Punch
Gel Snacks, Groovalicious Grape
Gel Snacks, Ice Blue Raspberry
Gel Snacks, Oh Yeah Orange
Gel Snacks, Soarin' Strawberry

Kozy Shack ⓘ
SmartGels (All)

Kroger
Mandarin Oranges in Orange Gelatin

Lakeview Farms
Gelatin (All)

Luisa's
Single Serve Gelatin (All)

Margarita's
Gelatin- Family Size (All)
Gelatin- Ring Molds (All)
Gelatin- Single Serve (All)

Meijer
Berry Blue Gelatin Dessert
Cherry Gelatin Dessert
Cranberry Gelatin Dessert
Grape Gelatin Dessert
Lime Gelatin Dessert
Orange Gelatin Dessert
Raspberry Gelatin Dessert
Strawberry Gelatin Dessert
Sugar Free Cherry Gelatin Dessert
Sugar Free Cranberry Gelatin Dessert
Sugar Free Lime Gelatin Dessert
Sugar Free Orange Gelatin Dessert
Sugar Free Raspberry Gelatin Dessert
Sugar Free Strawberry Gelatin Dessert
Unflavored Gelatin Dessert
Wild Strawberry Gelatin Dessert

Our Family
Cherry Gelatin
Lemon Gelatin
Lime Gelatin
Orange Gelatin
Raspberry Gelatin
Strawberry Banana Gelatin
Strawberry Gelatin
Sugar Free Cherry Gelatin

Sugar Free Lime Gelatin
Sugar Free Orange Gelatin
Sugar Free Raspberry Gelatin
Sugar Free Strawberry Banana Gelatin
Sugar Free Strawberry Gelatin

Publix
Mandarin Oranges in Gel
Sugar Free Raspberry & Orange Gelatin
Sugar Free Strawberry Gelatin

Real Desserts
Gelatin (All)

Senor Rico
Single Serve Gelatin (All)

Shaw's
Cherry Gelatin
Cherry Gelatin Mix
Lime Gelatin
Orange Gelatin
Orange Gelatin Mix
Raspberry Gelatin
Stawberry Banana Gelatin Mix
Strawberry Gelatin

Tropical Cheese
Gelatina Dessert

Valu Time (Brookshire)
Cherry Gelatin Dessert
Lemon Gelatin Dessert
Lime Gelatin Dessert
Orange Gelatin Dessert
Raspberry Gelatin Dessert
Strawberry Gelatin Dessert

Wegmans
Orange and Raspberry Gelatin Variety
Pack
Strawberry Gelatin
Sugar Free Cherry and Black Cherry
Gelatin
Sugar Free Orange and Raspberry
Gelatin
Sugar Free Strawberry Geltain

Winky Brand
Gelatin (All)

GUM

Bazooka Bubble Gum
Bazooka Bubble Gum (All)

Chicza
 Chicza (All)
Glee Gum
 Glee Gum (All Flavors)
Price Chopper
 Dubble Bubble

NUTS, SEEDS & MIXES

Aimee's Livin' Magic
 Organic Raw Brazil Nuts
 Organic Raw Hazelnuts
 Seeds of Longevity
 Spicy Pumps
 Sweet Livin' Walnuts
 Wild Naked Brazil Nuts
Almond Accents ⓘ 🍴
 Almond Accents (All BUT Roasted
 Garlic Caesar)
Arrowhead Mills
 Sesame Seeds, Mechanically Hulled
BHUJA
 Crunchy Seasoned Peas
 Fruit & Nut Mix
 Nut Mix
 Seasoned Almonds
 Seasoned Cashews
 Seasoned Peanuts
Blue Diamond Growers 🍴
 BOLD Blazin' Buffalo Wing Almonds
 BOLD Carolina BBQ Almonds
 BOLD Habanero BBQ Almonds
 BOLD Jalapeno Smokehouse Almonds
 BOLD Lime 'n Chili Almonds
 BOLD Salt & Black Pepper Almonds
 BOLD Salt & Vinegar Almonds
 Honey Roasted Almonds
 Lightly Salted Almonds (Low Sodium)
 Roasted Salted Almonds
 Smokehouse Almonds
 Whole Natural Almonds
Carrington
 Organic Flax Seed Products (All)
**Central Market Classics
(Price Chopper)**
 Almond, Cashew and Macadamia Nut
 Mix

 Honey Roasted Almonds
 Jumbo Honey Roasted Cashews
 Roasted and Salted Almonds
 Roasted and Salted Macadamia Nuts
 Slow Roasted Pecans
 Smoked Almonds
ChickPz ◊
 ChickPz Natural Roasted Chickpea
 Snacks (All)
David Seeds
 David Seeds (All Varieties)
DeLallo
 Pignoli Nuts ⓘ
Earth Family ◊
 Sea Salted Peanuts
Eden Foods
 All Mixed Up
 All Mixed Up Too
 Organic Pistachios, Shelled & Dry
 Roasted
 Organic Pumpkin Seeds, Dry Roasted
 & Salted
 Organic Spicy Pumpkin Seeds, Dry
 Roasted with Tamari
 Organic Tamari Roasted Almonds
 Organic Tamari Roasted Spicy Pumpkin
 Seeds
Equal Exchange ⓘ
 Almonds (All)
Fiona's Granola
 Chipotle Peanuts
 Chipotle Pecans
 Cinnamon Almonds
 Rosemary Hazelnuts
 Walnuts a L'Orange
Fire Dancer
 Fire Dancer Jalapeno Nuts (All)
Fisher Nuts ◊
 Almonds
 Butter Toffee Peanuts
 Cashews
 Chef's Naturals (All)
 Culinary Touch Almond/Cranberry
 Blend
 Culinary Touch Pecan/Cranberry/
 Orange Blend
 Culinary Touch Slivered Almonds

Culinary Touch Toasted Cashews
Culinary Touch Toasted Pine Nuts
Culinary Touch Walnut/Apple/
  Blueberry Blend
Dry Roasted Sunflower Kernels
Fusions Energy Blend Snack Mix
Fusions Ice Cream Sundae Snack Mix
Fusions Tropical Twist Snack Mix
Honey Roasted Peanuts (Oil Roasted,
  Can)
In-Shell Peanuts (All)
Macadamia Nuts
Mixed Nuts
Nature's Nut Mix
Party Peanuts
Pecans
Pine Nuts (Pignolas)
Pistachios
Salted In-Shell Sunflower Seeds
Spanish Peanuts
Sunflower Nuts/Seeds
Unsalted Golden Roast Peanuts
Walnuts

Food You Feel Good About (Wegmans)
In the Shell Unsalted Peanuts

Foods Alive ♟
Organic Raw Black Sesame Seed
Organic Raw Chia Seed
Organic Raw Golden Flax Seed
Organic Raw Hulled Hemp Seeds
Organic Raw Jungle Peanuts
Organic Raw Toasted Hemp Seeds with
  Salt

Fresh Gourmet ()
Sliced Almonds - Honey Roasted
Sliced Almonds - Toasted

Frito Lay ⓘ
Cashews
Deluxe Mixed Nuts
Dill Pickle Sunflower Seeds
Flamas Sunflower Seeds
Honey Roasted Peanuts
Hot Peanuts
Praline Pecans
Ranch Sunflower Seeds

Salted Peanuts
Sunflower Seed Kernels
Sunflower Seeds

Gerbs Pumpkin Seeds
Flax Seeds
Pumpkin Seeds
Sunflower Seeds

Giant
Cashews Halves and Pieces
Dry Roasted Hulled Sunflower Seeds
Dry Roasted Salted Peanuts
Dry Roasted Unsalted Peanuts
Mixed Nuts

Go Raw ✔
Go Raw (All)

Goya
Annatto Seeds
Breadfruit Nuts

Great Lakes International Trading ⓘ
Pine Nuts

Hail Merry
Hail Merry (All)

Herr's ()
Chocolate Covered Peanuts
Hickory Smoked Almonds
Honey Cashews
Honey Roasted Peanuts
Hot Peanuts
Roasted & Salted Natural Pistachios
Roasted & Salted Sunflower Seeds
Salted Cashews
Salted Peanuts
Swiss Mix

Hines Nut Company
Hines Nut Company (All)

Hoffman's ()
Chocolate Covered Nuts

Hy-Vee
Black Walnuts
English Walnut Pieces
English Walnuts
Natural Almonds
Natural Sliced Almonds
Pecan Halves
Pecan Pieces
Raw Spanish Peanuts

Salted Blanched Peanuts
Salted Spanish Peanuts
Slivered Almonds

Italian Classics (Wegmans)
Pine Nuts

Kaia Foods ✔
Pumpkin Seeds
Sunflower Seeds (All Flavors)

Karmic Krunch ✔
Karmic Krunch Gluten Free Snack Mix

Keenan Farms
Keenan Farms (All)

Koeze
Almonds
Classic Mixed Nuts
Colossal Cashews
Mixed Nuts with Macadamias
Peanuts
Pecans
Pistachios

Landgarten
Pumpkin & Chocolate Snack Mix
Pumpkin Seed Snack
Pumpkin Seed Snack, Dark Chocolate
Pumpkin Seed Snack, Milk Chocolate
Snack Mix
Soy & Chocolate Snack Mix
Soy Snack
Soy Snack, Dark Chocolate
Soy Snack, Milk Chocolate
Tamari Roasted Sicilian Almonds
Tamari Roasted Soy Beans Snack

Living Intentions
Gone Nuts! (All)
Super Seed (All)

Maisie Jane's
Almonds (All BUT Tamari Flavored)
Cashews (Flavored, Natural)
Macadamias, Chocolate
Pecans, Chocolate
Pistachios (Flavored, Natural)
Walnuts, Flavored

Meijer
Cashew Halves with Pieces
Cashew Halves with Pieces, Lightly Salted
Cashews, Whole

Deluxe Mixed Nuts
Mixed Nuts
Mixed Nuts, Lightly Salted
Nut Topping
Peanuts, Blanched
Peanuts, Blanched Lightly Salted
Peanuts, Butter Toffee
Peanuts, Dry Roasted
Peanuts, Dry Roasted Lightly Salted
Peanuts, Dry Roasted Unsalted
Peanuts, Honey Roasted
Peanuts, Hot & Spicy
Peanuts, Spanish
Pine Nuts
Sunflower Seeds
Sunflower Seeds, Salted in Shell

Mrs. May's Naturals
Crunches (All)

Munchies ⓘ
Flamin' Hot Peanuts
Honey Roasted Peanuts
Lime & Chili Flavored Almonds

Nature's Promise (Giant)
Organic Raw Cashews

Nature's Promise (Stop & Shop)
Organic Raw Cashews

Nut Harvest ⓘ
Natural Lightly Roasted Almonds
Natural Sea Salted Whole Cashews

Nutiva
Organic Shelled Hempseeds ⚱

O Organics ⌇
Cashews, Roasted & Salted
Mixed Nuts
Walnut Pieces and Halves

Olomomo Nut Company ⓘ
Olomomo Nut Company (All)

Oregon Dukkah ⓘ
Oregon Dukkah (All)

Oskri
Nuts and Seeds (All)

Our Family
Almonds, Blanched Slivered
Almonds, Natural Sliced
Pecan Halves
Walnut Pieces
Walnuts

Pastene
  Pignoli Nuts (Pine Nuts)
Planters ⌀
  Almonds, Nut-Rition Lightly Salted
  Almonds, Pumpkin Spice
  Almonds, Recipe Ready
  Almonds, Sliced
  Almonds, Slivered
  Almonds, Smoked
  Cashew Sesame Mix, Made With Pure
    Sea Salt
  Cashew Sesame Mix, Salt & Pepper Nut
    Mix Peanuts/Almonds/Cashews
  Cashews, Chocolate Covered
  Cashews, Chocolate Lovers Milk
    Chocolate
  Cashews, Deluxe Jumbo with Sea Salt
  Cashews, Deluxe Whole Honey Roasted
  Cashews, Deluxe Whole with Sea Salt
  Cashews, Dry Roasted
  Cashews, Halves & Pieces
  Cashews, Halves & Pieces Lightly Salted
  Cashews, Halves & Pieces Salted
  Cashews, Halves & Pieces with Pure Sea
    Salt
  Cashews, Halves And Pieces
  Cashews, Honey Roasted
  Cashews, Jumbo All Natural
  Cashews, Salted
  Cashews, Select Cashews Almonds &
    Pecans with Sea Salt
  Cashews, Whole
  Cashews, Whole Lightly Salted
  Crunchy Nut Bar, Carb Well Caramel
    Chocolate Crunch
  Crunchy Nut Bar, Carb Well Peanut
    Butter Crunch
  Hazelnuts, Chopped
  Honey Roasted/Sweet'n Crunchy/
    Cocktail, Holiday Selection
  Lightly Salted Almonds, Go-Nuts
  Lightly Salted Heart-Healthy Mix, Go-
    Nuts
  Macadamia, Cashew, Mix, & Almonds
    Select
  Macadamias, Chopped
  Macadamias, with Sea Salt

Mixed Nuts
Mixed Nuts, Deluxe Cashews, Almonds,
  Brazils, Hazelnuts & Pecans
Mixed Nuts, Deluxe Lightly Salted
Mixed Nuts, Deluxe with Sea Salt
Mixed Nuts, Honey Roasted
Mixed Nuts, Lightly Salted
Mixed Nuts, Unsalted
Nut-Rition Mix, Almonds
Nut-Rition Mix, Heart Healthy Mix
Nuts, Holiday Winter Spiced
Peanut Bar, Original
Peanut Butter, Creamy
Peanut Butter, Crunchy
Peanuts, Cocktail
Peanuts, Cocktail Lightly Salted
Peanuts, Cocktail Lightly Salted Made
  With Pure Sea Salt
Peanuts, Cocktail Party Pack
Peanuts, Cocktail Peanuts
Peanuts, Cocktail Raging Buffalo Wing
Peanuts, Cocktail Smoky Bacon
Peanuts, Cocktail Unsalted
Peanuts, Cocktail White Hot Wasabi
Peanuts, Cocktail with Sea Salt
Peanuts, Dry Roasted
Peanuts, Dry Roasted Honey Roasted
Peanuts, Dry Roasted Lightly Salted
Peanuts, Dry Roasted Lightly Salted
  with Sea Salt
Peanuts, Dry Roasted Unsalted
Peanuts, Dry Roasted with Sea Salt
Peanuts, Heat
Peanuts, Honey & Dry Roasted
Peanuts, Honey Roasted
Peanuts, Rich Roasted Whole In Milk
  Chocolate
Peanuts, Roasted In-Shell Salted
Peanuts, Salted
Peanuts, Sweet 'N Crunchy
Peanuts, Wicked Hot Chipotle
Pecan Chips, Recipe Ready
Pecan Halves, Halves
Pecan Halves, Recipe Ready
Pecan Lovers Mix, Pecan Lovers with
  Cashews & Pistachios
Pecan Pieces, Pieces

Pecan Pieces, Recipe Ready
Pepitas, Made With Pistachios Peanuts & Almonds
Pepitas, Roasted Salted
Pepitas, Wicked Hot Chipotle
Pine Nuts
Pistachio Lovers Mix, Pistachio Lovers Mix with Jumbo Cashews & Almonds
Pistachios, Dry Roasted
Spanish Peanuts, Redskin
Sunflower Kernels
Sunflower Kernels, Dry Roasted
Sunflower Seeds, Roasted & Salted
Sweet Roasts, Honey Roasted
Walnut Pieces, Recipe Ready
Walnuts
Walnuts, Black, Recipe Ready
Walnuts, Recipe Ready

Price Chopper
Almonds, Slivered
Bridge Mix
Double Dipped Peanuts
Hazelnuts, Chipped
Macadamias
Macadamias, Chopped
Pecan Halves
Pecans, Chopped
Pine Nut Pignoli
Salted Almonds
Walnut Chips
Walnut Halves
Walnuts Chipped
White Almonds

Publix
Jumbo Cashew
Virginia Peanuts

Rice River Farms ⓘ
Almonds, Blanched Slivered
Almonds, Dry Roasted
Almonds, Hickory Smoked
Almonds, Marcona
Almonds, Sliced
Almonds, Whole
Almonds, Whole Blanched
Brazil Nuts, Medium
Cashews, Raw Whole
Cashews, Whole Roasted Salted

Chestnuts, Whole
Chickpeas, Masala Roasted
Corn Nuts, Jumbo
Hazelnuts, Peeled
Hazelnuts, Whole
Macadamia Nuts
Peanuts, Honey Roasted
Pecan Halves
Pine Nuts
Pistachios, Roasted Salted in Shell
Pistachios, Shelled Raw
Poppy Seed, White
Pumpkin Seeds, Pepitas
Pumpkin Seeds, Roasted Salted
Sesame Seeds, Black
Sesame Seeds, Hulled White
Sesame Seeds, Toasted
Sesame Seeds, Tuxedo Blend
Sunflower Seeds, Hulled Raw
Sunflower Seeds, Roasted No Salt
Sunflower Seeds, Roasted Salted
Walnuts, Black (Pieces)
Walnuts, English

River Street Sweets
Glazed Pecans
Sugar & Spice Pecans

Ruth's Hemp Foods ✓
Raw Goodness Chia Seed
Soft Hemp

Sabritas ⓘ
Picante Peanuts
Salt & Lime Peanuts

Safeway ⌒
Almonds, Sliced
Almonds, Slivered
Almonds, Smoke Flavor
Chopped Pecans
Chopped Walnuts
Dry Roasted Chopped Macadamia Nuts
Mixed Nuts with Peanuts
Pecan Chips
Pecan Halves
Roasted and Salted Almonds
Shelled Walnuts
Walnut Pieces
Walnuts
Whole Almonds

Whole Natural Almonds
Whole Roasted and Salted Cashews

Safeway Select 🌀
Dry Roasted Macadamia Nuts with Sea
Salt Prepacked

Sahale Snacks ⓘ
Ksar Nut Blend
Soledad Nut Blend
Valdosta Nut Blend

Salba Smart
Ground Seed 🍸
Whole Seed 🍸

Schnucks
Almonds, Roasted Salted
Almonds, Smoked
Cashew Halves & Pieces, Low Salt
Cashews (Halves, Whole)
Deluxe Mixed Nuts
Macadamia Nuts
Mixed Nuts
Mixed Nuts, Low Salt
Peanuts, Dry Roasted
Peanuts, Dry Roasted Unsalted
Peanuts, Honey Roasted
Peanuts, Party
Peanuts, Spanish
Sunflower Kernels

Sensible Foods
Sensible Foods (All)

Snapdragon Pan-Asian Cuisine
Chili Lime Cashew Crunchies
Wasabi Cashew Crunchies

Spitz ⓘ
Chili Lime Sunflower Seeds
Cracked Pepper Sunflower Seeds
Dill Pickle Sunflower Seeds
Salted Sunflower Seeds
Seasoned Pumpkin Seeds
Seasoned Sunflower Seeds
Smoky BBQ Sunflower Seeds
Spicy Sunflower Seeds

Stop & Shop
Roasted Peanuts in Shell
Salted Cashews

Taza Chocolate
Chocolate Covered Nuts (All)

Trader Joe's
Almond Clusters
Cinnamon Almonds
Dark Chocolate Covered Almonds
Macadamia Nut Clusters (Seasonal)
Marcona Almonds (All)
Pecans Praline
Pumpkin Seeds And Pepitas
Raw and Roasted Nuts (All)
Sunflower Seeds
Yogurt Covered Almonds

Truson Organics
Roasted Soy Nuts (All)

Vons 🌀
Butter Toffee Peanuts
Cashew Halves and Pieces
Deluxe Mixed Nuts
Party Peanuts
Roasted and Salted Mixed Nuts
Whole Cashews

Wegmans
Almonds - Natural Whole
Almonds - Roasted & Salted
Cashews - Honey Roasted Whole
Cashews - Roasted Jumbo
Cashews - Roasted Salted Halves &
Pieces
Cashews - Roasted Whole Salted
Cashews - Roasted Whole Unsalted
Deluxe Mixed Nuts with Macadamia -
Roasted & Salted
Jumbo Cashew Mix with Almonds,
Pecans, and Brazils - Roasted
Lightly Salted Roasted Party Peanuts
Macadamia Nuts - Dry Roasted
Marcona Almonds - Roasted & Salted
Mixed Nuts with Peanuts - Roasted,
Lightly Salted
Party Mixed Nuts with Peanuts -
Roasted
Party Mixed Nuts with Peanuts -
Roasted, Salted
Party Peanuts - Roasted & Salted
Peanuts - Dry Roasted, Lightly Salted
Peanuts - Dry Roasted, Seasoned
Peanuts - Dry Roasted, Unsalted
Peanuts - Honey Roasted

Peanuts - Salted, In The Shell
Spanish Peanuts - Roasted
Virginia Peanuts - Salted
Virginia Peanuts - Salted Snack Packs

Wilderness Poets
Wilderness Poets (All)

Wine Nuts
Wine Nuts (All)

Yumnuts 🦷
Flavor Roasted Almonds
Flavor Roasted Cashews

POPCORN

479° Popcorn
Popcorn (All) ()

ACME
Microwave Butter Flavor Popcorn
Microwave Light Butter Popcorn
Microwave Low-Fat/Sodium Popcorn
Microwave Movie Theater Popcorn
White Popcorn
Yellow Popcorn

ACT II
Microwave Popcorn (All)

Albertsons
Microwave Popcorn Butter Flavor
Microwave Popcorn Kettle Corn
Microwave Popcorn Movie Theater
Unpopped Yellow Popcorn

Always Save
Buttered Popcorn
Cheese Popcorn
Microwave Butter Popcorn
White Cheddar Popcorn
Yellow Popcorn

Best Choice
Butter Microwave Popcorn
Extra Butter Microwave Popcorn
Fat Free Butter Popcorn
Giant Butter Popcorn
Lite Butter Microwave Popcorn
Microwave Kettle Corn
Natural Butter Popcorn
White Popcorn
Yellow Popcorn

Central Market (H-E-B)
Organic Microwavable Natural Popcorn
Organic Microwavable Popcorn Butter

Chester's ⓘ
Butter Flavored Puffcorn Snacks
Cheddar Cheese Flavored Popcorn
Cheese Flavored Puffcorn Snacks

Clearly Organic (Best Choice)
Butter Microwave Popcorn
Gourmet Popcorn
Natural Microwave Popcorn
White Cheddar Popcorn

Cracker Jack ⓘ
Original Caramel Coated Popcorn &
  Peanuts

Cub Foods
White Popcorn
Yellow Popcorn

Eden Foods
Organic Popcorn

Fastco (Fareway)
Caramel Corn
Cheese Popcorn
Popcorn

Flavorite (Cub Foods)
Microwave 94% Fat-Free Mini Bag
  Popcorn
Microwave Butter Popcorn
Microwave Kettle Corn Popcorn
White Popcorn
Yellow Popcorn

Food Club (Brookshire)
94% Fat Free Microwave Popcorn
Butter Microwave Popcorn
Crazy Butter Microwave Popcorn
Kettle Corn Microwave Popcorn
Lite Butter Microwave Popcorn
Natural Lite Microwave Popcorn
Yellow Popcorn

Food Club (Marsh)
Butter Microwave Popcorn
Crazy Butter Microwave Popcorn
Lite Butter Microwave Popcorn
Natural Microwave Popcorn

**Food You Feel Good About
(Wegmans)**
Yellow Popcorn

Full Circle (Schnucks)
Popcorn
White Cheddar Popcorn
Giant
Kapop Butter Microwave Popcorn
Kapop Ultimate Butter Microwave
Popcorn
Lite Butter Microwave Popcorn
Good Health Natural Products
Half-Naked Popcorn ()
Goya
Yellow Popcorn ()
Grandpa Po's
Grandpa Po's (All)
Haggen
Microwave Popcorn (Butter, Butter
Crazy, Butter Light, Kettle, Natural)
Popcorn
Halfpops
Halfpops (All)
Heaven Sent
Grow Your Family Healthy Caramel
Kettle Corn
Herr's ()
Cheese Hulless Popcorn
Chocolate Flavor Drizzled Caramel
Corn
Lite Popcorn
Low Sodium White Cheddar Popcorn
(Schools)
Original Hulless Popcorn
Original Popcorn
White Cheddar Popcorn
Hill Country Fare (H-E-B)
94% Fat Free Microwave Popcorn
Butter Flavor Microwave Popcorn
Kettle Microwave Popcorn
Lite Butter Microwave Popcorn
Natural Microwave Popcorn
Theatre Style Microwave Popcorn
Theatre Style Popcorn
White Popcorn
Yellow Popcorn
Hy-Vee
94% Fat Free Butter Microwave Popcorn
Butter Flavor No Salt Microwave
Popcorn

Butter Microwave Popcorn
Extra Butter Lite Microwave Popcorn
Extra Butter Microwave Popcorn
Kettle Microwave Popcorn
Light Butter Microwave Popcorn
Natural Flavor Microwave Popcorn
White Popcorn
Yellow Popcorn
Jewel-Osco
Microwave 94% Fat-Free Mini Bags
Popcorn
Microwave Butter Flavor Popcorn
Microwave Kettle Corn Popcorn
Microwave Light Butter Popcorn
Microwave Low-Fat/Sodium Popcorn
Microwave Movie Theater Popcorn
No Salt White Popcorn
No Salt Yellow Popcorn
Jolly Time
Better Butter
Blast O Butter
Blast O Butter Light
Butter-Licious
Butter-Licious Light
Crispy'n White
Crispy'n White Light
Healthy Pop 100 Calorie Butter Minis
Healthy Pop 100 Calorie Kettle Minis
Healthy Pop 94% Fat Free Butter Flavor
Healthy Pop 94% Fat Free Butter Flavor
Low Sodium
Healthy Pop 94% Fat Free Caramel
Apple
Healthy Pop 94% Fat Free Kettle Corn
Homemade
Kernel Corn, American's Best White
Kernel Corn, American's Best Yellow
Kernel Corn, White Pop Corn
Kernel Corn, Yellow Pop Corn
KettleMania
Mallow Magic
Sassy Salsa
The Big Cheez
White & Buttery
Kernel Season's ⓘ
Pre-Seasoned Popcorn

Kroger
Butter Popcorn
Cheese Popcorn
Gourmet White Cheddar Popcorn

Martin's Potato Chips
Popcorn Products (All)

Meijer
Caramel Corn
Cheese Popcorn
Chicago Style Popcorn
Popcorn
Popcorn, Giant Extra Butter
Popcorn, Microwave (Butter, Butter
Lite, Extra Butter, Extra Butter Lite,
Natural Lite)
Popcorn, Microwave 94% Fat Free
Popcorn, Microwave Butter 75% Fat
Free
Popcorn, Microwave Hot N' Spicy
Popcorn, Microwave Kettle Sweet &
Salty
Popcorn, Mini (Butter, Extra Butter,
Light Butter)
Popcorn, White
Popcorn, Yellow
Purple Cow Butter Popcorn
White Cheddar Popcorn

Meijer Naturals
Popcorn (Butter, Butter Light)
Popcorn, Double Butter

Meijer Organics
Popcorn, Organic (Butter, Natural)

Nature's Promise (Giant)
Organic Plain Microwave Popcorn

Nature's Promise (Stop & Shop)
Organic Plain Microwave Popcorn

Newman's Own Organics ⓘ
Pop's Corn, Butter Flavored
Pop's Corn, Light Butter
Pop's Corn, No Butter/No Salt

O Organics ᨏ
Organic Butter Flavored Microwave
Popcorn
Organic Lightly Salted Popcorn
Organic Microwave Popcorn
Organic White Cheddar Popcorn

O-Ke-Doke ⓘ
Butter Popcorn
Cheese Popcorn
Hot Cheese Popcorn
White Cheddar Popcorn
White Popcorn

Old Dutch Foods
Caramel Corn, Tub
Caramel Puffcorn
Cheese Popcorn
Northern Lites Fat Free Caramel Corn
Original Puffcorn
Popcorn
White Cheddar Popcorn

Oogie's ♟
Oogie's (All)

Orville Redenbacher's
Jar Popcorn (All BUT Crunch N Munch
& Poppycock)
Microwave Popcorn (All BUT Crunch
N Munch & Poppycock)

Our Family
94% Fat Free Microwave Popcorn
Butter Microwave Popcorn
Butter Microwave Popcorn, Lite
Microwave Kettle Corn
Natural Microwave Popcorn
Popcorn Kernels (Jar)
Theater Style Butter Microwave Popcorn

Pirate's Booty ⓘ
Pirate's Booty (All)

Popcorn Indiana ✓
Popcorn Indiana (All)

Publix
Deli Popcorn

Ricos ✓
Popcorn (All)

Safeway ᨏ
Extra Butter Microwave Popcorn
Microwave Kettle Corn Popcorn
White Popcorn Kernals
Yellow Popcorn Kernals

Sauce Goddess ✓
Moroccan Caramel Corn

Schnucks
Butter Popcorn, Microwave
Crazy Butter Popcorn

Extra-Butter Popcorn, Microwave
Lite Butter Popcorn, Microwave
White Popcorn
Yellow Popcorn

Shaw's
Microwave 94% Fat-Free Mini Bags Popcorn
Microwave Butter Popcorn
Microwave Kettle Corn Popcorn
Microwave Light Butter Flavor Popcorn
Microwave Light Butter Popcorn
Microwave Low-Fat/Sodium Popcorn
Microwave Movie Theater Popcorn
Natural Unpopped Popcorn

Smart Balance
Smart Balance (All)

Smartfood ⓘ
Kettle Corn Flavored Popcorn
Movie Theater Butter Flavored Popcorn
Reduced Fat White Cheddar Cheese Flavored Popcorn
White Cheddar Cheese Flavored Popcorn

Snyder's of Hanover ⓘ
Buttered Popcorn

Trader Joe's
Cranberry Nut Clusters Popcorn (Seasonal)
Fat Free Caramel Popcorn
Gourmet White Popcorn
Kettle Corn (Regular & Lite)
Lite Popcorn 50% Less Salt
Microwave Popcorn, 94% Fat Free
Organic Popcorn with Olive Oil
Organic Popping Corn
Reduced Guilt Popcorn
White Cheddar Popcorn

Utz ⚇
Popcorn (Butter, Cheese, White Cheddar)
Puff 'N Corn (Caramel, Cheese, Plain)

Valu Time (Brookshire)
Cheese Popcorn
Microwavable Popcorn (Butter, Lite Butter)

Valu Time (Marsh)
Cheese Popcorn

Valu Time (Schnucks)
Butter Popcorn
Chocolate Syrup
Lite Butter Popcorn
Movie Butter Popcorn

Vic's Gourmet Foods
Caramel Popcorn
Fat Free Caramel Popcorn
Half Salt White Popcorn
Kettle Corn
Lite Caramel Popcorn
Lite White Half Salt Popcorn
Lite White Popcorn
Lite Yellow Cheddar Cheese
Organic Cheese Popcorn
Organic Lite White Half Salt Popcorn
Regular Caramel Popcorn
White Cheddar Cheese
White Half Salt Popcorn
White Popcorn
Yellow Cheddar Cheese

Wegmans
Microwave Popcorn - 94% Fat Free Butter Flavor
Microwave Popcorn - Butter Flavor
Microwave Popcorn - Colossal Butter
Microwave Popcorn - Kettle Corn
Microwave Popcorn - Light Butter Flavor
Microwave Popcorn - Movie Theater Butter

Wild Harvest (ACME)
Microwave Light Butter Popcorn
Organic Microwave Popcorn

Wild Harvest (Albertsons)
100 Calorie Microwave Butter Popcorn
Organic Microwavable Butter Popcorn
Organic Microwavable Popcorn

Wild Harvest (Cub Foods)
Microwave 100 Cal Butter Popcorn
Organic Microwave Butter Popcorn
Organic Microwave Popcorn

Wild Harvest (Jewel-Osco)
Microwave 100 Calorie Butter Popcorn
Microwave Light Butter Popcorn
Organic Microwave Butter Popcorn
Organic Microwave Popcorn

Wise Snacks
- Butter Popcorn
- Hot Cheese Popcorn
- White Cheddar Popcorn
- White Cheddar Puffs

PORK SKINS & RINDS

Baken-Ets ⓘ
- Fried Pork Skins
- Hot 'N Spicy Flavored Pork Skins
- Hot 'N Spicy Flavored Fried Pork Cracklins
- Red Pepper Flavored Fried Pork Cracklin Strips
- Tangy BBQ Flavored Fried Pork Skins

Best Choice
- Jalapeno Pork Skins
- Plain Pork Skins
- Salsa Pork Skins
- Vinegar Pork Skins

Goya
- Chicharrones
- Hot & Spicy Chicharrones
- Pork Cracking Chicharrones

Herr's ⟨⟩
- Colossal Cracklins
- Cracklin Strips
- Hot & Spicy Colossal Cracklins
- Original Pork Rinds
- Red Pepper Cracklin Strips
- Smoked BBQ Pork Rinds

Hill Country Fare (H-E-B)
- BBQ Pork Rinds
- Hot & Spicy Cracklin Curls
- Hot & Spicy Pork Rinds
- Limon Chile Pork Rinds
- Original Cracklin Curls
- Pork Rinds
- Salt & Vinegar Pork Rinds

Valu Time (Brookshire)
- Pork Rinds

PRETZELS

Ener-G
- Pretzels

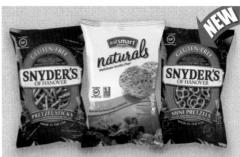
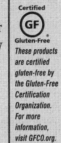
- Sesame Pretzel Rings
- Wylde Pretzels
- Wylde Sesame Pretzels

Glutino
- Chocolate Covered Pretzels
- Pretzel Sesame Rings
- Pretzel Sticks
- Pretzel Twists
- Yogurt Covered Pretzels

Mary's Gone Crackers
- Mary's Gone Crackers (All)

Snyder's of Hanover ⓘ
- Gluten-Free Pretzel Mini Pretzels
- Gluten-Free Pretzel Sticks
- Gluten-Free Pretzel Sticks (100 Calorie Packs)

PUDDING & PUDDING MIXES

ACME
- Butterscotch Pudding In Tabs
- Cherry Pudding Mix
- Chocolate Prepared Pudding

Chocolate Pudding
Fat-Free Chocolate Pudding
Instant Chocolate Pudding/Pie Filling
Pistachio Pudding/Pie Filling
Prepared Pudding Vanilla
Raspberry Pudding/Gelatin Mix
Sugar-Free Pudding/Pie Filling Vanilla
Vanilla Pudding/Pie Filling

Albertsons
Fat Free Chocolate Pudding
Instant Pudding, Vanilla
Vanilla Pudding & Pie Filling

Always Save
Instant Chocolate Pudding
Instant Lemon Pudding
Instant Vanilla Pudding

Angelica's Gelatina
Authentic Baked Flan
Rice Pudding

Best Choice
French Vanilla Instant Pudding
Lemon Instant Pudding
Pistachio Instant Pudding
Vanilla Instant Pudding

Bi Aglut
Bi Aglut (All)

Cub Foods
Chocolate Pudding
Vanilla Pudding

D'Gari
Flan

Dr. Oetker
Crème Brulee
Crème Caramel
Dark Chocolate Truffle Mousse
French Vanilla Mousse
Milk Chocolate Mousse
Organic Chocolate Pudding & Pie
  Filling
Organic Vanilla Pudding & Pie Filling
Original Chocolate Pudding
Original Vanilla Pudding
Shirriff Key Lime Pudding & Pie Filling
Shirriff Lemon Pudding & Pie Filling
Strawberry Mousse

Fastco (Fareway)
Instant Butterscotch Pudding

Instant Chocolate Pudding
Instant French Vanilla Pudding
Instant Lemon Pudding
Instant Milk Chocolate Pudding
Instant Pistachio Pudding
Instant Vanilla Pudding
Sugar Free Instant Butterscotch Pudding
Sugar Free Instant Chocolate Pudding
Sugar Free Instant Vanilla Pudding
Tapioca Pudding

Flavorite (Cub Foods)
Sugar-Free Chocolate Instant Pudding
Sugar-Free Vanilla Instant Pudding
Vanilla Instant Pudding

Food Club (Brookshire)
Banana Pudding Snack
Butterscotch Pudding Snack
Chocolate Fudge Pudding Snack
Chocolate Pudding Snack
Chocolate/Vanilla Swirl Pudding
Cook & Serve Chocolate Pudding
Cook & Serve Vanilla Pudding
Fat Free Chocolate Pudding Snack
Instant Banana Cream Pudding
Instant Butterscotch Pudding
Instant Chocolate Pudding
Instant Coconut Cream Pudding
Instant French Vanilla Pudding
Instant Lemon Pudding
Instant Pistachio Pudding
Instant Vanilla Pudding
Strawberry Banana Pudding Snack
Sugar Free & Fat Free Instant Vanilla
  Pudding
Sugar Free Chocolate Pudding with
  Calcium
Sugar Free Chocolate/Vanilla Swirl
  Pudding with Calcium
Sugar Free Instant Chocolate Pudding
Tropical Pudding Snack
Vanilla Pudding Snack

Food Club (Marsh)
Banana Pudding Snack
Butterscotch Pudding Snack
Chocolate Pudding (Refrigerated)
Chocolate Pudding Snack

Chocolate/Vanilla Swirl Pudding
  (Refrigerated)
Cook & Serve Butterscotch Pudding
Cook & Serve Chocolate Pudding
Cook & Serve Vanilla Pudding
Instant Banana Cream Pudding
Instant Butterscotch Pudding
Instant Chocolate Pudding
Instant Lemon Pudding
Instant Vanilla Pudding
Lite Fat Free Chocolate Pudding Snack
Sugar Free & Fat Free Instant Vanilla
  Pudding
Sugar Free Instant Chocolate Pudding
Tapioca Pudding Snack
Vanilla Pudding Snack

Food You Feel Good About (Wegmans)

Homestyle Chocolate Pudding
Homestyle Rice Pudding
Homestyle Tapioca Pudding

Giant

Chocolate Pudding Snack
Instant Chocolate Pudding
Instant Vanilla Pudding
Vanilla Pudding Snack

Goya

Flan ()
Majarete Arroz ()
Majarete Maiz ()
Tembleque ()

Great Value (Wal-Mart) 25

Banana Cream Instant Pudding & Pie
  Filling
Banana Cream Instant Pudding
Chocolate Family Size Instant Pudding
Chocolate Instant Pudding
French Vanilla Instant Pudding & Pie
  Filling
French Vanilla Instant Pudding
Pistachio Instant Pudding & Pie Filling
Pistachio Instant Pudding
Sugar Free Chocolate Instant Pudding
Sugar Free French Vanilla Instant
  Pudding
Vanilla Family Size Instant Pudding
Vanilla Instant Pudding & Pie Filling

Vanilla Instant Pudding

Handi Snacks Pudding ⌒

Pudding Doubles, Baskin Robbins
  Banana Split
Pudding Doubles, Baskin Robbins
  Chocolate Chip Cookie
Pudding Doubles, Baskin Robbins
  Chocolate Vanilla Sundae
Pudding Doubles, Baskin Robbins
  Fudge Rocky Road
Pudding, Banana
Pudding, Butterscotch
Pudding, Chocolate
Pudding, Rice
Pudding, Sugar Free Chocolate Reduced
  Calorie
Pudding, Sugar Free Creamy Caramel
  Reduced Calorie
Pudding, Sugar Free Vanilla Reduced
  Calorie
Pudding, Vanilla

Hill Country Fare (H-E-B)

Ready To Eat Banana Banana Pudding
  Cup
Ready To Eat Banana Chocolate
  Pudding Cup
Ready To Eat Banana Strawberry
  Pudding Cup
Ready To Eat Banana Tapioca Pudding
  Cup
Ready To Eat Banana Vanilla Pudding
  Cup

Hispania Foods

Flan (Caramel, Premium Baked Vanilla)

Hy-Vee

Chocolate Fudge Pudding Cups
Chocolate Pudding Cups
Fat Free Chocolate Pudding Cups
Instant Sugar Free Fat Free Chocolate
  Reduced Calorie Pudding
Instant Sugar Free Fat Free Vanilla
  Reduced Calorie Pudding
Tapioca Pudding Cups
Vanilla Pudding Cups

Jell-O ⌒

Pudding & Pie Filling, Cook & Serve
  Banana Cream

Pudding & Pie Filling, Cook & Serve Butterscotch

Pudding & Pie Filling, Cook & Serve Chocolate

Pudding & Pie Filling, Cook & Serve Chocolate Fudge

Pudding & Pie Filling, Cook & Serve Chocolate Sugar Free

Pudding & Pie Filling, Cook & Serve Coconut Cream

Pudding & Pie Filling, Cook & Serve Lemon

Pudding & Pie Filling, Cook & Serve Vanilla

Pudding & Pie Filling, Cook & Serve Vanilla Sugar Free

Pudding & Pie Filling, Instant Banana Cream

Pudding & Pie Filling, Instant Banana Cream Sugar Free & Fat Free

Pudding & Pie Filling, Instant Butterscotch

Pudding & Pie Filling, Instant Butterscotch Sugar Free & Fat Free

Pudding & Pie Filling, Instant Cheesecake

Pudding & Pie Filling, Instant Cheesecake Sugar Free & Fat Free

Pudding & Pie Filling, Instant Chocolate

Pudding & Pie Filling, Instant Chocolate Fudge

Pudding & Pie Filling, Instant Chocolate Fudge Sugar Free & Fat Free

Pudding & Pie Filling, Instant Chocolate Sugar Free & Fat Free

Pudding & Pie Filling, Instant Coconut Cream

Pudding & Pie Filling, Instant Devil's Food Fat Free

Pudding & Pie Filling, Instant French Vanilla

Pudding & Pie Filling, Instant Lemon

Pudding & Pie Filling, Instant Lemon Sugar Free & Fat Free

Pudding & Pie Filling, Instant Pistachio

Pudding & Pie Filling, Instant Pistachio Sugar Free & Fat Free

Pudding & Pie Filling, Instant Pumpkin Spice

Pudding & Pie Filling, Instant Vanilla

Pudding & Pie Filling, Instant Vanilla Sugar Free & Fat Free

Pudding & Pie Filling, Instant White Chocolate Fat Free

Pudding & Pie Filling, Instant White Chocolate Sugar Free & Fat Free

Pudding Snacks Creme Savers, Strawberries & Creme Swirled

Pudding Snacks, Chocolate Fudge Sundaes

Pudding Snacks, Chocolate Sugar Free Reduced Calorie

Pudding Snacks, Chocolate Vanilla Swirls Sugar Free Reduced Calorie

Pudding Snacks, Creamy Caramel Sugar Free

Pudding Snacks, Devil's Food & Chocolate Fat Free

Pudding Snacks, Double Chocolate Sugar Free

Pudding Snacks, Fat Free Chocolate

Pudding Snacks, Fat Free Chocolate Vanilla Swirls

Pudding Snacks, Fat Free Tapioca

Pudding Snacks, Original Chocolate

Pudding Snacks, Original Chocolate Vanilla Swirls

Pudding Snacks, Original Tapioca

Pudding Snacks, Original Vanilla

Pudding Snacks, Original with The Taste Of Oreo Cookies

Pudding Snacks, Sundae Toppers Vanilla With Caramel Topping

Pudding Snacks, Vanilla & Chocolate 100 Calorie Packs Fat Free

Pudding Snacks, Vanilla Caramel Sundaes 100 Calorie Packs Fat Free

Pudding Snacks, Vanilla Sugar Free

Pudding Sticks, X-Treme Chocolate

Pudding, Cook & Serve Tapioca Fat Free

Pudding, Sugar Free Rice Pudding Creme Brulee Reduced Calorie

Pudding, Sundae Toppers Chocolate
With Chocolate Topping
Rice Pudding, Americana Fat Free

Jewel-Osco
Butterscotch Prepared Pudding
Chocolate Instant Pudding
Chocolate Pudding & Pie Filling
Chocolate Pudding Cups
Fat-Free Chocolate Pudding
French Vanilla Instant Pudding Mix
Pistachio Instant Pudding Mix
Sugar-Free Vanilla Pudding
Vanilla Instant Pudding Mix
Vanilla Pudding & Pie Filling
Vanilla Pudding Cups

Junket
Pudding (All)

Kozy Shack ⓘ
Puddings (All)

La Crème
Mousse (All)

Lakeview Farms
Chocolate Créme Dessert
Chocolate Mousse
Chocolate Pudding
Peanut Butter Cup Mousse
Rice Pudding
Tapioca Pudding

Luisa's
Flan (Baked, Cream Cheese, Coconut)
Rice Pudding

Margarita's
Flan (Flan, Authentic Baked, Creamy)
Rice Pudding (Arroz Con Leche)

Meijer
Banana Pudding Snack
Butterscotch Pudding Snack
Chocolate Fudge Pudding Snack
Chocolate Pudding Snack
Cook & Serve Butterscotch Pudding
Cook & Serve Chocolate Pudding
Cook & Serve Vanilla Pudding
Fat Free Chocolate Pudding Snack
Instant Banana Cream Pudding
Instant Chocolate Pudding & Pie Filling
Instant Coconut Cream Pudding & Pie
Filling

Instant Fat Free & Sugar Free
Butterscotch Pudding
Instant Fat Free & Sugar Free Chocolate
Pudding
Instant Fat Free & Sugar Free Vanilla
Pudding
Instant French Vanilla Pudding & Pie
Filling
Instant Pistachio Pudding & Pie Filling
Instant Vanilla Pudding & Pie Filling
Premium Chocolate Peanut Butter
Pudding
Premium French Vanilla Pudding
Premium Orange Dream Pudding
Tapioca Pudding Snack
Vanilla Pudding Snack

Mori-Nu
Mates Pudding Mixes (Chocolate,
Vanilla) ()

NOH of Hawaii ()
Haupia Coconut Pudding

Our Family
Chocolate Pudding
Instant Banana Cream Pudding
Instant Butterscotch Pudding
Instant Chocolate Pudding
Instant Lemon Pudding
Instant Pistachio Pudding
Instant Sugar Free & Fat Free Chocolate
Pudding
Instant Sugar Free & Fat Free Vanilla
Pudding
Instant Vanilla Pudding
Vanilla Pudding

Prairie Farms
Holiday (Boiled) Custard

Price Chopper
Sugar Free Instant Butterscotch Pudding
Sugar Free Instant Chocolate Pudding
Sugar Free Instant Vanilla Pudding

Publix
Rice Pudding
Tapioca Pudding

Safeway ⌒
Ready To Eat Chocolate/Vanilla Multi
Pack Pudding Snack
Tapioca Pudding

Senor Rico
Flan (Caramel Cream, Creamy)
Pudding (Rice, Rice with Caramel, Sugar Free Rice, Tapioca)

Shaw's
Butterscotch Aspartame Pudding Pie Filling Mix
Chocolate Aspartame Pudding Pie Filling Mix
Chocolate Kosher Pudding & Pie Filling
Chocolate Pudding & Pie Filling
Chocolate Pudding Mix
Chocolate Sugar Pudding & Pie Filling Mix
Coconut Cream Sugar Pudding Pie & Filling Mix
Fat Free Chocolate Pudding
French Vanilla Pudding Mix
Kosher Cherry Gelatin
Kosher Raspberry Gelatin
Kosher Strawberry Gelatin
Lemon Sugar Pudding Pie & Filling Mix
Low Fat Chocolate Pudding
Low Fat Low Sodium Rice Pudding
Pistachio Sugar Pudding Pie & Filling Mix
Prepared Butterscotch Pudding
Prepared Chocolate Tub Pudding
Sugar Free Pudding
Tapioca Sugar Pudding Mix
Vanilla Aspartame Pudding & Pie Filling Mix
Vanilla Pudding & Pie Filling
Vanilla Pudding Mix
Vanilla Sugar Pudding Pie & Filling Mix
Vanilla Tub Pudding Prepared

Snack Pack
Pudding (All BUT Ones Containing Tapioca)

Stop & Shop
Chocolate Pudding Snacks
Vanilla Pudding Snack

Swiss Miss
Pudding (All BUT Ones Containing Tapioca)

Trader Joe's
Crème Brulee in Chocolate Cups
Puddings (Chocolate, Rice, Tapioca)

Tropical Cheese
Arroz Con Leche
Carmel Flan

Valu Time (Brookshire)
Instant Butterscotch Pudding
Instant Chocolate Pudding
Instant Vanilla Pudding

Vons ↶
Ready To Eat Butterscotch Pudding
Ready To Eat Chocolate Fudge Pudding
Ready To Eat Chocolate Pudding
Ready To Eat Tapioca Pudding
Ready To Eat Vanilla Pudding

Wegmans
Chocolate Pudding
Chocolate Vanilla Swirl Pudding
Fat Free Chocolate Pudding
Fat Free Chocolate Vanilla Swirl Pudding
Fat Free Vanilla Pudding
Sugar Free Chocolate Pudding
Sugar Free Chocolate Vanilla Swirl Pudding
Sugar Free Vanilla Pudding
Vanilla Pudding

Winky Brand
Pudding (All)

ZenSoy
ZenSoy Products (All)

RICE CAKES

Flavorite (Cub Foods)
Crunchy Rice Squares

Giant
White Cheddar Rice Cakes

H-E-B
Rice Squares

Kallo
Hint of Chili Jumbo Rice Cakes
Low Fat Thick Salted Rice Cakes
Mature Cheese & Chive Jumbo Rice Cakes
Mini Hint of Chili Rice Cakes
Mini Mature Cheese & Chive Rice Cakes
Organic Fairtrade Sesame Rice Cakes
Organic Fairtrade Unsalted Rice Cakes

Organic Thick No Salt Rice Cakes
Organic Thick Salted Rice Cakes
Organic Thick Sesame Salted Rice Cakes
Organic Thick Slice Savoury Rice Cakes
Organic Thin Dark Chocolate Rice Cakes
Organic Thin Milk Chocolate Rice Cakes
Organic Thin No Salt Rice Cakes
Sea Salt & Balsamic Rice Cakes
Sea Salt & Balsamic Vinegar Jumbo Rice Cakes
Sea Salt & Cracked Pepper Jumbo Rice Cakes

Lundberg Family Farms 〇
Brown Rice
Brown Rice (Salt Free)
Caramel Corn
Cinammon Toast
Eco-Farmed Apple Cinnamon
Eco-Farmed Brown Rice
Eco-Farmed Brown Rice (Salt Free)
Eco-Farmed Buttery Caramel
Eco-Farmed Honey Nut
Eco-Farmed Sesame Tamari
Eco-Farmed Toasted Sesame
Koku Seaweed
Mochi Sweet
Popcorn
Sesame Tamari
Sweet Green Tea with Lemon
Tamari with Seaweed
Wild Rice

Mother's ✓
Caramel Rice Cake
Plain Salted Rice Cake
Plain Unsalted Rice Cake
Salted Butter Rice Cake
White Cheddar Rice Cake

Publix
Lightly Salted Rice Cakes
Mini Caramel Rice
Mini Cheddar Rice
Mini Ranch Rice
Unsalted Rice Cakes
White Cheddar Rice Cakes

Quaker ✓
Gluten-Free Apple Cinnamon Large Rice Cakes

Gluten-Free Butter Popped Corn Large Rice Cakes
Gluten-Free Caramel Corn Large Rice Cakes
Gluten-Free Chocolate Crunch Large Rice Cakes
Gluten-Free Lightly Salted Large Rice Cakes
Gluten-Free Salt Free Large Rice Cakes
Gluten-Free White Cheddar Large Rice Cakes

Safeway 〜
Crispy Cheddar Mini Rice Cakes
Lightly Salted Rice Cakes
White Cheddar Rice and Corn Cakes

Schnucks
Caramel Corn Rice Cakes
Salted Rice Cakes
White Cheddar Rice Cakes

Stop & Shop
Multigrain Salt Free Rice Cakes
Plain Salt Free Rice Cakes

Trader Joe's
Lightly Salted Rice Cakes

TRAIL MIX

Aimee's Livin' Magic
Superhero Galactic Trail Mix

Best Choice
Oriental Trail Mix
Santa Fe Trail Mix

Brookfarm ⓘ
7 Mile Walkabout Mix
Mt. Bogong Walkabout Mix
Night Cap Range Walkabout Mix

El's Kitchen ✓
Medleys (All)

Enjoy Life Foods 〇 ✓
Beach Bash Seed and Fruit Mix
Mountain Mambo Seed and Fruit Mix

Fiona's Granola
Jungle Blend Trail Mix
Mountain Blend Trail Mix

Fisher Nuts ()
Fusions Trail Blazer Snack Mix

Frito Lay ⓘ
Nut & Chocolate Trail Mix
Nut & Fruit Trail Mix
Original Trail Mix
Gerbs Pumpkin Seeds
Trail Mix
Living Intentions
Sprouted Trail Mix (All)
Lydia's Organics ♒
Lydia's Organics (All)
Naturally Nutty
Naturally Nutty (All)
Nature's Promise (Giant)
Organic Cranberry and Walnut Mix
Nature's Promise (Stop & Shop)
Organic Cranberry and Walnut Mix
Nut Harvest ⓘ
Natural Nut & Fruit Mix
O Organics ᏉᎧ
Cranberry Harvest Trail Mix
Planters ᏉᎧ
Trail Mix, Fruit & Nut
Trail Mix, Fruit & Nut Mix
Trail Mix, Mixed Nuts & Raisins
Trail Mix, Nut & Chocolate Mix
Trail Mix, Nuts Seeds & Raisins
Publix
Party Time Mix
Rice River Farms ⓘ
Almond Trail Mix
Classic Trail Mix
Deluxe Nut Mix
Farmer's Market Mix
Rub With Love ⓘ
Gluten Free Snack Mix
Safeway ᏉᎧ
Autumn Mix
Safeway Select ᏉᎧ
Deluxe Trail Mix
Trader Joe's
Almonds, Cranberries, Pistachio &
Cherry Mix
Peanut Butter Cup Trax Mix
Simply Almonds, Cashews &
Cranberries Trek Mix
Simply the Best Trek Mix

Sweet, Savory & Tart Trek Mix
Tempting Trail Mix
Vons ᏉᎧ
Trail Mix with M&M Candies
Wilderness Poets
Wilderness Poets (All)

MISCELLANEOUS

Alpro Soya
Desserts (All)
Cerrone Cone ♒ ✓
Ice Cream Cone
Clearly Organic (Best Choice)
Corn Pops
Crunchies ⓘ
Dried Vegetables (All)
Goldbaum's
Ice Cream Cones (All)
Good Health Natural Products
Veggie Snax ⟨⟩
Goya
Buñuelos
Natillas
Ponche Almibar
Hy-Vee
Cherry Eucalyptus Flavor Drops
Honey Lemon Cough Drops
Menthol Cough Drops
Let's Do… ✓
Gluten-Free Ice Cream Cones
Gluten-Free Sugar Cones
Metamucil
Metamucil Capsules
Price Chopper
Wax Bottles
Trader Joe's
Brown Rice Marshmallow Treats
Green Bean Snacks
Roasted Seaweed Snack
Savory Thins (Original, Minis,
Edamame or Multiseed with Soy
Sauce)
V & V Supremo
Desserts (All)

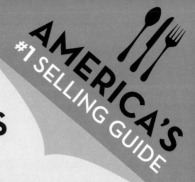
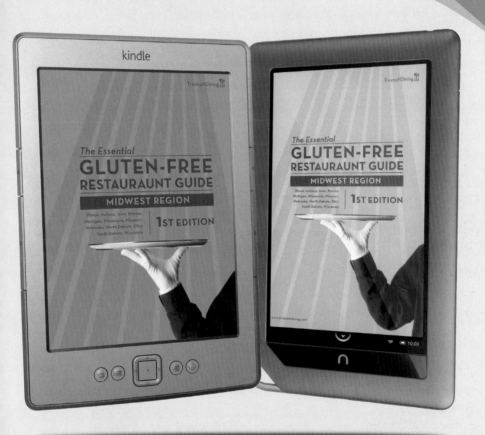

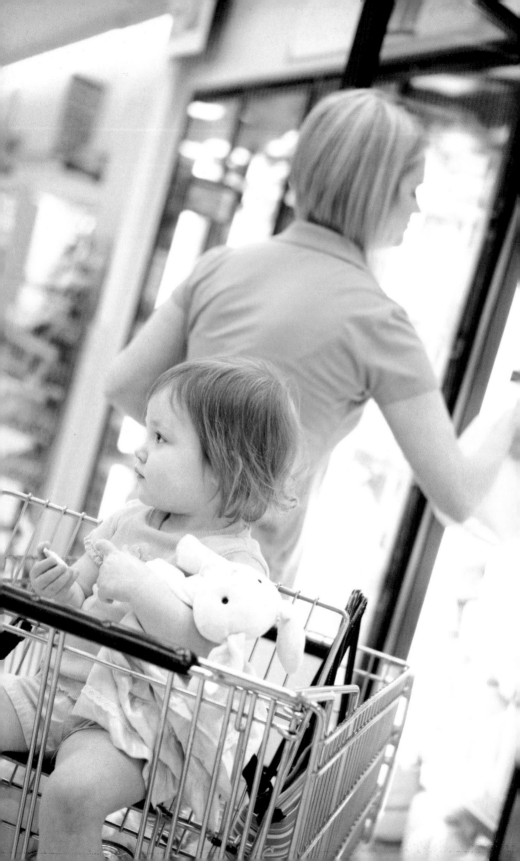

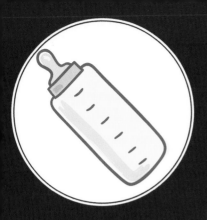

BABY FOOD & FORMULA

BABY FOOD

Beech Nut Baby Food
Apple Mango & Carrot
Apples & Bananas
Apples & Blueberries
Apples & Cherries
Apples & Chicken
Apples, Mango & Kiwi
Apples, Pears & Bananas
Applesauce
Apricots with Pears & Apples
Banana & Mixed Berries
Banana Apple Yogurt
Beef & Beef Broth
Carrots
Chicken & Chicken Broth
Chicken & Rice Dinner
Chicken Noodle Dinner
Chiquita Bananas
Chiquita Bananas & Strawberries
Corn & Sweet Potatoes
Country Garden Vegetables
Creamy Chicken Noodle Dinner
DHA Plus Apple Delight
DHA Plus Apples with Pomegranate
  Juice
DHA Plus Banana Supreme
DHA Plus Squash with Corn
DHA Plus Sweet Potatoes
Green Beans
Ham, Pineapple & Rice
Hearty Vegetable Stew
Homestyle Apples & Bananas
Homestyle Apples, Cherries & Plums

Homestyle Chiquita Bananas
Homestyle Cinnamon Raisins & Pears
Homestyle Green Beans & Potatoes
Homestyle Green Beans, Corn & Rice
Homestyle Peaches, Apples & Bananas
Homestyle Pears & Blueberries
Homestyle Rice Cereal & Pears
Homestyle Squash & Zucchini
Homestyle Sweet Corn & Rice
Homestyle Sweet Potatoes
Homestyle Turkey Rice Dinner
Homestyle Vegetable Medley with
  Turkey
Homestyle Vegetables & Chicken
Macaroni & Beef with Vegetables
Mango
Mixed Fruit Nibbles
Mixed Vegetables
Peaches
Pears
Pears & Green Beans
Pears & Pineapple
Pears & Raspberries
Peas & Carrots
Pineapple Glazed Ham
Rice Cereal
Rice Cereal & Apples with Cinnamon
Rice with Chiquita Bananas
Squash
Squash & Apples
Strawberry Fruit Nibbles
Sweet Corn Casserole
Sweet Potato & Turkey
Sweet Potato & Zucchini
Sweet Potatoes & Apples

Sweet Potatoes & Chicken
Tender Golden Sweet Potatoes
Tender Sweet Carrots
Tender Sweet Peas
Tender Young Green Beans
Turkey & Turkey Broth
Turkey Rice Dinner
Turkey Tetrazzini
Turkey Vegetable
Vegetable Beef
Vegetables & Chicken
White Cheddar Puffed Grain Baked
Snacks

Belle's Biscuits
Teething Biscuits (All)

Full Circle (Price Chopper)
Apple Apricot Baby Food
Apple Banana Baby Food
Mixed Vegetables Baby Food
Organic Carrot Baby Food
Organic Pears Baby Food
Sweet Potato Baby Food
White Lima Beans Baby Food

Full Circle (Schnucks)
Stage 1 Applesauce
Stage 1 Bananas
Stage 1 Carrots
Stage 1 Pears
Stage 1 Peas
Stage 1 Sweet Potatoes
Stage 2 Apple Apricot
Stage 2 Apple Banana
Stage 2 Apple Blueberry
Stage 2 Applesauce
Stage 2 Banana
Stage 2 Carrots
Stage 2 Mixed Vegetables
Stage 2 Pears
Stage 2 Peas & Brown Rice
Stage 2 Squash
Stage 2 Sweet Potato & Chicken
Stage 2 Sweet Potatoes
Stage 2 Vegetable Beef

Gerber
2ND FOODS Fruits in 4 oz – Apple
Blueberry / Manzana y Arándanos

2ND FOODS Fruits in 4 oz – Apple
Strawberry Banana / Manzana Fresa
Banana
2ND FOODS Fruits in 4 oz –
Applesauce
2ND FOODS Fruits in 4 oz – Bananas
2ND FOODS Fruits in 4 oz – Pears
2ND FOODS Meats – Beef & Beef
Gravy
2ND FOODS Meats – Chicken &
Chicken Gravy
2ND FOODS Meats – Ham & Ham
Gravy
2ND FOODS Meats – Turkey & Turkey
Gravy
2ND FOODS Vegetables in 4 oz –
Carrots
2ND FOODS Vegetables in 4 oz – Green
Beans
2ND FOODS Vegetables in 4 oz – Peas
2ND FOODS Vegetables in 4 oz –
Squash
2ND FOODS Vegetables in 4 oz – Sweet
Potatoes
DHA & Probiotic Cereal – Rice
GRADUATES FOR PRESCHOOLERS
Fruit Twists – Apple & Strawberry
GRADUATES FOR PRESCHOOLERS
Fruit Twists – Cherry Berry
GRADUATES FOR PRESCHOOLERS
Fruit Twists – Strawberry & Grape
GRADUATES FOR PRESCHOOLERS
Healthy Meals – Mixed Vegetables,
Chicken & Rice in Sauce with Carrots
GRADUATES FOR TODDLERS Fruit
Strips – Strawberry
GRADUATES FOR TODDLERS Fruit
Strips – Wildberry
GRADUATES FOR TODDLERS LIL'
ENTRÉES – Rice and Turkey in Gravy
GRADUATES FOR TODDLERS LIL'
STICKS – Chicken Sticks
GRADUATES FOR TODDLERS LIL'
STICKS – Meat Sticks
GRADUATES FOR TODDLERS LIL'
STICKS – Turkey Sticks

GRADUATES FOR TODDLERS MINI FRUITS – Apple

GRADUATES FOR TODDLERS MINI FRUITS – Banana Strawberry

GRADUATES Fruit & Veggie Melts Snack – Truly Tropical Blend

GRADUATES Fruit & Veggie Melts Snack – Very Berry Blend

GRADUATES Fruit Pick-Ups – Diced Apples

GRADUATES FRUIT SPLASHERS Single-Serve Drink Boxes – Apple Berry

GRADUATES FRUIT SPLASHERS Single-Serve Drink Boxes – Mixed Berry

GRADUATES Grabbers Squeezable Fruit - Apple, Mango & Strawberry

GRADUATES Grabbers Squeezable Fruit - Apple, Pear & Peach

GRADUATES Grabbers Squeezable Fruit - Banana Blueberry

GRADUATES Grabbers Squeezable Fruit & Veggies - Apple & Sweet Potato with Cinnamon

GRADUATES Grabbers Squeezable Fruit & Veggies - Pear & Squash

GRADUATES LIL' CRUNCHIES – Cinnamon Maple

GRADUATES LIL' CRUNCHIES – Garden Tomato

GRADUATES LIL' CRUNCHIES – Mild Cheddar

GRADUATES LIL' CRUNCHIES – Veggie Dip

GRADUATES Veggie Pick-Ups – Diced Carrots

GRADUATES WAGON WHEELS – Apple Harvest

GRADUATES WAGON WHEELS – Cheesy Carrot

GRADUATES Yogurt Blends Snack – Banana Vanilla

GRADUATES Yogurt Blends Snack – Mixed Berry

GRADUATES Yogurt Blends Snack – Strawberry Banana

GRADUATES YOGURT MELTS – Mixed Berries

GRADUATES YOGURT MELTS – Peach

GRADUATES YOGURT MELTS – Strawberry

Grain & Fruit Cereal – Rice & Apple

Grain & Fruit Cereal – Rice & Mixed Fruit

NatureSelect 1ST FOODS Fruits – Apples

NatureSelect 1ST FOODS Fruits – Bananas

NatureSelect 1ST FOODS Fruits – Peaches

NatureSelect 1ST FOODS Fruits – Pears

NatureSelect 1ST FOODS Fruits – Prunes

NatureSelect 1ST FOODS Vegetables – Carrots

NatureSelect 1ST FOODS Vegetables – Green Beans

NatureSelect 1ST FOODS Vegetables – Peas

NatureSelect 1ST FOODS Vegetables – Squash

NatureSelect 1ST FOODS Vegetables – Sweet Potatoes

NatureSelect 2ND FOOD Fruits – Bananas with Apples & Pears

NatureSelect 2ND FOODS Cereals – Apples & Mangos with Rice Cereal

NatureSelect 2ND FOODS Fruits – Apple Blueberry

NatureSelect 2ND FOODS Fruits – Apple Strawberry Banana

NatureSelect 2ND FOODS Fruits – Apples

NatureSelect 2ND FOODS Fruits – Apples & Cherries

NatureSelect 2ND FOODS Fruits – Apricot with Mixed Fruit

NatureSelect 2ND FOODS Fruits – Banana Mixed Berries

NatureSelect 2ND FOODS Fruits – Banana Orange Medley

NatureSelect 2ND FOODS Fruits – Banana Plum Grape

NatureSelect 2ND FOODS Fruits – Bananas

NatureSelect 2ND FOODS Fruits – Peaches

NatureSelect 2ND FOODS Fruits – Pear Pineapple

NatureSelect 2ND FOODS Fruits – Pears

NatureSelect 2ND FOODS Fruits – Prunes with Apples

NatureSelect 2ND FOODS Nutritious Dinners – Apples & Chicken

NatureSelect 2ND FOODS Nutritious Dinners – Chicken & Rice

NatureSelect 2ND FOODS Nutritious Dinners – Vegetable Beef

NatureSelect 2ND FOODS Spoonable Smoothies – Fruit Medley

NatureSelect 2ND FOODS Spoonable Smoothies – Hawaiian Delight

NatureSelect 2ND FOODS Spoonable Smoothies – Mango

NatureSelect 2ND FOODS Spoonable Smoothies – Peach Cobbler

NatureSelect 2ND FOODS Vegetables – Carrots

NatureSelect 2ND FOODS Vegetables – Garden Vegetables

NatureSelect 2ND FOODS Vegetables – Green Beans

NatureSelect 2ND FOODS Vegetables – Mixed Vegetables

NatureSelect 2ND FOODS Vegetables – Peas

NatureSelect 2ND FOODS Vegetables – Squash

NatureSelect 2ND FOODS Vegetables – Sweet Potatoes

NatureSelect 2ND FOODS Vegetables – Sweet Potatoes & Corn

NatureSelect 3RD FOODS Fruits - Apple, Banana & Peach

NatureSelect 3RD FOODS Fruits - Apple, Mango & Kiwi

NatureSelect 3RD FOODS Fruits – Apples

NatureSelect 3RD FOODS Fruits – Banana Strawberry

NatureSelect 3RD FOODS Fruits – Bananas

NatureSelect 3RD FOODS Fruits – Pears

NatureSelect 3RD FOODS Nutritious Dinners – Mixed Vegetables & Beef

NatureSelect 3RD FOODS Nutritious Dinners – Mixed Vegetables & Chicken

NatureSelect 3RD FOODS Nutritious Dinners – Mixed Vegetables & Turkey

NatureSelect 3RD FOODS Nutritious Dinners – Turkey, Rice & Vegetables

NatureSelect 3RD FOODS Spoonable Smoothies – Fruit Medley

NatureSelect 3RD FOODS Vegetables – Broccoli & Carrots with Cheese

NatureSelect 3RD FOODS Vegetables – Green Beans with Rice

NatureSelect 3RD FOODS Vegetables – Squash

NatureSelect 3RD FOODS Vegetables – Sweet Potatoes

Organic Smart Nourish 2ND FOODS Fruit & Vegetable – Apple Sweet Potato

Organic SmartNourish 1ST FOODS Fruits – Apples

Organic SmartNourish 1ST FOODS Fruits – Bananas

Organic SmartNourish 1ST FOODS Fruits – Pears

Organic SmartNourish 1ST FOODS Fruits – Prunes

Organic SmartNourish 1ST FOODS Vegetables – Carrots

Organic SmartNourish 1ST FOODS Vegetables – Sweet Peas

Organic SmartNourish 1ST FOODS Vegetables – Sweet Potatoes

Organic SmartNourish 2ND FOODS Fruit & Vegetable – Apple Sweet Potato

Organic SmartNourish 2ND FOODS Fruits – Apple Strawberry

Organic SmartNourish 2ND FOODS Fruits – Apples

Organic SmartNourish 2ND FOODS Fruits – Bananas

Organic SmartNourish 2ND FOODS Fruits – Pear & Wild Blueberry

Organic SmartNourish 2ND FOODS Fruits – Pears

Organic SmartNourish 2ND FOODS Purees – Apple Blackberry

Organic SmartNourish 2ND FOODS Purees – Apples & Summer Peaches

Organic SmartNourish 2ND FOODS Purees – Banana Mango

Organic SmartNourish 2ND FOODS Purees – Pear Raspberry

Organic SmartNourish 2ND FOODS Purees – Vegetable Risotto with Cheese

Organic SmartNourish 2ND FOODS Vegetables – Butternut Squash & Corn

Organic SmartNourish 2ND FOODS Vegetables – Carrots

Organic SmartNourish 2ND FOODS Vegetables – Green Beans

Organic SmartNourish 2ND FOODS Vegetables – Sweet Potatoes

Organic SmartNourish Single Grain Cereal – Brown Rice

Single Grain Cereal – Rice

SmartNourish 2ND FOODS Purees – Banana Pineapple Orange Medley

SmartNourish 2ND FOODS Purees – Spring Garden Vegetables with Brown Rice

Yogurt Blends Snack – Apple Cinnamon with Whole Grains

Yogurt Blends Snack – Banana

Yogurt Blends Snack – Blueberry with Whole Grains

Yogurt Blends Snack – Pear

Yogurt Blends Snack – Strawberry

Yogurt Blends Snack– Peach

Goya

Apple Baby Food

Apple/Pineapple Baby Food

Banana Baby Food

Fruit Cocktail Baby Food

Guava Baby Food

Mango Baby Food

Mixed Fruit Baby Food

Peach Baby Food

Pear Baby Food

Pineapple/Peach Baby Food

Prune Baby Food

Sweet Peas Baby Food

Tangerine Baby Food

Tropical Fruits Baby Food

Happy Baby

Baby Dhal & Mama Grain

Chick Chick

Easy Going Greens & Great Greens

Easy Organic Meals 1, Mango

Easy Organic Meals 1, Pear

Easy Organic Meals 2, Apple & Cherry

Easy Organic Meals 2, Apricot & Sweet Potato

Easy Organic Meals 2, Banana, Beet & Blueberry

Easy Organic Meals 2, Broccoli, Pear & Peas

Easy Organic Meals 2, Kiwi & Banana

Easy Organic Meals 2, Spinach/Mango/Pear

Easy Organic Meals 3, Amaranth Ratatouille

Easy Organic Meals 3, Beef Stew

Easy Organic Meals 3, Chick Chick

Easy Organic Meals 3, Gobble Gobble

Easy Organic Meals 3, Mama Grain

Easy Organic Meals 3, Super Salmon ()

Gluten Free Strawberry Baby Puffs ()

Gluten Free Sweet Potato Baby Puffs ()

Gobble Gobble & Paradise Puree

Happy Bellies Brown Rice Cereal

Happy Bellies MultiGrain Cereal ()

Happy Bellies Oatmeal Cereal ()

Happy Munchies, Broccoli, Kale and Cheddar Cheese

Happy Munchies, Cheddar Cheese with Carrot

HappyBites, Chicken Bites

HappyMelts, Organic Banana Mango
HappyMelts, Organic Mixed Berry
HappyMelts, Organic Strawberry
HappyTot, Apple & Butternut Squash
HappyTot, Banana/Mango/Peach
HappyTot, Banana/Peach/Prunes/
Coconut
HappyTot, Green Beans/Pears/Peas
HappyTot, Spinach/Mango/Pear
HappyTot, Sweet Potato/Apple/Carrots
Smarter Squash & Wiser Apple
Sweeter Potatoes & Purer Pears
Yes Peas & Thank You Carrots

Healthy Times
Baby Brown Rice Baby Cereal
Jar Baby Foods (All)

Hot Kid
Mum-Mum Baby Banana
Mum-Mum Baby Organic Original
Mum-Mum Baby Original
Mum-Mum Baby Vegetable
Mum-Mum Toddler Organic
OriginalMum-Mum Toddler Organic
Strawberry

Meijer
Chocolate
Little Fruit Apple
Little Fruit Strawberry Banana
Little Veggies Corn
Strawberry Diabetic Nutritional Drink
Strawberry Pediatric Nutritional Drink
Vanilla Diabetic Nutritional Drink
Vanilla Soy Pediatric Nutritional Drink
Vanilla with Fiber Pediatric Nutritional
Drink

O Organics ᕲ
Chicken For Baby Stage 2
Stage 1 Baby Food Organic Applesauce
Stage 1 Baby Food Organic Bananas
Stage 1 Baby Food Organic Pears
Stage 1 Baby Food Organic Sweet
Potatoes
Stage 2 Baby Food Organic Apple
Apricot
Stage 2 Baby Food Organic Apple Wild
Blueberry

Stage 2 Baby Food Organic Applesauce
Stage 2 Baby Food Organic Mixed
Vegetables
Stage 2 Baby Food Organic Peach Rice
Banana
Stage 2 Baby Food Organic Pears
Stage 2 Baby Food Organic Peas and
Brown Rice
Stage 2 Baby Food Organic Prunes
Stage 2 Baby Food Organic Squash
Stage 2 Baby Food Organic Summer
Vegetables
Stage 2 Baby Food Organic Sweet
Potatoes
Toddler Gummi Fruit Snacks

BABY JUICE & OTHER DRINKS

Beech Nut Baby Food
Apple Juice
Apple Pomegranate Juice
DHA Plus Yogurt Blends with Juice
(Mixed Berry, Tropical Fruit)
Good Morning Chiquita Banana Juice
with YogurtPear Blueberry Juice
Spring Water with Added Fluoride
White Grape Juice
White Grape Peach Juice

Bright Beginnings
Soy Pediatric Nutrition Drink

Gerber ᕲ
GRADUATES FOR PRESCHOOLERS
Juice Treats – Fruit Medley
GRADUATES FOR PRESCHOOLERS
Juice Treats – Tropical
GRADUATES FRUIT SPLASHERS
Beverage – Grape
GRADUATES FRUIT SPLASHERS
Beverage – Strawberry Kiwi
GRADUATES FRUIT SPLASHERS
Beverage – Tropical
GRADUATES Lil' Water
GRADUATES SMART SIPS Dairy
Beverage – Plain
GRADUATES SMART SIPS Dairy
Beverage – Strawberry

GRADUATES SMART SIPS Dairy
Beverage – Vanilla

Harvest Juice – Apple Carrot Juice
Blend

Harvest Juice – Mango Puree, Pineapple
& Carrot Juice Blend

NatureSelect 100% Fruit Juice – Apple

NatureSelect 100% Fruit Juice – Apple
Juice Blend (Apple Grape)

NatureSelect 100% Fruit Juice – Apple
Prune

NatureSelect 100% Fruit Juice – Banana
Juice Blend (Apple Banana)

NatureSelect 100% Fruit Juice – Mixed
Fruit

NatureSelect 100% Fruit Juice – Pear

NatureSelect 100% Fruit Juice – White
Grape

NatureSelect 3RD FOODS Nutritious
Dinners – Mixed Vegetables & Beef

NatureSelect 3RD FOODS Nutritious
Dinners – Mixed Vegetables &
Chicken

NatureSelect 3RD FOODS Nutritious
Dinners – Mixed Vegetables & Turkey

NatureSelect 3RD FOODS Nutritious
Dinners – Turkey, Rice & Vegetables

Organic 100% Juice – Apple

Organic 100% Juice – Pear

Happy Baby
SUPER Banana
SUPER Cinnamon
SUPER Pom, Apple and Peach
SUPER Pumpkin and Orange with
Mangosteen
SUPER Yumberry and Apple

Hy-Vee
Mother's Choice Infant Water
Mother's Choice Infant Water with
Fluoride

Meijer
Bright Beginnings Soy Vanilla
Follow On with DHA
Gentle Protein with DHA
Gluco Burst Arctic Cherry

Gluco Burst Chocolate Diabetic
Nutritional Drink

Gluco Burst Strawberry Diabetic
Nutritional Drink

Gluco Burst Vanilla Diabetic Nutritional
Drink

Lactose Free with DHA

Milk with DHA

Soy with DHA

Vanilla Pediatric Nutritional Drink

Mom to Mom ⌒
Pediatric Electrolyte Fruit Flavor
Pediatric Electrolyte Grape
Pediatric Electrolyte Unflavored

Our Family
Pediatric Electrolyte Apple
Pediatric Electrolyte Fruit Flavor
Pediatric Electrolyte Grape Flavor
Pediatric Electrolyte Regular

PediaSure
PediaSure (All Flavors)
PediaSure with Fiber - Vanilla

Schnucks
Infant Water
Kids Drinking Water

Wegmans
Pediatric Drink - Chocolate
Pediatric Drink - Strawberry
Pediatric Drink - Vanilla
Pediatric Drink - Vanilla with Fiber

FORMULA

Bright Beginnings
Infant Formulas (All)

Enfagrow
Gentlease Toddler
Premium Older Toddler Vanilla Drink
Premium Toddler
Soy Toddler

Enfamil
EnfaCare
Enfalyte
Enfamil 5% Glucose in Water
Enfamil A.R.
Enfamil Water

Enfaport
Gentlease
Human Milk Fortifier Powder
Lipil
Premature Lipil
Premium Infant
Premium Newborn
Prosobee
RestFull

Mead Johnson
Infant Formulas (All)
Pediatric Products (All)

Meijer
Regular Term Formula
Soy Term Formula

Nutramigen
Nutramigen
Nutramigen AA
Nutramigen with Enflora LGG

PediaSure
PediaSure Enteral Formula - Vanilla

Pregestimil
Pregestimil

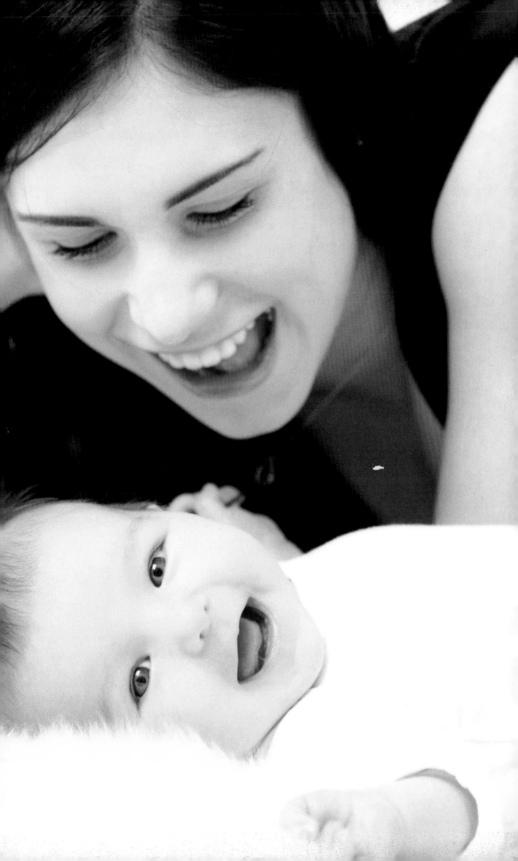

FAN GLUTENFREE TASTIC

Why are we calling attention to the fact that Jones All Natural Sausage contains no gluten and none of the ingredients hidden in other brands? Because we thought you'd like to know. It's just pork, salt and spices—has been for over 120 years. Plus our sausage is frozen so it's always fresh. Always fantastic.

Visit **jonesdairyfarm.com/glutenfree** for great recipes and special savings.

No nitrites

No MSG

No artificial flavors

Find us on Facebook!

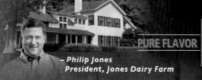

— **Philip Jones**
President, Jones Dairy Farm

PURE FLAVOR SIMPLE PLEASURE

GF

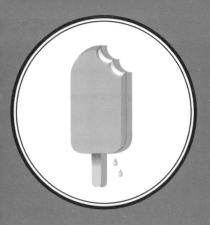

FROZEN FOODS

BEANS

Albertsons
  Cut Green Beans
  Whole Blackeyed Peas
Always Save
  Green Beans, Cut
Best Choice
  Baby Lima Beans
  Butter Beans
  Green Beans, French Style
  Green Beans, Whole
  Steamed Cut Green Beans
Clearly Organic (Best Choice)
  Green Bean Steamer
Cub Foods
  Baby Lima Beans
  French Cut Green Beans
  Green Beans
Fastco (Fareway)
  Green Beans, Cut
  Green Beans, Whole
FLAV.R.PAC
  Baby Lima Beans
  Green Beans, Cut
  Green Beans, French Cut
  Green Beans, Whole
Flavorite (Cub Foods)
  Baby Lima Beans
  Individually Quick Frozen Steamables
    Green Beans
  Speckled Butter Beans
Food Club (Brookshire)
  Baby Lima Beans
  Green Beans, Cut

  Green Beans, French Cut
  Green Beans, Whole
Food Club (Marsh)
  Baby Lima Beans
  Green Beans, Cut
  Green Beans, French Cut
  Green Beans, Whole
  Steamin' Easy, Cut Green Beans Steamin'
    Easy, French Cut Green Beans
Food You Feel Good About
(Wegmans)
  Baby Lima Beans
  Fordhook Lima Beans
  Green Beans, French Style
  Green Beans, Whole
Genuardi's ⌀
  Fordhook Lima Beans
Giant
  Baby Lima Beans
  Blue Lake Green Beans, Whole
  Green Beans, Cut
  Harvest Choice French Style Green
    Beans
Goya
  Baby Lima Beans
  Fava Beans
  Green Beans, Cut
Great Value (Wal-Mart) 🔲25
  Green Beans, Cut
  Green Beans, Cut (Microwavable)
Green Giant
  Valley Fresh Steamers - Cut Green
    Beans
  Valley Fresh Steamers - Select Whole
    Green Beans

Haggen
- Green Beans (Cut, French Style, Whole, Whole Petite)
- Lima Beans, Baby

Hanover Foods
- Baby Lima Beans
- Blue Lake Cut Green Beans
- Blue Lake French Green Beans
- Blue Lake Whole Green Beans
- Fordhook Lima Beans
- Golden Beans, Whole
- Green Beans, Cut
- Green Beans, Italian Cut
- Green Beans, Petite
- Green Beans, Whole

Hy-Vee
- Baby Lima Beans
- Green Beans, French Cut

Jewel-Osco
- Baby Lima Beans
- Cut Green Beans Steamables
- Fordhook Lima Beans
- French Style Sliced Green Beans
- Italian Cut Green Beans

Market Day
- Green Beans, Gourmet

Meijer Organics
- Green Beans (Cut, French Cut, French Style, Italian Cut, Steamer)
- Lima Beans (Baby, Fordhook)

Nature's Promise (Giant)
- Organic Cut Green Beans

Our Family
- Green Beans, Cut Steamable
- Lima Beans

Publix
- Green Beans - Cut
- Green Beans - French Cut
- Lima Beans - Baby
- Lima Beans - Fordhook
- Special Butter Beans

Schnucks
- Green Beans, Cut
- Green Beans, French Cut
- Lima Beans, Baby

Seapoint Farms
- Edamame, Grab N Go (Pods, Shelled) (All)
- Edamame, Ready to Eat Salted Pods (All)
- Edamame, Shelled (All)
- Organic Edamame (Pods, Shelled)

Stop & Shop
- Green Beans, Cut
- Green Beans, French Style

Thrifty Maid (Winn-Dixie)
- Green Beans, Cut
- Peas, Sweet Green

Valu Time (Marsh)
- Green Beans, Cut

Vons ⤶
- Baby Lima Beans
- Green Beans, Cut
- Pinto Beans
- Small Red Beans

Wegmans
- Green Beans - Cut
- Green Beans - Italian
- Green Beans
- Micro Baby Lima Beans

Westpac
- Baby Lima Beans
- Green Beans, Cut
- Green Beans, French Cut
- Speckled Butter Beans

Winn-Dixie
- Butter Beans
- Green Beans (Cut, French Style Sliced, Italian, Whole)
- Lima Beans (Baby, Fordhook, Petite, Speckled)
- Organic Green Beans, Cut
- Steamable Green Beans, Cut

COOKIE DOUGH

French Meadow Bakery
- Gluten-Free Chocolate Chip Cookie Dough

Gilbert's Goodies ⓘ ✓
- Cookie Dough

WOW Baking 🔸
Cookie Dough (All)

DOUGH

Chebe 🔸
Bread Sticks
Ciabatta Rolls
Original Cheese Rolls
Tomato-Basil Breadsticks

FROZEN YOGURT

Broughton
Sugar Free Fat Free Vanilla Frozen
Yogurt Mix ⟨⟩
Gifford's Ice Cream ⓘ
Black Raspberry with Chocolate Chips
Cappuccino
Chocolate Peanut Butter Cup
Low Fat No Sugar Added Butter Pecan
Moose Tracks
No Fat No Sugar Added Black
Raspberry
No Fat No Sugar Added Vanilla with
Raspberry Swirl
Hiland Dairy
Frozen Yogurt (Chocolate, Strawberry,
Vanilla)
Hood
Chocolate Fat Free Frozen Yogurt
Maine Blueberry & Sweet Cream Fat
Free Frozen Yogurt
Mocha Fudge Fat Free Frozen Yogurt
Strawberry Banana Fat Free Frozen
Yogurt
Strawberry Fat Free Frozen Yogurt
Vanilla Fat Free Frozen Yogurt
Mayfield Dairy
Chocolate Light Frozen Yogurt ⟨⟩
Peach Light Frozen Yogurt ⟨⟩
Praline Pecan Light Frozen Yogurt ⟨⟩
Vanilla Light Frozen Yogurt ⟨⟩
Oberweis Dairy
Chocolate Yogurt
French Vanilla Yogurt

Our Family
Strawberry Frozen Yogurt
Vanilla Frozen Yogurt
Perry's Ice Cream ⓘ
Chocolate Almond Yogurt
Fat Free Peach Yogurt
Fat Free Vanilla Yogurt
Peanut Butter Chip Yogurt
Raspberry Truffle Yogurt
Prairie Farms
Chocolate Frozen Yogurt
Steak N Shake Frozen Yogurt
Strawberry Frozen Yogurt
Vanilla Frozen Yogurt
Publix
Black Cherry Premium Low Fat Frozen
Yogurt
Butter Pecan Premium Low Fat Frozen
Yogurt
Chocolate Premium Low Fat Frozen
Yogurt
Neapolitan Premium Low Fat Frozen
Yogurt
Peach Premium Low Fat Frozen Yogurt
Peanut Butter Cup Premium Low Fat
Frozen Yogurt
Strawberry Premium Low Fat Frozen
Yogurt
Vanilla Orange Premium Low Fat
Frozen Yogurt
Vanilla Orange Premium Low Fat
Frozen Yogurt, No Sugar Added
Vanilla Premium Low Fat Frozen Yogurt
Safeway Select 〰
Black Cherry Chocolate Chip Fat Free
Frozen Yogurt
Chocolate Fat Free Frozen Yogurt
Vanilla Fat Free Frozen Yogurt
Sweet Scoops ⓘ
Frozen Yogurt (All BUT Coffee Cookies
and Cream)
Turkey Hill
Chocolate Marshmallow Frozen Yogurt
Fudge Ripple Frozen Yogurt
Neapolitan Frozen Yogurt
Peach Melba Frozen Yogurt (Limited
Edition)

PomBlueberry Chocolate Truffle Frozen
Yogurt (Limited Edition)
Vaniila Bean Frozen Yogurt
Yasso Frozen Greek Yogurt ⓘ
Yasso Frozen Greek Yogurt (All)

Fruit

Best Choice
Blackberries
Blueberries
Cherries
Cherries (Individually Quick Frozen)
Mango Chunks
Mixed Berries
Mixed Fruit
Mixed Fruit (Individually Quick Frozen)
Peaches (Individually Quick Frozen)
Raspberries
Rhubarb
Sliced Peaches
Sliced Strawberries
Sliced Strawberries with Splenda
Strawberries (Individually Quick
Frozen)
Strawberries, Whole
Clearly Organic (Best Choice)
Blueberries
Mixed Berries
Raspberries
Whole Strawberries
FLAV.R.PAC
Blueberries
Deluxe Berry Mix
Marion Blackberries
Red Raspberries
Sliced Strawberries
Strawberries, Whole
Food Club (Brookshire)
100% Grape Cocktail
Berry Medley
Blackberries
Blueberries
Dark Sweet Cherries
Freestone Peaches
Fruit Punch
Grapefruit Concentrate

Lemonade
Mango Chunks
Mixed Fruit
Red Raspberries
Sliced Peaches
Sliced Strawberries
Strawberries, Whole
Wild Blueberries
Food Club (Marsh)
Berry Medley
Blackberries Individually Quick Frozen
Blueberries
Blueberries Individually Quick Frozen
Cherries, Dark Sweet
Peach Slices, Individually Quick Frozen
Raspberries, Red, Individually Quick
Frozen
Sliced Strawberries
Strawberries Whole
Strawberries Whole, Individually Quick
Frozen
**Food You Feel Good About
(Wegmans)**
Sweet Cherries
Full Circle (Schnucks)
Blueberries
Raspberries
Strawberries
Genuardi's
Berry Mix
Dark Sweet Pitted Cherries
Peaches, Sliced
Red Raspberries
Giant
Harvest Choice Berry Medley
Harvest Choice Blackberries
Harvest Choice Blueberries
Harvest Choice Dark Sweet Cherries
Harvest Choice Red Raspberries
Harvest Choice Sliced Peaches
Mango Chunks (Frozen)
Unsweetened Whole Strawberries
Goya
Ponche Mix Frozen Fruit
Great Value (Wal-Mart) 25
Berry Medley
Sliced Strawberries

Haggen
- Berry Medley
- Blackberries
- Blueberries
- Mixed Fruit Medley
- Peaches, Sliced
- Raspberries
- Raspberries, Red with Heavy Syrup
- Strawberries (Sliced, Whole)

Hill Country Fare (H-E-B)
- Strawberries & Cream
- Strawberries in Syrup

Hy-Vee
- Blueberries (Unsweetened)
- Cherry Berry Blend (Unsweetened)
- Red Raspberries (Unsweetened)
- Sliced Strawberries
- Whole Strawberries

Market Day
- Fruit Singles

Meijer
- Berry Medley
- Blackberries
- Cherries (Dark Sweet, Tart)
- Mango (Chunks, Sliced)
- Mixed Fruit
- Pineapple (Chunks)
- Triple Berry Blend
- Tropical Fruit Blend

Meijer Organics
- Blueberries
- Peaches (Sliced)
- Raspberries (Individual, Whole)
- Strawberries (Sliced, Individual) (Meijer Organic)

Nature's Promise (Giant)
- Organic Mangos
- Organic Raspberries
- Organic Whole Strawberries

Nature's Promise (Stop & Shop)
- Organic Raspberries

O Organics
- Organic Mango
- Organic Wild Blueberries

Our Family
- Berry Medley
- Blackberries
- Blueberries
- Dark Sweet Cherries
- Mango Chunks
- Mixed Fruit
- Raspberries (Individually Quick Frozen)
- Red Raspberries in Sugar Syrup
- Strawberries (Individually Quick Frozen)
- Strawberries, Sliced
- Strawberries, Sliced Splenda Sweetened
- Strawberries, Sliced Sugar Sweetened

Publix
- Blackberries
- Blueberries
- Cherries - Dark Sweet
- Cranberries
- Mixed Berries
- Mixed Fruit
- Peaches - Sliced
- Raspberries
- Strawberries - Sliced, Sweetened
- Strawberries - Whole

Safeway
- Unsweetened Whole Blueberries
- Unsweetened Whole Strawberries
- Whole Blackberries

Schnucks
- Berries Supreme
- Blackberries, Whole
- Blueberries, Whole
- Dark Sweet Cherries
- Fancy Mixed Fruit
- Mango Chunks
- Pineapple Chunks
- Red Raspberries, Whole
- Rhubarb, Cut
- Strawberries (Sliced, Whole)
- Strawberries, Sliced (Individually Quick Frozen)

Stahlbush Island Farms ⓘ
- Stahlbush Island Farms (All BUT Black Barley & Wheat Berries)

Stop & Shop
- Sliced Strawberries
- Unsweetened Whole Strawberries

Trader Joe's
- Chile Mango Fruit Floes

Frozen Fruits (All)
Fruit Floes
Valu Time (Brookshire)
Sliced Strawberry
Vons 〰
Strawberries, Sliced Sweetened
Wegmans
Berry Medley
Blackberries
Blueberries
Raspberries
Raspberries with Sugar
Sliced Peaches
Sliced Strawberries - Light (With Aspartame)
Sliced Strawberries with Sugar
Strawberries
Westpac
Sliced Strawberries
Winn-Dixie
Berry Medley
Blackberries
Blueberries
Dark Sweet Cherries
Mango Chunks
Mixed Fruit
Peaches, Sliced
Red Raspberries
Strawberries (No Sugar Added, Sugar Added)
Strawberries, Whole
Wyman's
Wyman's (All)

ICE CREAM

Agave Dream
Ice Cream (All)
Almond-licious Ice Supreme
ICE Supreme (All Flavors)
Always Save
Chocolate Ice Cream
French Vanilla Ice Cream
Lowfat Vanilla Ice Cream
Neapolitan Ice Cream
Strawberry Ice Cream
Vanilla Ice Cream

Vanilla Orange Ice Cream
Vanilla/Fudge Ice Cream
Always Save (Price Chopper)
Vanilla Ice Cream
Arctic Zero ⓘ
Ice Cream (All)
Berkeley Farms
Banana Split ()
Caramel ()
Chocolate Chip ()
Chocolate ()
French Vanilla ()
Mint Chip ()
Moose Tracks ()
Neapolitan ()
Pistachio ()
Rocky Road ()
Strawberry ()
Tin Roof Sundae ()
Vanilla ()
Best Choice
Chocolate Chip
Chocolate Ice Cream
Churn Butter Pecan
Churn Moose Track
Churn Vanilla
Country Vanilla
Neapolitan
No Sugar Vanilla
Premium Almond Fudge
Premium Belgium Chocolate
Premium Butter Pecan
Premium Candy Corn
Premium Chocolate Marshmallow
Premium French Vanilla
Premium Vanilla
Premium Vanilla Bean
Rocky Road
Strawberry/Cream
Tin Roof
Vanilla
Vanilla/Chocolate
Broughton
10% Chocolate Ice Cream Mix
6% Ice Cream Mix
Black Raspberry ()
Butter Pecan ()

Cherry Nut ()
Cherry Vanilla ()
Chocolate Almond ()
Chocolate Chip ()
Chocolate ()
Chocolate Ice Cream Cups ()
Country Love Chocolate Chip ()
Country Love Chocolate ()
Country Love Fudge Marble ()
Country Love Lowfat Fudge Ripple ()
Country Love Lowfat Neapolitan ()
Country Love Lowfat Vanilla ()
Country Love Neapolitan ()
Country Love Strawberry ()
Country Love Vanilla ()
Country Love Vanilla Orange ()
Death By Chocolate ()
Maplehurst Chocolate ()
Maplehurst Neapolitan ()
Maplehurst Vanilla ()
Mint Chocolate Chip ()
Moose Track ()
Nutty Buddy ()
Orange Pineapple ()
Peanut Butter ()
Peanut Caramel Crunch ()
Premium Black Cherry ()
Premium Butter Pecan ()
Premium Cherry Nut ()
Premium Chocolate ()
Premium Death By Chocolate ()
Premium Moose Tracks ()
Premium Peanut Butter ()
Premium Peanut Caramel Crunch ()
Premium Rocky Road ()
Premium Vanilla Bean ()
Premium Vanilla ()
Strawberry ()
Strawberry Ice Cream Cups ()
Sugar Free Fat Free Vanilla ()
Superman ()
Vanilla Bean ()
Vanilla ()
Vanilla Ice Cream Cups ()
White Chocolate Raspberry ()

Bud's of San Francisco
Bittersweet Chocolate

Brown Cow Palace
French Vanilla
Kona Chip
Mint Chip
Rocky Road
Vanilla
Vanilla Bean

Ciao Bella ⓘ
Gelato Pints (All BUT Malted Milk Ball,
Key Lime Graham, Maple Ginger
Snap, Belgian Chocolate Smores, and
Hazelnut Biscotti)

Clemmy's Ice Cream
Ice Cream (All)

Creamland Dairies
Adobe Double Fudge ()
Bernalillo Banana Split ()
Chama Chocolate Chip ()
Choco Canyon Chocolate ()
Desert Mountain Chocolate Almond ()
Fiesta Mexican Chocolate ()
Old Mesilla Butter Pecan ()
Old Town Neapolitan ()
Pecos Praline Pecan ()
Rio Grande Rocky Road ()
Route 66 Vanilla ()
White Sands French Vanilla ()

Eating Right ∿
Mocha Cappucino Ice Cream
Pomegranate Ice Cream
Vanilla Ice Cream

Fastco (Fareway)
Cherry Nut Ice Cream
Chocolate Chip Ice Cream
Chocolate Ice Cream
English Toffee Ice Cream
Fast Tracks Ice Cream
Fudge Revel Ice Cream
Mint Chip Ice Cream
Neapolitan Ice Cream
New York Vanilla Ice Cream
Strawberry Ice Cream
Tin Roof Sundae
Vanilla Ice Cream

Full Circle (Schnucks)
Butter Pecan Ice Cream
Chocolate Ice Cream

Neapolitan Ice Cream
Vanilla Ice Cream

Gandy's ⓘ
Ice Cream (All BUT Cookies and Cream
& Chocolate Chip Cookie Dough) ◊

Giant
Andes Crème de Menthe Ice Cream
Light Churn Style Moosetrack Ice
Cream
Light Churn Style Vanilla Ice Cream
Moosetracks Ice Cream
Premium Chocolate Ice Cream
Premium Chocolate, Vanilla &
Strawberry Ice Cream
Premium French Vanilla Ice Cream
Premium Mint Chocolate Chip Ice Cream
Premium Real Chocolate Moosetracks
Ice Cream
Premium Vanilla Ice Cream
Vanilla Ice Cream Cups

Gifford's Ice Cream ⓘ
Black Raspberry
Butter Pecan
Butterscotch Vanilla
Camp Coffee
Caramel Caribou
Cherry Amaretto Chip
Cherry Vanilla
Chocolate
Chocolate Chip
Chocolate Rainforest Crunch
French Vanilla
Maine Black Bear
Maine Deer Tracks
Maine Maple Walnut
Maine Wild Blueberry
Mint Chocolate Chip
Moose Tracks
Old Fashioned Vanilla
Peanut Butter Cup
Pink Peppermint Stick
Pistachio Nut
Pumpkin
Smurf (Cotton Candy)
Strawberry
Toasted Coconut
Vanilla Bean

Haggen
Black Cherry Chunk
Caramel Vanilla
French Vanilla
Mint Chocolate Chip
Mocha Almond Fudge
Neapolitan
Organic Vanilla
Rocky Road
Strawberry
Tin Roof Sundae

Heaven Sent
Heaven Sent Non Dairy Frozen Dessert
(All Flavors)

Hiland Dairy
Chocolate Ice Cream
French Vanilla Ice Cream
Ice Cream Cups (Chocolate, Strawberry,
Vanilla)
Real Vanilla Ice Cream
Reduced Fat Ice Cream Mix (4% and 5%
Vanilla & Chocolate)
Vanilla Bean Ice Cream
Vanilla Ice Cream

Hood
Chocolate
Chocolate Chip
Classic Trio
Creamy Coffee
Fudge Twister
Golden Vanilla
Maple Walnut
Natural Vanilla Bean
New England Creamery Ice Cream,
Black Raspberry Sherbert
New England Creamery Ice Cream,
Boston Vanilla Bean
New England Creamery Ice Cream,
Light Chocolate Chip
New England Creamery Ice Cream,
Light Coffee
New England Creamery Ice Cream,
Light Martha's Vineyard Black
Raspberry
New England Creamery Ice Cream,
Light Vanilla

New England Creamery Ice Cream, Maine Blueberry & Sweet Cream

New England Creamery Ice Cream, Martha's Vineyard Black Raspberry

New England Creamery Ice Cream, Orange Sherbert

New England Creamery Ice Cream, Rainbow Sherbert

New England Creamery Ice Cream, Rhode Island Lighthouse Coffee

New England Creamery Ice Cream, Vermont Maple Nut

New England Creamery Ice Cream, Wildberry Sherbert

Patchwork

Red Sox Ice Cream, Grand Slam Vanilla Strawberry

Horizon Organic
Ice Cream (All BUT Ice Cream Sandwiches)

It's Soy Delicious
Almond Pecan Soy Ice Cream
Awesome Chocolate Soy Ice Cream
Chocolate Almond Soy Ice Cream
Chocolate Peanut Butter Soy Ice Cream
Green Tea Soy Ice Cream
Raspberry Soy Ice Cream
see also So Delicious Dairy Free
Vanilla Soy Ice Cream

Junket
Ice Cream Mixes (All)

Laloo's
Goat Milk Ice Cream (All)

Lindy's Homemade
Gelato (All)

Living Harvest ⓘ ✔
Tempt Frozen Dessert

Louis Trauth Dairy
Banana Split ()
Birthday Cake ()
Black Walnut ()
Brown Cow ()
Butter Pecan ()
Candy Bar ()
Chocolate Chip ()
Chocolate ()
Chocolate Marshmallow ()

Chocolate Ripple ()
Extreme Moose Tracks ()
Homemade Vanilla ()
Lemon ()
Mint Chocolate Chip ()
Moose Tracks ()
Neapolitan ()
Peppermint Stick ()
Snow Cream ()
Strawberry ()
Turtle Tracks ()
Vanilla & Chocolate ()
Vanilla Bean ()
Vanilla ()

Lucerne (Safeway) ✑
Chocolate Chip Ice Cream
Chocolate Ice Cream
Creamery Fresh Ice Cream - Dutch Chocolate
Creamery Fresh Ice Cream - Fresh Mint
Creamery Fresh Ice Cream - Vanilla
Creamery Fresh Ice Cream Cup Butter Pecan
Creamery Fresh Ice Cream Cup Mint Chocolate Chip
Creamery Fresh Ice Cream Cup Vanilla
French Vanilla Ice Cream
Low Fat Vanilla Ice Cream
Mint Chocolate Chip Ice Cream
Mint Chocolate Chip Low Fat Ice Cream
Neapolitan Ice Cream
Ole Vanilla Ice Cream
Orange Sherbet and Vanilla Ice Cream
Ranch Pecan Ice Cream
Rocky Road Ice Cream
Strawberry Ice Cream
Vanilla Ice Cream

Luna & Larry's Coconut Bliss ⓘ ✔
Coconut Bliss (All)

Mayfield Dairy
Banana Split ()
Birthday Cake ()
Black Walnut ()
Brown Cow ()
Butter Pecan ()
Candy Bar ()
Chocolate Almond ()

Chocolate Chip ()
Chocolate ()
Chocolate Marshmallow ()
Chocolate Ripple ()
Classic Vanilla Ice Cream Swirled with
    Cherries ()
Creamier Churn Black Cherry Chunk ()
Creamier Churn Black Walnut ()
Creamier Churn Butter Pecan ()
Creamier Churn Chocolate ()
Creamier Churn No Sugar Added Butter
    Pecan ()
Creamier Churn No Sugar Added
    Chocolate ()
Creamier Churn No Sugar Added
    Vanilla ()
Creamier Churn Vanilla Bean ()
Double Chocolate Chip ()
Extreme Moose Tracks ()
French Vanilla ()
Homemade Vanilla ()
Lemon ()
Mint Chocolate Chip ()
Moose Tracks ()
Neapolitan ()
Peppermint Stick ()
Pomegranate Medley ()
Rocky Road ()
Snow Cream ()
Strawberry ()
Sweet Butter Flavored Ice Cream ()
Turtle Tracks ()
Vanilla & Chocolate ()
Vanilla Bean ()
Vanilla ()

Meadow Gold
Premium Birthday Cake Ice Cream ()
Premium Chocolate Ice Cream ()
Premium Kona Coffee Ice Cream ()
Premium Macadamia Nut Ice Cream ()
Premium Mint Chocolate Chip Ice
    Cream ()
Premium Neapolitan Ice Cream ()
Premium Rocky Road Ice Cream ()
Premium Vanilla Ice Cream ()

Meijer
Birthday Cake

Black Cherry
Blue Moon
Bordeaux Cherry
Butter Pecan
Candy Bar Swirl
CandyBar Overload
Carb Conquest Chocolate
Carb Conquest Vanilla
Cherry Fudge
Chocolate
Chocolate Chip
Chocolate MooseTracks
Chocolate Thunder
Churned Light Butter Pecan
Churned Light Chocolate
Churned Light Chocolate MooseTracks
Churned Light French Vanilla
Churned Light MooseTracks
Churned Light Neapolitan
Churned Light Vanilla
Combo Cream
Cotton Candy Confetti
Dulce De Leche
Fat Free No Sugar Added Caramel Pecan
    Crunch with Splenda
Fat Free No Sugar Added Vanilla with
    Splenda
French Vanilla
Fudge Swirl
Golden Vanilla
Heavenly Hash
Light Neapolitan
Macadamia Island Fudge
Mint Chocolate Chip
Mint MooseTracks
MooseTracks
Neapolitan
No Sugar Added Fat Free Vanilla
No Sugar Added Light Butter Pecan
No Sugar Added Light Butter Pecan
    with Splenda
No Sugar Added Light Chocolate Chip
No Sugar Added Light Vanilla with
    Splenda
Orange Vanilla
Peanut Butter Fudge
Peppermint

Praline Pecan
Scooperman
Strawberry
Strawberry Cheesecake
Tin Roof Ice Cream
Totally Awesome Strawberry
Vanilla
Vanilla Bean

Meijer Gold
Caramel Toffee Swirl
Double Nut Chocolate
Georgian Bay Butter Pecan
Peanut Butter Fudge Swirl
Peanut Butter Fudge Tracks
Thunder Bay Cherry
Victorian Vanilla

Oak Farms Dairy
Butter Pecan ()
Chocolate ()
Homemade Vanilla ()
Strawberry ()
Toffee Ice Cream Bars ()
Vanilla ()
Vanilla Ice Cream Bars ()

Oberweis Dairy
Black Cherry
Black Walnut
Brandy
Butter Brickle
Butter Pecan
Chocolate
Chocolate Almond
Chocolate Chip
Chocolate Chocolate Chip
Chocolate Marshmallow
Chocolate Peanut Butter
Cinnamon
Coffee
Cotton Candy
Dark Chocolate
Dulce de Leche
Egg Nog
Lowfat Chocolate
Lowfat Chocolate Marshmallow
Lowfat Strawberry
Lowfat Vanilla
Mango Pomegranate

Mint Chocolate Chip
No Sugar Added Chocolate
No Sugar Added Vanilla
Peach
Peppermint
Pistachio
Pumpkin
Rocky Road
Rum Raisin
Strawberry
Udderly Truffles
Vanilla
Vanilla Soft Serve

Organic Nectars
Cashewtopia (All)

Organicville
Ice Cream (All) 🙂 ✓

Our Family
Chocolate Chip Ice Cream
Chocolate Ice Cream
Chocolate Marshmallow Ice Cream
Chocolate Sundae Ice Cream
Chocolate-Vanilla Ice Cream
Maple Nut Ice Cream
Neapolitan Ice Cream
New York Vanilla Ice Cream
Orange Dream Ice Cream
Orange Twist Ice Cream
Strawberry Sundae Ice Cream
Vanilla Ice Cream

Perry's Ice Cream ⓘ
Birthday Bash
Bittersweet Sinphony
Black Cherry
Black Cherry Grande
Black Raspberry
Bubblegum
Butter Almond Crunch
Butter Pecan
Butterscotch Swirl
Caramel Cashew
Caramel Cup Craze
Caramel Praline Turtle
Chocolate
Chocolate Almond
Chocolate Custard
Chocolate Panda Paws

Chunky Chocolate Chip
Coconut Almond Fudge
Coconut Mango Swirl
Cotton Candy
Death By Chocolate
Fireball
Fool's Gold
French Roast Coffee
French Vanilla
Heavenly Hash
Kahlua Almond Amaretto
Mango
Maple Walnut
Midnight Orange
Mint Chip
Mint Ting-a-Ling
Muddy Sneakers
NSA Light Butter Pecan
NSA Light Panda Paws
Orange Blossom
Orange Pineapple
Panda Paws
Parkerhouse
Peanut Butter Cup
Peanut Butter Fudge
Peanut Butter Swirl
Pistachio Nut
Raspberry Swirl
Red Velvet
Rocky Mountain Raspberry
Rum Raisin
Sprinkle Cone
Strawberry
Strawberry Cheesecake
Super Hero
Vanilla
Vanilla Custard
Vanilla/Chocolate Twist
White Lightning

PET Milk
Banana Split ()
Birthday Cake ()
Bittmore Vanilla ()
Black Sweet Cherry ()
Black Walnut ()
Brown Mule ()
Butter Pecan ()

Cherry Vanilla ()
Chocolate ()
Chocolate Marshmallow ()
Chocolate Moose Tracks ()
Country Churn Black Sweet Cherry ()
Country Churn Butter Pecan ()
Country Churn Moose Tracks ()
Country Churn Vanilla ()
Double Fudge Swirl ()
French Vanilla ()
Heavenly Hash ()
Mint Chocolate Chip ()
Moose Tracks ()
Neapolitan ()
Peach Frozen Yogurt ()
Praline Pecan ()
Pralines and Cream ()
Strawberries N' Cream ()
Strawberry ()
Turtle Tracks ()
Vanilla & Chocolate ()
Vanilla Bean ()
Vanilla ()
Vanilla Orange ()

Prairie Farms
4% and 5% Reduced Fat Ice Cream
  Mixes (Chocolate, Vanilla)
Belgian Chocolate Ice Cream
Chocolate Chip Ice Cream
Chocolate Ice Cream
French Vanilla Ice Cream
Mint Chip Ice Cream
Neapolitan Ice Cream
Steak N Shake High and Low Butterfat
  Ice Cream
Vanilla Bean Ice Cream
Vanilla Ice Cream
Vanilla Ice Cream Mixes (6%, 10%, 14%)
Vanilla Orange Ice Cream

Prestige (Winn-Dixie)
Chocolate Almond Ice Cream
Chocolate Ice Cream
Vanilla Ice Cream

Price Chopper
Butterscotch Whirl Ice Cream
Clear Value Vanilla Ice Cream
Fudge Swirl Ice Cream

Jr. Pops No Sugar
Mint Chip Ice Cream
Vanilla /Chocolate Ice Cream
Vanilla Ice Cream

Price's Creameries
Banana Nut ( )
Banana Split ( )
Butter Pecan ( )
Cherry Vanilla ( )
Chocolate Chip ( )
Chocolate Cups ( )
Chocolate ( )
Chocolate Peanut Butter Cup ( )
French Vanilla ( )
Orange Cream Bars ( )
Praline Pecan ( )
Strawberry Cups ( )
Strawberry ( )
Vanilla Cups ( )
Vanilla Neapolitan ( )

Publix
Banana Split Premium Ice Cream
Black Jack Cherry Premium Ice Cream
Buckeye's & Fudge Premium Limited
  Edition Ice Cream
Butter Pecan Premium Homemade Ice
  Cream
Butter Pecan Premium Ice Cream
Butter Pecan Premium Light Ice Cream
Caramel Mountain Tracks Premium
  Limited Edition Ice Cream
Cherry Nut Premium Ice Cream
Chocolate Almond Premium Ice Cream
Chocolate Cherish Passion Premium Ice
  Cream
Chocolate Chip Premium Ice Cream
Chocolate Ice Cream
Chocolate Low Fat Ice Cream
Chocolate Marshmallow Swirl Ice
  Cream
Chocolate Premium Ice Cream
Chocolate Premium Light Ice Cream
Coffee Almond Fudge Premium Light
  Ice Cream
Coffee Premium Ice Cream
Dulce de Leche Premium Ice Cream

Egg Nog Premium Limited Edition Ice
  Cream
French Silk Duo Premium Limited
  Edition Ice Cream
French Vanilla Premium Ice Cream
Fudge Royal Ice Cream
Fudge Royal Low Fat Ice Cream
Heavenly Hash Premium Ice Cream
Maple Walnut Premium Limited Edition
  Ice Cream
Mint Chocolate Chip Premium Ice
  Cream
Monkey Business Premium Limited
  Edition Ice Cream
Neapolitan Ice Cream
Neapolitan Low Fat Ice Cream
Neapolitan Premium Ice Cream
Neapolitan Premium Light Ice Cream
Otter Paws Premium Ice Cream
Peanut Butter Goo Goo Premium Ice
  Cream
Peppermint Stick Premium Limited
  Edition Ice Cream
Rum Raisin Premium Limited Edition
  Ice Cream
Santa's White Christmas Premium Ice
  Cream
Strawberry Premium Homemade Ice
  Cream
Strawberry Premium Ice Cream
Strawberry Premium Light Ice Cream
Vanilla Ice Cream
Vanilla Low Fat Ice Cream
Vanilla Premium Homemade Ice Cream
Vanilla Premium Ice Cream
Vanilla Premium Light Ice Cream
Vanilla Strawberry Ice Cream

Purely Decadent Dairy Free
Cherry Nirvana Soy Ice Cream
Chocolate Obsession Soy Ice Cream
Cookie Dough (Gluten Free) Soy Ice
  Cream
Dulce De Leche Soy Ice Cream
Mint Chocolate Chip Soy Ice Cream
Mocha Almond Fudge Soy Ice Cream
Peanut Butter Zig Zag Soy Ice Cream
Pomegranate Chip Soy Ice Cream

Praline Pecan Soy Ice Cream
Purely Vanilla Soy Ice Cream
see also So Delicious Dairy Free
Turtle Trails Soy Ice Cream

Purity Dairies
Butter Pecan Ice Cream
Chocolate Ice Cream
Homemade Vanilla Ice Cream
Neapolitan Ice Cream
Strawberry Ice Cream
Vanilla Bean Ice Cream
Vanilla Ice Cream

Reed's
Ginger Ice Cream

Rice Dream
Cocoa Marble Fudge
Neapolitan
Vanilla

Safeway Select
Alaskan Classics Moose Tracks Ice
Cream Cups
Bananas Foster Ice Cream
Black Walnut Ice Cream
Butter Pecan Ice Cream
Chocolate Covered Strawberry Ice
Cream
Chocolate Ice Cream
Chocolate Toffee Mocha Ice Cream
Churned Light Butter Pecan Ice Cream
Churned Light French Vanilla Ice
Cream
Churned Light Strawberry Ice Cream
Coconut Caramel Flan Ice Cream
Coconut Pineapple Premium Ice Cream
Denali Caramel Caribou Ice Cream
Denali Chocolate Moose Tracks Ice
Cream
Denali Moose Tracks Ice Cream
Dulche De Leche Premium Ice Cream
Extreme Moose Tracks Ice Cream
Fleur De Sel Ice Cream
French Salted Caramel Ice Cream Cup
French Vanilla Ice Cream
French Vanilla Light Ice Cream
Homestyle Vanilla Ice Cream
Java Chip Ice Cream
Java Chip Ice Cream Cup

Light Caribou Caramel Ice Cream
Light Chocolate with Moose Tracks
Fudge Ice Cream
Light Vanilla with Moose Tracks Fudge
Ice Cream
Mint Chocolate Chip Ice Cream
Mint Chocolate Chip Light Ice Cream
Mint Cup Moosetracks Ice Cream
Peanut Butter Cup Ice Cream
Peppermint Chocolate Chunk Ice
Cream
Premium Chocolate Ice Cream
Pure Vanilla Ice Cream
Rocky Road Ice Cream
Rocky Road Light Ice Cream
Salted Caramel Butter Pecan Ice Cream
Strawberry Ice Cream
Vanilla Bean Churned Light Ice Cream
Vanilla Ice Cream
Vanilla Light Ice Cream

Schnucks
Light Vanilla Ice Cream
Vanilla Ice Cream (Bucket)

Schnucks Select
Black Cherry Ice Cream
Butter Pecan Ice Cream
Chunky Chocolate Chip Ice Cream
Churned Butter Pecan Ice Cream
Churned Vanilla Ice Cream
French Vanilla Ice Cream
Mint Chocolate Chip Ice Cream
Peanut Butter Crunch Ice Cream
Peppermint Ice Cream
Vanilla Ice Cream
White Thunder Ice Cream

Shamrock Farms
Ice Cream (All BUT Grand Butter
PeCanyon and Coyote Cookies 'n
Cream)

Simply Enjoy (Giant)
Coconut Gelato

Simply Enjoy (Stop & Shop)
Chocolate Ice Cream
Coconut Gelato
Strawberry Ice Cream
Vanilla Ice Cream

So Delicious Dairy Free

Coconut Milk Ice Cream, Cherry Amaretto
Coconut Milk Ice Cream, Chocolate
Coconut Milk Ice Cream, Chocolate Peanut Butter Swirl
Coconut Milk Ice Cream, Coconut
Coconut Milk Ice Cream, Coconut Almond Chip
Coconut Milk Ice Cream, Cookie Dough (Gluten Free)
Coconut Milk Ice Cream, German Chocolate
Coconut Milk Ice Cream, Green Tea
Coconut Milk Ice Cream, Mint Chip
Coconut Milk Ice Cream, Mocha Almond Fudge
Coconut Milk Ice Cream, No Sugar Added Butter Pecan
Coconut Milk Ice Cream, No Sugar Added Chocolate
Coconut Milk Ice Cream, No Sugar Added Mint Chip
Coconut Milk Ice Cream, No Sugar Added Toasted Almond Chip
Coconut Milk Ice Cream, No Sugar Added Vanilla Bean
Coconut Milk Ice Cream, Passionate Mango
Coconut Milk Ice Cream, Pomegranate Chip
Coconut Milk Ice Cream, Swiss Almond
Coconut Milk Ice Cream, Turtle Trails
Coconut Milk Ice Cream, Vanilla Bean
Organic Soy Ice Cream, Butter Pecan
Organic Soy Ice Cream, Chocolate Peanut Butter
Organic Soy Ice Cream, Chocolate Velvet
Organic Soy Ice Cream, Creamy Vanilla
Organic Soy Ice Cream, Dulce De Leche
Organic Soy Ice Cream, Mint Marble Fudge
Organic Soy Ice Cream, Mocha Fudge
Organic Soy Ice Cream, Neapolitan
Organic Soy Ice Cream, Strawberry

Stop & Shop

Light Churn Style Moosetrack Ice Cream
Light Churn Style Vanilla Ice Cream
Premium Mint Chocolate Chip Ice Cream

Straus Family Creamery

Ice Cream (All)

Talenti ✓

Gelato (All BUT Caramel Cookie Crunch Gelato)

Tillamook

Banana Split Ice Cream ⓘ
Black Walnut Ice Cream ⓘ
Bubble Gum Ice Cream ⓘ
Caramel Butter Pecan Ice Cream ⓘ
Caramel Pecan Praline Ice Cream ⓘ
Chocolate Ice Cream ⓘ
Chocolate Peanut Butter Ice Cream ⓘ
Cinnamon Banana Bliss Ice Cream ⓘ
Coffee Almond Fudge Ice Cream ⓘ
Espresso Mocha Ice Cream ⓘ
French Vanilla Ice Cream ⓘ
Mint Chocolate Chip Ice Cream ⓘ
Mountain Huckleberry Ice Cream ⓘ
Old Fashioned Vanilla Ice Cream ⓘ
Oregon Black Cherry Ice Cream ⓘ
Oregon Strawberry Ice Cream ⓘ
Peaches and Cream Ice Cream ⓘ
Peppermint Candy Ice Cream ⓘ
Pumpkin Ice Cream ⓘ
Rocky Road Ice Cream ⓘ
Root Beer Float Ice Cream ⓘ
Tillamook Mudslide Ice Cream ⓘ
Udderly Chocolate Ice Cream ⓘ
Udderly Peanutbutterly Ice Cream ⓘ
Vanilla Bean Ice Cream ⓘ
White Licorice Ice Cream ⓘ
Wild Mountain Blackberry Ice Cream ⓘ

Trader Joe's

Coconut Milk Non-Dairy Ice Cream (Chocolate & Strawberry)
Mango Vanilla Ice Cream Bars
Soy Creamy Cherry Chocolate Chip
Soy Creamy Organic Vanilla

Super Premium Ice Cream (French Vanilla, Mint Chocolate, Ultra Chocolate)

Turkey Hill
All Natural Recipe, Cherry Vanilla
All Natural Recipe, Chocolate
All Natural Recipe, Coffee
All Natural Recipe, Mint Chocolate Chip
All Natural Recipe, Vanilla Bean
All Natural Recipe, Vanilla Chocolate & Butter Almond
Banana Split Premium Ice Cream
Black Cherry Premium Ice Cream
Black Raspberry Premium Ice Cream
Butter Pecan Premium Ice Cream
Choco Mint Chip Premium Ice Cream
Chocolate Marshmallow Premium Ice Cream
Chocolate Peanut Butter Cup Premium Ice Cream
Chocolate Premium Ice Cream
Chunky Peanut Butter Premium Ice Cream
Colombian Coffee Premium Ice Cream
Dutch Chocolate Premium Ice Cream
Eagle's Touchdown Sundae Premium Ice Cream
Egg Nog Premium Ice Cream (Seasonal)
French Vanilla Premium Ice Cream
Fudge Ripple Premium Ice Cream
Gertrude Hawk Box of Chocolate Premium Ice Cream
Homemade Vanilla Premium Ice Cream
Individual Selection, Moose Tracks
Individual Selections, Vanilla Bean
Light Ice Cream, Bavarian Espresso
Light Ice Cream, Chocolate Nutty Moose Tracks
Light Ice Cream, Moose Tracks
Light Ice Cream, Vanilla Bean
Moose Tracks Stuff'd Ice Cream
Neapolitan Premium Ice Cream
No Sugar Added, Cherry Fudge Ripple
No Sugar Added, Cool White Mint
No Sugar Added, Dutch Chocolate
No Sugar Added, Moose Tracks
No Sugar Added, Vanilla Bean

Nutty Chocolate Moose Tracks Stuff'd Ice Cream
Orange Cream Swirl Premium Ice Cream
Original Vanilla Premium Ice Cream
Peaches 'N Cream Premium Ice Cream (Seasonal)
Peanut Butter Ripple Premium Ice Cream
Raspberry Cream Swirl Premium Ice Cream (Limited Edition)
Rocky Road Premium Ice Cream
Rum Raisin Premium Ice Cream
Strawberries and Cream Premium Ice Cream
Vanilla & Chocolate Premium Ice Cream
Vanilla Bean Premium Ice Cream
Vanilla Swiss Almond Premium Ice Cream (Limited Edition)
Venice Premium Ice Cream, Cherry Lemon
Venice Premium Ice Cream, Mango
Venice Premium Ice Cream, Pomegranate Blueberry with Acai

Valu Time (Marsh)
Chocolate Chip Ice Cream
Chocolate Ice Cream
Fudge Swirl Ice Cream
Neapolitan Ice Cream
Rainbow Sherbet
Strawberry Swirl Ice Cream
Vanilla Ice Cream

Valu Time (Schnucks)
Vanilla Bucket
Vanilla Square

Wegmans
All Natural Chocolate
All Natural Coffee Explosion
All Natural French Vanilla
All Natural Mint Chocolate Chip
All Natural Neopolitan Ice Cream
All Natural Vanilla
All Natural Vanilla Fudge
Black Raspberry
Café Latte with Whipped Cream Flavored Ripple Coffee

Chocolate
Chocolate Chip
Chocolate Marshmallow
Chocolate/Vanilla Ice Cream
Crème De Menthe
Egg Nog Flavored
French Roast Coffee
French Vanilla
Hazelnut Chip Coffee
Heavenly Hash
Low Fat Cappuccino Chip
Low Fat Chocolate Indulgence
Low Fat Mint Chip
Low Fat Praline Pecan
Low Fat Raspberry Truffle
Low Fat Vanilla
Maple Walnut
Neapolitan
Peak of Perfection Black Cerry
Peak of Perfection Mango
Peanut Butter Cup
Peanut Butter Sundae
Peanut Butter Swirl
Pistachio Vanilla Swirl
Premium Chocolate Caramel
Premium Mint Chocolate Chip
Premium Peanut Butter Cup
Premium Pistachio
Premium Strawberry
Raspberry Cashew Swirl
Strawberry
Super Premium Butter Pecan
Super Premium Cherry Armagnac
Super Premium Chocolate
Super Premium Coconut Mango
Super Premium Creamy Caramel
Super Premium Crème Brulee
Super Premium Dark Chocolate
Super Premium French Roast
Super Premium Hazelnut Chip
Super Premium Jamocha Almond Fudge
Super Premium Peanut Butter & Jelly
Super Premium Rum Raisin
Super Premium Vanilla
Tin Roof
Vanilla
Vanilla Ice Cream with Orange Sherbet

Vanilla Raspberry Sorbet

Winn-Dixie
Classic Chocolate Ice Cream
Classic Neapolitan Ice Cream
Classic Strawberry Ice Cream
Classic Vanilla Ice Cream

JUICE & JUICE DRINKS

Always Save
Apple Juice
Lemonade
Orange Juice

Best Choice
100% Grape Juice
Apple Juice
Lemonade
Limeade
Orange Juice
Orange Juice with Calcium
Orange Juice, Country Style
Orange Juice, Pulp Free

Cub Foods
Frozen Apple Juice
Frozen Orange Juice
Orange Calcium Frozen Juice
Orange Country Style Frozen Juice
Pink Lemonade Frozen Juice

Fastco (Fareway)
Orange Juice

Food Club (Brookshire)
Orange Concentrate
Orange Concentrate, Hi Pulp
Orange Concentrate, No Pulp
Orange Concentrate, With Calcium
Pink Lemonade

Food Club (Marsh)
Apple Concentrate
Lemonade
Orange Concentrate
Orange Concentrate, No Pulp
Orange with Calcium
Pink Lemonade

Food You Feel Good About (Wegmans)
Apple Juice Concentrate
Orange Juice Concentrate

Orange Juice Concentrate Country Style

Giant
Sunrise Valley Lemonade
(Concentrated)
Sunrise Valley Orange Juice with
Calcium (Concentrated)
Sunrise Valley Pink Lemonade
(Concentrated)

Great Value (Wal-Mart)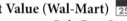
Concentrate Pulp Free Orange Juice
Concentrated 100% Grape Juice
Concentrated Apple Juice
Concentrated Country Style Orange
Juice
Concentrated Florida Grapefruit Juice
Concentrated Fruit Punch
Concentrated Grape Juice Drink
Concentrated Lemonade
Concentrated Limeade
Concentrated Orange Juice
Concentrated Orange Juice with
Calcium
Concentrated Pink Lemonade

Hy-Vee
Apple Juice Concentrate
Fruit Punch Concentrate
Grape Juice Cocktail Concentrate
Lemonade Concentrate
Limeade Concentrate
Orange Juice Concentrate
Orange Juice Concentrate, Calcium
Added
Pink Lemonade Concentrate

Mayfield Dairy
Green Fruit Punch
Red Fruit Punch

Meijer
Apple Juice Concentrate
Fruit Punch Concentrate
Grape Juice Concentrate
Grapefruit Juice Concentrate
Lemonade Concentrate
Limeade Concentrate
O.J. Concentrate (with Calcium, High
Pulp, Pulp Free)
Pink Lemonade Concentrate
White Grape Juice Cocktail Concentrate

Publix
Concentrated Orange Juice

Sambazon
Sambazon (All)

Shaw's
Apple Juice
Cranberry Juice
Cranberry Raspberry Juice
Fruit Punch Juice Concentrate
Orange Juice
Pink Lemonade Concentrate
Purple Vitamin C Grape Juice Cocktail
White Lemonade Concentrate

Valu Time (Marsh)
Orange Juice Concentrate

Valu Time (Schnucks)
Lemonade
Orange Juice
Orange Juice Concentrate No Pulp
Orange Juice Concentrate with Calcium

Vons ᏪᎤ
Lemonade

Wegmans
Apple Juice with Calcium
Fruit Punch Concentrate
Grape Juice Cocktail Concentrate
Lemonade Concentrate
Limeade Concentrate
Orange Juice Concentrate with Calcium
Pink Lemonade Concentrate

MEAT

Always Save
Beef Patties

Bell & Evans ⓘ ✓
Buffalo Style Wings
Chicken Burgers
Fully Cooked Grilled Chicken Breasts
Gluten-Free Breaded Chicken Breasts
Gluten-Free Breaded Chicken Nuggets
Gluten-Free Breaded Chicken Patties
Gluten-Free Breaded Chicken Tenders
Gluten-Free Breaded Italian Chicken
Patties
Gluten-Free Garlic Parmesan Breaded
Chicken Breast

Honey BBQ Style Wings

Best Choice
80% Lean Beef Patty
80% Patty Box
Individually Quick Frozen Chicken
  Breast Tenders
Individually Quick Frozen Chicken
  Wings

Bubba Burger
Bubba Burgers (All)

Byron's ⓘ
Pork BBQ

Coleman Natural ⓘ
Gluten Free Chicken Breast Nuggets

Cub Foods
Boneless Skinless Chicken Breasts
Party Wings

Empire Kosher
Chicken Drumsticks
Chicken Leg Quarters
Chicken Split Breasts
Chicken Thighs
Chicken Wing Drumettes
Frozen Boneless Skinless Breast
Ground Turkey
Rock Cornish Broiler
Whole Turkey
Whole Turkey Breast

Geisha
Cooked Shrimp
Cooked Tail Off Shrimp
Imitation Crab
Peeled and Deveined Shrimp
Raw White Shrimp

Giant
1st & 2nd Wing Sections Chicken
  Wingettes
Peppered Bacon

Jennie-O Turkey Store
Ground Seasoned Turkey
Ground Turkey
Turkey Burgers

Market Day
All Beef Hot Dogs
Baby Back Ribs
Baby Back Ribs, Fully Cooked with
  Sauce

Bacon Slices, Fully Cooked
Bacon Wrapped Pork Tournedos
Bacon Wrapped Ranch Steaks
BBQ Pulled Pork
Beef Brisket with Sauce
Beef Patties, 1/4 lb.
Beef Stew Meat
Chicken Breast Strips, Seasoned
Chicken Tenderloins, Diced
ChicNSteakes
Filet of Sirloin
Ground Beef, 85% Lean
Ham, Boneless Sliced Petite
Ham, Spiral Sliced
Mahi Mahi Naked Fillets
Naked Haddock Fillets
Peruvian Bay Scallops
Pork Chops, Boneless
Pork Flat Iron
Rack of Pork Roast
Ranch Steaks
Salmon, Seasoned
Salmon, Wild Alaskan Grilled
Shrimp, Garlic & Herb
Shrimp, Jumbo Party with Sauce
Shrimp, Large
Sirloin Roast, Marinated
Tilapia Fillets
Turkey Breast Roast
Turkey Breast, Oven Ready Boneless
Turkey Sausage Links, Fully Cooked
Turkey Tournedos
Vidalia Onion Burgers
Vienna Corned Beef
Whole Beef Flat Iron
Whole Pork Tenderloins

Meijer
Turkey Breast, Young

Mountaire
Mountaire (All)

Philly-Gourmet ⓘ
Pure Beef Homestyle Patties
Pure Beef Sandwich Steaks
Pure Beef Thick & Beefy Homestyle
  Patties

Publix
Boneless Skinless Chicken Breasts

Boneless Skinless Chicken Cutlets
Chicken Breast Tenderloins
Chicken Wingettes
Quaker Maid Meats ⓘ
Pure Beef Sandwich Steaks (All)
Safeway 〰
Buffalo Wings
Chicken Breast Boneless Skinless Valu
Pack
Shelton's ⓘ
Chicken Franks
Smoked Chicken Franks
Smoked Turkey Franks
Turkey Breakfast Sausage
Turkey Burgers
Turkey Franks
Turkey Italian Sausage
Turkey Sausage Patties
Simply Enjoy (Giant)
Beef Tenderloins Wrapped with Black
Peppered Bacon
Steak-umm ⓘ
Patties (Original, Sweet Onion)
Sliced Steaks
Trader Joe's
Chili Lime Chicken Burgers
Wegmans
Chicken Wings
Jumbo Buffalo Style Chicken Wings
Wellshire Farms
Beef Hamburgers
Chicken Bites
Turkey Burgers

NOVELTIES

Arctic Zero ⓘ
Novelties (All)
Best Choice
Fudge Bar
Ice Cream Bar
Jr. Pops
Orange Cream Bar
Tropical Pops
Broughton
Flintstone Fred Push Up ◐
Flintstone Rainbow Push Up ◐

Good Humor Bullet Fireckracker ◐
Good Humor Cream Bars ◐
Good Humor Fudge Bars ◐
Good Humor Juice Scribblers ◐
Good Humor Nicktoon's Sponge Bob ◐
Good Humor Pops (Cherry, Grape,
Orange) ◐
Good Humor Push Up's ◐
Good Humor Rainbow Pop ◐
Good Humor Sugar Free Fudge Bars ◐
Good Humor Sugar Free Popsicles ◐
Budget Saver
Ice Cream Pops (All)
Chunks O' Fruti
Frozen Fruit Bars (All)
Concord Foods
Chocolate Banana Pop
Creamies
Creamies (All)
Creamland Dairies
Banana Pops ◐
Brown Cow ◐
Fudge Bars ◐
Ice Cream Bars ◐
Lowfat Ice Cream Bars ◐
Orange Cream Bars ◐
Toffee Bars ◐
Twin Pops, Assorted Flavors ◐
Del Monte ⓘ
Fruit Chillers (Cups or Freeze & Eat
Tubes)
Diana's Banana Babies ⚇
Diana's Banana Babies (All)
Fastco (Fareway)
Fudge Bars
Glacier Bars
Orange Push Pops
Sundae Cups
Twin Pops, Assorted
Fat Boy Ice Cream
Peppermint Sundae
Sundaes Vanilla Dipped in Chocolate
Toffee Crunch
Food Club (Brookshire)
Banana Pops
Ice Cream Bars
Juice Pops

Junior Pops (Cherry, Grape, Orange)
No Sugar Added Junior Fudge Pops
Orange Cream Bars
Red, White, Blue Pops
Sundae Cup Variety
Turbo Tubes
Vanilla Cups

Food Club (Marsh)
Fudge Bars

Food You Feel Good About (Wegmans)
Juice Bars Variety Pack (Orange, Lime, & Raspberry)

Gaga's SherBetter ⓘ ✓
SherBetter (All)

Glutenfreeda ⓘ 👄
Ice Cream Sandwiches (All)

Hiland Dairy
Chocolate Coated Vanilla Flavored Ice Cream Bars
Old Recipe Bars
Reduced Fat Ice Cream Bars

Hood
Fudge Stix
Hoodsie Cups
Hoodsie Pops
Hoodsie Sundae Cups
Ice Cream Bar
Kids Karnival Stix
Orange Cream Bar

ICEE
Freezer Bars (All)

Lindy's Homemade
Italian Ice (All)

Louis Trauth Dairy
Banana Pop
Brown Cow Junior
Brown Cow Juniors Light
Brown Cows
Cream Bars
Fudge Bars
Fudge Stix
Light Fruit Stix
Light Fudge Stix
Pop Stix
Real Fruit Stix
Snow Cream Stix

Sour Pop

Lucerne (Safeway) ⌇
Natural Fudge Ice Cream Bars
Orange Ice Cream Bars
Root Beer Float Light Ice Cream Bars
Toffee Brittle Ice Cream Bars
Vanilla Sundae Ice Cream Bars
Watchin Carbs Fudge Bars
Watchin Carbs Ice Cream Bars

Luigi's Real Italian Ice
Luigi's Real Italian Ice (All)

Market Day
Frozen Fruit Pops
Fruit with Purpose

Mayfield Dairy
Banana Pops
Brown Cow Junior
Brown Cow Junior Light
Brown Cows
Cream Bars
Fruit Bars
Fudge Bars
Fudge Stix
Pop Stix
Snow Cream Sticks
Sour Pops
Toffee Bars

Meadow Gold
Chocolate Fudge Bars
Orange Dream Bars
Root Beer Float Bars
Toffee Bars
Twin Pops

Meijer
Dream Bars
Fudge Bars (No Sugar Added)
Gold Bars
Ice Cream Bars
Juice Stix
Orange Glider
Party Pops (Assorted, Cherry, Grape, No Sugar Added, Orange)
Red White and Blue Pops
Toffee Bars
Twin Pops

Minute Maid
Frozen Lemonade Products (All)

Juice Bars (Cherry, Grape, Orange)

North Star
Fudge Bars

Oak Farms Dairy
Banana Pops
Cherry Pops
Fudge Bars
Grape Pops
Orange Dream Bars
Orange Pops

Our Family
Crunch Bars
Dream Bars
Fudge Bars
Juice Bars
Junior Pops
Patriot Pops
Twin Pops

PET Milk
Assorted Pops
Banana Pops
Brown Mules
Cream Bars
Fudge Bars

PhillySwirl
PhillySwirl (All)

Prairie Farms
Chocolate Coated Vanilla Flavored Ice
  Cream Bars
Chocolate Ice Cream Cups
Old Recipe Bars
Reduced Fat Ice Cream Bars
Strawberry Ice Cream Cups
Vanilla Ice Cream Cups

Price Chopper
Fudge Pop No Sugar

Price's Creameries
Assorted Twin Pops
Banana Pops
Brown Cow Juniors
Fudge Bars
Ice Cream Bars ( )
Krispy Bars
Reduced Fat Bars
Toffee Bars
Turtle Tracks

Publix
Banana Pops
Cream Pops
Fudge Bar
Fudge Sundae Cups
Ice Cream Bar
Ice Cream Squares
No Sugar Added Fudge Pops
No Sugar Added Ice Cream Bars
Orange, Cherry and Grape Junior Ice
  Pops
Red White and Blue Junior Ice Pops
Toffee Bar
Twin Pops
Vanilla Cups

Safeway
Astro Pops
Coconut Cream Fruit Bars
Freezer Pops
Party Pride Fudge Ice Cream Bars

Schnucks
Fudge Bars
Ice Cream Bars
Junior Pops
No Sugar Added Fudge Bars
Orange Cream Bars
Tropical No Sugar Added Pops

So Delicious Dairy Free
Agave Fruit Bar, Orange Passion
Agave Fruit Bar, Raspberry
Agave Fruit Bar, Strawberry
Coconut Milk Ice Cream, Coconut
  Almond Bar
Coconut Milk Ice Cream, Fudge Minis
  Bar
Coconut Milk Ice Cream, No Sugar
  Added Fudge Bar
Coconut Milk Ice Cream, No Sugar
  Added Vanilla Bar
Coconut Milk Ice Cream, Vanilla Bar
Creamy Orange Bar
Kidz Assorted Fruit Pops
Organic Soy Ice Cream, Creamy Fudge
  Bar

Sweet Nothings
Fudge Bar

Trader Joe's
Four Fruit Frenzy Bars
Gone Bananas Chocolate Dipped
Banana Bites
Valu Time (Brookshire)
Tropical Ice Pops
Twin Pops
Wegmans
Assorted Fruity Pops - Cherry, Orange,
& Grape Flavors
Assorted Sugar Free Fruity Pops -
Cherry, Orange, & Grape Flavors
Cherry with Dark Chocolate Ice Cream
Bars
Fudge Bars
Fudge Bars No Sugar Added
Ice Cream Bars
Ice Pops Twin Stick
Peanut Butter Candy Sundae Cups
Peanut Butter Cup Sundae Cups
Vanilla & Dark Chocolate Premium Ice
Cream Bars
Whole Fruit
Fruit Bars
Winn-Dixie
Banana Pops
Fudge Bars

PIZZA & CRUSTS

Against the Grain
Pesto Pizza
Three-Cheese Pizza
Amy's Kitchen ✓
Rice Crust Cheese Pizza
Rice Crust Spinach Pizza
Single Serve Non-Dairy Rice Crust
Cheeze Pizza
Single Serve Rice Crust Margherita
Pizza
Single Serve Rice Crust Roasted
Vegetable Pizza
Better Bread
Pizza (All)
Chebe
Pizza Crust

Conte's Pasta ✓
Gluten Free Margherita Pizza
Gluten Free Mushroom Florentine Pizza
Gluten Free Prebaked Pizza Shell
Domata Living Flour ✓
Gluten Free Pizza
Foods by George
Pizza
Pizza Crusts
Gluten Free Harvest, A
A Gluten Free Harvest (All)
Glutino
BBQ Chicken Pizza
Duo Cheese Pizza
Pepperoni Pizza
Premium Pizza Crusts
Spinach & Feta Pizza
Spinach Soy Cheese Brown Rice Crust
Pizza
Three Cheese Pizza with Brown Rice
Crust
Udi's Gluten Free Foods ✓
Margherita Frozen Pizza
Three Cheese Frozen Pizza
Uncured Pepperoni Frozen Pizza

POTATOES

57th Street Grille
Cheddar & Bacon Potato Skins
Always Save
French Fries
Best Choice
Crinkle Cut Potatoes
Crispy Crowns
Hashbrown Patty
Potatoes O'Brien
Regular Cut French Fries
Shoestring Potatoes
Shredded Hashbrowns
Southern Style Hashbrowns
Steakhouse Fries
Tater Puffs
Diner's Choice
Diner's Choice (All)
Dr. Praeger's ✓
Potato Littles

Sweet Potato Littles
Sweet Potato Pancakes
Fastco (Fareway)
French Fries
Fries, Crinkle
Golden Taters
Shredded Hash Browns
Southern Style Hash Browns
Flavorite (Cub Foods)
Cut Okra
French Fries
Golden Crowns
Hash Brown Patty
Shoestring Fries
Southern Style Hash Browns
Steak Fries
Tater Puffs
Food Club (Brookshire)
French Fried Potatoes
French Fries, Crinkle Cut
Hashbrown Patties
Potato Crowns
Potatoes O'Brien
Regular French Fries
Shoestring Fries
Shredded Hash Browns
Southern Style Hashbrowns
Steak Fries
Tater Treats
Food Club (Marsh)
French Fries
French Fries, Crinkle Cut
Hash Brown Patties
Hashbrowns, Southern Style
Potatoes O'Brien
Shredded Potato Hash Browns
Steak Fry
Tater Treats
Genuardi's ✍
Crinkle Cut French Fried Potatoes
Giant
Steak Fries
Goya
French Fries, Crinkle Cut
French Fries, Shoe String
French Fries, Straight Cut

Market Day
Baby Baked Potatoes
Baked Potatoes
Four Cheese Potatoes
Mashed Potato Patties
Quick 'N' Crispy Shoestring French
Fries
Meijer
French Fries (Crinkle Cut, Quickie
Crinkles, Seasoned, ShoeString, Steak
Cut)
Green Potato (Cheese and Herbs)
HashBrowns (Patty, Shredded, Southern
Style, Western Style)
Tater Tots
Tater Treats
Ore-Ida
ABC Tater Tots
Cottage Fries
Country Fries
Country Inn Classics Hash Browns,
Peppers & Onions
Country Inn Classics Hash Browns,
Savory Seasoned
Country Inn Classics Hash Browns,
Sour Cream & Chives
Country Style Hashbrowns
Country Style Steak Fries
Crispers
Crunch Time Classics Straight Cut
Extra Crispy Crinkle Cut
Extra Crispy Easy Golden Crinkles
Fast Food Fries
French Fries
Golden Crinkles
Golden Fries
Golden Patties
Golden Twirls
Pixie Crinkles
Potatoes O'Brien
Roasted Garlic & Parmesan
Roasted Original
Shoestrings
Southern Style Hash Browns
Steak Fries
Steam n' Mash Cut Russets
Steam n' Mash Cut Sweet Potatoes

Steam n' Mash Garlic Seasoned Potatoes
Sweet Potato Fries
Tater Tots (All Varieties)
Waffle Fries

Our Family
Hashbrowns
Potatoes (Crinkle Cut, Regular Cut)
Shoe String Potatoes
Steak Fries
Tater Puffs

Publix
Crinkle Cut Fries
Golden Fries
Shoestring Fries
Southern Style Hash Browns
Steak Fries
Tater Bites
Tater Puffs

Safeway
Country Style Hash Brown Potatoes

Shaw's
Crinkle Cut French Fries
Grade A French Fries, Wedge
Grade A Shoestring French Fries
Shred Golden Potato
Southern Style Hash Browns
Straight Cut French Fries
Tater Treat

Shoppers Value (Cub Foods)
Crinkle Cut French Fries
Shoestring Potatoes

Smart Ones
Broccoli & Cheddar Potatoes

Stop & Shop
French Fried Potatoes
Tater Bites

Trader Joe's
Handsome Cut Potato Fries
Trader Potato Tots

Valu Time (Brookshire)
French Fries, Regular
Shoestring Potatoes

Valu Time (Marsh)
French Fries, Regular

Vons
Crinkle Cut French Fried Potatoes
Regular Cut French Fries

Shoestring Potatoes
Steak Cut French Fried Potatoes

Wegmans
Country Style Hashbrowns
Crinkle Cut Potatoes
Hash Browns
Hash Browns O'Brien
Steak Cut Grade A Thick Sliced Potatoes
Straight Cut Potatoes
Tater Puffs

PREPARED MEALS & SIDES

Amy's Kitchen ✓
Asian Noodle Stir-Fry
Baked Ziti Bowl
Black Bean Enchilada Whole Meal
Black Bean Tamale Verde
Black Bean Vegetable Enchilada
Brown Rice & Vegetables Bowl
Brown Rice, Black-Eyed Peas & Veggies Bowl
Cheese Enchilada
Cheese Enchilada Whole Meal
Cheese Tamale Verde
Cream of Rice Hot Cereal Bowl
Dairy Free Rice Macaroni & Cheeze
Enchilada Verde Whole Meal
Garden Vegetable Lasagna
Gluten Free Cheddar Burrito
Gluten Free Non Dairy Burrito
Indian Mattar Paneer
Indian Mattar Tofu
Indian Palak Paneer
Indian Paneer Tikka
Indian Vegetable Korma
Kids Baked Ziti Meal
Light & Lean Black Bean & Cheese Enchilada
Light & Lean Roasted Polenta
Light & Lean Soft Taco Fiesta
Light & Lean Sweet & Sour Bowl
Light in Sodium Black Bean Vegetable Enchilada
Light in Sodium Brown Rice & Vegetables Bowl
Light in Sodium Indian Mattar Paneer

Light in Sodium Mexican Casserole
Bowl
Light in Sodium Shepherd's Pie
Mexican Casserole Bowl
Mexican Tamale Pie
Mexican Tofu Scramble
Rice Mac & Cheese
Roasted Vegetable Tamale
Santa Fe Enchilada Bowl
Shepherd's Pie
Teriyaki Bowl
Thai Stir-Fry
Tofu Scramble
Tortilla Casserole & Black Beans Bowl

Chung's ⓘ
Chung's For 2 - Sweet 'N Sour Chicken

Coleman Natural ⓘ
Gourmet Chicken Meatballs, Italian
Parmesan
Gourmet Chicken Meatballs, Pesto
Parmesan
Gourmet Chicken Meatballs, Spinach,
Fontina Cheese, and Roasted Garlic
Gourmet Chicken Meatballs, Sun-Dried
Tomato Basil Provolone

Conte's Pasta 🍴 ✓
Gluten Free Cheese Lasagna Microwave
Meal
Gluten Free Cheese Ravioli
Gluten Free Cheese Ravioli Microwave
Meal
Gluten Free Gnocchi
Gluten Free Gnocchi Microwave Meal
Gluten Free Pierogi, Potato & Onion
Gluten Free Pierogi, Potato, Cheese &
Onion
Gluten Free Spinach & Cheese Ravioli
Gluten Free Stuffed Shells
Gluten Free Stuffed Shells Microwave
Meal

Contessa ⓘ
Chicken Fried Rice
Dragon Tail Shrimp
Honey Roasted Shrimp
Jambalaya
Paella
Sesame Chicken

Shanghai Stir Fry Vegetables
Shrimp on the Bar-B
Shrimp Scampi
Tikka Masala Shrimp

Culinary Circle (Jewel-Osco)
Chicken Tikka Masala

Delimex
Chipotle Beef Rice Bowl
CORN Taquitos (All)
Santa Fe Style Chicken Rice Bowl
Tamales (All)

Don Miguel
Bean & Cheese Crispy Tacos
Chicken & 2 Mexican Cheese Mini Taco
Chicken and Cheese Mini Taco
Chicken Taquitos
Chipotle Chicken Mini Taco
El Charrito Queso Enchilada Dinner
Shredded Beef Steak Taquitos
Shredded Beef Taquitos
Steak & Green Chile Mini Taco

Dr. Praeger's ✓
Broccoli Littles
Potato Crusted Fillet Fish Sticks
Potato Crusted Fish Fillets
Potato Crusted Fishies
Spinach Littles

FLAV.R.PAC
Rice Stir Fry
Vegetable Stir Fry

Gluten Free Café
Asian Noodles
Fettuccini Alfredo
Lemon Basil Chicken
Pasta Primavera

Gluten Free Harvest, A
A Gluten Free Harvest (All)

Glutenfreeda ⓘ 🍴
Burritos (All)

Glutino
Chicken Pad Thai
Chicken Penne Alfredo
Chicken Pomodoro
Chicken Ranchero
Macaroni & Cheese
Penne Alfredo

Goya
- Baked Plantain/Horneado
- Broccoli & Cheese ()
- Classic Entrees - Rice with Chicken
- Cuban Tamales
- Rellenitos de Platano
- Spanish Omelet/ Tortilla Española
- Tamal de Papa
- Tamal Negro
- Tamales Colorados
- Tamales de Arroz
- Tamalitos de Cambray
- Tamalitos de Chipilin
- Tamalitos de Elote
- Tamalitos de Loroco
- Toston Cup

Jimmy Dean ᠔
- Ham & Cheese Omelets
- Sausage & Cheese Omelets
- Three Cheese Omelets

Kettle Cuisine ⓘ ✔
- Angus Beef Steak Chili with Beans

- Chicken Chili with White Beans
- Chicken Soup with Rice Noodles
- New England Clam Chowder
- Organic Mushroom and Potato Soup
- Roasted Vegetable Soup
- Southwestern Chicken and Corn Chowder
- Thai Curry Chicken Soup
- Three Bean Chili
- Tomato Soup with Garden Vegetables

Mama Lucia ⓘ
- Fully Cooked Sausage Meatballs

Market Day
- Breakfast Skillet
- Chicken Tortilla Soup
- Mini Cheese Omelets
- Praline Sweet Potato Casserole
- Shrimp Scampi
- Swiss and Mushroom Burgers

Night Hawk Foods
- Steak 'n Corn
- Steak 'n Taters

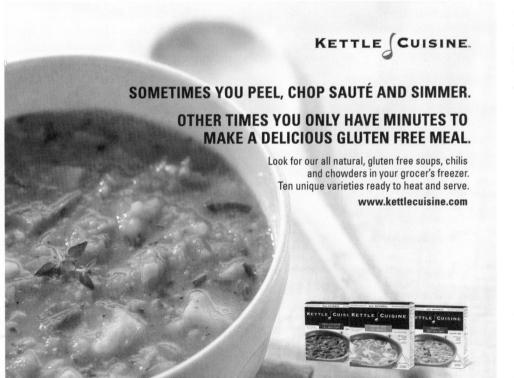

O Organics 〰
Organic Black Bean Enchiladas
Organic Cheese Enchiladas
Rosina ⓘ
Rosina Sausage Meatballs
Safeway 〰
Salmon Fillet, Raw (Value Pack)
Swai Fillet, Raw (Value Pack)
Tilapia Fillet, Raw
Whiting Fillets
SeaPak ⓘ
Shrimp Scampi
Skyline Chili ⓘ
Frozen Chili (All)
Smart Ones
Chicken Santa Fe
Cranberry Turkey Medallions
Lemon Herb Chicken Piccata
Santa Fe Rice & Beans
Sol Cuisine ✓
Falafel with Sauce
Tabatchnick Fine Foods
Balsamic Tomato & Rice Soup
Black Bean Soup
Cabbage Soup
Corn Chowder
Cream of Broccoli Soup
Cream of Spinach Soup
Creamed Spinach
Lentil Soup
New England Potato Soup
No Salt Split Pea Soup
Old Fashioned Potato Soup
Southwest Bean Soup
Split Pea Soup
Vegetarian Chili
Wilderness Wild Rice Soup
Yankee Bean Soup
Trader Joe's
Shepherds Pie (Beef)
Tamales (Cheese, Beef, Chicken)
Taquitos (Black Bean, Chicken)
Wellshire Farms
Kids Dino Shaped Chicken Bites

SAUSAGE

Wellshire Farms
Chicken Apple Sausage Links

SHERBET & SORBET

Agave Dream
Sorbets (All)
Berkeley Farms
Rainbow Sherbet ()
Best Choice
Orange Sherbet
Rainbow Sherbet
Broughton
Lime Sherbet ()
Orange Sherbet Cups ()
Orange Sherbet ()
Rainbow Sherbet ()
Fastco (Fareway)
Orange Sherbet
Rainbow Sherbet
Raspberry Sherbet
Food Club (Brookshire)
Sorbet (Cherry, Peach, Strawberry)
(Shelf Stable)
Food Club (Marsh)
Cherry Lemon Sherbet
Lime Sherbet
Orange Sherbet
Pineapple Sherbet
Rainbow Sherbet
Raspberry Sherbet
Gaga's SherBetter ⓘ ✓
SherBetter (All)
Gifford's Ice Cream ⓘ
Orange Sherbet
Rainbow Sherbet
Red Raspberry Sorbet
Haggen
Orange Sherbet
Rainbow Sherbet
Red Raspberry Sherbet
Hiland Dairy
Sherbet (All Flavors)
Hood
Sherbet (All)

Jolly Llama
SqueezeUps (All)

Lindy's Homemade
Sorbet (All)

Louis Trauth Dairy
Lime Sherbet ()
Orange Sherbet ()
Pineapple Sherbet ()
Rainbow Sherbet ()

Mayfield Dairy
Lime Sherbet ()
Orange Sherbet ()
Pineapple Sherbet ()
Rainbow Sherbet ()

Meadow Gold
Orange Sherbet
Rainbow Rapture Sherbet
Sherbet Party Cups

Meijer
Cherry Sherbet
Lemon Berry Twirl Sherbet
Lime Sherbet
Orange Sherbet (In Plastic Container)
Pineapple Sherbet
Rainbow Sherbet
Raspberry Sherbet

Oak Farms Dairy
Lime Sherbet ()
Orange Sherbet ()
Orange Sherbet Treats ()
Strawberry Sherbet ()

Oberweis Dairy
Lemon Sorbet
Mango Pomegranate Sorbet
Orange Sherbet
Raspberry Sherbet

Our Family
Coolers A Go Go Freeze & Eat Fruit
Sorbet, Cherry
Coolers A Go Go Freeze & Eat Fruit
Sorbet, Raspberry
Coolers A Go Go Freeze & Eat Fruit
Sorbet, Strawberry
Coolers A Go Go Freeze & Eat Fruit
Sorbet, Strawberry Banana
Lime Sherbet
Orange Sherbet

Rainbow Sherbet

Perry's Ice Cream ⓘ
Lemon Sorbet
Orange Sherbet
Rainbow Sherbet
Raspberry Sorbet
Watermelon Sherbet

Prairie Farms
Sherbet (All Flavors)

Price Chopper
Orange Sherbet
Rainbow Sherbet
Raspberry Sherbet

Price's Creameries
Lime Sherbet ()
Mango Sherbet ()
Orange Sherbet ()
Pineapple Sherbet ()
Rainbow Sherbet ()
Sherbet Cups (Lime or Orange Flavor) ()

Publix
Cool Lime Sherbet
Exotic Fruit Medley Sherbet
No Sugar Added Sunny Orange Sherbet
Peach Mango Passion Sherbet
Rainbow Dream Sherbet
Raspberry Blush Sherbet
Sunny Orange Sherbet
Tropic Pineapple Sherbet
Tropical Swirl Sherbet

Purity Dairies
Sherbet

Safeway Select ⤳
Berry Patch Low Fat Sherbet
Fat Free Chocolate Sorbet
Fat Free Lemon Sorbet
Fat Free Mango Sorbet
Fat Free Raspberry Sorbet
Key Lime Low Fat Sherbet
Mandarin Orange Low Fat Sherbet
Pineapple Raspberry and Orange Low
Fat Sherbet
Strawberry Sorbet
Swiss Orange Sherbet

Sambazon
Sambazon (All)

Schnucks
- Lemon Sherbet
- Lime Sherbet
- Orange Sherbet
- Pineapple Sherbet
- Rainbow Sherbet
- Raspberry Sherbet

Simply Enjoy (Giant)
- Mango Sorbetto

Simply Enjoy (Stop & Shop)
- Mango Sorbetto

So Delicious Dairy Free
- Coconut Water Sorbet, Hibiscus
- Coconut Water Sorbet, Lemonade
- Coconut Water Sorbet, Mango
- Coconut Water Sorbet, Raspberry

Talenti ✓
- Sorbetto (All BUT Caramel Cookie Crunch Gelato)

Tillamook
- Orange Sherbet ⓘ

Trader Joe's
- Pomegranate Blueberry Sherbet
- Sorbet (All)

Turkey Hill
- Fruit Rainbow Sherbet
- Orange Grove Sherbet

Wegmans
- Green Apple Sorbet
- Lemon Sorbet
- Raspberry Sorbet

Whole Fruit
- Sorbet

VEGETABLES

Albertsons
- Broccoli Cuts
- Broccoli Floret
- Brocolli/Carrot/Chestnut Blend Stir Fry
- Brussels Sprouts
- Carrots Crinkle Cut
- Cauliflower
- Chopped Broccoli
- Chopped Spinach Box
- Corn On The Cob
- Fiesta Blend Mixed Vegetables
- Green Peas Whole
- Mixed Stew Vegetables
- Mixed Vegetable Blend
- Peas N' Carrots
- Spinach Leaf Veggies
- Sugar Snap Mixed Vegetables Stir Fry
- Vegetable Blend Stir Fry
- Vegetable Mix Crinkle Cut
- Whole Kernel Corn
- Winter Mix Vegetable Blend

Allens
- Frozen Vegetables (All BUT Breaded/ Battered Items & Sauce Items)

Always Save
- Broccoli, Chopped
- Corn, Cob
- Corn, Cut
- Mixed Vegetables
- Peas

Best Choice
- Baby Carrots, Whole
- Baby Okra, Whole
- Blackeye Peas
- Broccoli Florets
- Broccoli Spears (Individually Quick Frozen)
- Broccoli, Chopped
- Broccoli, Cut
- Broccoli/Carrots/Water Chesnuts
- Brussel Sprouts
- California Mix
- Cauliflower
- Cob Corn
- Collard Greens
- Corn, Cut
- Country Style Vegetables
- Crinkle Cut Carrots
- Crowder Peas
- Japanese Blend
- Mix Vegetables
- Mustard Green
- Okra, Cut
- Peas
- Petite Peas
- Santa Fe Blend
- Steamed Broccoli Florets
- Steamed Cut Corn

Steamed Green Peas
Steamed Mix Vegetables
Stew Vegetables
Stir Fry Vegetables
Sweet White Corn
Tuscan Blend
Winter Mix

Clearly Organic (Best Choice)

Broccoli Florets Steamer
Cut Corn Steamer
Edamame Steamer
Green Peas Steamer
Mixed Vegetables Steamer

Cub Foods

Cantonese Stir Fry Vegetables
Chopped Spinach
Corn
Corn On The Cob
Crinkle Cut Carrots
Cut Corn
Cut Green Beans
Cut Leaf Spinach
Green Peas
Individually Quick Frozen Steamable
   Frozen Corn
Individually Quick Frozen Steamable
   Frozen Green Beans
Individually Quick Frozen Steamable
   Frozen Mix Vegetables
Individually Quick Frozen Steamable
   Frozen Peas
Japanese Stir Fry Vegetables
Leaf Spinach
Mini Ear Corn On The Cob
Mixed Vegetables
Peas

Fastco (Fareway)

Broccoli Florets
Broccoli Stir Fry
Broccoli, Cut
Broccoli/Cauliflower/Carrot
Brussels Sprouts
California Blend
Carrots, Crinkle
Cauliflower
Corn, Cut
Green Peas

Italian Blend
Leaf Spinach, Cut
Lima Beans
Mandarin Stir Fry
Mixed Vegetables
Oriental Blend
Peas & Carrots
Petite Peas
White Corn
Winter Blend

FLAV.R.PAC

Asparagus Cut Spears
Asparagus Stir Fry
Baby Carrots, Whole
Baby Okra, Whole
Blackeye Peas
Broccoli Cut Spears
Broccoli Normandy
Broccoli Spears
Broccoli, Chopped
Carrots, Crinkle Cut
Cauliflower Florets
Corn on the Cob
Corn, Whole Kernel
Country Trio
Dinner Vegetables
Flavor Fiesta
Grande Classics Caribbean Blend
Grande Classics Normandy Blend
Green Peas
Gumbo Mix
Leaf Spinach
Leaf Spinach, Cut
Mediterranean Vegetables
Mixed Vegetables
Okra, Cut
Oriental Vegetables
Peas and Carrots
Petite Peas
Ranchero Blend
Seasoning Blend
Southwest Blend
Speckled Butter Beans
Spinach, Chopped
Squash, Cooked
Stew Vegetables
Sugar Snap Pea Stir Fry

Sugar Snap Peas
Super Sweet White Corn
Turnip Greens, Chopped
Vegetable Soup Mix

Flavorite (Cub Foods)
Asparagus Spears
Blackeyed Peas
Chopped Green Peppers
Chopped Mustard Greens
Corn On The Cob
Crowder Peas
Cut Corn
Cut Kernels Corn
Green Peas
Individually Quick Frozen Steamables
   Corn
Individually Quick Frozen Steamables
   Mix Vegetables
Individually Quick Frozen Steamables
   Peas
Leaf Spinach
Peas
Petite Peas
Squash
Whole Baby Carrots

Food Club (Brookshire)
Baby Broccoli Florets
Blackeye Peas
Broccoli Cuts
Broccoli Spears
Broccoli, Chopped
Brussel Sprouts
Brussel Sprouts Petite
California Style Vegetables
Carrots, Crinkle Cut
Cauliflower Florets
Chopped Turnip Greens
Chuck Wagon Corn
Collards, Chopped
Corn on Cob
Corn, Whole Kernel
Crowder Peas
Florentine Vegetables
Green Peas
Gumbo Mix
Leaf Spinach, Cut
Mixed Vegetables

Mustard Greens, Chopped
Okra, Cut
Okra, Whole
Parisian Style Vegetables
Peas and Carrots
Petite Cut Corn
Petite Green Peas
Purple Hull Peas
Spinach, Chopped
Stew Mix Vegetables
Stir Fry Vegetables
Super Sweet Cob
Turnip Greens with Turnips
Turnip, Chopped
Vegetables for Soup

Food Club (Marsh)
Broccoli Baby Florets
Broccoli Cuts
Broccoli, Chopped
Brussel Sprouts
Carrots, Crinkle Cut
Carrots, Whole Baby
Cauliflower Florets
Corn On Cob
Corn, Whole Kernel
Green Peas
Green Peas, Petite
Mixed Vegetables
Onions, Diced
Peas & Carrots
Spinach, Chopped
Spinach, Cut Leaf
Steamin' Easy, Broccoli Cuts
Steamin' Easy, California Style
Steamin' Easy, Florentine
Steamin' Easy, Green Peas
Steamin' Easy, Mixed Vegetables
Steamin' Easy, Peas & Carrots
Steamin' Easy, Whole Kernel Corn
Sugar Snap Peas
Vegetable Stir Fry
Vegetables, California Style
Vegetables, Florentine
Vegetables, Italian
White Corn, Super Sweet

Food You Feel Good About (Wegmans)
Carrots, Potatoes, Celery, & Onions
Crinkle Cut Carrots
Far East Stir-Fry Vegetables
Green Beans, Broccoli, Onions, & Mushrooms
Mixed Vegetables
Spinach, Cut Leaf
Sugar Snap Peas
Sweet Petite Peas

Full Circle (Schnucks)
Corn, Whole
Green Beans, Cut
Mixed Vegetables
Peas
Steamable Mixed Vegetables
Steamable Peas

Genuardi's
Broccoli Cuts

Giant
Broccoli, Cauliflower & Carrots
Broccoli, Corn & Red Peppers
Carrots, Crinkle Cut
Harvest Choice Broccoli Florets
Harvest Choice Cauliflower Florets
Harvest Choice Chopped Onions
Harvest Choice Chopped Spinach
Harvest Choice Cut Broccoli
Harvest Choice Mixed Vegetables
Harvest Choice Peas & Carrots
Harvest Choice Super Sweet White Corn
Harvest Choice Sweet Peas
Harvest Choice Vegetables for Soup
Harvest Choice Vegetables for Stew
Mixed Peppers Strips
Okra, Cut
Petite Peas
Spinach Leaf
Spinach, Chopped
SteamReady Asparagus Spears
SteamReady Broccoli and Cauliflower
SteamReady Brussels Sprouts
Succotash
Sugar Snap Peas
Sweet Corn, Whole Kernel
Sweet Peas

Zucchini, Sliced

Goya
Broccoli Florets
Carrots, Sliced
Choclo
Choclo 2 pcs
Corn, Cut
Large Ears Corn-Cob
Leaf Spinach, Cut
Mini Ears Corn-Cob
Mixed Vegetables
Okra, Cut
Peas and Carrots
Spinach, Chopped
Steam Best - California Blend
Steam Best - Mixed Vegetables
Steam Best - Whole Kernel Corn
Steam Best - Winter Blend
Sweet Peas
Viandas Para Sancocho
Yuca Frita

Great Value (Wal-Mart) 25
Asparagus Spears, All Green Extra Long
Broccoli & Cauliflower
Broccoli Cuts
Broccoli Florets
Broccoli, Cauliflower, & Carrots
Broccoli, Cut
California Style Vegetable Mix
Cauliflower
Corn On The Cob
Corn On The Cob, Cut
Diced Carrots, Microwavable
Golden Corn, Whole Kernel (Microwavable)
Golden Sweet Corn, Whole Kernel No Salt Added
Leaf Spinach, Cut
Mixed Vegetables
Seasoned Mixed Garden Medley
Sweet Peas, Microwaveable
Vegetable Medley

Green Giant
Valley Fresh Steamers - Broccoli Cuts
Valley Fresh Steamers - Chopped Broccoli

Valley Fresh Steamers - Extra Sweet
Niblets Corn
Valley Fresh Steamers - Mixed
Vegetables
Valley Fresh Steamers - Niblets Corn
Valley Fresh Steamers - Select Baby
Sweet Peas
Valley Fresh Steamers - Select Broccoli
Florets
Valley Fresh Steamers - Select Sugar
Snap Peas
Valley Fresh Steamers - Select White
Shoepeg Corn
Valley Fresh Steamers - Sweet Peas

Haggen
Broccoli (Cuts, Florets)
Brussel Sprouts
California Blend
Corn (No Salt Added, Super Sweet,
Whole Kernel)
Country Vegetable Trio
Fiesta Style Vegetables
Green Peas (Petite, Regular)
Mixed Vegetables
Spinach, Chopped
Stir Fry Vegetables
Winter Mix Vegetables

Hanover Foods
Asparagus Spears
Broccoli & Cauliflower Blend
Broccoli Cuts
Broccoli Florets
Broccoli Florets Petite
Broccoli, Water Chestnuts, Red Peppers,
Yellow Peppers
Brussel Sprouts Petite
California Blend
Carrots, Sliced
Carrots, Whole Baby
Cauliflower Clusters
Green Peppers, Diced
Oriental Blend
Petite Peas
Snow Peas
Spinach, Cut Leaf
Sugar Snap Peas
Sweet Peas

White Sweet Corn

Hatch
Chile (All)

Hy-Vee
Broccoli Cuts
Broccoli Florets
Broccoli, Chopped
Brussels Sprouts
California Mix
Carrots, Crinkle Cut
Cauliflower Florets
Corn on the Cob
Corn on the Cob, Mini
Cream Style Golden Corn
Fiesta Blend
Golden Corn, Cut
Italian Blend
Leaf Spinach
Mixed Vegetables
Oriental Vegetables
Spinach, Chopped
Sweet Peas
Winter Mix

Jewel-Osco
Chopped Spinach
Corn On The Cob
Crinkle Cut Carrots
Cut Corn
Cut Leaf Spinach
Cut Okra
Green Peas Steamables
Leaf Spinach
Mixed Vegetable Blend
Petite Pearl Onions
Stew Vegetables
Super Sweet White Cut Corn
Western Vegetable Blend
Whole Green Beans
Whole Green Peas
Whole Kernel Corn
Whole Okra
Whole Petite Peas

Market Day
"Extra Young" Tiny Peas
Asparagus Spears
Baja Roasted Corn Blend
Broccoli Florets

Corn, Supersweet
Kyoto Blend
Nantucket Island Blend
Prince Edward Vegetable Medley
Stir-Fry Blend
Sweet Potato Medley
Yin Yang Vegetable Blend
Yukon Gold Potato & Vegetable Blend

Meijer
Artichoke (Quarters)
Broccoli Cuts Steamer
Brussel Sprouts
California Blend Steamer
California Style Vegetables
Carrots (Crinkle Cut, Whole Baby)
Cauliflower Florets
Chinese Pea Pods
Collards (Chopped)
Corn (Fire Roasted, Original, White Sweet)
Edamame (Soy Beans)
Fiesta Vegetables
Fire Roasted Mukimame Blend
Fire Roasted Southwestern Blend
Florentine Vegetables
Florets (California)
Green Asparagus (Spears)
Green Bell Peppers (Diced)
Green Peppers (Chopped)
Green Vegetable Mix with Potato
Italian Vegetables
Mexican Vegetables
Mixed Vegetable Steamer
Mixed Vegetables (Organic)
Okra (Chopped, Whole)
Onions (Chopped)
Onions (Diced)
Oriental Blend Steamer
Oriental Vegetables
Parisian Vegetables
Peas (Green, Organic, Petite)
Peas and Carrots
Squash (Cooked, Winter)
Stew Mix Vegetables
Stir Fry Vegetables
Sweet Corn Steamer
Tuscan Blend Vegetables

Vegetable Stew
Whole Corn Kernels (Golden, Original)
Whole Onion Ring
Winter Blend Steamer

Meijer Organics
Broccoli (Chopped, Cuts, Florets, Spears)
Corn Cob(Mini Ear, Original)
Spinach (Chopped, Cut, Leaf) (Meijer Organic)

Nature's Promise (Giant)
Organic Asparagus Spears
Organic Cut Spinach Leaf
Organic Cut Yellow Corn
Organic Edamame in the Pod (Frozen)
Organic Green Peas
Organic Mini Broccoli Spears
Organic Mixed Vegetables

Nature's Promise (Stop & Shop)
Organic Asparagus Spears
Organic Cut Green Beans
Organic Cut Spinach Leaf
Organic Cut Yellow Corn
Organic Edamame in the Pod (Frozen)
Organic Green Peas
Organic Mixed Vegetables
Organic Whole Green Beans

O Organics
Organic Chopped Spinach
Organic Golden Cut Corn
Organic Haricots Verts
Organic Petite Broccoli Florets

Ore-Ida
Chopped Onions

Our Family
Broccoli Cuts
Broccoli Cuts with California Blend
Broccoli Florets
Broccoli Stir Fry
Broccoli, Cut Steamable
Brussels Sprouts
California Blend
California Blend Vegetables, Steamable
Carrots, Crinkle Cut
Cauliflower
Corn
Corn on the Cob

Corn, Whole Kernel Steamable
Mixed Vegetables
Mixed Vegetables, Steamable
Oriental Stir Fry
Oriental Vegetables
Peas
Peas & Carrots
Peas, Steamable
Rhubarb
Spinach, Chopped
Spinach, Leaf
Winter Blend Vegetables, Steamable

Publix
Alpine Blend
Broccoli - Chopped
Broccoli - Cuts
Broccoli - Spears
Brussels Sprouts
California Blend
Carrots - Crinkle Cut
Carrots - Whole Baby
Cauliflower
Collard Greens - Chopped
Corn - Cut
Corn On The Cob
Del Oro Blend
Field Peas with Snap
Green Peppers - Diced
Gumbo Mix
Italian Blend
Japanese Blend
Mixed Vegetables
Okra - Cut
Okra - Whole Baby
Onions - Diced
Peas - Blackeye
Peas - Butter
Peas - Crowder
Peas - Green
Peas - Petite
Peas - Purple Hull
Peas
Peas and Carrots
Rhubarb
Roma Blend
Soup Mix with Tomatoes
Spinach - Chopped

Spinach - Cut Leaf
Spinach - Leaf
Squash - Cooked
Squash - Yellow Sliced
Succotash
Turnip Greens - Chopped
Turnip Greens with Diced Turnips

Schnucks
Broccoli (Chopped, Cut, Spears)
Brussels Sprouts
California Vegetable Blend
Carrots (Crinkle Cut, Whole Baby)
Cauliflower Florets
Corn
Corn, Mini Cob
Corn, Whole Kernel Gold
Florentine Blend
Green Peas
Green Peppers
Mixed Vegetables
Peas
Peas & Carrots
Spinach, Chopped
Spinach, Cut Leaf
Stew Vegetables
Vegetable Stir Fry

Seapoint Farms
Eat Your Greens Organic Veggie Blend
Garden Blend Veggies
Oriental Blend Veggies

Shoppers Value (Cub Foods)
Whole Kernel Corn

Stahlbush Island Farms ⓘ
Stahlbush Island Farms (All BUT Black Barley & Wheat Berries)

Stop & Shop
Broccoli and Cauliflower, Cut
Broccoli Florets
Broccoli Spears
Broccoli, Cauliflower and Carrots
Broccoli, Cut
Brussels Sprouts
Carrots, Crinkle Cut
Cauliflower Florets
Corn, Cut
Green Peas
Mixed Vegetables

Okra, Cut
Onions, Chopped
Peas & Carrots
Petite Green Peas
Rancho Fiesta Blend Vegetables
Spinach Leaf, Cut
Spinach, Chopped

Thrifty Maid (Winn-Dixie)
Mixed Vegetables

Trader Joe's
Frozen Vegetables (All)

Valu Time (Brookshire)
Corn, Whole Kernel
Green Peas
Mini Corn Cobs
Mixed Vegetables

Valu Time (Marsh)
Corn, Whole Kernel
Mixed Vegetables
Peas, Green

Valu Time (Schnucks)
Corn, Whole Kernel
Mixed Vegetables
Peas

Vons ⌒
Blackeye Peas
Collard Greens, Chopped
Corn on the Cob, Mini
Corn, Cut
Green Split Peas
Mixed Vegetables
No Salt Green Peas
Okra, Cut
Onions, Chopped
Peas
Peas and Carrots
Spinach, Chopped
Stew Vegetables
Stir Fry Blends
Stir Fry Vegetables with Asparagus

Wegmans
Artichoke Hearts - Halves & Quarters
Asian Stir Fry
Baby Carrots
Broccoli - Chopped
Broccoli - Spears

Broccoli Cuts & Cauliflower Florets
Broccoli Cuts
Broccoli Cuts, Cauliflower Florets, &
   Carrots
Brussels Sprouts
Brussels Sprouts in Butter Sauce
Cauliflower Florets
Corn - Whole Kernel
Corn - Whole Kernel in Butter Sauce
Corn on the Cob
Mixed Vegetables
Peas
Peas with Pearl Onions
Pepper & Onion Mix
Petite Peas in Butter Sauce
Santa Fe Mix
Southern Mix
Spinach - Chopped
Spinach - Whole Leaf
Spinach in Cream Sauce
Spring Mix
Stir Fry Vegetables-Hong Kong
Zucchini, Carrots, Cauliflower, Baby
   Lima Beans & Italian Style Green
   Beans

Westpac
Asparagus Cut Spears
Baby Okra, Whole
Blackeye Peas
Broccoli Cut Spears
Broccoli Florets
Broccoli Normandy
Broccoli, Chopped
Broccoli-Cauliflower
Brussels Sprouts
Carrots, Crinkle Cut
Cauliflower
Collard Greens, Chopped
Corn on the Cob
Corn, Whole Kernel
Dinner Vegetables
Green Peas
Gumbo Mix
Leaf Spinach, Cut
Mediterranean Vegetables
Mixed Vegetables

Mustard Greens, Chopped
Okra, Cut
Oriental Vegetables
Peas & Carrots
Petite Peas
Ranchero Blend
Seasoning Blend
Southern Style Stew Vegetables
Southwest Blend
Spinach, Chopped
Stew Vegetables
Sugar Snap Peas
Super Sweet White Corn
Vegetable Soup Mix

Winn-Dixie
Broccoli (Chopped, Cuts, Florets, Spears)
Brussels Sprouts
Carrots (Crinkle Cut, Whole Baby)
Cauliflower
Collard Greens, Chopped
Corn on the Cob (Mini, Regular)
Green Peppers, Diced
Mixed Vegetables
Mustard Greens
Okra (Cut, Whole)
Onions, Diced
Organic Green Peas
Organic Mixed Vegetables
Organic Yellow Corn, Cut
Pearl Onions
Peas & Carrots
Peas, Butter
Peas, Crowder
Peas, Field with Snaps
Peas, Green
Peas, Petite Green
Spinach (Chopped, Cut Leaf)
Squash, Yellow
Steamable Broccoli, Cut
Steamable Mixed Vegetables
Steamable Sweet Green Peas
Steamable Yellow Corn, Cut
Succotash
Turnip Greens (Chopped, with Turnips)
White Corn, Cut
Yellow Corn, Cut

World Classics (Schnucks)
Asparagus
Haricots Verts
Shoepeg Corn
Snap Peas
Snow Peas

VEGETARIAN MEAT

Creative Chef
Tofettes Brazilian
Tofettes Hot & Spicy
Tofettes Jamaican Jerk
Tofettes Lemon Garlic
Sol Cuisine ✓
BBQ Tofu Ribs

VEGGIE BURGERS

Amy's Kitchen ✓
Bistro Veggie Burger
Sonoma Veggie Burger
Dr. Praeger's ✓
Gluten-Free California Veggie Burger
Sol Cuisine ✓
Mushroom Rice Burger
Original Burger
Spicy Bean Burger
Vegetable Burger
Veggie Breakfast Patties
Sunshine Burger ⛨ ✓
Barbecue Organic Sunshine Burger
Breakfast Organic Sunshine Burger
Falafel Organic Sunshine Burger
Garden Herb Organic Sunshine Burger
Original Natural Sunshine Burger
South West Organic Sunshine Burger

WAFFLES & FRENCH TOAST

Nature's Path ⓘ ✓
Buckwheat Wildberry Waffles
Homestyle Waffles
Mesa Sunrise Waffles
Trader Joe's
Wheat Free Toaster Waffles

Van's Natural Foods ⓘ ✓
Wheat-Gluten Free Apple Cinnamon Waffles
Wheat-Gluten Free Blueberry Waffles
Wheat-Gluten Free Buckwheat Waffles
Wheat-Gluten Free Cinnamon French Toast Sticks
Wheat-Gluten Free Flax Waffles
Wheat-Gluten Free Minis Totally Natural Waffles
Wheat-Gluten Free Totally Natural

WHIPPED TOPPINGS

Always Save
Whipped Topping
Best Choice
Extra Creamy Whipped Topping
Lite Whipped Topping
Whipped Topping
Fastco (Fareway)
Fat Free Topping
Whipped Topping
Food Club (Brookshire)
Extra Creamy Whipped Topping
Fat Free Whipped Topping
Lite Whipped Topping
Whipped Cream Aerosol
Whipped Topping
Food Club (Marsh)
Extra Creamy Whipped Topping
Fat Free Whipped Topping
Lite Whipped Topping
Whipped Topping
Giant
Lite Non Dairy Whipped Topping
Whipped Topping
Great Value (Wal-Mart) 25
Fat Free Whipped Topping
Light Whipped Topping
Whipped Topping
Hy-Vee
Extra Creamy Whipped Topping
Fat Free Whipped Topping
Lite Whipped Topping
Whipped Topping

Meijer
Whipped Topping (Extra Creamy, Fat Free, Lite)
Safeway ⌇
Non Dairy Whipped Topping
Schnucks
Fat Free Whipped Topping
Light Whipped Topping
Whipped Topping
Valu Time (Brookshire)
Whipped Topping
Wegmans
Fat Free Whipped Topping
Lite Whipped Topping
Whipped Topping

MISCELLANEOUS

Goya
Arañitas/Plantain Hashbrown
Maduros
Tostones
Perfect Puree, The ⓘ
Perfect Puree, The (All)

Boar's Head

DID YOU KNOW?

All Boar's Head meats, cheeses and condiments are GLUTEN FREE.

Talk to us at:

boarshead.com

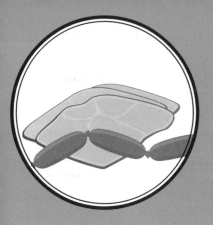

MEAT

BACON

ACME
Original Cooked Bacon
Albertsons
Pre-Cooked Bacon, Original
Always Save
Sliced Bacon
Beeler's 🏅
Beeler's (All)
Best Choice
Cooked Bacon
Low Sodium Smoked Bacon
Sliced Smoked Bacon
Stack Pack Bacon
Thick Slice Bacon
Coleman Natural ⓘ
Uncured Hickory Smoked Bacon
Cub Foods
Pre-Cooked Bacon
Dak
Bacon (All)
Dietz & Watson ✓
Canadian Bacon
Gourmet Imported Bacon
Pancetta
Pancetta Hunk
Eating Right 〰
Turkey Bacon
Farmer John
Center Cut Bacon
Ends and Pieces Bacon
Maple Ends & Pieces Bacon
Old Fashioned Maple Table Brand
Bacon

Premium Applewood Bacon
Premium Cracked Peppercorn Bacon
Premium Low Sodium Bacon
Premium Old Fashioned Maple Bacon
Premium Regular Smoked Bacon
Premium Thick Sliced Bacon
Table Brand Bacon
Thick Smoked Bacon
Fastco (Fareway)
Bacon
Food Club (Brookshire)
Precooked Pork Bacon Strips
Regular L-Board Bacon
Thick L-Board Bacon
Giant Eagle
Bacon
Center Cut Bacon
Center Cut Sliced Bacon
Fully Cooked Bacon
Low Salt Bacon
Low Sodium Bacon
Peppered Bacon
Regular Sliced Bacon
Thick Bacon
Thick Sliced Bacon
Godshall's ⓘ
Canadian Turkey Bacon
Chicken Bacon
Maple Turkey Bacon Sliced
Peppered Turkey Bacon
Sliced Beef Bacon
Turkey Bacon
Great Value (Wal-Mart) 📅
Hickory Fully Cooked Bacon
Hickory Smoked Bacon

Lower Sodium Bacon
Peppered Bacon

Haggen
Bacon (Low Sodium, Sliced, Thick Sliced)

Hatfield ()
Applewood Smoked Bacon
Classic Bacon
Reduced Sodium Bacon
Sliced Bacon

Hempler Foods Group ⓘ
Canadian Bacon
Pepper Bacon
Regular Bacon
Uncured Bacon

Hormel
Black Label Bacon
Canadian Style Bacon
Fully Cooked Bacon
Microwave Bacon

Jennie-O Turkey Store
Extra Lean Turkey Bacon
Regular Turkey Bacon

Jewel-Osco
Cooked Bacon

Jimmy Dean ᐧᐧ
Bacon Breakfast Skillets
Breakfast Bowls: Bacon, Eggs, Potatoes and Cheddar Cheese
Hickory Smoked Bacon Slices
Lower Sodium Premium Bacon
Maple Bacon Slices
Original Premium Bacon
Thick Sliced Hickory Smoked Bacon
Thick Sliced Maple Bacon
Thick Sliced Premium Bacon

Jones Dairy Farm
Canadian Bacon Slices
Cherry Hardwood Smoked Sliced Bacon
Old Fashioned Slab Bacon
Regular Sliced Bacon
Thick Sliced Bacon

Kunzler ⸸
Bacon (All)

Meijer
Bacon
Canadian Bacon

Center Cut Bacon
Low Sodium Bacon
Pre-Cooked Thick Sliced Bacon
Thick Sliced Bacon
Turkey Bacon

Nature's Basket (Giant Eagle)
Bacon

Oscar Mayer ᐧᐧ
Bacon, Center Cut Original
Bacon, Center Cut Thick Sliced
Bacon, Lower Sodium
Bacon, Maple
Bacon, Naturally Hardwood Smoked
Bacon, Naturally Hardwood Smoked Thick Cut
Bacon, Smoked Uncured
Bacon, Super Thick Cut Applewood Smoked
Ready to Serve Bacon, Bacon Fully Cooked
Ready to Serve Bacon, Bacon Thick Cut Fully Cooked
Ready to Serve Bacon, Canadian Bacon Fully Cooked
Ready to Serve Bacon, Real Bacon Bits
Ready to Serve Bacon, Real Bacon Recipe Pieces
Roast Beef Cold Cuts, Slow Roasted 96% Fat Free
Turkey Bacon, Lower Sodium with Sea Salt
Turkey Bacon, Smoked Cured 50% Less Fat

Our Family
Bacon
Double Smoked Bacon
Lower Sodium Bacon
Maple Bacon

Petit Jean
Petit Jean (All)

Plumrose ✓
Plumrose (All)

Price Chopper
Vermont Smoke & Cure Maple Cure Bacon

Publix
Bacon (All Varieties)

Range Brand
Bacon

Safeway 〰
Applewood Smoked Bacon, Thick Sliced
Fully Cooked

Safeway Select 〰
Regular Sliced Bacon
Thick Sliced Bacon

Shaw's
Cooked Bacon

Shoppers Value (ACME)
Sliced Smoked Bacon

Shoppers Value (Albertsons)
Sliced Smoked Bacon

Shoppers Value (Cub Foods)
Sliced Smoked Bacon

Shoppers Value (Jewel-Osco)
Sliced Smoked Bacon

Smithfield Foods ⓘ
Bacon (All)

Smith's
Smith's (All)

Sugardale
Bacon (All)

Superior's
Low Salt Bacon
Regular Sliced Bacon
Thick Sliced Bacon
Thin Sliced Bacon

Trader Joe's
Turkey Bacon
Uncured Bacon
Uncured Bacon Ends & Pieces

Valu Time (Marsh)
Tux Bacon

Wellshire Farms
Beef Bacon
Bulk Slab Pork Bacon
Bulk Sliced Pepper Bacon
Canadian Style Bacon Nugget
Classic Sliced Dry Rubbed Bacon
Classic Sliced Turkey Bacon
Classic Sliced Turkey Peppered Bacon
Dry Rubbed Applewood Smoked Bacon
Dry Rubbed Bacon Ends & Pieces
Frozen Layout Applewood Bacon
Fully Cooked Hickory Smoked Bacon

Irish Brand Bacon
Organic Dry Rubbed Bacon
Organic Turkey Bacon
Pancetta Bacon
Sliced Apple Wood Dry Rub Bacon
Sliced Bacon
Sliced Canadian Style Bacon
Sliced Canadian Style Turkey Bacon
Sliced Dry Rubbed Applewood Bacon
Sliced Maple Bacon
Sliced Pancetta Bacon
Sliced Peppered Dry Rub Bacon
Thick Range Sliced Dry Rubbed Bacon
Thick Sliced Dry Rubbed Bacon
Turkey Peppered Bacon
Whole Pancetta Bacon

Winn-Dixie
Hickory Sweet Lower Sodium Bacon
Hickory Sweet Sliced Bacon
Hickory Sweet Thick Sliced Bacon
Hickory Sweet Thin Sliced Bacon

Zeigler ()
Bacon
Stack Pack Bacon
Thick Sliced Bacon

BEEF

ACME
Roast Beef Tub

Always Tender
Non-Flavored Fresh Beef
Peppercorn Flavored Fresh Beef

Angus Pride
Meat (All)

Beeler's 🍴
Beeler's (All)

Best Choice
91% Lean Beef Patty
Thin Slice Beef

Buddig 🍴 25
Buddig Original – Beef
Buddig Original – Corned Beef
Buddig Original – Pastrami

Cajun Prize (Manda) ⓘ
Cooked Roast Beef

Cajun Rite (Manda) ⓘ
Cooked Roast Beef

Chef Master (Manda) ⓘ
Cooked Roast Beef

Cub Foods
Roast Beef Tub

DeLallo
Corned Beef Top Round
Roast Beef Top Round

Di Lusso
Beef

Dietz & Watson ✓
California Style Corned Beef
Choice Top Round Roast Beef
Classic Top Round Dried Beef
Corned Beef Brisket
Corned Beef-Cap Off-Top Round
Italian Style Roast Beef
London Broil Roast Beef
Oven Roasted Roast Beef Medium
Oven Roasted Roast Beef Rare
Premium Angus Roast Beef
Premium Homestyle Roast Beef
Roast Beef
Seasoned Prime Rib of Beef with Juices
Top Round London Broil Roast Beef
Top Round Roast Beef Medium
Top Round Roast Beef Rare
U.S.D.A. Choice Eye Round Roast Beef
USDA Pepper Choice Eye Round Roast Beef

D'Italia (Manda) ⓘ
Italian Style Roast Beef

Eating Right ⌒
Roast Beef

Extra Value ⓘ
Extra Value Beef Patties (1.5 lb & 5 lb boxes)

Farmer John
Roast Beef Natural Meats

Fastco (Fareway)
Smoked Beef

Four Star (Manda) ⓘ
Cooked Corned Beef
Cooked Roast Beef

Full Circle (Schnucks)
Beef Patties

Giant Eagle
Pulled Beef with BBQ Sauce
Ribs
Roast Beef Tub
Seasoned Shredded Beef with BBQ Sauce

Goya
Corned Beef

Great Value (Wal-Mart) 25
100% Pure Beef Patties (75/25)
100% Pure Beef Patties (80/20)
100% Pure Beef Patties (85/15)
Beef Philly Steak
Thinly Sliced Seasoned Roast Beef

GreenWise Market (Publix)
Beef Back Ribs
Beef Cubed Steak
Beef for Stew
Bottom Round
Bottom Round Steak
Brisket Flat
Chuck Eye Steak
Chuck Roast, Boneless
Chuck Short Ribs
Chuck Short Ribs, Boneless
Chuck Steak, Boneless
Eye Round
Eye Round Steak
Flank Steak
Flap Meat
Flat Iron Steak
Ground Chuck
Ground Chuck for Chili
Ground Chuck Patties
Ground Round
Inside Skirt Steak
Outside Skirt Steak
Porterhouse Steak
Rib Eye Roast, Boneless
Rib Eye Steak, Bone-In
Rib Eye Steak, Boneless
Rib Roast
Round Cubes
Rump Roast
Shoulder Roast, Boneless
Shoulder Steak
Sirloin Flap Meat

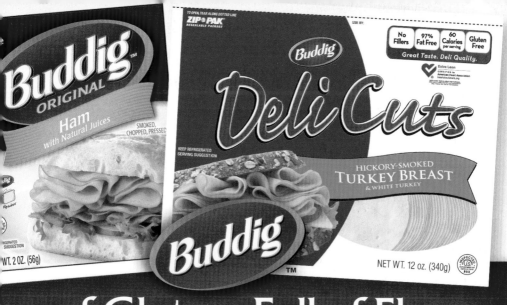

ee of Gluten. Full of Flavor.

o gluten free with Buddig and Old Wisconsin.® Buddig Original and Deli Cuts are
eat-tasting, naturally high in protein and low in fat. Deli Cuts are certified by the
erican Heart Association® to display their heart-check mark, making them an even
er way to help you control your diet. Old Wisconsin products offer a wide range
ardwood-smoked beef and turkey meat snacks to fit your lifestyle. Enjoy naturally
n free lunchmeat and snacks with the Buddig and Old Wisconsin family of products.*
uddig.com and oldwisconsin.com to learn more or visit your local grocery retailer.

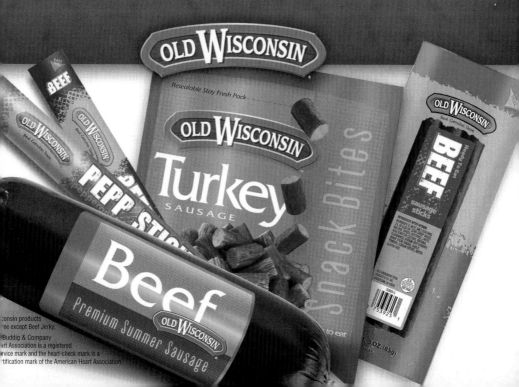

Sirloin for Kabobs
Sirloin for Stir Fry
Sirloin Tip Roast
Sirloin Tip Side Steak
Sirloin Tip Steak
Strip Steak Boneless
T-Bone Steak
Tenderloin Roast
Tenderloin Steak
Top Blade Roast, Boneless
Top Blade Steak
Top Round
Top Round for Stir Fry
Top Round London Broil
Top Round Steak
Top Round Steak, Thin Sliced
Top Sirloin Filet Steak
Top Sirloin Steak, Boneless
Tri Tip Roast
Tri Tip Steaks

Hatfield ()
Roast Beef

H-E-B
Cajun Roast Beef
Mesquite Smoked Roast Beef
Mesquite Smoked Roast Beef, Pre-Sliced
Seasoned Roast Beef
Seasoned Roast Beef, Pre-Sliced

Hebrew National
Hebrew National (All BUT Franks in a Blanket)

Hempler Foods Group ⓘ
Uncured Gray Corned Beef

Jewel-Osco
Roast Beef Tub

Kunzler
Roast Beef (Presliced, Whole)

Louisiana Pride (Manda) ⓘ
Cooked Roast Beef

Manda ⓘ
Cooked Corn Beef (Brown Label)
Cooked Roast Beef (Manda Supreme Gold Label)
Italian Style Roast Beef (Manda Supreme Gold Label)

Meijer
80/20 Ground Beef

83/17 Ground Chuck
85/15 Ground Round
90/10 Ground Sirloin
96/4 Extra Lean Ground Beef
Ground Beef Chuck, Fine
Ground Beef, Fine
Ground Chuck (Flavor Seal)

Old Neighborhood
Old Neighborhood (All)

Oscar Mayer
Carving Board Roast Beef, Cured Slow Roasted

Petit Jean
Petit Jean (All)

Plumrose ✓
Plumrose (All)

Price Chopper
Pearl Gray Corned Beef Brisket
Scallopini

Private Selection (Kroger)
Corned Beef
Roast Beef

Publix
Beef Pot Roast with Home-Style Gravy, Fully Cooked
Corned Beef (Pre-Packed Sliced Deli Lunch Meats)
Ground Round Patties
Premium Certified Beef

Ranchers Reserve
Beef Chuck Short Rib Flanked Style Boneless
Beef Cube Steak
Beef Flank Steak
Beef for Stew
Beef for Stew Tenderized
Beef Loin New York Strip Steak Boneless Extreme Value
Beef Loin New York Strip Steak Thin Boneless
Beef Petite Tender Cracked Pepper
Beef Petite Tender Roasted Garlic
Beef Ribeye Roast Bone In
Beef Ribeye Roast Boneless
Beef Ribeye Steak Boneless Thin
Beef Round Tip Steak Cap Off
Beef Round Tip Steak Cap Off Thin

Beef Top Round London Broil Extreme Value

Saag's ⓘ
Saag's (All BUT British Bangers & Marzenbier Brats)

Sausages by Amylu ⓘ
Burgers by Amylu (All)
Meatballs by Amylu (All)

Schnucks
Beef Tips
Pot Roast

Shady Brook Farms
Beef (All BUT Italian Style Beef Meatballs, Rosemary, Garlic & Chardonnay Seasoned Sirloin Tri-Tip, and Sizzling Ginger Sirloin Tri-Tip)

Skylark
Skylark (All)

Smith's
Smith's (All)

Tallgrass Beef Company
Bone-In Prime Rib
Boneless Prime Rib
Burger Patties
Chuck Roast
Coulotte Steak
Fajita Meat
Filet Mignon
Flat Iron Steak
Ground Beef
Hanger Steak
N.Y. Strip Steak
Osso Bucco
Rib Eye Steak
Sirloin Steak
Stew Meat
Tenderloin Tips
Tri-Tip Steak
Whole Tenderloin
Whole Untrimmed Brisket

Thumann's ✓
All Natural Black Angus Cooked Corned Beef Round
All Natural Black Angus Pastrami Round
All Natural Black Angus Top Round Choice Capless

Beef Tongue
Beef Top Round London Broil
Bottom Roast Beef
Cajun Style Beef Top Round London Broil
Cap Corned Beef
Capless Roast Beef
Cooked Brisket
Cooked Corned Beef Round, Capless
Cooked Corned Beef Round, Split
Cooked Corned Beef Round, Top
Corned Beef Bottom
First Cut Corned Beef, Cooked
First Cut Corned Beef, Raw
Fresh Cooked Brisket
Hamburger & Beef Patties
Italian Style Roast Beef, Capless
No Fat Beef
No Fat Beef Special
Raw Corned Beef Brisket
Ripple Roast Beef
Roast Beef Top, Large
Roast Beef Top, Small
Special Chop Beef
Special Chop Beef Bag
Top Round

Trader Joe's
Fully Cooked & Seasoned Prime Rib of Beef
Unprocessed Raw Meat (All)

Wellshire Farms
Corned Beef Brisket
Corned Beef Round
Corned Beef Whole
Shredded Beef in Barbeque
Sliced Corned Beef
Sliced Roast Beef
Whole Roast Beef

BOLOGNA

Best Choice
Beef Bologna
Regular Bologna

Dietz & Watson ✓
Beef Bologna
Bologna

Gourmet Lite Bologna

Empire Kosher
Turkey Bologna Slices

Farmer John
Bologna Lunch Meats

Fastco (Fareway)
Ring Bologna

Food Club (Brookshire)
Bologna
Thick Bologna

Giant Eagle
All Meat Bologna

Hatfield ⟨⟩
Beef Bologna
German Brand Bologna
Hatfield Bologna
Ring Bologna

Hebrew National
Hebrew National (All BUT Franks in a
Blanket)

Hempler Foods Group ⓘ
Bologna
German Bologna
Uncured Bologna

Hill Country Fare (H-E-B)
Meat Bologna

Johnsonville
Hearty Beef Ring Bologna
Original Ring Bologna

Kunzler ⛾
Ring Bologna (Garlic, Non-Garlic, Old
Fashion, Plain)

Norbest ⓘ
Turkey Bologna Lunchmeat

Old Neighborhood
Old Neighborhood (All)

Old Wisconsin ⓘ 25
Ring Bologna

Oscar Mayer ∿
Bologna Cold Cuts, 98% Fat Free
Bologna Cold Cuts, Beef
Bologna Cold Cuts, Beef Light
Bologna Cold Cuts, Beef Thick Cut
Bologna Cold Cuts, Beef Thin Sliced
Bologna Cold Cuts, Bologna
Bologna Cold Cuts, Garlic Made with
Chicken & Pork

Bologna Cold Cuts, Light
Bologna Cold Cuts, Light Beef
Bologna Cold Cuts, Made with Chicken
& Pork
Bologna Cold Cuts, Thick Cut
Bologna Cold Cuts, Thick Cut Made
with Chicken & Pork
Bologna Cold Cuts, Thin Sliced
Bologna Cold Cuts, Turkey Lower Fat

Our Family
Beef Bologna
Bologna
Garlic Bologna
German Bologna
Thick Bologna

Publix
Beef Bologna (Pre-Packed Sliced Deli
Lunch Meats)
German Bologna (Pre-Packed Sliced
Deli Lunch Meats)

Saag's ⓘ
Saag's (All BUT British Bangers &
Marzenbier Brats)

Seltzer's
Lebanon Bologna (All)

Shoppers Value (ACME)
Shaved Bologna

Shoppers Value (Albertsons)
Beef Bologna
Bologna
Shaved Bologna
Thick Sliced Bologna

Shoppers Value (Cub Foods)
Beef Bologna
Bologna
Shaved Bologna
Thick Sliced Bologna

Shoppers Value (Jewel-Osco)
Beef Bologna
Bologna
Shaved Bologna

Smith's
Smith's (All)

Superior's
Bologna
Chub Bologna
Cleveland Bologna

Garlic Bologna
Thick Bologna

Thumann's ✓
Angle Cut Bologna
Beef Bologna
Chub Bologna
Garlic Bologna
Ham Bologna
Jumbo Bologna
Long Bologna
Lower Sodium Bologna
Old Fashioned Bologna
Red Bologna
Ring Bologna
Thick Bologna

Valu Time (Brookshire)
Bologna
Think Sliced Bologna

Wellshire Farms
Old Fashioned Deli Beef Bologna
Sliced Beef Bologna
Sliced Turkey Bologna

Zeigler ()
Garlic Bologna
Original Recipe Sliced Bologna
Original Recipe Thick Sliced Bologna
Seasoned To Please Bologna
Sliced Bologna
Thick Sliced Bologna

CHICKEN

ACME
Chicken Breast

Al Fresco All Natural
Chicken Franks (All)
Chicken Meatballs (All)

Allen Family Foods, Inc.
Chicken (All)

Bell & Evans ⓘ ✓
Fresh Chicken (All)

Best Choice
Boneless Skinless Chicken Breast
Thin Slice Chicken

Buddig 🍴 25
Buddig Original – Chicken
Deli Cuts – Rotiserrie Chicken

Fix Quick – Chicken

Coleman Natural ⓘ
Bone-in Skin-on Chicken Thigh
Boneless Skinless Chicken Breast
Boneless Skinless Chicken Thigh
Drummettes
Drumsticks
Fresh for the Freezer Chicken
Organic Bone-in Skin-on Chicken Thigh
Organic Boneless Skinless Chicken Breast
Organic Boneless Skinless Chicken Thigh
Organic Chicken Breast Tenders
Organic Chicken Wings, Buffalo Style
Organic Drummettes
Organic Drumsticks
Organic Fresh For the Freezer Chicken
Organic Mild Italian Chicken Sausage
Organic Split Breast
Organic Whole Chicken
Organic Wings
Split Breast
Whole Chicken
Wings

Dak
Premium Oven Roasted Chicken Breast (All)

Di Lusso
Chicken

Dietz & Watson ✓
Buffalo Style Chicken Breast
Gourmet Breast of Chicken
Honey Barbecue Breast of Chicken
Momma Dietz Chicken Parmigiana
Rotisserie Breast of Chicken

Domata Living Flour 🍴 ✓
Gluten Free Boneless Chicken Wings

Empire Kosher
Boneless Skinless Chicken Breasts
Chicken Drumsticks
Chicken Leg Quarters
Chicken Split Breasts
Chicken Thighs
Cut Up Chicken, 8 Piece
Fully Cooked BBQ Chicken

Organic Boneless Skinless Breasts
Organic Chicken Drumsticks
Organic Whole Broiler Chicken
Quartered Broiler Chicken
Ready to Roast Garlic & Herb Chicken
Whole Broiler Chicken

Food Club (Brookshire)
Chicken Breast
Chicken Party Wings
Chicken Tenders

Giant Eagle
Boneless Chicken Breast Strips
Boneless Skinless Chicken Breast
Iff Boneless Breast
Iff Boneless Breast Tender
Iff Chicken Wings
Pulled Chicken with BBQ Sauce
Shredded Chicken Breast with BBQ
Sauce
Thin Sliced Boneless Chicken Breast
Thin Sliced Chicken Breast
Whole Chicken Leg

Great Value (Wal-Mart) 25
100% Natural Boneless Skinless Chicken
Breasts
Boneless Skinless Chicken Breast Fillets
Chicken Drumsticks
Chicken Thighs
Chicken Wing Drumettes
Chicken Wing Sections

GreenWise Market (Publix)
Boneless Chicken Breast
Boneless Chicken Thighs
Chicken Cutlet
Chicken Drummettes
Chicken Drumsticks
Chicken Fillet
Chicken Sausage, Herb and Tomato
Chicken Sausage, Hot Italian
Chicken Sausage, Mild Italian
Chicken Tenderloin
Chicken Thighs
Chicken Wings
Ground Chicken
Skinless Chicken Drumsticks
Skinless Chicken Thighs
Split Chicken Breast

Whole Chicken

Harvestland
Fresh All Natural Chicken Parts
Fresh All Natural Chickens
Frozen Chicken Breasts (Individually
Wrapped)
Frozen Fully Cooked Grilled Breast
Strips

H-E-B
Rotisserie Flavored Chicken Breast
Seasoned Cilantro Lime Chicken Breast
Seasoned Italian Style Chicken Breast
Seasoned Lemon Herb Chicken Breast
Seasoned Southwest Style Chicken
Breast
Seasoned Sweet Chile Chicken Breast

Mountaire
Mountaire (All)

Nature's Basket (Giant Eagle)
Boneless Chicken Breast
Boneless Skinless Chicken Thigh
Chicken Drumstick
Chicken Tenders
Chicken Thigh
Chicken Wings
Iff Chicken
Split Chicken Breast

Original Brat Hans, The ⓘ
Aged Parmesan & Fennel Chicken
Meatballs
Buffalo Style Chicken Meatballs
Chipotle Pepper & Cheddar Chicken
Meatballs
Florentine with Spinach & Fontina
Cheese Chicken Burger
Jalapeno & Sharp Cheddar Chicken
Burger
Pesto Parmesan Chicken Burger
Pesto Parmesan Chicken Meatballs
Pineapple Teriyaki Chicken Meatballs
Spinach, Fontina, & Roasted Garlic
Chicken Meatballs
Uncured Bacon & Cheddar Chicken
Burger

Oscar Mayer ✎
Carving Board Chicken Breast,
Rotisserie Seasoned

Our Family
Premium Chicken Breast

Perdue
Buffalo Style Jumbo Chicken Wings
Carving Chicken Breast, Oven Roasted
Grilled Chicken Breast Strips, All
Natural
Ground Breast of Chicken
Ground Chicken Burgers
Honey BBQ Jumbo Chicken Wings
Hot and Spicy Jumbo Chicken Wings
Individually Frozen Chicken Breasts
Individually Frozen Chicken
Tenderloins
Individually Frozen Chicken Wings
Perfect Portions Boneless Skinless
Chicken Breast, All Natural
Perfect Portions Boneless Skinless
Chicken Breast, Roasted Garlic with
White Wine
Perfect Portions Boneless Skinless
Chicken Breat, Herb and Pepper
Perfect Portions Boneless Skinless
Chicken Breat, Italian Style
Rotisserie Chicken, Barbecue
Rotisserie Chicken, Chesapeake
Seasoned
Rotisserie Chicken, Italian
Rotisserie Chicken, Lemon Pepper
Rotisserie Chicken, Oven Roasted
Rotisserie Chicken, Smoky Peppercorn
Rotisserie Chicken, Toasted Garlic
Rotisserie Chicken, Tuscany Herb
Roasted
Sauce N Toss Buffalo Style Chicken
Wings
Sauce N Toss Honey Barbecue Chicken
Wings
Short Cuts Carved Chicken Breast
Grilled, Southwestern Style
Short Cuts Carved Chicken Breast,
Honey Roasted
Short Cuts Carved Chicken Breast,
Original Roasted
Short Cuts Carved Chicken Breast,
Roasted Garlic with White Wine
Sliced Chicken Breast, Oil Fried

Price Chopper
Drums
Drums Jumbo
Jumbo Whole Wings
Necks
Thighs
Whole Wing

Publix
All Natural Fresh Chicken

Rocky Jr. ⓘ
Bone-In Skin-On Chicken Thigh
Boneless Skinless Chicken Thigh
Chicken Breast Tenders
Drummettes
Drumsticks
Split Breast
Whole Chicken
Wings

Rocky the Range ⓘ
Whole Chicken

Rosie Organic ⓘ
Bone-In Skin-On Chicken
Boneless Skinless Chicken Thigh
Chicken Breast Tenders
Drummettes
Drumsticks
Split Breast
Whole Chicken
Wings

Safeway ⌒
Chicken Breast Boneless Skinless
Extreme Value

Schnucks
White Chicken Chunks

Shady Brook Farms
Chicken

Thumann's ✓
All Natural Oven Roasted Gourmet
Chicken Breast
All Natural Oven Roasted Hickory
Smoked Chicken Breast
Oven Roasted Chicken Breast, Barbeque
Style
Oven Roasted Chicken Breast, Buffalo
Style
Oven Roasted Premium Chicken Breast,
Browned in Oil

Trader Joe's
Just Chicken, Plain
Unprocessed Raw Meat (All)
Wellshire Farms
Oven Roasted Chicken Breast
Shredded Chicken in Barbeque Sauce

DELI MEATS

ACME
Fully Cooked Pork Luncheon Meat
Albertsons
Deli 98% Fat Free Ham Premium
Deli Chopped Ham
Deli Cooked Ham
Deli Fat Free Ham Premium
Deli Fat Free Oven Roasted Turkey
Breast
Deli Ham Low Sodium
Deli Honey Ham
Deli Individual Chicken Rotisserie
Breast
Deli Individual Honey Ham
Deli Individual Honey Smoked Turkey
Deli Individual Honey Smoked Turkey
Breast
Deli Individual Oven Roasted Turkey
Deli Individual Oven Roasted Turkey
Breast
Deli Individual Smoked Ham
Deli Individually Baked Honey Ham
Shaved
Ham Tub Refill Brown Sugar
Luncheon Meat
Roast Beef Tub
Roasted Turkey Tub Refill
Best Choice
Pickle Loaf
Boar's Head
Meat (All)
Buddig
Deli Cuts – Honey Roasted Turkey
Deli Cuts – Oven-Roasted Turkey
Deli Cuts – Smoked Turkey
Deli Cuts – Pastrami
Deli Cuts – Roast Beef
Deli Cuts – Baked Honey Ham

Deli Cuts – Brown Sugar Baked Ham
Deli Cuts – Smoked Ham
Columbus Salame
Deli Meats (All)
Cub Foods
Thin Sliced Cooked Ham Lunchmeat
Dak
Premium Deli Ham (All)
Sliced Turkey Ham (All)
Dietz & Watson ✓
Beef Bologna
BF Braunschweiger Liverwurst
BF Braunschweiger Liverwurst, NC
Black Forest Beerwurst
Black Forest Smoked Ham
Blutwurst
Bologna
Braunschweiger Liverwurst
Buffalo Style Chicken Breast
Capocollo Hot
Capocollo Sweet
Classic Deluxe Loaf
Classic Peppered Loaf
Genoa Salami
Gourmet Lite Cooked Ham
Hamcola
Head Cheese
Honey Roll
Lunch Roll
Mortadella
Mortadella Hunk
Mortadella with Pistachios
New York Style Pastrami Brisket
Olive Loaf
P&P Loaf
Pastrami-Bottom Round
Pickle and Pimiento Loaf
Souse Roll
Southern Fried Breast of Chicken
Spiced Beef Pastrami
Spiced Luncheon Meat
Eating Right
Chicken Breast Oven Roasted Deli Style
Luncheon Meat
Pastrami
Empire Kosher
Turkey Pastrami

Turkey Pastrami Slices

Farmer John
Cotto Salami
Ham Roll
Headcheese
Mission Loaf
Original Premium Liverwurst
Premium Braunschweiger
Premium Liverwurst with Bacon
Premium Oven Roasted Turkey Breast

Food Club (Brookshire)
Turkey Breast 97% Fat Free
Turkey Ham 95% Fat Free

Four Star (Manda) ⓘ
Big Cajun Hog Head Cheese
Pastrami/Cooked Pastrami

Giant
Regular Sliced Top Round Roast Beef
Thin Sliced Buffalo Chicken Breast
Thin Sliced Oven Roasted Chicken
    Breast
Thin Sliced Top Round Roast Beef (Deli)

Giant Eagle
Bavarian Ham
Brown Sugar Ham Off the Bone
Honey Ham
Honey Ham, Tub
Honey Turkey Breast, Tub
Italian Style Ham
Maple Ham
Oven Roasted Turkey Breast, Tub
Peppered Ham
Smoked Ham, Tub
Smoked Turkey Breast, Tub
Virginia Ham

Godshall's ⓘ
Turkey Liverwurst Chub

Goya
Luncheon Meat
Luncheon Meat- All Pork

Hatfield ⓞ
Liverwurst
Liverwurst Chunks
Original Loaf
Pickle & Pimiento Loaf

H-E-B
All Natural Honey Ham Lunchmeat

All Natural Oven Roasted Chicken
    Breast Lunchmeat
All Natural Roast Beef Lunchmeat
Black Forest Ham Tub
Brown Sugar Ham Tub
Hard Salami Tub
Honey Ham Tub
Honey Turkey Tub
Mesquite Smoked Ham Tub
Mesquite Smoked Turkey Tub
Oven Roasted Turkey Tub
Peppered Turkey Tub
Roast Beef Tub
Rotissere Chicken Tub

Hebrew National
Deli Meats (All BUT Franks in a
    Blanket)

Hempler Foods Group ⓘ
Head Cheese
Uncured Braunschweiger

Hill Country Fare (H-E-B)
Cajun Roast Beef
Peppered Turkey
White Meat Turkey

Hillshire Farms ⌇
Deli Select Brown Sugar Baked Ham
    Water Added
Deli Select Club Sandwich Variety Pack
Deli Select Ham Sandwich Variety Pack
    Water Added
Deli Select Honey Ham Water Added
Deli Select Honey Roasted Turkey
    Breast
Deli Select Mesquite Smoked Turkey
    Breast
Deli Select Oven Roasted Chicken
    Breast Caramel Colored
Deli Select Oven Roasted Turkey Breast
Deli Select Pastrami With Up To 15% Of
    A Curing & Flavoring Solution
Deli Select Premium Hearty Slices
    Honey Roasted Turkey Breast
Deli Select Premium Hearty Slices Oven
    Roasted Turkey Breast 1lb Family Size
    Caramel Colored

Deli Select Premium Hearty Slices Oven Roasted Turkey Breast Caramel Colored

Deli Select Premium Hearty Slices Signature Honey Ham Water Added

Deli Select Premium Hearty Slices Virginia Brand Baked Ham Water Added – Caramel Colored – Made in Kentucky

Deli Select Roast Beef With Up To 33% Of A Curing & Flavoring Solution

Deli Select Smoked Ham Water Added

Deli Select Smoked Turkey Breast

Deli Select Sub Sandwich Variety Pack

Deli Select Ultra Thin Brown Sugar Baked Ham Water Added

Deli Select Ultra Thin Cracked Black Pepper Turkey Breast

Deli Select Ultra Thin Hard Salami

Deli Select Ultra Thin Honey Ham Water Added

Deli Select Ultra Thin Honey Roasted Turkey Breast

Deli Select Ultra Thin Mesquite Smoked Turkey Breast

Deli Select Ultra Thin Oven Roasted Turkey Breast

Deli Select Ultra Thin Oven Roasted Turkey Breast 1lb Family Size

Deli Select Ultra Thin Pastrami With Up to 15% of a Curing & Flavoring Solution

Deli Select Ultra Thin Roast Beef Containing up to 10% of a Flavoring Solution, Caramel Colored

Deli Select Ultra Thin Rotisserie Seasoned Chicken Breast Oven Browned with Caramel Color

Deli Select Ultra Thin Smoked Ham Water Added

Turkey Polska Kielbasa Links

Ultra Thin Lower Sodium Honey Roasted Turkey Breast

Ultra Thin Lower Sodium Oven Roasted Turkey Breast 99% FAT FREE

Variety Pack Honey Roasted Turkey Breast & Smoked Ham Water Added

Variety Pack Oven Roasted Turkey Breast & Honey Ham Water Added

Hormel

Luncheon Meat

Natural Choice - Brown Sugar Deli Ham

Natural Choice - Canadian Bacon

Natural Choice - Cooked Deli Ham

Natural Choice - Fully Cooked Sausage Patties

Natural Choice - Grilled Chicken Strips

Natural Choice - Hard Salami (Uncured)

Natural Choice - Honey Deli Ham

Natural Choice - Honey Deli Turkey

Natural Choice - Hot Dogs (Uncured)

Natural Choice - Mesquite Turkey

Natural Choice - Oven Roasted Chicken Strips

Natural Choice - Oven Roasted Deli Turkey

Natural Choice - Peppered Turkey Breast

Natural Choice - Pepperoni (Uncured)

Natural Choice - Roast Beef

Natural Choice - Rotisserie Style Deli Chicken Breast

Natural Choice - Smoked Deli Ham

Natural Choice - Smoked Deli Turkey

Natural Choice - Smoked Ring Sausage

Natural Choice - Uncured Bacon

Jennie-O Turkey Store

Deli Chicken Breast - Buffalo Style

Deli Chicken Breast - Mesquite Smoked

Deli Chicken Breast - Oven Roasted

Jewel-Osco

97% Fat-Free Cooked Ham Lunchmeat

98% Fat-Free Premium Ham Lunchmeat

Fat-Free Ham Lunchmeat

Ham Lunchmeat

Low Salt 98% Fat-Free Ham NJ Lunchmeat

Jones Dairy Farm

Braunschweiger, Sandwich Size Slices

Chub Braunschweiger, Bacon & Onion

Chub Braunschweiger, Light

Chub Braunschweiger, Mild & Creamy

Chub Braunschweiger, Regular

Chunk Braunschweiger, Light
Chunk Braunschweiger, Regular
Old Fashioned Cured Ham, Deli Slices
Sliced Braunschweiger, Cracker Size
Slices
Sliced Braunschweiger, Sandwich Size
Slices

Kunzler ⚱

Braunschweiger (Liverwurst)
Lunch Meats (All BUT Ham Loaf &
Macaroni & Cheese Loaf)
Meadows Mush
Pan Pudding

Land O'Frost ⓘ

Lunchmeats (All BUT Taste Escapes
Lemon Pepper Chicken)

Manda ⓘ

Hog Head Cheese (Yellow Label)
Pastrami/Cooked Pastrami (Brown
Label)

Meijer

Beef, Sliced Chipped Meat
Chicken Sliced, Chipped Meat
Cooked Ham, Sliced 97% Fat Free
Corned Beef Sliced, Chipped Meat
Ham, Sliced Chipped Meat
Honey Ham 97% Fat Free
Pastrami, Sliced Chipped Meat
Turkey Breast, 97% Fat Free (Zip Pouch)
Turkey, Sliced Chipped Meat

Nature's Promise (Giant)

Deli Black Forest Ham, Thin Sliced
Deli Oven Roasted Turkey Breast,
Regular Sliced
Deli Oven Roasted Turkey Breast, Thin
Sliced
Deli Roasted Chicken Breast, Regular
Sliced
Deli Roasted Chicken Breast, Thin
Sliced

Norbest ⓘ

Turkey Pastrami Lunchmeat

Norwestern

Deli Turkey - Hickory Smoked
Deli Turkey - Oven Roasted

Oscar Mayer ⌇

Braunschweiger Cold Cuts, Authentic
Liver Sausage
Deli Fresh Combos, The American,
Ham Honey/Roast Beef Cured
Deli Fresh Combos, The Classic, Turkey
Breast Oven Roasted/Ham Smoked
Deli Fresh Combos, The Honey, Turkey
Breast Honey Smoked/Ham Honey
98% Fat Free
Deli Fresh Ham, Black Forest Shaved
98% Fat Free
Deli Fresh Ham, Brown Sugar Shaved
98% Fat Free
Deli Fresh Ham, Honey Shaved 98% Fat
Free
Deli Fresh Ham, Smoked Shaved
Deli Fresh Ham, Smoked Shaved 98%
Fat Free
Deli Fresh Ham, Virginia Brand Shaved
97% Fat Free
Deli Fresh Roast Beef, Cured French
Dip Flavored
Deli Fresh Roast Beef, Slow Roasted
Cured Slow Roasted
Deli Fresh Salami, Beef
Deli Fresh Shaved/Sliced, Barbecue
Seasoned Shaved 98% Fat Free
Deli Fresh Shaved/Sliced, Honey
Roasted 97% Fat Free
Deli Fresh Shaved/Sliced, Oven Roasted
97% Fat Free
Deli Fresh Shaved/Sliced, Rotisserie
Seasoned Shaved 98% Fat Free
Deli Fresh Turkey Breast, Honey
Smoked Shaved 98% Fat Free
Deli Fresh Turkey Breast, Mesquite
Shaved 98% Fat Free
Deli Fresh Turkey Breast, Oven Roasted
Shaved
Deli Fresh Turkey Breast, Oven Roasted
Shaved 98% Fat Free
Deli Fresh Turkey Breast, Smoked
Shaved
Deli Fresh Turkey Breast, Smoked
Shaved 98% Fat Free

Jamon De Pierna Cold Cuts, 98% Libre De Grasa

Liver Cheese Cold Cuts

Sub Kit Cold Cuts, Ham & Beef Salami

Sub Kit Cold Cuts, Ham & Turkey

Sub Kit Cold Cuts, Ham & Turkey Breast

Variety Pak Cold Cuts, Ham & Turkey Breast

Variety Pak Cold Cuts, Ham/Turkey Breast/Canadian Style Bacon

Variety Pak Cold Cuts, Turkey Breast 96% Fat Free

White Chicken Cold Cuts Homestyle Oven Roasted

Our Family

Braunschweiger

Deli Thin Cooked Ham (Tub)

Deli Thin Honey Ham (Tub)

Deli Thin Honey Turkey (Tub)

Deli Thin Oven Roasted Turkey (Tub)

Pickle and Pimento Loaf

Spiced Loaf

Perdue

Deli Dark Turkey Pastrami, Hickory Smoked

Deli Pick Up Sliced Turkey Ham, Honey Smoked

Deli Pick Ups Sliced Turkey Breast, Golden Brown

Deli Pick Ups Sliced Turkey Breast, Honey Smoked

Deli Pick Ups Sliced Turkey Breast, Mesquite Smoked

Deli Pick Ups Sliced Turkey Breast, Oven Roasted

Deli Pick Ups Sliced Turkey Breast, Smoked

Deli Turkey Bologna

Deli Turkey Breast, Oil Browned

Deli Turkey Ham, Hickory Smoked

Deli Turkey Salami

Ground Chicken

Plainville Farms

Deli Meat (All)

Primo Taglio (Safeway)

Hickory Smoked Turkey Vacuum Pack

Oven Roasted Turkey Vacuum Pack

Prosciutto Vacuum Pack

Roasted Oven Turkey

Sliced Italian Dry Salame

Sliced Pancetta Vacuum Pack

Publix

Apple Wood Smoked Rotisserie Chicken

Barbecue Flavored with Barbecue Seasoning and Sauce Rotisserie Chicken

Barbecue Flavored with Barbecue Seasoning Rotisserie Chicken

Beef Bottom Round Roast (Pre-Packed Sliced Deli Lunch Meats)

Cooked Ham (Pre-Packed Sliced Deli Lunch Meats)

Extra Thin Sliced Honey Ham (Pre-Packed Sliced Deli Lunch Meats)

Extra Thin Sliced Oven Roasted Turkey Breast (Pre-Packed Sliced Deli Lunch Meats)

Extra Thin Sliced Smoked Turkey Breast (Pre-Packed Sliced Deli Lunch Meats)

Fully Cooked Turkey, Whole

Hard Salami - Reduced Fat (Pre-Packed Sliced Deli Lunch Meats)

Honey Kut Ham (Pre-Packed Sliced Deli Lunch Meats)

Lemon Pepper Flavored with Lemon & Herb Seasoning Rotisserie Chicken

Low Salt Ham (Pre-Packed Sliced Deli Lunch Meats)

Olive Loaf (Pre-Packed Sliced Deli Lunch Meats)

Original Roasted Rotisserie Chicken

Peppered Beef (Pre-Packed Sliced Deli Lunch Meats)

Pickle & Pimento Loaf (Pre-Packed Sliced Deli Lunch Meats)

Smoked Turkey (Pre-Packed Sliced Deli Lunch Meats)

Spanish Style Pork (Pre-Packed Sliced Deli Lunch Meats)

Sweet Ham (Pre-Packed Sliced Deli Lunch Meats)

Tavern Ham (Pre-Packed Sliced Deli Lunch Meats)

Turkey Breast (Pre-Packed Sliced Deli
Lunch Meats)

U.S.D.A. Choice Cooked Beef Bottom
Round Roast

Virginia Brand Ham (Pre-Packed Sliced
Deli Lunch Meats)

Saag's ⓘ
Saag's (All BUT British Bangers &
Marzenbier Brats)

Shaw's
Cooked Ham Lunchmeat
Honey Ham Lunchmeat
Luncheon Meat
Oven Roasted Lunchmeat
Oven Roasted Turkey Lunchmeat
Premium Ham Lunchmeat
Sliced Pepperoni Lunchmeat

Shoppers Value (ACME)
Luncheon Loaf

Shoppers Value (Albertsons)
Luncheon Loaf

Shoppers Value (Cub Foods)
Luncheon Loaf

Shoppers Value (Jewel-Osco)
Luncheon Loaf

Skylark
Skylark (All)

Smithfield Foods ⓘ
Lunchmeat (All)

Smith's
Smith's (All)

Stop & Shop
98% Fat Free Regular Sliced Oven
Roasted Chicken Breast

98% Fat Free Thin Sliced Oven Roasted
Chicken Breast

99% Fat Free Regular Sliced Buffalo
Chicken Breast (Deli)

99% Fat Free Thin Sliced Buffalo
Chicken Breast

Regular Sliced Cured Honey Ham
Regular Sliced Honey Turkey Breast
Regular Sliced Italian Roast Beef
Regular Sliced Premium Cooked Ham
Regular Sliced Premium Corned Beef
Regular Sliced Premium Ham
Regular Sliced Premium Pastrami

Regular Sliced Rare Cooked Roast Beef
Regular Sliced Smoked Turkey Breast
Regular Sliced Turkey Breast
Regular Sliced Virginia Ham
Thin Sliced Cured Honey Ham
Thin Sliced Honey Turkey Breast
Thin Sliced Italian Roast Beef
Thin Sliced Premium Cooked Ham
Thin Sliced Premium Corned Beef
Thin Sliced Premium Ham
Thin Sliced Premium Pastrami
Thin Sliced Rare Cooked Roast Beef
Thin Sliced Smoked Turkey Breast
Thin Sliced Turkey Breast
Thin Sliced Virginia Ham

Sugardale
Chopped Deli Ham
Deli Bacon, Canadian Bacon
Deli Bacon, Sliced Slab Meat
Deli Ham, Cooked
Deli Loaves, Cleveland Bologna
Deli Loaves, Emberdale Bologna
Deli Loaves, Leona Bologna
Deli Loaves, Old Fashioned Jumbo
Bologna
Deli Loaves, Premium Bologna
Lunch Meat (All)
Virginia Classic Deli Ham

Thumann's ✓
Blood & Tongue Loaf
Braunschweiger - Chub Yellow Casing
Liverwurst
Braunschweiger - Fresh Liverwurst
Braunschweiger - Smoked Liverwurst
Braunschweiger - White Casing
Liverwurst
Braunschweiger - Yellow Casing
Liverwurst
Chub Smoked Liverwurst
First Cut Pastrami
Head Cheese
Luncheon Loaf
Old Fashioned Head Cheese
Olive Loaf
Oval Minced
Pastrami
Pastrami Bottom

Pickle & Pimento Loaf

Wellshire Farms
Black Forest Deli Ham
Pastrami Brisket
Pastrami Navel
Pastrami Round
Pork Liverwurst
Sliced Pastrami
Turkey Liverwurst
Virginia Brand Deli Ham
Virginia Sliced Deli Ham

Zeigler ◔
Chunk Souse
Country Brand Souse
Deli Ham Slices
Deli Tub Cooked Ham
Deli Tub Smoked Ham
Deli Tub Smoked Honey Ham
Deli Tub Smoked Honey Turkey
Deli Tub Smoked Turkey
Hot Chunk Souse
Hot Country Brand Souse
Sliced Country Brand Souse
Sliced Hot Country Brand Souse
Sliced Olive Loaf
Sliced Pickle Loaf

HAM & PROSCIUTTO

ACME
Honey Ham
Smoked Ham

Albertsons
97% Fat Free Cooked Ham
98% Fat Free Honey Ham Baked
Boneless Honey Ham, Sliced
Honey Ham Tub Refill
Honey Ham Wafer Sliced
Premium Ham

Beeler's ⚇
Beeler's (All)

Best Choice
Cooked Ham
Honey Ham
Smoked Ham
Thin Slice Ham
Tub Honey Ham

Tub Smoked Ham

Buddig ⚇ 25
Buddig Original – Brown Sugar Ham
Buddig Original – Ham
Buddig Original – Honey Ham
Fix Quick – Smoked Ham

Cajun Prize (Manda) ⓘ
Spicy Cajun Ham

**Central Market Classics
(Price Chopper)**
Bone In Extra Smoked Ham
Boneless Extra Smoked Ham
Boneless Honey Ham Slices
Boneless Sliced Ham
Boneless Smoked Quarter Ham
Boneless Spiral Sliced Extra Smoked
  Ham
Reduced Sodium Extra Smoked Ham
  Steak

Chef Master (Manda) ⓘ
Boneless Ham & Water Product
Honey Cured Ham
Virginia Brand Smoked Ham

Cub Foods
98% Fat-Free Baked Honey Ham
98% Fat-Free Premium Ham
Fat-Free 97% Cooked Ham
Thin Sliced Cooked Ham Lunchmeat
Thin Sliced Honey Ham Lunch Meat

Cure 81
Ham and Ham Steaks

Dak
Canned Ham (All)
Premium Sliced Ham (All)

DeLallo
10% Deli Cooked Ham
Boneless Prosciutto
Capicola, Cooked (Hot, Sweet)
Capicola, Home Style (Hot, Sweet)
Oven Roasted Rosemary Ham

Di Lusso
Ham

Dietz & Watson ✓
Black Forest Brand Deep Smoked Ham
Black Forest Cooked Ham
Black Forest Cured Honey Ham
Black Forest Smoked Ham Half

Branded Cooked Ham
Branded Cooked Ham Half
Breakfast Ham Fillets
Brown Sugar and Molasses Ham
Brown Sugar and Molasses Ham Steak
Cajun Ham
Chef Carved Ham
Chopped Ham
Classic Ham
Classic Ham Half
Classic Tiffany Ham
Classic Tiffany Ham Half
Cooked Ham
Cooked Ham Round
Golden Recipe Honey Cured Dinner
  Ham, Half
Golden Recipe Honey Cured Dinner
  Ham, One Quarter
Golden Recipe Honey Cured Dinner
  Ham, Whole
Gourmet Lite VA Ham Decorated
Gourmet Lite VA Ham Low Salt
Ham Capocolla
Ham Cubes
Hickory Smoked Chef Carved Ham
Honey Cured Ham Steak
Honey Cured Tavern Ham
Imported Cooked Ham
Imported Tavern Ham
Maple Cured Ham Steak
Maple Glazed Ham
Our Traditional Ham Steaks
Pepper Ham
Pepper Ham Half
Prosciutto
Prosciutto American Style
Prosciutto Classico
Prosciutto Hunk
Prosciutto, Shelf Stable
Rosemary Ham
Semi Boneless Smoked Ham
Semi Boneless Smoked Ham Half
Smoked Maple Ham
Square Red Pepper Ham
Tomato Basil Ham
Virginia Baked Ham
Virginia Brand Ham

Eating Right ✍
  Honey Ham
Farmer John
  Black Forest Ham Lunch Meats
  Brown Sugar & Honey Ham Lunch
    Meats
  Canless Honey Ham Boneless Ham
    (Glaze Packets Contain Wheat)
  Clove Ham Steaks
  Golden Tradition Boneless Ham
  Golden Tradition Premium Black Forest
    Boneless Ham
  Golden Tradition Premium Brown
    Sugar and Honey Boneless Ham
  Golden Tradition Premium Original
    Whole and Half Boneless Ham
  Maple Ham Steaks
  Original Ham Steaks
  Pee Wee Half Boneless Ham
  Pineapple & Mango Ham Steaks
  Premium Butt and Shank Portions
    Bone-In Ham
  Premium Gold Wrap Bone-In Ham
  Premium Half Bone-In Ham
  Premium Honey Ham Natural Meats
  Premium Sliced Ham Steaks Bone-In
    Ham
  Premium Spiral Sliced Bone-In Ham
  Premium Spiral Sliced Half Bone-In
    Ham
  Sliced Cooked Ham Lunch Meats
  Smoked Ham Natural Meats
  Smoked Ham Steaks
  Whole Bone-In Ham (Glaze Packets
    Contain Wheat)
Fastco (Fareway)
  1/2 Spiral Ham
  1/4 Boneless Ham
  Bone-In Ham
  Boneless 1/2 Ham
  Boneless Ham
  Ham Chops
  Ham Large Bone-In
  Ham Steaks
  Ham Tub
  Mini Boneless Ham
  Spiral Ham

Food Club (Brookshire)
Chopped Fat Free Ham
Cooked Ham Water Added 96% Fat Free
Honey Ham Water Added 96% Fat Free
Imported Sliced Ham 98% Fat Free

Four Star (Manda) ⓘ
Honey Cured Ham
Old Fashioned Ham
Smoked Ham

Giant Eagle
4x6 Cooked Ham
Black Forest Ham Tub
Boneless Maple Ham
Brown Sugar Ham Tub
Ground Ham
Half Boneless Ham
Half Semi Boneless Ham
Pastrami Tub
Preglazed Spiral Half Ham
Quarter Boneless Ham
Whole Boneless Ham
Whole Boneless Maple N/J
Whole Semi Boneless Ham

Great Value (Wal-Mart) 🔲
97% Fat Free Baked Ham
97% Fat Free Cooked Ham
97% Fat Free Honey Ham
Sliced Chopped Ham
Sliced Turkey Ham
Thinly Sliced Smoked Ham
Thinly Sliced Smoked Honey Ham

Hatfield ()
Black Forest Dinner Ham
Breakfast Ham Slices
Brown Sugar Mustard Ham Steak
Canadian Ham Slices
Classic Boneless Ham (Half, Quarter,
 Reduced Sodium, Whole)
Classic Ham Steak
Hickory Smoked Ham Steak
Honey Dinner Ham
Honey Ham Steak
Imported Brand Cooked Ham
Maple Ham Steak
Peppered Ham
Premium Cooked Ham
Semi-Boneless Ham (Half, Whole)

Simply Tender Fresh Ham Filet
Skinless and Shankless Ham (Half,
 Whole)
Sweet Brown Sugar Ham Steak
Tavern Ham
Traditional Dinner Ham
Virginia Brand Ham

H-E-B
45% Lower Sodium Honey Ham
Applewood Smoked Ham
Black Forest Ham
Bourbon Glazed Ham
Brown Sugar Ham
Honey Mesquite Ham
Old Fashioned Ham Off the Bone
Premium Sliced Ham with Natural
 Juices

Hempler Foods Group ⓘ
Apple Honey Ham
Black Forest Ham
Bone in Ham
Boneless Ham
Raspberry Ham
Semi-Boneless Ham
Uncured Boneless Ham
Uncured Ham Hocks

Hill Country Fare (H-E-B)
Chopped Ham
Cooked Ham

Hillshire Farms ᕙ
Baked Honey Cured Ham Boneless Half,
 Water Added
Brown Sugar Cured Ham Bone-In Half,
 With Natural Juices – Caramel Color
 Added
Brown Sugar Cured Spiral Sliced Ham
 Bone–In, With Natural Juices –
 Caramel Color Added
Honey Cured Spiral Sliced Ham Bone–
 In Half, With Natural Juices
Smoked Ham Bone-In Half, With
 Natural Juices
Smoked Ham Bone-In Whole, Water
 Added
Smoked Spiral Sliced Ham Bone–In,
 With Natural Juices

Ultra Thin Lower Sodium Honey Ham with Natural Juices
Ultra Thin Lower Sodium Smoked Ham with Natural Juices

Hormel
Black Label Chopped Ham
Cubed Ham
Diced Ham
Ham Patties
Ham Steaks
Julienne Ham

Jewel-Osco
4 Boneless Ham Slices
Boneless Ham Steak Slice
Honey Deli Ham
Sugarless Boneless Honey Half Ham

Jimmy Dean
Breakfast Bowls: Ham, Eggs, Potatoes and Cheddar Cheese
D-Lights Ham Breakfast Bowl
Ham Breakfast Skillets

Jones Dairy Farm
Dainty Ham
Deli Style Honey & Brown Sugar Slicing Ham, Cured
Family Ham (Half, Whole)
Ham Slices
Ham Steaks
Old Fashioned Cured Whole Ham, Hickory Smoked
Whole Fully Cooked Hickory Smoked Ham
Whole Fully Cooked Semi-Boneless Ham

Kunzler
Hams (All)

Manda
Cooked Ham (Yellow Label)
Cooked Ham for Seasoning, Pre-Diced (Yellow Label)
Honey Cured Ham (Manda Supreme Gold Label)
Honey Cured Ham (Yellow Label)
Smoked Boneless Ham & Water Product (Yellow Label)
Smoked Ham (Brown Label)

Smoked Ham (Manda Supreme Gold Label)
Smoked Ham (Yellow Label)

Meijer
Double Smoked Ham
Honey Roasted Ham

Norbest
Ham Turkey

Old Neighborhood
Old Neighborhood (All)

Oscar Mayer
Carving Board Ham, Slow Cooked
Ham Cold Cuts, Baked Cooked 96% Fat Free
Ham Cold Cuts, Boiled 96% Fat Free
Ham Cold Cuts, Chopped
Ham Cold Cuts, Cooked 96% Fat Free
Ham Cold Cuts, Honey 96% Fat Free
Ham Cold Cuts, Lower Sodium 96% Fat Free
Ham Cold Cuts, Natural Smoked
Ham Cold Cuts, Smoked 98% Fat Free

Our Family
Bone-In Ham, Water Added (Half, Steaks, Whole)
Boneless Ham Steaks
Boneless Round Half Ham, Water Added
Boneless Round Whole Ham
Chopped Ham
Cooked Ham
Ham & Water Ham
Honey Ham
Pre-Sliced Ham
Spiral Sliced Half Ham Natural Juice

Perdue
Carving Turkey Ham, Honey Smoked
Slicing Turkey Ham

Petit Jean
Petit Jean (All)

Plumrose
Plumrose (All)

Price Chopper
Carve 'n Serve Boneless Half Ham
Carve 'n Serve Boneless Ham
Cumberland Gap Semi Boneless Half Ham

Cumberland Gap Semi Boneless Whole Ham
Fat Free Boneless Single Ham Steak
Ham Steaks

Private Selection (Kroger)
Hickory Smoked Ham
Honey Ham

Publix
Hickory Smoked Ham, Semi-Boneless, Fully Cooked
Honey Cured Bone-In Ham - Brown Sugar Glazed
Honey Cured Bone-In Ham - with Brown Sugar Glaze Mix Packet
Honey Cured Boneless Ham - with Brown Sugar Glaze

Saag's ⓘ
Saag's (All BUT British Bangers & Marzenbier Brats)

Safeway 〰
Ham Brown Sugar Honey 95% Fat Free
Ham Cooked Water Added 95% Fat Free
Ham Hickory Smoked Butt Half
Ham Honey 97% Fat Free Tub
Ham Shank Hickory Smoked

Safeway Select 〰
Ham Half Boneless
Honey Ham Half Boneless

Shaw's
Shaved Honey Ham
Smoked Ham Tub

Shoppers Value (ACME)
Ham

Shoppers Value (Albertsons)
Ham

Shoppers Value (Cub Foods)
Ham

Shoppers Value (Jewel-Osco)
Ham

Smithfield Foods ⓘ
Boneless Hams (All)
Spiral Hams (All BUT Honey or BBQ Marinated)

Smith's
Smith's (All)

Sugardale
Ham (All)
Hamcola

Superior's
Easy Carve Boneless Ham (Whole, Half, Quarter, or Sliced)
Prestige Old Fashioned Cooked Ham
Semi-Boneless Ham (Half or Whole)
Tavern Boneless Hams (Whole, Half, or Quarter)
Tavern Ham Slices
Village Tavern Ham, Bavarian
Village Tavern Ham, Brown Sugar
Village Tavern Ham, Cajun
Village Tavern Ham, Honey
Village Tavern Honey Half Ham

Thumann's ✓
All Natural Black Forest Brand Ham
Black Forest Brand Ham
Bone and Tied Ham
Bone in Smoked Short Shank
Bone in Smoked Short Shank Virginia Ham
Boneless Fully Cooked Smoked Ham
Boneless Fully Cooked Smoked Virginia Ham
Brown Sugar Coated Cooked Ham
Chef's Slice Ham
Easy Slice Spiral Cut Ham
Flat Smoked Ham
Honey Cured Baby Baked Ham
Honey Cured Baked Ham
Jersey Made Hot Ham
Jersey Made Oblong Ham
Natural Casing Hot Ham
Our Ham-O-Collo Cooked Hot Ham
Our Hot Ham
Oven Roasted Fresh Ham, Homestyle
Ready to Eat Hot Ham
Ripple Hot Ham
Ripple Proscuittini
Round Proscuitto
Short Cut Deluxe Coed Ham- Baby
Short Cut Deluxe Coed Ham- Lower Sodium
Short Cut Deluxe Coed Ham- Prague Shaped

Short Cut Deluxe Coed Ham- Small Round Shape

Short Cut Deluxe Coed Ham- Square Shape

Short Cut Deluxe Cooked Ham- Tear Drop Shape

Small Round Smoked Ham

Wally Oblong Box Ham

Wally Oblong Ham

Wally Pear Shape Ham

Wally Pear Shape Ham Box

Wally Square Ham

Trader Joe's

Prosciutto Di Italia

Valu Time (Brookshire)

Ham and Water 35%

Turkey Ham- 95% Fat Free

Wegmans

Cooked Ham Thin Sliced with Natural Juices

Smoked Ham Thin Sliced with Natural Juices

Smoked Honey Ham Thin Sliced with Natural Juices

Wellshire Farms

Black Forest Boneless Half Ham

Black Forest Boneless Ham Nugget

Black Forest Quarter Ham

Bulk Tavern Ham

Glazed Boneless Half Ham

Old Fashioned Traditional Boneless Half Ham

Old Fashioned Traditional Boneless Whole Ham

Semi Boneless Half Ham

Semi Boneless Whole Ham

Sliced Black Forest Ham

Sliced Breakfast Ham

Sliced Tavern Ham

Sliced Turkey Ham

Sliced Virginia Brand Boneless Ham Steak

Sliced Virginia Brand Deli Ham

Smoked Ham Hocks

Smoked Ham Shanks

Sunday Breakfast Ham

Turkey Ham Halves

Turkey Ham Nuggets

Turkey Ham Steak

Uncured Turkey Ham

Virginia Brand Boneless Ham Steak

Virginia Brand Buffet Ham

Virginia Brand Honey Ham Nugget

Virginia Brand Quarter Ham

Virginia Uncured Deli Ham

Whole Turkey Ham

Zeigler ()

4x6 Cooked Ham

4x6 Honey Ham

Black Pepper Ham

Buffet Ham

Cooked Ham

Finest Baked Ham

Finest Baked Ham Slices

Pre-Sliced Boneless Ham

Red Pepper Ham

Smoked Ham Halves

Tender Smoked Ham

Whole Baked Ham

Whole Finest Baked Ham

HOT DOGS & FRANKS

ACME

Beef Franks

Franks

Ball Park 🐑

Angus Beef Franks - Bun Size

Angus Beef Franks - Lower Fat Full Taste

Angus Beef Franks - Original

Ball Park SINGLES Beef Franks

Ball Park SINGLES Franks Made with Turkey, Pork & Beef

Beef Franks

Bun Size Beef Franks - Deli Style

Bun Size Beef Franks - Original

Bun Size Franks Made with Turkey, Pork & Beef

Bun Sized Smoked White Turkey Franks

Cheese Franks Made with Turkey, Pork & Beef

Deli Style Beef Franks

Fat Free Beef Franks

Fat Free Franks Made with Turkey, Pork & Beef
Franks Made with Turkey, Pork & Beef
Hearty Beef Franks
Jumbo Beef Franks
Lite Beef Franks
Lite Franks Made with Turkey, Pork & Beef
Turkey Franks

Beeler's
Beeler's (All)

Big City Reds
Beef Hot Dogs

Coleman Natural ⓘ
Beef Hot Dog
Beef-Pork Frank

Dietz & Watson ✓
Beef Franks
Grillers
Meat Franks

Empire Kosher
Chicken Franks
Turkey Franks

Farmer John
Dodger Dogs
Premium Beef Franks
Premium Jumbo Beef Franks
Premium Jumbo Meat Wieners
Premium Meat Wieners
Premium Quarter Pounder Beef Franks

Fastco (Fareway)
Jumbo Hot Dogs
Natural Casing Hot Dogs

Food Club (Brookshire)
All Beef Franks
Bun Length Hot Dogs
Jumbo Hot Dogs

Hatfield ()
Authentic Deli Style Beef Frank
Beef Franks
Cheese Franks
Classic Franks
Jumbo Franks
Phillies Beef Frank
Phillies Franks
Reduced Sodium Franks

Hebrew National
Hebrew National (All BUT Franks in a Blanket)

Hillshire Farms
Lit'l Beef Franks

Honeysuckle White
Honeysuckle White (All BUT Asian Grilled Marinated Turkey Strips, Beer Smoked Turkey Bratwurst Fully Cooked, Italian Style Meatballs, Cajun Fried Turkey, and Teriyaki Turkey Breast Tenderloins)

Jennie-O Turkey Store
Turkey Franks

Kayem
Kayem (All)

Kunzler
Hot Dogs/Franks (All)

Old Neighborhood
Old Neighborhood (All)

Old Wisconsin ⓘ 25
Natural Casing Wieners

Original Brat Hans, The ⓘ
Uncured German Style Wiener

Oscar Mayer
Hot Dogs, Beef Classic Franks Bun-Length
Hot Dogs, Beef Franks Natural Smoked Uncured
Hot Dogs, Beef Franks XXL Premium
Hot Dogs, Beef Light Franks
Hot Dogs, Bun-Length Turkey Franks
Hot Dogs, Classic 98% Fat Free Wieners
Hot Dogs, Classic Beef Franks
Hot Dogs, Classic Bun-Length Turkey Franks
Hot Dogs, Classic Bun-Length Wieners
Hot Dogs, Classic Cheese Dogs
Hot Dogs, Classic Cheese Turkey Franks
Hot Dogs, Classic Light Wieners
Hot Dogs, Classic Turkey Franks
Hot Dogs, Classic Wieners Made with Turkey & Chicken/Pork
Hot Dogs, Premium Beef & Cheddar Franks
Hot Dogs, Premium Beef Franks

Hot Dogs, Premium Jalapeno &
   Cheddar Franks
Hot Dogs, Selects Angus Beef Bun
   Length Franks
Hot Dogs, Selects Angus Beef Franks
Hot Dogs, Selects Hardwood Smoked
   Turkey Franks
Hot Dogs, Selects Premium Beef Franks
Hot Dogs, Selects Premium Franks
Hot Dogs, Turkey Franks
Hot Dogs, Wieners

Our Family
All Beef Hot Dogs
Cocktail Smokies
Hot Dogs
Jumbo Franks
Natural Casing Wieners

Price Chopper
Beef Franks
Franks
Pork and Beef Medium Franks
State National All Beef Skinless
State National Skinless Beef Hot Dog

Publix
Beef Franks
Beef Hot Dogs
Meat Franks
Meat Hot Dogs

Rocky Dogs ⓘ
Chicken Hot Dogs

Roger Wood
Roger Wood (All)

Saag's ⓘ
Saag's (All BUT British Bangers &
   Marzenbier Brats)

Sabrett ⓘ
All Beef Frankfurters
Pork & Beef Frankfurters

Safeway Select ⌇
Meat Franks

Shoppers Value (ACME)
Meat Franks

Shoppers Value (Albertsons)
Beef Franks
Meat Franks

Shoppers Value (Cub Foods)
Meat Franks

Shoppers Value (Jewel-Osco)
Beef Franks
Meat Franks

Smith's
Smith's (All)

Sugardale
Wieners (All)

Superior's
Beef Frankies
Big As Bunz Hot Dogs
Frankies
Hot Dogs

Tallgrass Beef Company
Beef Hot Dogs

Tanka
Tanka Dogs

Thumann's ✓
4-1 Franks
All Beef Package Franks
All Natural Pork & Beef Frankfurters
Cocktail Franks
Natural Casing Franks
Pushcart Hots
Pushcart Skinless Franks

Trader Joe's
All Natural Uncured Chicken Hot Dogs
Uncured All Beef Hot Dogs

Valu Time (Brookshire)
Bun Length Hot Dog
Cheese Dogs
Hot Dogs
Jumbo Hot Dogs

Wegmans
Beef Hot Dogs - Skinless
Cocktail Hot Dogs - Skinless
   Frankfurters
Hot Dogs - Combo Pack
Lite Red Hot Dogs - Skinless
Red Hot Dogs - Skinless
Uncured Beef Hot Dogs-Skinless
Uncured Hot Dogs - Skinless

Wellshire Farms
4XL Big Beef Franks
Cheese Frank

GFS Sliced Pepperoni is GF

Chicken Franks
Cocktail Franks
Old Fashioned Beef Franks
Old Fashioned Beef Hot Dogs
Original Deli Frank
Premium Beef Hot Dog
Turkey Franks
Zeigler ()
Dinner Franks
Hot Dog Party Pack
Jumbo Franks
Original Recipe Wieners
Zeigler Hot Dog
Zeigler Wieners

Meat Alternatives

El Burrito
Pepperoni Crumbles
Soy Ground
Soyrizo
SoyTaco
Franklin Farms ⓘ
Chick'n Nuggets
Veggiballs
Veggiburger
Veggidogs
Frieda's
Soyrizo
Soytaco
Konjac Foods
Konjac Vegetarian Shrimp
LightLife ⓘ
Tofu Pups
Manna Soy
Manna Soy Gourmet Meat Alternative
    (All Flavors)
Pulmuone Wildwood ⚇
Veggie Burgers
Soyrizo
Soyrizo
SoyTaco
SoyTaco

Pepperoni

ACME
Original Pepperoni
Albertsons
Original Pepperoni
Turkey Pepperoni
Cub Foods
Pepperoni
Sliced Pepperoni Turkey
DeLallo
Pepperoni (Sliced, with Cheese)
Sandwich Pepperoni Whole
Dietz & Watson ✓
Slicing Pepperoni
Twinstick Pepperoni
Giant Eagle
Pepperoni Stick
Premium Sliced Sandwich Pepperoni
Sliced Pizza Pepperoni
Sliced Prepackaged Pepperoni
Sliced Prepackaged Turkey Pepperoni
Haggen
Pepperoni, Pillow Pack
Hempler Foods Group ⓘ
Uncured Pepperoni
Hormel   *Sams is Hormel*
Pepperoni
Turkey Pepperoni
Jewel-Osco
Original Pepperoni
Turkey Pepperoni
Oscar Mayer *GF*
Pepperoni Slices Cold Cuts
Shaw's
Pepperoni Turkey
Sugardale
Pepperoni (All)
Sandwich Pepperoni
Wegmans
Italian Style Pepperoni - Sliced
Italian Style Pepperoni - Sticks
Wellshire Farms
Dried Pepperoni Stick
Original Matt's Select Pepperoni Sticks
Pillow Pack Pepperoni
Sliced Pepperoni

Sliced Uncured Pepperoni
Whole Pepperoni

PORK

Albertsons
Pork
Always Tender
Apple Bourbon Flavored Fresh Pork
Bourbon Maple Flavored Fresh Pork
Brown Sugar Maple Flavored Fresh Pork
Citrus Flavored Fresh Pork
Honey Mustard Flavored Fresh Pork
Lemon-Garlic Flavored Fresh Pork
Mediterranean & Olive Oil Flavored
  Fresh Pork
Mesquite BBQ Flavored Fresh Pork
Mesquite Flavored Fresh Pork
Non-Flavored Fresh Pork
Onion-Garlic Flavored Fresh Pork
Original Flavored Fresh Pork
Peppercorn Flavored Fresh Pork
Roast Flavor Flavored Fresh Pork
Sun-Dried Tomato Flavored Fresh Pork
Beeler's
Beeler's (All)
Coleman Natural
Hampshire Pork Baby Back Ribs
Hampshire Pork Chops
Hampshire Pork Loin
Hampshire Pork St. Louis Ribs
Hampshire Pork Tenderloins
Dietz & Watson
Boneless Smoked Pork Chops
Canadian Center Cut Pork Spare Ribs
Classic Boneless Smoked Pork Shoulder
  Butt (Cello)
Classic Pork Shoulder Butt (Plain)
Cuban Roast Pork
Italian Style Cooked Roast Pork
Roasted Sirloin of Pork
Farmer John
California Natural Back Ribs
California Natural Bone-In Butt Roast
California Natural Bone-In Pork Loin
California Natural Bone-In Pork Picnic
California Natural Boneless Loin

California Natural Boneless Pork Butt
California Natural Boneless Pork Picnic
California Natural Boneless Pork
  Shoulder
California Natural Boneless Pork Sirloin
California Natural Case Ready Pork
  Chops
California Natural Ground Pork
California Natural Pork Cushion
California Natural Spareribs
California Natural St. Louis Style
  Spareribs
California Natural Tenderloins
Carefree Cookin' Pork, Boneless Leg
Carefree Cookin' Pork, Boneless Pork
  Loin
Carefree Cookin' Pork, Boneless Sirloin
Carefree Cookin' Pork, Picnics
Carefree Cookin' Pork, Pork Butt
Carefree Cookin' Pork, Pork Cushion
Carefree Cookin' Pork, Riblets
Carefree Cookin' Pork, Ribs
Carefree Cookin' Pork, Spareribs
Carefree Cookin' Pork, St. Louis Style
  Spareribs
Carefree Cookin' Pork, Tenderloins
Flavorite (Cub Foods)
Pork
Giant Eagle
Baby Back Pork Ribs
Pulled Pork with BBQ Sauce
Shredded Pork with BBQ Sauce
Hatfield ()
All Natural Pork Shoulder Roast
  (Picnic)
BBQ Center Cut Thick Chops
Boardwalk Style Pork Roll
Cooked Roast Pork
Garden Herb Pork Roast
Italian Center Cut Thick Chops
Italian Loin Filet
Italian Style Pork Roast
Italian Tenderloin
Lemon & Garlic Loin Filet
Oven Roasted Center Cut Thick Chops
Oven Roasted Loin Filet
Peppercorn Center Cut Thick Chops

Peppercorn Tenderloin
Pork Roll 1 Lb
Precooked Baby Back Ribs
Simply Tender Boneless Pork Loin Fillet
Simply Tender Boneless Sirloin Roast
Simply Tender Portions Traditional
  Pork Chop
Simply Tender Tenderloin Filet
Tangy Pork Roll

H-E-B
Fully Cooked Sliced Smoked Pork Loin

Hormel
Pickled Pigs Feet, Hocks & Tidbits

Kunzler ♀
Pork BBQ

Manda ⓘ
Tasso Cajun Spicy Pork (Yellow Label)

Our Family
Ground Pork
Pork Burger

Publix
All Natural Fresh Pork

Roger Wood
Roger Wood (All)

Saag's ⓘ
Saag's (All BUT British Bangers &
  Marzenbier Brats)

Schnucks
Pork Roast

Smithfield Foods ⓘ
Fresh Unflavored Pork (All)

Thumann's ✓
Ripple Roast Pork
Small Pork Butt
Smoked Shanks

Trader Joe's
Baby Back Pork Ribs
Unprocessed Raw Meat (All)

Wellshire Farms
Pork Baby Back Ribs
Pork Maple Fully Cooked Sausage
  Patties
Pork Tasso
Shredded Pork in Barbeque Sauce

SALAMI

ACME
Hard Salami Tub

Albertsons
Hard Salami Tub

Best Choice
Cotto Salami

Columbus Salame
Salame (All)

Cub Foods
Hard Salami Tub

DeLallo
Genoa Salami Half
Sopressata, Large Half (Hot, Sweet)
Sopressata, Small (Hot, Sweet)

Dietz & Watson ✓
Baby Genoa
Baby Genoa Pepper Salame
Beef Cooked Salami
Cooked Salami
Genoa Salami Whole
Hard Salami
Hot and Zesty Salame
Hot Soppressata
Landjaeger
Milano Salame Paper Wrap
Mini Salame
Soppressata
Sweet Soppressata

Empire Kosher
Turkey Salami Slices

Food Club (Brookshire)
Salami

Giant Eagle
Hard Salami Tub
Premium Genoa Salami
Premium Sliced Hard Salami
Sliced Prepackaged Hard Salami

Goya
Cervero Salchichon Colombiano
Higueral Popular- Black
Higueral Salami- Red
Mallita Salami
Salami
Salchichon Dominicano

Hatfield ()
Hatfield Salami
Hebrew National
Hebrew National (All BUT Franks in a Blanket)
Hempler Foods Group ⓘ
Cooked Salami
Uncured Cooked Salami
Hormel
Hard Salami
Norbest ⓘ
Turkey Salami Lunchmeat
Oscar Mayer ⌒
Cotto Salami Cold Cuts
Cotto Salami Cold Cuts, 97% Fat Free
Cotto Salami Cold Cuts, Beef
Cotto Salami Cold Cuts, Oven Roasted & White Chicken
Cotto Salami Cold Cuts, Thin Sliced
Salami Cold Cuts, Hard
Our Family
Salami
Saag's ⓘ
Saag's (All BUT British Bangers & Marzenbier Brats)
Shaw's
Hard Salami Tub
Shoppers Value (ACME)
Salami
Shoppers Value (Albertsons)
Salami
Shoppers Value (Cub Foods)
Salami
Shoppers Value (Jewel-Osco)
Salami
Smith's
Smith's (All)
Sugardale
Genoa Salami
Hard Salami
Salami (All)
Superior's
Cooked Salami
Paradise Cooked Salami
Thumann's ✓
Cooked Salami

Trader Joe's
Busseto Premium Genoa Salami
Tropical Cheese
Salami Especial
Salami Original
Salami Popular
Salami Superior
Wellshire Farms
Chub Black Peppered Salami
Chub Genoa Salami
Chub Herb Salami
Chub Original Salami
Sliced Black Pepper Salami
Sliced Genoa Salami
Sliced Hard Salami
Sliced Herb Salami
Sliced Original Salami
Sliced Sopressata
Sopressata Stick
Whole Black Pepper Salami
Whole Genoa Salami
Whole Hard Salami
Whole Herb Salami
Whole Original Salami
Whole Sopressata

SAUSAGE

Al Fresco All Natural
Chicken Sausages (All)
Always Save
Meat Wieners
Roll Sausage, Hot
Roll Sausage, Regular
Beeler's ⌇
Beeler's (All)
Best Choice
Ground Italian Sausage
Italian Sausage
Original Bratwurst
Original Sausage
Premium Sausage, Hot
Sage Sausage
Big City Reds
Polish Sausage Links
Coleman Natural ⓘ
Artichokes & Olives Chicken Sausage

All Bob Evans is gluten-free except Beer Bratwurst

Bratwurst
Mild Italian Chicken Sausage
Organic Apple Chicken Sausage
Organic Spinach & Feta Chicken
Sausage
Organic Sun-Dried Tomato & Basil
Chicken Sausage
Polish Kielbasa
Spicy Andouille Chicken Sausage
Spicy Chipotle Chicken Sausage
Spicy Cilantro Chicken Sausage
Spicy Italian Chicken Sausage
Spinach & Feta Cheese Chicken Sausage
Sun-Dried Tomato and Basil Chicken
Sausage
Sweet Apple Chicken Sausage

Conecuh Sausage Company
Smoked Sausage

Di Lusso
Dry Sausage

Dietz & Watson ✓
Beef Summer Sausage
Cacciatore
Gourmet Chicken Sausages
Hot & Mild Sausage
Hot Abruzzese
Krakow Sausage
Mini Chorizo
Natural Casing Franks & Sausages
Sweet Abruzzese
Sweet Sopressata

Evergood Fine Foods ⓘ
Sausage Products (All BUT British
Bangers)

Farmer John
Firehouse Hot Roll Breakfast Sausage
Links & Patties
Hot Louisiana Smoked Dinner Sausage
Jalapeno Pepper Premium Rope Dinner
Sausage
Jalapeno Pepper Premium Smoked
Dinner Sausage
Old Fashioned Maple Skinless Breakfast
Sausage Links & Patties
Original Roll Breakfast Sausage Links &
Patties

Original Skinless Breakfast Sausage
Links & Patties
Premium Beef Rope Dinner Sausage
Premium Original Chorizo Breakfast
Sausage Links & Patties
Premium P C Links Lower Fat Breakfast
Sausage Links & Patties
Premium Polish Dinner Sausage
Premium Pork Rope Dinner Sausage
Premium S C Links Breakfast Sausage
Links & Patties
Premium Sausage Patties Lower Fat
Breakfast Sausage Links & Patties
Premium Spicy Hot Chorizo Breakfast
Sausage Links & Patties
Premium Traditional Chorizo Breakfast
Sausage Links & Patties
Quick Serve Fully Cooked Breakfast
Sausage Links & Patties
Red Hots Extra Premium Smoked
Dinner Sausage

Fastco (Fareway)
80% Pork Patties
Brat Patties
Pork & Bacon Pattie
Summer Sausage
Summer Sausage Sticks
Turkey Sausage
Turkey Summer & Cheese Sausage
Turkey Summer Jalapeno & Cheese
Sausage
Turkey Summer Sausage

Fortuna's ⓘ
Dry Sausages (All)
Fresh Sausages (All)

Giant Eagle
Beef Polska Kielbasa
Beef Summer Sausage
Breakfast Sausage Maple Links
Breakfast Sausage Original Links
Breakfast Sausage Original Patties
Fully Cooked Sausage Links
Fully Cooked Sausage Patties
Maple Sausage Links
Original Sausage Links
Original Sausage Patties
Original Sausage Roll

Polska Kielbasa
Polska Kielbasa Links
Pork and Beef Polska Kielbasa
Savory Sausage Roll
Smoked Pork and Beef Sausage
Smoked Sausage
Smoked Sausage Link, Cheese
Smoked Sausage Link, Chili Cheese and
  Onion
Smoked Sausage Link, Jalapeno and
  Cheese
Zesty Hot Sausage Roll

Goya
Chorizos
El Mino Chorizon
Savoy Sausages
Vienna Sausages

Great Value (Wal-Mart) 25
Fully Cooked Beef Breakfast Patties
Fully Cooked Maple Pork Sausage
  Patties
Fully Cooked Original Pork Sausage
  Patties
Fully Cooked Sausage Links
Fully Cooked Spicy Pork Sausage Patties
Hot Pork Sausage
Mild Pork Sausage
Sage Pork Sausage

Hatfield ()
Bratwurst Links
Country Links
Country Sausage Roll
Hot Italian Rope Sausage
Hot Italian Sausage Links
Jumbo Country Links
Kielbasa Loops
Pennsylvania Dutch Rope Sausage
Pepper and Onion Sausage Links
Phillies Hot Beef Sausage
Phillies Mild Beef Sausage
Smoked Sausage Loops
Sweet Italian Rope Sausage
Sweet Italian Sausage Links

H-E-B
Andouille Chicken Sausage
Chicken Sausage - Fajita
Chicken Sausage - Pablano & Cheddar

Lean Smoked Sausage
Premium Beef Ring Sausage
Premium Cheese Smoked Sausage Ring
Premium Jalapeno Cheddar Smoked
  Sausage
Premium Jalapeno Smoked Sausage
  Ring
Premium Original Pork/Beef Sausage
Premium Pork & Beef Sausage Ring
Premium Sausage Beef
Premium Sausage Beef Link
Premium Sausage Cheese Link
Premium Sausage Jalapeno
Premium Sausage Jalapeno Link
Premium Sausage Mesquite Link
Premium Sausage Pork/Beef Link
Sausage On A Stick
Smoked Sausage - Garlic Ring

Hebrew National
Hebrew National (All BUT Franks in a
  Blanket)

Hempler Foods Group ⓘ
Andouille
Bockwurst
Bratwurst
Brauschweiger
Breakfast Sausage
Chorizo
Franks
Garlic Sausage
German Sausage
Hot Links
Italian Sausage
Kielbasa
Knockwurst
Linguisa
Polish
Potato Sausage
Salami
Smoked Garlic
Summer Sausage
Uncured Beef Wieners
Uncured Bratwurst
Uncured Veal Bratwurst
Veal Bratwurst
Wieners

Hill Country Fare (H-E-B)
- Beef Cocktail Smoked Sausage
- Beef Sausage
- Beef Smoked Sausage
- Cheese Smoked Sausage
- Cocktail Smoked Sausages
- Mesquite Smoked Sausage
- Polish Sausage
- Polish Smoked Sausage
- Red Hot Links
- Sausage with Cheese
- Skinless Beef Smoked Sausage
- Skinless Polish Smoked Sausage
- Skinless Smoked Sausage
- Smoked Sausage
- Smokey Links

Hillshire Farms
- Beef Lit'l Smokies Beef Smoked Sausage
- Beef Polska Kielbasa
- Beef Smoked Sausage
- Beef Smoked Sausage with Chile Peppers
- Beef Summer Sausage
- Cheddar Lit'l Smokies Smoked Sausage with Cheddar Cheese, Made with Pork, Turkey and Beef
- Hardwood Chicken Smoked Sausage
- Hot & Spicy Italian Style Smoked Sausage
- Hot Smoked Sausage Hot Smoked Sausage
- Italian Style Smoked Sausage Made with Pork, Turkey and Beef
- Lite Polska Kielbasa Made with Turkey, Pork, Beef
- Lite Smoked Sausage Made with Turkey, Pork, Beef
- Lit'l Polskas Smoked Polish Sausage, Made with Pork, Turkey and Beef
- Lit'l Smokies Smoked Sausage, Made with Pork, Turkey and Beef
- Lit'l Wieners Made with Pork, Turkey & Beef
- Polska Kielbasa
- Polska Kielbasa Made with Pork, Turkey and Beef

- Smoked Sausage Made with Pork, Turkey and Beef
- Smoked Sausage with Chile Peppers
- Smoked Sausage with Wisconsin Cheese
- Smoked Sausage with Wisconsin Cheese Made with Pork, Turkey and Beef
- Smoked, Cured, and Fully Cooked Bratwurst
- Summer Sausage
- Turkey Li'l Smokies Made with Turkey Smoked Sausage
- Turkey Polska Kielbasa
- Turkey Smoked Sausage
- Turkey Smoked Sausage with Pepper Jack Cheese Links
- Yard-O-Beef

Honeysuckle White
- Honeysuckle White (All BUT Asian Grilled Marinated Turkey Strips, Beer Smoked Turkey Bratwurst Fully Cooked, Italian Style Turkey Meatballs, Italian Style Meatballs, and Teriyaki Turkey Breast Tenderloins)

Hormel
- Crumbled Sausage
- Smokies

Jennie-O Turkey Store
- Breakfast Lover's Turkey Sausage
- Extra Lean Smoked Kielbasa Turkey Sausage
- Extra Lean Smoked Turkey Sausage
- Fresh Breakfast Sausage - Maple Links
- Fresh Breakfast Sausage - Mild Links
- Fresh Breakfast Sausage - Mild Patties
- Fresh Dinner Sausage - Hot Italian
- Fresh Dinner Sausage - Lean Turkey Bratwurst
- Fresh Dinner Sausage - Sweet Italian

Jimmy Dean
- All Natural Regular Pork Sausage
- Breakfast Bowls: Sausage, Eggs, Potatoes and Cheddar Cheese
- Heat 'N Serve Maple Sausage Links
- Heat 'N Serve Sausage Links
- Heat 'N Serve Sausage Links, Hot
- Heat 'N Serve Sausage Patties
- Hot Hearty Sausage Crumbles

Hot Sausage Patties
Maple Links
Maple Patties
Maple Sausage Links
Maple Sausage Patties
Original Hearty Sausage Crumbles
Original Links
Original Patties
Original Sausage Links
Original Sausage Patties
Premium Pork Hot Sausage
Premium Pork Italian Sausage
Premium Pork Light Sausage
Premium Pork Mild Country Sausage
Premium Pork Regular Sausage
Premium Pork Sage Sausage
Sandwich Size Sausage Patties
Sausage Breakfast Skillets
Turkey Hearty Sausage Crumbles
Turkey Sausage Links
Turkey Sausage Patties

Johnsonville

All Natural Hot Italian Ground Sausage
All Natural Mild Italian Ground Sausage
All Natural Sweet Italian Ground Sausage
Beddar with Cheddar
Beef Deli Bites
Beef Hot Links
Beef Summer Sausage
Brat Patties
Brown Sugar and Honey Breakfast Sausage
Cheddar Bratwurst
Cheddar Cheese Breakfast Sausage
Chili Cheese Smoked Sausage
Chorizo Sausage
Four Cheese Italian Sausage
Garlic Summer Sausage
Hot Italian Sausage
Hot 'n Spicy Bratwurst
Hot Sausage Roll
Irish O'Garlic Sausage
Jalapeno with Cheese Sausage
Mild Country Roll
Mild Italian Sausage
New Orleans Brand
Old World Summer Sausage
Original Bratwurst
Original Breakfast Patties
Original Breakfast Sausage
Original Deli Bites
Original Recipe Summer Sausage
Regular Sausage Roll
Salami Deli Bites
Smoked Beef Bratwurst
Smoked Bratwurst
Smoked Polish
Smoked Turkey Sausage
Smoked Turkey with Cheddar Sausage
Stadium Style Brats
Sweet Italian Sausage
Vermont Maple Syrup Breakfast Patties
Vermont Maple Syrup Breakfast Sausage

Jones Dairy Farm

Hearty Pork Sausage Links
Light Pork Sausage & Rice Links
Light Sausage & Rice Links, Precooked
Little Link Pork Sausage
Little Link Turkey Sausage
Made From Beef Sausage Links, Precooked
Maple Little Link Pork Sausage
Maple Sausage Links, Precooked
Maple Sausage Patties, Precooked
Mild Sausage Links, Precooked
Mild Sausage Patties, Precooked
Original Pork Roll Sausage
Pork & Uncured Bacon Sausage Links, Precooked
Pork Sausage Patties
Spicy Sausage Links, Precooked
Turkey Sausage Links, Precooked

Kunzler

Fresh Sausages (All)
Smoked Sausages (All)

Little Sizzlers

Original Sausage Links and Patties

Manda ⓘ

Andouille Sausage (Yellow Label)
Country Brand Smoked Sausage (Yellow Label)
Deli Style Smoked Sausage (Manda Supreme Gold Label)

Deli Style Smoked Sausage (Yellow Label)
Excello Ham Sausage (Yellow Label)
Kielbasa (Yellow Label)
Smoked Sausage Made with Beef (Hot, Mild) (Yellow Label)
Smoked Sausage Made with Pork (Garlic, Green Onion, Hot, Mild) (Yellow Label)

Odom's Tennessee Pride
Extra Mild Sausage Roll ()
Open-Face Sausage Links ()
Open-Face Sausage Patties ()

Old Neighborhood
Old Neighborhood (All)

Old Wisconsin ⓘ 25
Festival Bratwurst
Polish Kielbasa
Smoked Sausage with Cheddar

Original Brat Hans, The ⓘ
Knockwurst with Garlic
Mild Italian Chicken Sausage
Organic Apple Chicken Sausage
Organic Bratwurst Chicken Sausage
Organic Breakfast Links Chicken Sausage
Organic Spinach & Feta Cheese Chicken Sausage
Organic Sweet Italian Chicken Sausage
Original Bratwurst
Shaboygan Style Bratwurst
Skinless Chicken Breakfast Links
Spicy Andouille Chicken Sausage
Spicy Chipotle Chicken Sausage
Spicy Cilantro Chicken Sausage
Spicy Italian Chicken Sausage
Spinach & Feta Cheese Chicken Sausage
Sun-Dried Tomato & Basil Chicken Sausage
Sweet Apple Chicken Sausage
Weisswurst with Parsley

Oscar Mayer
Summer Sausage Cold Cuts, Beef
Summer Sausage Cold Cuts, Summer Sausage

Our Family
Bratwurst

Maple Breakfast Links
Polish Sausage
Roll Sausage
Smoked Sausage
Summer Sausage

Perdue
Seasoned Fresh Lean Turkey Sausage, Sweet Italian
Turkey Breakfast Sausage

Perri
Hot Italian Ground Sausage
Hot Italian Sausage
Sweet Italian Ground Sausage
Sweet Italian Sausage

Petit Jean
Petit Jean (All)

Price Chopper
Hot Italian Sausage
Polska
Smoked Sausage
Sweet Italian Sausage
Vermont Smoke & Cure Summer Sausage

Publix
Fresh Bratwurst
Fresh Chorizo
Fresh Italian Sausage, Hot
Fresh Italian Sausage, Mild
Fresh Turkey Italian Sausage, Hot
Fresh Turkey Italian Sausage, Mild

Roger Wood
Roger Wood (All)

Saag's ⓘ
Saag's (All BUT British Bangers & Marzenbier Brats)

Sausages by Amylu ⓘ
Sausages by Amylu (All)

Silva Sausage
Fresh Uncooked Sausage (All BUT Morcella Blood Sausage)
Linguica & Chorizo (All BUT Morcella Blood Sausage)
Smoked Chicken Sausage (All BUT Morcella Blood Sausage)
Specialty Sausage (All BUT Morcella Blood Sausage)

Skylark
Skylark (All)

Smith's
Smith's (All)

Superior's
Polish Sausage
Smoked Sausage

Tallgrass Beef Company
Beef Bratwurst
Beef Smoked Sausage

Thrifty Maid (Winn-Dixie)
Mild Pork Sausage

Thumann's ✓
Bratwurst
Hog Casing Sausage
Italian Hot Sausage
Italian Sausage Hot Package
Italian Sausage Sweet Package
Italian Sweet Sausage
Kielbasi Loaf
Kielbasi Natural Smoke Flavor
Knockwurst
Pre-Cooked Bratwurst
Pre-Cooked Sausage
Sausage Patties
Sheep Casing Sausage

Trader Joe's
Sausage (All)

Tropical Cheese
Chorizo
Farmer Sausage

V & V Supremo
Chorizo Products (All)

Wellshire Farms
Aged Provolone Chicken Sausage
Andouille Sausage
Apple Chicken Sausage
Artichoke Calamata Chicken Sausage
Chicken Apple Fully Cooked Skinless
Sausage Links
Chicken Sausage with Peppers &
Onions
Chorizo Sausage
Dried Chorizo Stick
Feta Cheese and Spinach Chicken
Sausage

Fully Cooked Chicken Apple Sausage
Patties
Linguica Sausage
Mild Italian Dinner Links
Morning Maple Turkey Breakfast Link
Sausage
Original Fully Cooked Sausage Patties
Original Fully Cooked Skinless Sausage
Links
Original Style Brown and Serve Links
Polska Kielbasa
Pork Maple Fully Cooked Skinless
Sausage Links
Roasted Red Pepper & Garlic Chicken
Sausage
Sliced Dried Chorizo
Spicy Italian Chicken Sausage
Sun Dried Tomato Chicken Sausage
Sunrise Maple Fully Cooked Skinless
Sausage Links
Turkey Andouille Sausage
Turkey Kielbasa
Turkey Maple Fully Cooked Sausage
Patties
Turkey Maple Fully Cooked Skinless
Sausage Links
Whole Chorizo

Zeigler ()
Cheesy Bratwurst
Hot Zeigler Finest Pork Sausage
Mild Zeigler Finest Pork Sausage
Plantation Style Smoked Sausage
Smoked Bratwurst
Smoked Polish Links
Smoked Sausage
Southern Style Smoked Sausage

SEAFOOD

Arctic Shores (ACME)
Cooked Shrimp
Count Individually Quick Frozen Raw
Shrimp
EZ Raw Shrimp
Flounder Fillets
Individually Quick Frozen EZ Peel Raw
Shrimp

King Crab Legs
Orange Roughy Fillets
Raw Peeled/Deveined Shrimp
Raw Shrimp
Tail Off Cooked Shrimp
Whiting Fillets

Arctic Shores (Albertsons)
Cod Fillets
Cooked Shrimp
Cooked Shrimp Tail Off
count
Flounder Fillets
King Crab Legs
Orange Roughy Fillets
Raw Shrimp
Salmon Fillets
Shrimp Peeled/Deveined
Tilapia Fillets
Whiting Fillets

Arctic Shores (Cub Foods)
Cod Fillets
Cooked Shrimp
Individually Quick Frozen EZ Peel Raw
   Shrimp
Individually Quick Frozen Raw Shrimp
Salmon Fillets
Tail Off Cooked Shrimp
Tilapia Fillets

Arctic Shores (Jewel-Osco)
Cod Fillets
Cooked Large Shrimp
Cooked Peeled Shrimp
Cooked Shrimp
EZ Raw Shrimp
Flounder Fillets
Individually Quick Frozen EZ Peel Raw
   Shrimp
Individually Quick Frozen Raw Shrimp
King Crab Legs
Orange Roughy Fillets
Raw Peeled/Deveined Shrimp
Raw Shrimp
Salmon Fillets
Tail Off Cooked Shrimp
Tilapia Fillets
Whiting Fillets

Best Choice
Cooked Shrimp
Shrimp
Shrimp Ring

Food Club (Brookshire)
Cooked Shrimp
Indiviual Quick Freeze EZ-Peel Shrimp
Pink Salmon
Red Sockeye Salmon

Food You Feel Good About (Wegmans)
Alaskan Halibut Fillets, Wild Caught
Chilean Sea Bass Fillets, Wild Caught
Lobster Tails
Mahi Mahi Portions, Wild Caught
Pacific Cod Fillets, Wild Caught
Sockeye Salmon Fillets, Wild Caught
Yellowfin Tuna Steaks, Wild Caught

Full Circle (Schnucks)
Cod Fillets
Cooked Shrimp
Keta Salmon Fillets
Mahi Mahi Fillets
Raw EZ Shrimp
Raw Peeled & Deveined Shrimp
Swordfish Steaks
Wild Halibut Steaks
Yellowfin Steaks

Goya
Boneless Pollock Bag
Cod Boneless in Bag
Cod in Cello Bag
Jack Mackerel
Pollock Fillets Choice Box
Pollock Fillets in Bag

Great Value (Wal-Mart) 25
Alaskan Pink Salmon

Meijer
Atlantic Salmon
Atlantic Salmon, Asian Sesame Garlic
Atlantic Salmon, Black Pearl
Atlantic Salmon, Cedar Wrap
Atlantic Salmon, Fillet
Atlantic Salmon, Kabob
Atlantic Salmon, Steak
Atlantic Salmon, White Wine
Atlantic Salmon, Whole

Bay Scallops
Black Cod
Black Grouper
Black Tip Shark
Blue Marlin
Catfish
Catfish Fillet
Catfish Lemon Pepper Fillet
Catfish Nugget
Catfish Steak
Catfish, Cajun
Cobia Fillet
Cod Fillet
Cod, Stuffed
Coho Salmon
Coho Salmon Fillet
Coho Salmon Steak
Easy Peel Shrimp
Flounder Dress
Grass Carp Wheel Dress
Grouper Fillet
Haddock Fillet
Hake Fillet
Halibut
Halibut Fillet
Halibut Roast
Halibut Steak
Imitation Crab Chunk
Imitation Crab Flake
Imitation Crab Legs
Imitation Crab Shredded
Imitation Lobster Meat
Key West Pink Shrimp
Lake Smelt
Lake Trout Dressed Fresh
Lake Trout Fillet
Lake Trout Steak
Lobster, Live
Mackerel Dress
Mahi Mahi
Mahi Mahi Whole
Marlin Steak
Monkfish Fillet
Mullet Wheel
Ocean Perch Fillet
Opah Fillet
Oysters, Shelled

Oysters, West Coast
Pollock Fillet
Rainbow Trout Dressed
Rainbow Trout Fillet
Red Snapper
Salmon Fillet with Bourbon
Salmon Kabobs
Salmon Maple BBQ
Salmon Milano
Salmon Stuffed Fillet
Salmon Stuffed PinWheel
Salmon, Garlic Wine Herb
Sauger Fillet
Sea Bass Dress Stripe
Sea Bass Fillet
Sea Scallops
Shrimp
Skate Fillet
Snapper Dress
Snapper Fillet
Sockeye Fillet
Sockeye Salmon Dress
Sockeye Salmon Roast
Sockeye Salmon Steak
Soft Shell Crab
Sole Fillet
Sole Stuffed
Steelhead Trout Fillet
Stone Crab Claws Cooked
Sun Fish Blue Gill Dress
Sun Fish Blue Gill Fillet
Swordfish Cold Smoke Steak
Swordfish Kabob
Swordfish Loin
Tilapia Bourbon Fillet
Tilapia Garlic and Wine
Tilapia Maple BBQ
Turbot
Wahoo Fillet
Walleye Dressed Fresh
Walleye Fillet
White Bass
White Bass Dressed
White Bass Dressed Medium
White Bass Fillet Medium
White Perch Fillet
Whitefish Dress

Whitefish Fillet
Yellow Lake Perch Fillet
Yellowfin Tuna
Yellowfin Tuna Loin

Price Chopper
Gluten Free Cod
Gluten Free Haddock
Gluten Free Halibut

Star of the Sea Seafood ⓘ
Gluten Free Crab Cake
Stuffed Flounder

Trader Joe's
Cod Provençale
Crabmeat
Marinated Ahi Tuna Steaks
Pink Salmon-Boneless, Skinless
Plain Seafood (All)
Premium Salmon Patties
Salmon Burger
Seasoned Mahi Mahi Fillets
Smoked Salmon
Uncooked, Uncured Bacon Wrapped Mahi Fillets

Tropical Cheese
Tropical Pollock Fillet

Valu Time (Brookshire)
Pink Salmon

Vita Foods ⓘ
Jim Beam Barbecue Seasoned Atlantic Salmon
Jim Beam Barbecue Smoked Atlantic Salmon
Jim Beam Original Seasoned Atlantic Salmon
Jim Beam Original Smoked Atlantic Salmon
Vita Classic Atlantic Nova
Vita Classic Hot Smoked Atlantic Salmon
Vita Classic Hot Smoked Atlantic Salmon Pepper
Vita Classic Hot Smoked Wild Sockeye
Vita Classic Peppered Atlantic Nova
Vita Classic Presliced Atlantic Salmon Sides
Vita Gold Wild Coho
Vita Gold Wild Sockeye
Vita Marinated Atlantic Salmon
Vita Presliced Atlantic Nova Salmon
Vita Royal Taste Wild Nova Salmon
Vita Salmon Bits
Vita Sliced Smoked Atlantic Nova Salmon
Vita Sliced/Smoked Wild Lox Salmon
Vita Sliced/Smoked Wild Nova Salmon
Vita Smoke Salted Cracked Peppercorn Wild Salmon
Vita Smoke Salted Lemon Pepper Wild Salmon
Vita Smoked Atlantic Salmon (Honey)

Wegmans
Atlantic Salmon Fillets, Farm Raised
Orange Roughy Fillets, Wild Caught
Swordfish Steaks, Wild Caught
Tilapia Fillets, Farm Raised

TOFU & TEMPEH

Azumaya ⓦ
Tofu (All)

Eden Foods
Dried Tofu

Frieda's
Tofu

Godshall's ⓘ
Turkey Scrapple

House Foods ⓘ
Tofu (All BUT Agedashi Tofu)

LightLife ⓘ
Flax Tempeh
Garden Vegetable Tempeh
Soy Tempeh
Wild Rice Tempeh

Mori-Nu
Silken Tofu (All) ⓦ

Nasoya
Nasoya (All)

Nature's Promise (Giant)
Organic Extra Firm Tofu
Organic Firm Tofu

Nature's Promise (Stop & Shop)
Organic Extra Firm Tofu
Organic Firm Tofu

O Organics ⌇
Cubed Tofu
Firm Organic Tofu

Pulmuone Wildwood ⌇
Plain Sprouted Tofu Products (NOT
Baked or Smoked Tofu)

Sol Cuisine ✓
Tofu (All)

Trader Joe's
Organic Sprouted Tofu
Tofu (Organic Firm or Extra Firm)
Tofu Veggie Burger

Turtle Island Foods ⓘ
Coconut Curry Marinated Tempeh
Strips
Organic Five-Grain Tempeh
Organic Soy Tempeh
Spicy Veggie Tempeh

Vitasoy
Tofu (All)

Wegmans
Extra-Firm Tofu
Organic Extra Firm Tofu
Organic Firm Tofu

TURKEY

ACME
Honey Smoked Turkey
Oven Roasted Turkey
Pepperoni Turkey

Al Fresco All Natural
Turkey Breast (All)

Albertsons
Honey Turkey Wafer Sliced
Mesquite Turkey Tub Refill
Oven Roasted Turkey Wafer Sliced
Turkey Breast

Best Choice
Oven Roasted Turkey Breast
Sliced Honey Turkey
Thin Slice Turkey
Tub Turkey, Original
Tub Turkey, Smoked

Buddig ⌇ 25
Buddig Original – Honey Roasted
Turkey

Buddig Original – Mesquite Turkey
Buddig Original – Oven Roasted Turkey
Buddig Original – Turkey
Fix Quick – Turkey

Cajun Prize (Manda) ⓘ
Spicy Turkey Breast

Cub Foods
Fat-Free 98% Oven Roasted Turkey
Breast
Fat-Free Oven Roasted Turkey Breast
Thin Sliced Honey Smoked Turkey
Lunch Meat
Thin Sliced Turkey Breast Lunch Meat

Dak
Premium Sliced Turkey Breast (All)

DeLallo
Gold Classic Turkey
Turkey Breast, Smoked
Turkey Breast, Swirled Pepper
Turkey, Oven Roasted Heart Shape

Di Lusso
Turkey

Dietz & Watson ✓
Applewood Smoked Turkey Breast
Bacon Lovers Turkey Breast
BF Chef Carved Smoked Turkey
Black Forest Smoked Turkey Breast
Black Forest Turkey Breast
Black Forest Turkey Small
Black Pepper Turkey Breast
Butter Basted Turkey Breast
Cajun Turkey Breast
Carving Ready Turkey Breast
Chef Carved Turkey Breast
Chipotle Pepper Turkey
Fire Roasted Turkey Breast
Glazed Honey Cured Turkey Breast
Gourmet Gold'n Brown Turkey Breast
Gourmet Lite Turkey Breast
Gourmet Lite Turkey Breast, No Salt
Added
Herb Lemon Butter Turkey
Herb Roasted Turkey Breast
Honey Mustard Turkey Breast
Italian Style Turkey Breast
London Broil Turkey Breast
Maple and Honey Turkey Breast

Mesquite Turkey Breast
Oven Classic Turkey Breast
Oven Roasted Turkey Breast
Pepper and Garlic Turkey Breast
Roasted Turkey
Santa Fe Turkey Breast
Slow Roasted Turkey Breast
Smoked Julienne Turkey Strips
Smoked Peppercorn Turkey Breast
Smoked Turkey Breast Fillets
Turkey Ham

Eating Right 〰
Oven Roasted Turkey Breast
Smoked Turkey Breast

Empire Kosher
All Natural Turkey Breast with Skin
Fully Cooked BBQ Turkey
Ground Turkey
Half Turkey Breast
Honey Smoked Turkey Breast
Oven Prepared Turkey Breast Slices
Skinless All Natural Turkey Breast
Skinless Oven Turkey Breast
Skinless Smoked Turkey Breast
Smoked Turkey Breast Slices
Turkey Drumsticks
Turkey Tenders
Turkey Thighs
White Ground Turkey
Whole Turkey

Farmer John
Turkey Natural Meats

Fastco (Fareway)
Ground Turkey
Honey Smoked Turkey

Food Club (Brookshire)
95% Fat Free Turkey Ham
97% Fat Free Turkey Breast

Giant Eagle
4x6 Honey Turkey Breast
4x6 Oven Roasted Turkey Breast
Oven Roasted Turkey Breast Tub
Peppered Turkey Breast Tub

Godshall's ⓘ
Maple Flavored Smoked Turkey Ham
Smoked Honey Turkey Ham
Smoked Turkey Ham

Great Value (Wal-Mart) 🔳25
Fat Free Turkey Breast
Sliced Fat Free Smoked Turkey Breast
Sliced Fat Free Turkey Breast
Sliced Honey Turkey Breast
Thinly Sliced Oven Roasted Turkey
  Breast
Thinly Sliced Smoked Turkey Breast

Harvestland
Fresh Ground Turkey
Fresh Turkey
Fresh Turkey Burgers
Frozen Turkey Burgers

H-E-B
Cajun Turkey Breast
Fajita Turkey Breast
Fried Breast of Turkey
Honey Smoked Turkey Breast
Maple Turkey Breast
Mesquite Smoked Turkey Breast
Mesquite Smoked Turkey Breast, Pre-
  Sliced
Oven Roasted Turkey Breast
Peppercorn Turkey Breast
Salsa Turkey Breast
Sun Dried Tomato Turkey Breast

Hempler Foods Group ⓘ
Smoked Boneless Turkey Breast
Turkey Breast (Whole and Presliced)
Turkey Ham (Regular & Black Forest)

Honeysuckle White
Honeysuckle White (All BUT Asian
  Grilled Marinated Turkey Strips,
  Beer Smoked Turkey Bratwurst Fully
  Cooked, Italian Style Meatballs,
Cajun Fried Turkey, and Teriyaki
  Turkey Breast Tenderloins)

Hormel
Julienne Turkey

Jennie-O Turkey Store
Flavored Tenderloins - Applewood
  Smoked
Flavored Tenderloins - Garlic & Red
  Pepper
Flavored Tenderloins - Lemon-Garlic
Flavored Tenderloins - Roast Flavor
Flavored Tenderloins - Tequila Lime

Flavored Tenderloins - Traditional Herb
Fresh Ground Turkey - Extra Lean
Fresh Ground Turkey - Italian
Fresh Ground Turkey - Lean
Fresh Ground Turkey - Taco Seasoned
Fresh Lean Turkey Patties
Fresh Tray - Breast Slices
Fresh Tray - Breast Strips
Fresh Tray - Tenderloins
Grand Champion - Hickory Smoked Turkey Breast
Grand Champion - Homestyle Pan Roasted Turkey Breast
Grand Champion - Honey Cured Turkey Breast
Grand Champion - Mesquite Smoked Turkey Breast
Grand Champion - Oven Roasted Turkey Breast
Grand Champion - Tender Browned Turkey Breast
Hickory Smoked Turkey Breast - Cracked Pepper
Hickory Smoked Turkey Breast - Garlic Pesto
Hickory Smoked Turkey Breast - Honey Cured
Hickory Smoked Turkey Breast - Sun Dried Tomato
Natural Choice - Oven Roasted Turkey Breast
Natural Choice - Peppered Turkey Breast
Natural Choice - Tender Browned Turkey Breast
Oven Ready Turkey - Garlic & Herb
Oven Ready Turkey - Homestyle
Oven Ready Turkey (The Gravy Packet MAY contain gluten)
Oven Ready Turkey Breast (The Gravy Packet MAY contain gluten)
Oven Roasted Turkey Breast
Pan Roasts with Gravy - White
Pan Roasts with Gravy - White/Dark Combo

Prime Young Turkey (Fresh or Frozen) (The Gravy Packet MAY contain gluten)
Refrigerated Quarter Turkey Breasts - Cajun-Style
Refrigerated Quarter Turkey Breasts - Cracked Pepper
Refrigerated Quarter Turkey Breasts - Hickory Smoked
Refrigerated Quarter Turkey Breasts - Honey Cured
Refrigerated Quarter Turkey Breasts - Oven Roasted
Refrigerated Quarter Turkey Breasts - Sun-Dried Tomato
Refrigerated Turkey Ham
Smoked Turkey Breast - Hickory
Smoked Turkey Breast - Honey Cured
Smoked Turkey Breast - Mesquite
Smoked Turkey Wings & Drumsticks
So Easy - Slow Roasted Turkey Breast
Turkey Breast - Apple Cinnamon
Turkey Breast - Garlic Peppered
Turkey Breast - Honey Maple
Turkey Breast - Honey Mesquite
Turkey Breast - Hot Red Peppered
Turkey Breast - Italian Style
Turkey Breast - Maple Spiced
Turkey Breast - Mesquite Smoked
Turkey Breast - Oven Roasted
Turkey Breast - Peppered
Turkey Breast - Smoked
Turkey Breast - Smoked Peppered
Turkey Breast - Tender Browned
Turkey Breast - Tomato Basil

Jewel-Osco
Honey Smoked Deli Turkey
Oven Roasted Deli Turkey
Oven Roasted Deli Turkey Breast
Oven Roasted Fat-Free 98% Turkey Breast

Jimmy Dean 〰
D-Lights Turkey Sausage Breakfast Bowl

Manda ⓘ
Honey Cured Turkey Breast (Manda Supreme Gold Label)

Meijer
Hen Turkey
Hen Turkey, Fresh
Hickory Smoked Turkey Breast
Honey Roasted Turkey Breast
Tom Turkey
Tom Turkey, Fresh
Turkey Basted with Timer
Turkey Breast, Fresh
Turkey Breast, Frozen
Turkey, Fresh Natural

Meijer Gold
Hen Turkey
Tom Turkey

Norbest ⓘ
Turkey (All)

Old Neighborhood
Old Neighborhood (All)

Oscar Mayer
Carving Board Turkey Breast, Oven
Roasted
Turkey Breast Cold Cuts, Honey
Smoked & White Turkey
Turkey Breast Cold Cuts, Mesquite
Smoked & White Turkey
Turkey Breast Cold Cuts, Natural Oven
Roasted
Turkey Breast Cold Cuts, Oven Roasted
& White Turkey
Turkey Breast Cold Cuts, Oven Roasted
& White Turkey 96% Fat Free
Turkey Breast Cold Cuts, Oven Roasted
98% Fat Free
Turkey Breast Cold Cuts, Smoked &
White Turkey 96% Fat Free
Turkey Breast Cold Cuts, Smoked &
White Turkey 98% Fat Free
Turkey Breast Cold Cuts, Smoked 98%
Fat Free
Turkey Breast Cold Cuts, White Oven
Roasted 95% Fat Free
Turkey Ham Cold Cuts, Smoke Flavor
Added
Turkey Ham Cold Cuts, Turkey Ham

Our Family
Smoked Turkey Breast
Turkey Breast

Perdue
Bourbon Peppercorn Pan Roasted
Turkey Breast
Carving Classic Pan Roasted Turkey
Breast
Carving Classic Pan Roasted Turkey
Breast, Honey Smoked
Carving Classics Pan Roasted Turkey
Breast, Cracked Pepper
Carving Turkey Breast, Hickory
Smoked
Carving Turkey Breast, Honey Smoked
Carving Turkey Breast, Mesquite
Smoked
Carving Turkey Breast, Oven Roasted
Carving Whole Turkey
Fresh Ground Turkey Breast
Fresh Lean Ground Turkey
Ground Turkey Burgers
Health Sense Turkey Breast Fat Free
Reduced Sodium, Oven Roasted
Rotisserie Turkey Breast
Short Cuts Carved Turkey Breast, Oven
Roasted
Tender and Tasty Products
Whole Turkeys (Seasoned with Broth)

Petit Jean
Petit Jean (All)

Plainville Farms
Fresh Meat (All)

Price Chopper
Ground Turkey Breast
Ground Turkey Patties
Turkey Chops

Private Selection (Kroger)
Honey Smoked Turkey Breast
Oven Roasted Turkey

Publix
Fresh Young Turkey Breast
Fresh Young Turkey, Whole
Fully Cooked Smoked Turkey Breast
Fully Cooked Smoked Turkey, Whole
Fully Cooked Turkey, Breast
Ground Turkey
Ground Turkey Breast

Roger Wood
Roger Wood (All)

Saag's ⓘ
- Saag's (All BUT British Bangers & Marzenbier Brats)

Seltzer's
- Smoked Turkey Breast ()

Shady Brook Farms
- Turkey (All BUT Asian Grill Marinated Turkey Strips, Beer Smoked Turkey Brats, Italian Style Turkey Meatballs, and Teriyaki Turkey Breast Tenderloin)

Shaw's
- Honey Smoked Turkey
- Oven Roasted 98% Fat-Free Turkey Breast

Shoppers Value (ACME)
- Turkey

Shoppers Value (Albertsons)
- Turkey

Shoppers Value (Cub Foods)
- Turkey

Shoppers Value (Jewel-Osco)
- Turkey

Thumann's ✓
- All Natural Oven Roasted Gourmet Turkey Breast
- All Natural Oven Roasted Hickory Smoked Turkey Breast
- Golden Roasted Filet of Turkey, Cajun Style
- Golden Roasted Filet of Turkey, Caramel Color Skinless
- Golden Roasted Filet of Turkey, Cracked Pepper & Paprika Coated
- Golden Roasted Filet of Turkey, Honey & Molasses Coated
- Golden Roasted Filet of Turkey, Italian Style
- Golden Roasted Filet of Turkey, Lemon Pepper Coated
- Golden Roasted Filet of Turkey, Lower Sodium
- Golden Roasted Filet of Turkey, Mesquite Smoked
- Golden Roasted Filet of Turkey, Pastrami Seasoning
- Golden Roasted Filet of Turkey, Rotisserie Flavor
- Golden Roasted Filet of Turkey, Santa Fe Style
- Golden Roasted Gourmet Turkey
- Golden Roasted Skinless Filet of Turkey, Hickory Smoked
- Golden Roasted Skinless Filet of Turkey, Hickory Smoked (Catering)
- Oven Roasted Premium Turkey Breast
- Petite Filet of Turkey, Hickory Smoked (Skinless, Skin-On)
- Premium White Fillet of Turkey
- Premium White Fillet of Turkey - Skinless

Trader Joe's
- Mesquite Smoked Turkey Breast, Sliced
- Unprocessed Raw Meat (All)

Valu Time (Brookshire)
- Turkey Breast- 97% Fat Free

Wegmans
- Oven Roasted Turkey Breast - Thin Sliced
- Smoked Honey Turkey Breast - Thin Sliced
- Smoked Turkey Breast - Thin Sliced

Wellshire Farms
- Oven Roasted Turkey Breast
- Sliced Roasted Turkey Breast
- Sliced Smoked Turkey Breast
- Spicy Turkey Tom Tom Snack Sticks
- Turkey Snack Stick

Zeigler ()
- 4x6 Roast Turkey Breast
- 4x6 Smoked Turkey Breast
- Half Smoked Turkey Breast
- Pecan Smoked Turkey

MISCELLANEOUS

Hatfield ()
- Home Style Meat Loaf

Meijer
- Buffalo Fillet
- Buffalo Wheel
- Frozen Duckling

Perdue
Rotisserie Oven Stuffed Roaster
Rotisserie Oven Stuffed Roaster Breast
Seasoned Oven Ready Cornish Hen
Seasoned Oven Ready Roaster
Seasoned Oven Ready Roaster Bone In
   Breast
Thumann's ✓
Liverwurst Cap
Trader Joe's
Seasoned Rack Of Lamb

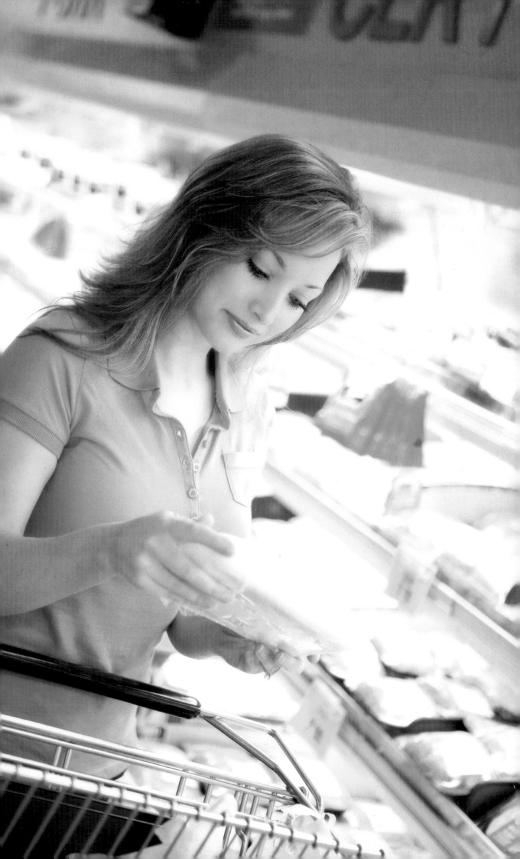

FREE NEWSLETTER

Symbols Summary   gf = gluten-free

 GF Lines or Facility; or
No chance of cross-contamination

 Gluten Testing is performed

 Gluten-Free based on review of ingredient label
(as no GF list was provided)

 Gluten-Free based on last year's list (use caution, as information
may be out of date)

 Procedures to mitigate Cross-Contamination are in place,
although there are shared facilities or equipment

 Cross-Contamination is possible; or, made with "gluten-free
ingredients" (with no specific mention of GF status by the
company)

No Icon. The company reported that the product is gluten-free
but provided no further context.

For the full key, see page 19 >>

THE GLUTEN-FREE DIET:
AN EASY REFERENCE INGREDIENTS TABLE

✓	Gluten-Free
✗	NOT Gluten-Free
?	Maybe - depends on manufacturer

Need a refresher on the gluten-free diet? These grains are safe: rice, soy, corn, potatoes, tapioca, buckwheat, arrowroot, amaranth, millet, quinoa, sorghum and teff. When plain, you can also eat: fruits, vegetables, milk, meat, eggs, beans, oil, wine, and distilled alcohols like vodka and gin.

As for what's off limits, "no wheat, rye, barley and oats*" in practice means, no (wheat) flour, pasta, croutons, bread, cookies, and "hidden" gluten sources like soy sauce, beer, and licorice. (But don't despair, there ARE specialty GF versions of these products in this guide!) Beyond these basics, even the most experienced shopper can stumped by mysterious ingredients like "guar gum."

We hope this ingredient list will make label-reading easier than ever, for both new and experienced GF shoppers!

Ingredient		Ingredient		Ingredient	
Agar-Agar	✓	Einkorn	✗	Mustard Flour	?
Alcohol, Distilled	✓	Farina	✗	Natural Colors	✓
Algin	✓	Flax	✓	Natural Flavors	✓
Annatto	✓	Fructose	✓	Polysorbates	✓
Arabic Gum	✓	Fumaric Acid	✓	Psyllium	✓
Artificial Colors	✓	Gelatin	✓	Rennet	✓
Artificial Flavoring	✓	Glucose	✓	Rice Malt	✓
Ascorbic Acid	✓	Glucose Syrup	✓	Rice Syrup	?
Aspartame	✓	Glutamic Acid	✓	Rum	✓
Baking Powder	?	Glutinous Rice	✓	Saccharin	✓
Beer	✗	Glycerides	✓	Seitan	✗
Beta Carotene	✓	Glycol	✓	Semolina	✗
BHA	✓	Graham Flour	✗	Silicon Dioxide	✓
BHT	✓	Guar Gum	✓	Sodium Benzoate	✓
Bulgur	✗	Gum Arabic	✓	Sodium Nitrate	✓
Calcium Disodium EDTA	✓	Hydrolyzed Corn Protein	✓	Sodium Nitrite	✓
Caprylic Acid	✓	Hydrolyzed Soy Protein	✓	Sodium Sulphite	✓
Caramel Color	✓	Hydrolyzed Wheat Protein	✗	Sorbate	✓
Carboxymethylcellulose	✓	Inulin	✓	Sorbic Acid	✓
Carnauba Wax	✓	Invert Sugar	✓	Sorbitol	✓
Carob Bean	✓	Kamut	✗	Soy Sauce	✗
Carrageenan	✓	Lactic Acid	✓	Spelt	✗
Casein	✓	Lactose	✓	Starch (on labels, this refers to cornstarch)	✓
Cellulose Gum	✓	Lecithin	✓	Stevia	✓
Citric Acid	✓	Malic Acid	✓	Sucralose	✓
Corn Gluten	✓	Malt (e.g., malt extract, malt flavoring, malt vinegar)	✗	Sucrose	✓
Corn Syrup	✓	Maltitol	✓	Sulfites	✓
Corn Syrup Solids	✓	Maltodextrin	✓	Tabbouleh	✗
Cornstarch	✓	Maltose	✓	Tartaric Acid	✓
Couscous	✗	Mannitol	✓	Triticale	✗
Cream of Tartar	✓	Matzo (matzoh)	✗	Vanilla Extract	✓
Dextrimaltose	✗	Molasses	✓	Vanilla Flavoring	✓
Dextrins	?	Mono and Diglycerides	✓	Vanillin	✓
Dextrose	✓	Monosodium Glutamate (MSG)	✓	Vinegar (All EXCEPT malt)	✓
Durum	✗			Vodka	✓
				Wheat Bran	✗
				Wheat Germ	✗
				Whey	✓
				Wine	✓
				Xanthan Gum	✓
				Xylitol	✓
				Yeast (All EXCEPT brewer's yeast)	✓

*See page 14 for a profile on "gluten-free" o

This ingredient table was created in collaboration with Shelley Case, B.Sc., RD, registered dietitian and aut. of **Gluten-Free Diet: A Comprehensive Resource Guide**. She is a member of the medical advisory boa of the Celiac Disease Foundation and Gluten Intolerance Group. For more in-depth information about gluten-free diet, ingredients, labeling laws and healthy eating, please visit **www.glutenfreediet.ca**.